Council on Ethical and Judicial Affairs

Code of Medical Ethics

Current Opinions with Annotations

2004–2005 Edition

Annotations prepared by the
Southern Illinois University Schools of Medicine and Law

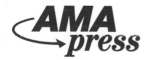

AMA press

AMA Press
Vice President, Business Products: Anthony J. Frankos
Publisher: Michael Desposito
Director, Production and Manufacturing: Jean Roberts
Senior Acquisitions Editor: Marsha Mildred
Developmental Editor: Carol Brockman
Director, Marketing: J. D. Kinney
Marketing Manager: Elizabeth Kerr
Senior Production Coordinator: Boon Ai Tan
Senior Print Coordinator: Ronnie Summers

Code of Medical Ethics:
Current Opinions with Annotations, 2004-2005 Edition

Additional copies of this book may be ordered from the American Medical Association.
For order information, call toll-free 800 621-8335.
Mention product number OP632304.

ISBN 1-57947-561-2

BP25:04-P-031:8/04

Contents

1.00 Introduction

2.00 Opinions on Social Policy Issues

3.00 Opinions on Interprofessional Relations

4.00 Opinions on Hospital Relations

5.00   Opinions on Confidentiality, Advertising, and Communications Media Relations

6.00   Opinions on Fees and Charges

7.00   Opinions on Physician Records

8.00   Opinions on Practice Matters

9.00   Opinions on Professional Rights and Responsibilities

10.00   Opinions on the Patient-Physician Relationship

Appendix

Index to Opinions

Table of Cases

Table of Articles

Preface

This edition of *Code of Medical Ethics: Current Opinions with Annotations* of the Council on Ethical and Judicial Affairs replaces all previous editions and includes Opinions based on Reports adopted through December 2003. It is one component of the American Medical Association (AMA)'s *Code*; the other components are the Principles of Medical Ethics, and the Reports of the Council on Ethical and Judicial Affairs. The Principles precede the Opinions in this volume. Reports are available separately.

The Principles of Medical Ethics are the primary component of the *Code*. They establish the core ethical principles from which the other components of the *Code* are derived. Most recently, the Principles were revised in 2001.

The Code of Medical Ethics: Current Opinions with Annotations reflects the application of the Principles of Medical Ethics to more than 175 specific ethical issues in medicine, including health care rationing, genetic testing, withdrawal of life-sustaining treatment, and family violence. Much as courts of law elaborate on constitutional principles in their holdings, the Council develops the meaning of the Principles of Medical Ethics in its opinions. Accordingly, each Opinion is followed by one or more roman numerals that identify the Principle(s) from which the Opinion is derived.

Each Opinion is also followed by a list of annotations reflecting citations to the opinion in judicial rulings and the medical, ethical, and legal literature.

The Reports—from which many of the opinions are derived—discuss the rationale behind the Council's Opinions, providing a detailed analysis of the relevant ethical considerations.

It is necessary to consult all three components of the AMA's *Code of Medical Ethics* to determine the Association's positions on ethical issues. In addition, the AMA's House of Delegates periodically issues statements on ethical issues. These statements are contained in the AMA's electronic policy database, the *PolicyFinder*. Because the Council on Ethical and Judicial Affairs is responsible for determining the AMA's positions on ethical issues, statements by the House of Delegates should be construed as the view of the House of Delegates but not as the ethics policy of the Association.

Medical ethics involve the professional responsibilities and obligations of physicians. Behavior relating to medical etiquette or custom is not addressed in the *Code*. The Opinions which follow are intended as guides to responsible professional behavior.

No one Principle of Medical Ethics can stand alone or be individually applied to a situation. In all instances, it is the overall intent and influence of the Principles of Medical Ethics which shall measure ethical behavior for the physician. Council Opinions are issued under its authority to interpret the Principles of Medical Ethics and to investigate general ethical conditions and all matters pertaining to the relations of physicians to one another and to the public.

The Code of Medical Ethics is published biennially. New Opinions, which are issued twice a year at the AMA's meetings of the House of Delegates, are available through the Council on Ethical and Judicial Affairs' Web site (http://www.ama-assn.org/go/ceja) and through the *PolicyFinder*. The Council on Ethical and Judicial Affairs encourages comments and suggestions for future editions of this publication.

Council on Ethical and Judicial Affairs

History

The Oath of Hippocrates, a brief statement of principles, has come down through history as a living statement of ideals to be cherished by the physician. This Oath was conceived some time during the period of Grecian greatness, probably in the fifth century B.C. It protected rights of the patient and appealed to the inner and finer instincts of the physician without imposing sanctions or penalties on him or her. Other civilizations subsequently developed written principles, but the Oath of Hippocrates (Christianized in the tenth or eleventh century A.D. to eliminate reference to pagan gods) has remained in Western Civilization as an expression of ideal conduct for the physician.

The most significant contribution to Western medical ethical history subsequent to Hippocrates was made by Thomas Percival, an English physician, philosopher, and writer. In 1803, he published his Code of Medical Ethics. His personality, his interest in sociological matters, and his close association with the Manchester Infirmary led to the preparation of a scheme of professional conduct relative to hospitals and other charities from which he drafted the code that bears his name.

At the first official meeting of the American Medical Association (AMA) at Philadelphia in 1847, the two principal items of business were the establishment of a code of ethics and the creation of minimum requirements for medical education and training. Although the Medical Society of the State of New York and the Medico-Chirurgical Society of Baltimore had formal written codes of medical ethics prior to this time, it is clear the AMA's first adopted Code of Ethics was based on Percival's Code.

In general, the language and concepts of the original Code drafted by Isaac Mays, MD and John Bell, MD and adopted by the Association in 1847 remained the same throughout the years. There were revisions, of course, which reflected the temper of the times and the eternal quest to express basic concepts with clarity. Major revisions did occur in 1903, 1912, 1947, and 1994.

In December 1955, an attempt was made to distinguish medical ethics from matters of etiquette. A draft of a two-part code seeking to accomplish this was submitted to the House of Delegates at that time but was not accepted. This proposal was, in effect, a separation of then existing statements found in the Principles into two categories. Little or no change was made in the language of the 48 sections of the Principles.

Subsequently, in June 1956, a seemingly radical proposal was submitted to the House of Delegates for consideration. This proposal, a short version of the Principles, was discussed at the December 1956 session of the House after wide publication and broad consideration among members of the medical profession. It was postponed for final consideration until the June 1957 meeting of the House of Delegates, when the short version was adopted.

The format of the Principles adopted in June 1957 is a change from the format of the Principles promulgated by Percival in 1803 and accepted by the Association in 1847. Ten short sections, preceded by a preamble, succinctly express the fundamental concepts embodied in the present (1955) Principles, according to the report of the Council on Constitution and Bylaws. That Council assured the House of Delegates in its June 1957 report that "every basic principle has been preserved; on the other hand, as much as possible of the prolixity and ambiguity which in the past obstructed ready explanation, practical codification and particular selection of basic concepts has been eliminated."

In 1977, the Judicial Council recommended to the House of Delegates that the AMA Principles of Medical Ethics be revised to clarify and update the language, to eliminate reference to gender, and to seek a proper and reasonable balance between professional standards and contemporary legal standards in our changing society. Given the desire of the Judicial Council for a new version of the Principles to be widely accepted and accurately understood, in 1978 the Judicial Council recommended that a special committee of the House be appointed to consider such a revision. This was done in 1980, and the House of Delegates adopted the revision of the AMA Principles of Medical Ethics at its Annual Meeting in June 1980. In June 2001, the House adopted further revisions, adding two new Principles.

In June 1985, the Judicial Council became the Council on Ethical and Judicial Affairs.

Guide to Use
of Annotations

Over the years, the American Medical Association (AMA) Principles of Medical Ethics and the *"The Code of Medical Ethics: Current Opinions with Annotations"* of the Council on Ethical and Judicial Affairs have emerged as an important source of guidance for responsible professional medical behavior, as well as the primary compendium of medical professional value statements in the United States.

The Opinions included in this volume are derived from two sources. The Council may issue Opinions directly at any time, usually during the Annual and Interim meetings of the AMA House of Delegates. Other Opinions are derived from the conclusions or recommendations of longer reports of the Council that are available from the AMA. Many of the Reports from which Opinions are derived are also published in peer-reviewed medical journals.

In this volume, an Opinion that is derived from a longer Report is followed by a citation to that Report and, if applicable, in a peer-reviewed medical journal. Opinions that are issued directly rather than derived from Reports are followed by information giving the date of issuance or most recent revision. For some of the older Opinions, however, this information is not available.

The impact of the Principles and Opinions has been significant. In this regard, attorneys and judges have shown an increasing willingness to look to the Principles and Opinions as a predicate for legal advocacy and decision-making in matters of health care law and litigation.

Against this backdrop of increasing reliance on the Principles and Opinions, these annotations have been prepared. They are designed to provide a research and reference tool for practitioners, scholars, jurists, and others who seek ready access to the Principles and Opinions in their work.

The annotations include summaries of all reported court decisions and selected state attorney general opinions that make substantive reference to the Principles or Opinions. Additionally, the annotations summarize selected articles from the medical, legal, and ethical literature.

These materials were gathered on the basis of carefully structured searches of a variety of computerized research services including WESTLAW®, LEXIS Publishing™, and MEDLINE®. Further, more generalized review of various medical and legal journals resulted in evaluation of approximately 3500 articles. The annotations are inclusive through December 2003.

The annotations have been prepared to maximize their usefulness as reference and research tools. After a brief synopsis of the facts and legal issues, each case annotation focuses on the court's reference to the Principle(s) or Opinion(s) and the role it played in the decision. In addition to the particular source referred to by the court, case annotations include, where necessary, a cross-reference to the relevant provision(s) of the present version of the Principles and Opinions.

Journal annotations provide a general summary of the subject article, along with an indication of the specific Principle(s) or Opinion(s) referenced therein. Again, a cross-reference feature is included. For convenience, consistent terminology is used in the journal annotations. When an author generally refers to the Principle or Opinion, the term *references* is used. When a Principle or Opinion is cited, this term is used. Finally, if an author directly quotes from a Principle or a Current Opinion, then the annotation so indicates.

With respect to both case and journal annotations, specific page references are provided to identify where the Principle(s) or Current Opinion(s) are discussed. This feature is intended to facilitate efficient use of these annotations. A Table of Cases and a Table of Articles also have been compiled to further enhance the usefulness of this compendium.

It is important to recognize that the Principle(s) and Opinion(s) have a long and evolving history. Many of the cases included herein refer to older versions of the Principles and Opinions, some of which have been eliminated or have changed considerably over the years. Nonetheless, these cases may be valuable to the user. Efforts were made to identify the most appropriate provisions of the present Principles and Opinions to which to assign these cases. However, in some instances the correspondence is not exact and the user will need to review carefully the particular case under consideration with respect to the user's specific interests.

The annotators would like to express appreciation to Melanie Basham, Keleigh Biggins, Frank Choi, Michelle Dillon, Charles Ellington, Elizabeth Foster, Roberto Hernandez, Jean Kirchner, Elizabeth Lingle, Alisha Logan, Laura McMullen, Michele Miller, Thomas Morrow, Holly Noyes, Jo Powers, Susan Tedrick, Elizabeth Valencia, and Christopher White, who provided valuable research, editing, and other assistance on this project. Finally, we owe a special debt of thanks to Pamela Graham, Bonnie Miller, and Susan Williams of the Southern Illinois University School of Law who handled the difficult task of entry of annotations into the database with skill and enthusiasm.

This project was supported by a grant from the American Medical Association.

Annotators

Theodore R. LeBlang, JD
Southern Illinois University
School of Medicine
Department of Medical Humanities

Frank G. Houdek, JD, MLS
Southern Illinois University
School of Law

April 2004

W. Eugene Basanta, JD, LLM
Southern Illinois University
School of Law

Connie Poole, AMLS
Southern Illinois University
School of Medicine
Department of Information and
Communication Sciences

American Medical Association
Principles of Medical Ethics

Preamble

The medical profession has long subscribed to a body of ethical statements developed primarily for the benefit of the patient. As a member of this profession, a physician must recognize responsibility to patients first and foremost, as well as to society, to other health professionals, and to self. The following Principles adopted by the American Medical Association are not laws, but standards of conduct which define the essentials of honorable behavior for the physician.

I. A physician shall be dedicated to providing competent medical care, with compassion and respect for human dignity and rights.

II. A physician shall uphold the standards of professionalism, be honest in all professional interactions, and strive to report physicians deficient in character or competence, or engaging in fraud or deception, to appropriate entities.

III. A physician shall respect the law and also recognize a responsibility to seek changes in those requirements which are contrary to the best interests of the patient.

IV. A physician shall respect the rights of patients, colleagues, and other health professionals, and shall safeguard patient confidences and privacy within the constraints of the law.

V. A physician shall continue to study, apply, and advance scientific knowledge, maintain a commitment to medical education, make relevant information available to patients, colleagues, and the public, obtain consultation, and use the talents of other health professionals when indicated.

VI. A physician shall, in the provision of appropriate patient care, except in emergencies, be free to choose whom to serve, with whom to associate, and the environment in which to provide medical care.

VII. A physician shall recognize a responsibility to participate in activities contributing to the improvement of the community and the betterment of public health.

VIII. A physician shall, while caring for a patient, regard responsibility to the patient as paramount.

IX. A physician shall support access to medical care for all people.

Adopted June 1957; revised June 1980; revised June 2001.

American Medical Association
Principles of Medical Ethics

Preamble

The medical profession has long subscribed to a body of ethical statements developed primarily for the benefit of the patient. As a member of this profession, a physician must recognize responsibility to patients first and foremost, as well as to society, to other health professionals, and to self. The following Principles adopted by the American Medical Association are not laws, but standards of conduct which define the essentials of honorable behavior for the physician.

Haw. 1995 After physician was convicted of attempted first degree sexual abuse and kidnapping, the civil court affirmed the Board of Medical Examiner's decision to suspend him from practicing medicine for one year. In challenging Board's action, physician argued, among other things, that convictions were not related to his qualifications, functions, or duties as a physician. The court disagreed with all of physician's points of error on appeal. In considering physician's claim that convictions were not related to his duties as a physician, the court referred to the Preamble as reflecting a duty to the public generally. *Loui v. Board of Medical Examiners*, 78 Haw. 21, 889 P.2d 705, 714.

Ind. 1991 Plaintiff sued physician for injuries caused by physician's patient as the result of medication administered by the physician. Weighing (1) the relationship between the parties, (2) the reasonable foreseeability of harm to the injured party, and (3) public policy, the court held that a physician generally owes no duty to unknown third parties who may be injured by the physician's treatment of a patient. Concurring opinion quoted the Preamble which mandates that a physician "recognize responsibility...to society" arguing that there is no absolute immunity to third-party suits. *Webb v. Jarvis*, 575 N.E.2d 992, 998.

N.J. 1979 In wrongful death action against a psychiatrist whose patient murdered plaintiff's decedent, the court concluded, in accord with Principle 9 (1957) [now Principle IV], that a psychiatrist may owe a duty to warn potential victims of possible danger from psychiatrist's patient despite the general emphasis on confidentiality. The court also noted the Preamble and Principles 1 and 3 (1957) [now revised Preamble, Principle I and Opinion 5.05] in discussing the psychiatrist-patient relationship. *McIntosh v. Milano*, 168 N.J. Super. 466, 403 A.2d 500, 510, 512-13.

Journal 2003 Examines policy options for integration of traditional and modern medicine. Concludes that solid cross-sectoral linkages between different traditions can stabilize an integrated health care system. Quotes Preamble and Opinion V. Holliday, *Traditional Medicines in Modern Societies: An Exploration of Integrationist Options through East Asian Experience*, 28 J. Med. & Phil. 373, 387 (2003).

Journal 2002 Explores the implications of withholding medical treatment when abortion results in a live birth. Concludes that, in these situations, abortive parents and physicians should not solely decide the child's best interest. Quotes Preamble, Principles I and III, and Opinions 2.035, 2.20, and 2.215. Casagrande, *Children Not Meant to Be: Protecting the Interests of the Child When Abortion Results in Live Birth*, 6 Quinnipiac Health L.J. 19, 44, 45, 47-48 (2002).

Journal 2002 Considers the dilemma of informed consent in the context of prescribing psychotropic medication to patients with mental illness and mental retardation. Recognizes the need for substituted decisionmaking in certain situations. Concludes that legislation would help address this issue. Quotes Preamble, Principles I, III, IV, VIII, and IX, and Opinion 8.08.

O'Sullivan & Borcherding, *Informed Consent for Medication in Persons with Mental Retardation and Mental Illness*, 12 Health Matrix 63, 75, 86, 87, 88 (2002).

Journal 2002 Discusses legal and medical policies that protect confidentiality in the physician-patient relationship. Concludes that reducing the current level of privacy protection would jeopardize health care. Quotes Preamble and Opinions 2.136, 5.05, and 10.01. References Principles VIII and IX. Sciarrino, *Ferguson v. City of Charleston: "The Doctor Will See You Now, Be Sure to Bring Your Privacy Rights in With You!"* 12 Temp. Pol. & Civ. Rts. L. Rev. 197, 213, 215, 220, 221, 222 (2002).

Journal 2000 Examines the increased prominence of medical ethics in light of various changes in medicine and society. Concludes with observations regarding how "preventive ethics" can enhance patient care. Quotes Preamble. Nandi, *Ethical Aspects of Clinical Practice*, 135 Arch. Surg. 22, 23 (2000).

Journal 2000 Examines current laws prohibiting discrimination in the context of access to health care, placing emphasis on people with HIV/AIDS. Considers the implications of *Bragdon v. Abbott*. Concludes that everyone should be entitled to health care in the absence of an acceptable justification for its denial. Quotes Preamble, Principle VI, and Opinion 9.131. *Shepherd, HIV, the ADA, and the Duty to Treat*, 37 Hous. L. Rev. 1055, 1061, 1083-84 (2000).

Journal 1999 Asserts that patient autonomy is closely linked to patient-doctor discourse. Proposes a constitutional framework for evaluating how governmental regulations may interfere with such discourse. Concludes by emphasizing the importance of protecting the quality of doctor-patient discourse. Quotes Preamble and Opinion 8.03. Gatter, *Protecting Patient-Doctor Discourse: Informed Consent and Deliberative Autonomy*, 78 Or. L. Rev. 941, 956 (1999).

Journal 1998 Argues that the doctrine of informed consent should not be abandoned. Explains why informed consent is needed. Suggests that even if physicians cannot determine patients' best interests, they can determine patients' reasonable interests. Quotes Preamble. White & Zimbelman, *Abandoning Informed Consent: An Idea Whose Time Has Not Yet Come*, 23 J. Med. Phil. 477, 496 (1998).

Journal 1997 Examines noncompetition clauses in the medical field. Reviews policy concerns and historical and common-law analyses of agreements not to compete. Posits that, the more commercialized the medical profession becomes, the more noncompetition clauses infringe upon the physician-patient relationship and patients' rights. Quotes Opinions 9.02 and 9.06. Cites Preamble and Opinion 6.11. Comment, *Noncompetition Clauses in Physician Employment Contracts in Oregon*, 76 Or. L. Rev. 195, 204-06 (1997).

Journal 1997 Considers principles of confidentiality in the physician-patient relationship. Notes the current trend emphasizing public reporting obligations of physicians to protect members of society. Emphasizes need for balance between patient rights and societal interests. Quotes Principle IV and Opinion 5.05. References Preamble. Jozefowicz, *The Case Against Having Professional Privilege in the Physician-Patient Relationship*, 16 Med. & L. 385, 386-87, 391 (1997).

Journal 1997 Discusses the need for balance between business ethics and medical ethics in the context of managed care. Explores two models for integrating ethics and managed care. Proposes the adoption of a collective responsibility model to improve quality of care. Quotes Principles I, II, III, IV, and V. Cites Preamble. References Opinion 8.13. Regan, *Regulating the Business of Medicine: Models for Integrating Ethics and Managed Care*, 30 Colum. J.L. & Soc. Probs. 635, 651, 656, 657 (1997).

Journal 1996 Considers the impact of gag clauses on the physician-patient relationship. Undertakes an extensive legal, ethical, and policy analysis. Concludes that gag clauses are violative of legal and ethical principles. Quotes Principles II, V, and VI, and Fundamental Elements (1). Cites Preamble. Martin & Bjerknes, *The Legal and Ethical Implications of Gag Clauses in Physician Contracts*, XXII Am. J. Law & Med. 433, 465-66 (1996).

Journal 1996 Considers prearraignment forensic evaluations. Notes the prohibition against use of such evaluations. Examines underlying ethical precepts. Observes that principles of beneficence are misapplied to forensic psychiatry in this context. Advocates a new ethical framework. Quotes Preamble. References Principle IV and Opinion 5.05. Ornish, Mills, & Ornish, *Prearraignment Forensic Evaluations: Toward a New Policy*, 24 Bull. Am. Acad. Psychiatry Law 453, 454, 469 (1996).

Journal 1995 Examines the metaphor of physicians as fiduciaries. Considers how the law holds physicians accountable in this regard. Quotes Preamble. Cites Opinion 8.03 (1986) [now Opinion 8.032]. Rodwin, *Strains in the Fiduciary Metaphor: Divided Physician Loyalties and Obligations in a Changing Health Care System*, XXI Am. J. Law & Med. 241, 246, 250 (1995).

Journal 1994 Reviews the evolution of the physician-patient relationship, with attention to patient autonomy. Examines the changing health care delivery environment. Quotes Preamble, Principles I, II, III, IV, V, and VI, Fundamental Elements (1) and (2), and Opinions 1.02 and 8.07 (1981) [now Opinion 8.08]. Cites Opinion 1.01. Szczygiel, *Beyond Informed Consent*, 21 Ohio N.U.L. Rev. 171, 217, 218, 220, 225, 226, 256 (1994).

Journal 1993 Discusses ethical issues that may arise in the context of caring for the critically ill. Emphasizes the need for organization of patient care when multiple providers are involved. Quotes Preamble. Bruening, Andrew, & Smith, *Concurrent Care: An Ethical Issue for Family Physicians*, 36 J. Fam. Practice 606, 607 (1993).

Journal 1991 Examines the informed consent doctrine and how it was broadened in *Moore v. Regents of the University of California*. Concludes that, in California, under *Moore*, a physician must disclose to patients any economic or research interest he or she might have in the patient's medical treatment. Quotes Preamble. Guise, *Expansion of the Scope of Disclosure Required Under the Informed Consent Doctrine: Moore v. The Regents of the University of California*, 28 San Diego L. Rev. 455, 462 (1991).

Journal 1990 Discusses the moral dilemma in deciding whether to withdraw artificial nutrition and hydration from a patient and the appropriate role of the judiciary. Concludes that judicial decisions do not represent the moral viewpoint of society and that moral pronouncements should not be made in the courtroom. Quotes Preamble, Principles I, II, III, IV, V, VI, and VII, and Opinion 2.20. Peccarelli, *A Moral Dilemma: The Role of Judicial Intervention in Withholding or Withdrawing Nutrition and Hydration*, 23 John Marshall L. Rev. 537, 539, 540, 541 (1990).

I.
A physician shall be dedicated to providing competent medical care, with compassion and respect for human dignity and rights.

10th Cir. 2001 Plaintiffs, former employees of a public medical center, brought suit against medical director under 42 U.S.C. § 1983, based upon medical director's racially and sexually harassing actions and statements. The district court awarded compensatory and punitive damages against the medical director. Affirming the award of damages, the court quoted Principles I and IV and concluded that the medical director's behavior impacted not only plaintiffs, but the overall public health. *Nieto v. Kapoor*, 268 F.3d 1208, 1223 n. 12.

D. Kan. 1995 Plaintiff, an occupational medicine physician, alleged that defendant-medical group wrongfully discharged him in violation of public policy and in breach of the implied covenant of good faith and fair dealing. Defendant complained that plaintiff consistently granted excess time off to patients. Even though defendant warned plaintiff that he would be terminated if he continued this practice, plaintiff refused to comply stating that he was ethically obligated to serve the best interests of his patients. Plaintiff claimed that to place the defendant's interests above his legal and ethical duties to his patients would violate public policy as set out by statute and the Principles of Medical Ethics, with apparent reference to Principle I. Since plaintiff failed to show that defendant's practice caused harm to patients or deviated from accepted standards, the court disregarded plaintiff's public policy exception to the employment-at-will doctrine and granted defendant's motion for summary judgment. *Aiken v. Business & Indus. Health Group*, 886 F. Supp. 1565, 1571.

N.J. 1979 In wrongful death action against a psychiatrist whose patient murdered plaintiff's decedent, the court concluded, in accord with Principle 9 (1957) [now Principle IV], that a psychiatrist may owe a duty to warn potential victims of possible danger from psychiatrist's patient despite the general emphasis on confidentiality. The court also noted the Preamble and Principles 1 and 3 (1957) [now revised Preamble, Principle I and Opinion 5.05] in discussing the psychiatrist-patient relationship. *McIntosh v. Milano*, 168 N.J. Super. 466, 403 A.2d 500, 510, 512-13.

Ohio 2000 Hospital sought court order permitting administration of antipsychotic medication to an involuntarily committed mentally ill patient without consent. The court said that forced medication is permitted in certain instances, including where medical personnel determine that patients present an imminent risk of harm to themselves or others. Quoting Principle I, the court found that placing such authority in a physician's hands is appropriate. Because the treating physician testified the patient did not pose a risk, the court ruled forced medication could not be required on this basis. *Steele v. Hamilton County Cmty. Mental Health Bd.*, 90 Ohio St. 3d 176, 736 N.E.2d 10, 18.

Ohio 1991 State medical board revoked license of physician who had consensual sexual relations with his patient. The court upheld the board's ruling that this violated Principles I, II and IV. Dissenting judge, citing AMA Council on Ethical and Judicial Affairs, Sexual Misconduct in the Practice of Medicine, 266 JAMA 2741 [now Opinion 8.14], argued that until 1991, the AMA did not clearly deem sexual contact with a patient unethical. *Pons v. Ohio State Medical Bd.*, 66 Ohio St. 3d 619, 623, 625, 614 N.E.2d 748, 752, 753.

Ohio App. 1999 Physician appealed trial court's affirmation of state medical board's decision to suspend his medical license because the physician engaged in sexual relationships with mothers of his pediatric patients. On appeal the physician claimed that he was denied due process because physicians were not adequately notified that having sexual relations with parents of pediatric patients was unethical. The physician also claimed that the board had not presented adequate evidence that AMA Principles I and IV extend to the parents of pediatric patients. The court quoted Principles I and IV, and stated that medical experts who testified were of the opinion that having sexual relationships with parents of pediatric patients constituted ethical violations. *Gladieux v. Ohio State Medical Board*, 1999 WL 770959, *2, *4.

Journal 2003 Considers the legal, medical, and ethical issues of physician-patient confidentiality in disclosure of paternity. Concludes that a balancing test should be applied to making determinations regarding disclosure of paternity. Quotes Principles I, IV, and V, and Opinions 1.02, 5.055, and 10.01. Cites Principle II and Opinion 5.05. Richards & Wolf, *Medical Confidentiality and Disclosure of Paternity*, 48 S.D. L. Rev. 409, 411, 412, 413 (2003).

Journal 2002 Explores the implications of withholding medical treatment when abortion results in a live birth. Concludes that, in these situations, abortive parents and physicians should not solely decide the child's best interest. Quotes Preamble, Principles I and III, and Opinions 2.035, 2.20, and 2.215. Casagrande, *Children Not Meant to Be: Protecting the Interests of the Child When Abortion Results in Live Birth*, 6 Quinnipiac Health L.J. 19, 44, 45, 47-48 (2002).

Journal 2002 Analyzes the expanded use of the Civil False Claims Act in prosecuting health care fraud. Concludes that, in enforcing the law, government must balance its promises to beneficiaries, health care providers, and the public. Quotes Principles I, II, and IV. Krause, *"Promises to Keep": Health Care Providers and the Civil False Claims Act*, 23 Cardozo L. Rev. 1363, 1365 (2002).

Journal 2002 Considers the dilemma of informed consent in the context of prescribing psychotropic medication to patients with mental illness and mental retardation. Recognizes the need for substituted decisionmaking in certain situations. Concludes that legislation would help address this issue. Quotes Preamble, Principles I, III, IV, VIII, and IX, and Opinion 8.08. O'Sullivan & Borcherding, *Informed Consent for Medication in Persons with Mental Retardation and Mental Illness*, 12 Health Matrix 63, 75, 86, 87, 88 (2002).

Journal 2002 Examines the origin and dynamics of the scope-of-practice laws governing health care providers. Concludes that the current system is not working and offers recommendations for change. Quotes Principles I and II. Safriet, *Closing the Gap Between Can and May in Health-Care Providers' Scopes of Practice: A Primer for Policymakers*, 19 Yale J. on Reg. 301, 311 (2002).

Journal 2001 Discusses the physician unionization debate with emphasis on the perspective of physicians. Concludes that physicians' arguments against managed care articulate a moral claim in favor of collective bargaining rights. Quotes Principle I. Fine, *Exploitation of the Elite: A Case for Physician Unionization*, 45 St. Louis L. J. 207, 207 (2001).

Journal 2000 Examines the AMA Code of Ethics. Explores historical developments. Concludes that professional ethical principles meaningfully affect the conduct of physicians and make a difference to the patients and the public they serve. Cites Principle I. Baker & Emanuel, *The Efficacy of Professional Ethics: The AMA Code of Ethics in Historical and Current Perspective*, 30 Hastings Center Rep. S13, S14 (July/Aug. 2000).

Journal 2000 Considers the rules governing expert testimony. Explores professional ethical standards affecting expert witnesses and concludes that codes of ethics have not succeeded in eliminating biased expert testimony. Recommends creation of an organization to assist courts in obtaining reliable expert witness testimony. Quotes Principle III and Opinion 6.01. Cites Principles I, II, and V and Opinions 1.02 and 9.07. Murphy, *Expert Witnesses at Trial: Where are the Ethics? 14 Geo. J. Legal Ethics 217, 231-32 (2000).*

Journal 1999 Analyzes the federal rules of evidence from a feminist perspective. Proposes a new "apology" evidence rule to serve as an exception to the general rule that statements by party-opponents are admissible during trial. Suggests that physicians who commit medical errors may ease patients' anger by apologizing. The new evidence rule would permit physicians to be more forthcoming in this regard. Quotes Principles I and II. Orenstein, *Apology Excepted: Incorporating a Feminist Analysis into Evidence Policy Where You Would Least Expect It, 28 S.W. U. L. Rev. 221, 264 (1999).*

Journal 1998 Explores the impact of managed care on the health care system. Discusses legal and ethical conflicts that have arisen and emphasizes the need to balance the interests of patients with the integrity of the system. Quotes Principle I. Field, *New Ethical Relationships Under Health Care's New Structure: The Need for a New Paradigm, 43 Vill. L. Rev. 467, 468 (1998).*

Journal 1998 Discusses managed care and the expansion of physicians' duties under such programs. Focuses on the current legal standard of care for physicians. Proposes that physicians who are mandated by managed care organizations to provide services performed by specialists, be held to the same standard of care as other physicians who are required to deliver those services. Quotes Principle I. Friedland, *Managed Care and the Expanding Scope of Primary Care Physicians' Duties: A Proposal to Redefine Explicitly the Standard of Care, 26 J. Law, Med. & Ethics 100, 104 (1998).*

Journal 1998 Examines the United States Supreme Court's decision in *Zinermon v. Burch* in relation to other Supreme Court decisions regarding the role of the courts in mental health treatment determinations. Argues that the government must strike a balance between the duty to care for the mentally ill and the duty to respect individual liberty. Provides approaches legislatures could adopt regarding mental health issues. References Principles I and III. Nidich, *Zinermon v. Burch and Voluntary Admissions to Public Hospitals: A Common Sense Proposal for Compromise, 25 N. Ky. L. Rev. 699, 710 (1998).*

Journal 1997 Discusses the practice of physician deselection by managed care organizations. Suggests that deselection harms the physician-patient relationship and creates a conflict of interest. Argues that solutions to deselection should consider effects on the patient rather than on the physician. Quotes Principle III. Cites Principle I and Opinions 8.05 and 8.13. Liner, *Physician Deselection: The Dynamics of a New Threat to the Physician-Patient Relationship, 23 Am. J. Law & Med. 511, 513, 527 (1997).*

Journal 1997 Discusses the need for balance between business ethics and medical ethics in the context of managed care. Explores two models for integrating ethics and managed care. Proposes the adoption of a collective responsibility model to improve quality of care. Quotes Principles I, II, III, IV, and V. Cites Preamble. References Opinion 8.13. Regan, *Regulating the Business of Medicine: Models for Integrating Ethics and Managed Care, 30 Colum. J.L. & Soc. Probs. 635, 651, 656, 657 (1997).*

Journal 1996 Discusses the trend toward conserving resources expended on health care by withholding services absent a showing of necessity. Claims that the high standard of care physicians owe patients is jeopardized by medical treatment decisions based on coverage concerns. Concludes that the legal structure regarding health care plans should be changed. Quotes Preamble, Principles I, II, III, IV, V, VI, and VII and Opinion 2.03. Hirshfeld & Thomason, *Medical Necessity Determinations: The Need for a New Legal Structure, 6 Health Matrix 3, 8-9 (1996).*

Journal 1995 Examines the rights of health care professionals to refuse to participate in patient care on the basis of conscientious objection. Suggests steps that health care facilities may take when dealing with health care professionals who object to participating in patient care. Quotes Principles I and VI and Opinions 1.02, 2.035, and 9.055. Dellinger & Vickery, *When Staff Object to Participating In Care, 28 J. Health & Hospital Law 269, 272, 276 (1995).*

Journal 1994 Considers whether an exception should be made to physician-patient confidentiality that would allow a physician to reveal parental medical history to a child. Concludes that such an exception would not completely erode physician-patient confidentiality. Quotes Principles IV, Fundamental Elements (4), and Opinion 5.05. Cites Principle I and Fundamental Elements (1). Friedland, *Physician-Patient Confidentiality: Time to Re-Examine a Venerable Concept in Light of Contemporary Society and Advances in Medicine, 15 J. Legal Med. 249, 257, 264, 276 (1994).*

Journal 1994 Argues that physician aid-in-dying should be protected by the US Constitution and that patients should have a federal cause of action to challenge prohibitive state statutes. Considers how such a cause of action might affect public policy. Quotes Principles I and III. References Opinion 2.06. Note, *Toward a More Perfect Union: A Federal Cause of Action for Physician Aid-In-Dying*, 27 U. Mich. J.L. Ref. 521, 538 (1994).

Journal 1994 Reviews the evolution of the physician-patient relationship, with attention to patient autonomy. Examines the changing health care delivery environment. Quotes Preamble, Principles I, II, III, IV, V, and VI, Fundamental Elements (1) and (2), and Opinions 1.02 and 8.07 (1981) [now Opinion 8.08]. Cites Opinion 1.01. Szczygiel, *Beyond Informed Consent*, 21 Ohio N.U.L. Rev. 171, 217, 218, 220, 225, 226, 256 (1994).

Journal 1993 Discusses physicians' duty to disclose to patients medical treatment alternatives that are not readily available. Proposes that based on the historical development and legal requirements of the informed consent doctrine, physicians should be required to inform patients of nonreadily available alternatives or face liability for breach of such obligation. Quotes Principles I, II, III, IV, and V and Opinion 8.08. Note, *Informed Choice: Physicians' Duty to Disclose Nonreadily Available Alternatives*, 43 Case W. Res. L. Rev. 491, 491, 498-99, 508, 509 (1993).

Journal 1990 Discusses the moral dilemma in deciding whether to withdraw artificial nutrition and hydration from a patient and the appropriate role of the judiciary. Concludes that judicial decisions do not represent the moral viewpoint of society and that moral pronouncements should not be made in the courtroom. Quotes Preamble, Principles I, II, III, IV, V, VI, and VII, and Opinion 2.20. Peccarelli, *A Moral Dilemma: The Role of Judicial Intervention in Withholding or Withdrawing Nutrition and Hydration*, 23 John Marshall L. Rev. 537, 539, 540, 541 (1990).

Journal 1986 Observes that the AMA policy on capital punishment expressly forbids psychiatrists from making determinations of competency for execution. Compares the psychiatrist's determination of competency for execution to the behavior of Nazi physicians, and condemns as inherently dishonest any therapy not grounded in the patient's best interests. References Principle I and Opinion 2.06. Sargent, *Treating the Condemned to Death*, 16 Hastings Center Rep. 5, 5 (Dec. 1986).

II. A physician shall uphold the standards of professionalism, be honest in all professional interactions, and strive to report physicians deficient in character or competence, or engaging in fraud or deception, to appropriate entities.

Cal. App. 1956 Physician-petitioner sought mandamus against local medical association whose bylaws provided for the expulsion of any member who violated the Principles. Petitioner had been expelled under the provision for alleged violation of Principles Ch. III, Art IV, Sec.4 (1947) [now Opinions 9.04 and 9.07] for making disparaging statements regarding another physician in a report used in judicial proceedings. In holding that application of the provision to petitioner was contrary to public policy, the court noted that the physician's statements had been made at the request of a civil litigant and enjoyed a statutory testimonial privilege. Further, the court found that the American Medical Association's right to formulate ethical principles did not extend to defining the duties of witnesses. Expulsion was also based on petitioner's critical comments about other physicians overheard by their patients in violation of Principles Ch. III, Art. IV, Sec.1 (1947) [now Principle II and Opinion 9.04]. The court found application of this Principle under the circumstances reasonable and not contrary to public policy. *Bernstein v. Alameda-Contra Costa Medical Ass'n*, 139 Cal. App. 2d 241, 293 P.2d 862, 863, 863 nn.1, 2 865 nn.4, 6, 866, 866 n.8, 867.

Fla. App. 1995 The court considered the issue of the effect of § 455.241(2) of the Florida Statutes on right of defense in a medical malpractice action to engage in ex parte communications with plaintiff's non-party treating physician. The court held that a 1988 amendment to § 455.241(2) negated the applicability of the statute to medical malpractice cases. The dissent, citing *Petrillo v. Syntex Laboratories, Inc.*, 148 Ill. App. 3d 581, 499 N.E.2d 952 (1986), quoted Principles II and IV and Opinions 5.05, 5.06, and 5.08 as strong public policy support for its position that ex parte communications should be barred altogether. *Castillo-Plaza v. Green*, 655 So. 2d 197, 206 n.4.

Ill. App. 1986 Defense attorney in product liability suit was held in contempt of court for conducting ex parte discussions with plaintiff-patient's treating physician without patient's consent and contrary to authorized methods of discovery. The court held that the strong public policy favoring physician-patient confidentiality articulated in Principles II and IV and Opinions 5.05, 5.06, 5.07, and 5.08 justified a rule against such ex parte discussions. Further, the court held that the public has the right to rely on physicians to faithfully execute their ethical obligations. *Petrillo v. Syntex Laboratories, Inc., 148 Ill. App. 3d 581, 499 N.E.2d 952, 957, 958, 959.*

Ky. App. 1978 Plaintiff-physician attempted to enjoin defendant medical society from expelling him for actions contrary to a variety of Principles, the most relevant to his alleged unethical behavior being Principle 4 (1957) [now Principles II and III]. After reviewing the procedures followed by the medical society in considering the evidence pertaining to the charges, the court affirmed judgment dismissing the action, concluding that plaintiff was not deprived of due process. *Kirk v. Jefferson County Medical Soc'y, 577 S.W.2d 419, 421.*

Md. App. 1993 State Board of Physician Quality Assurance received a complaint that psychiatrist was having a romantic relationship with a former patient. When, as part of its investigation, the Board subpoenaed psychiatrist's records, patient raised the constitutional right to privacy. The court held that the state's interest in investigating possible disciplinary action against psychiatrist outweighed patient's constitutional right to privacy. The court cited Principle II as a potential basis to justify the Board's investigation of possible unprofessional conduct by physician. *Dr. K. v. State Board of Physician Quality Assur., 98 Md. App. 103, 632 A.2d 453, 456, cert. denied, 334 Md. 18, 637 A.2d 1191 (1994), and cert. denied, 115 S. Ct. 75, 130 L. Ed. 29 (1994).*

Mass. 1955 Plaintiff-physician was charged under state licensing statute by defendant-board with conspiracy and fee-splitting. Both parties sought a declaratory judgment as to whether the defendant-board had jurisdiction to determine plaintiff's guilt or innocence. In holding that the board was qualified to determine if plaintiff's actions constituted gross misconduct under the statute, the court referred to Principles Ch.I, Secs.1 and 6 (1947) [now Principle II and Opinion 6.02] delineating, in part, limitations on payment for medical services. These provisions, the court said, reflected the medical profession's understanding of its peculiar obligations. *Forziati v. Board of Registration in Medicine, 333 Mass. 125, 128 N.E.2d 789, 791.*

Mich. App. 1968 Physician was properly dismissed from hospital staff for violating Principle 4 (1957) [now Principle II and Opinion 9.11] when on numerous occasions physician vilified other physicians, swore and screamed in the hospital, and quarreled with staff and hospital visitors. *Anderson v. Board of Trustees of Caro Community Hosp., 10 Mich. App. 348, 159 N.W.2d 347, 348-50.*

Minn. 1970 Defendant-physician appealed order to answer interrogatories, claiming that a medical malpractice plaintiff is prohibited from compelling expert testimony from a defendant to prove a charge of malpractice without calling other medical witnesses. In holding that a defendant could be compelled to provide expert medical opinion in response to interrogatories, the court quoted Principle 1 (1957) [now Principle II and Opinion 8.12] for the proposition that physicians owe a duty of disclosure to their patients. *Anderson v. Florence, 288 Minn. 351, 181 N.W.2d 873, 880, 880 n.7.*

N.Y. Sup. 1965 Physician sued publishing company to bar insertion of advertisement for baby and child care products in physician's book, seeking declaration that book contract was void to the extent that it allowed inclusion of such an advertisement. Physician asserted that the advertisement was contrary to public policy, citing Opinions and Reports of the Judicial Council Sec. 5, Para. 29 (1965) [now Opinion 5.02] which stated that a doctor should not lend his name to any product. In rejecting the physician's claim, the court was willing to give careful consideration to the Association's view but concluded that it did not, in itself, constitute an expression of public policy. *Spock v. Pocket Books, Inc., 48 Misc. 2d 812, 266 N.Y.S.2d 77, 79.*

Ohio 1991 State medical board revoked license of physician who had consensual sexual relations with his patient. The court upheld the board's ruling that this violated Principles I, II, and IV. Dissenting judge, citing AMA Council on Ethical and Judicial Affairs, Sexual Misconduct in the Practice of Medicine, 266 JAMA 2741 [now Opinion 8.14], argued that until 1991, the AMA did not clearly deem sexual contact with a patient unethical. *Pons v. Ohio State Medical Bd., 66 Ohio St. 3d 619, 623, 625, 614 N.E.2d 748, 752, 753.*

Ohio 1980 A physician, charged with violating the state medical licensing statute by distributing controlled substances without a proper license and writing prescriptions for narcotics in the name of one person when they were intended for another, challenged the state medical board's decision to suspend his license and place him on two years probation. Under the statute, a physician could be disciplined for various activities including violation of any provision of a code of ethics of a national professional organization such as the American Medical Association. The board found in part that the physician's actions violated Principles 4 and 7 (1957) [now Principles II and III and Opinions 8.06 and 9.04]. The trial court reversed, holding that the board had insufficient evidence for its decision, and the court of appeals affirmed. On appeal, the supreme court held that expert testimony was not required at a hearing before a medical licensing board because they were experts and could determine for themselves whether the Principles had been violated. *Arlen v. State, 61 Ohio St. 2d 168, 399 N.E.2d 1251, 1252, 1253-54.*

Journal 2003 Considers the legal, medical, and ethical issues of physician-patient confidentiality in disclosure of paternity. Concludes that a balancing test should be applied to making determinations regarding disclosure of paternity. Quotes Principles I, IV, and V, and Opinions 1.02, 5.055, and 10.01. Cites Principle II and Opinion 5.05. Richards & Wolf, *Medical Confidentiality and Disclosure of Paternity, 48 S.D. L. Rev. 409, 411, 412, 413 (2003).*

Journal 2003 Uses public policy arguments to support a preponderance standard for medical license revocations in situations involving false testimony by a medical expert witness. Concludes that medical licensing boards can more effectively protect the public by using a preponderance standard. Quotes Principles II, III, and IV, and Opinions 1.02 and 9.07. Widmer, *South Dakota Should Follow Public Policy and Switch to the Preponderance Standard for Medical License Revocation After In Re the Medical License of Dr. Reuben Setliff, M.D., 48 S.D. L. Rev. 388, 396-97, 402 (2003).*

Journal 2002 Discusses therapeutic jurisprudence and the importance of trust in the structure of health care law. Concludes that understanding trust provides tools to formulate responses to new ethical, legal, and policy challenges. Quotes Principle Ch. I, Art. I, Sec. 4 (1847) [now Principle II and Opinion 8.12]. Hall, *Law, Medicine, and Trust, 55 Stan. L. Rev. 463, 471 (2002).*

Journal 2002 Analyzes the expanded use of the Civil False Claims Act in prosecuting health care fraud. Concludes that, in enforcing the law, government must balance its promises to beneficiaries, health care providers, and the public. Quotes Principles I, II, and IV. Krause, *"Promises to Keep": Health Care Providers and the Civil False Claims Act, 23 Cardozo L. Rev. 1363, 1365 (2002).*

Journal 2002 Explores the development and current status of collective bargaining and unionization in the medical profession. Concludes that, because collective bargaining traditionally addresses conditions of employment, a focus on patient care will be difficult to ensure. References Principle II. Levy, *Collective Bargaining in the Elite Professions–Doctors' Application of the Labor Law Model to Negotiations with Health Plan Providers, 13 U. Fla. J.L. & Pub. Pol'y 269, 277 (2002).*

Journal 2002 Examines the origin and dynamics of the scope-of-practice laws governing health care providers. Concludes that the current system is not working and offers recommendations for change. Quotes Principles I and II. Safriet, *Closing the Gap Between Can and May in Health-Care Providers' Scopes of Practice: A Primer for Policymakers, 19 Yale J. on Reg. 301, 311 (2002).*

Journal 2002 Considers the case of Ferguson v. City of Charleston. Concludes that the Supreme Court's rationale in that case reflects insights from feminist legal theory. Quotes Opinion 10.01. Cites Principles II and IV. Taslitz, *A Feminist Fourth Amendment?: Consent, Care, Privacy, and Social Meaning in Ferguson v. City of Charleston, 9 Duke J. Gender L. & Pol'y 1, 18, 19 (2002).*

Journal 2001 Discusses whether or not the medical profession needs a policy on honesty. Reviews ethical codes and concludes they fail to offer physicians with meaningful guidance about what constitutes "the truth" and when and how to disclose it. Quotes Principle II and Opinions 8.12 and 10.01. DeVita, *Honestly, Do We Need a Policy on Truth? 11 Kennedy Inst. Ethics J. 157, 158 (2001).*

Journal 2001 Compares and contrasts certain ethical positions articulated by the legal and medical professions. Concludes that both professions generally agree on ethical principles, but sometimes differ in the manner of implementation. Quotes Principle II. Cites Opinion 5.02. Needell, *Legal Ethics in Medicine: Are Medical Ethics Different from Legal Ethics? 14 St. Thomas L. Rev. 31, 35, 50 (2001).*

Journal 2000 Considers whether government regulators should allow managed care organizations to cover the costs of alternative treatments. Concludes that legislation should be more attentive to its consumer protection role. Quotes Principle II. Boozang, *Is the Alternative Medicine? Managed Care Apparently Thinks So, 32 Conn. L. Rev. 567, 606 (2000).*

Journal 2000 Considers the rules governing expert testimony. Explores professional ethical standards affecting expert witnesses and concludes that codes of ethics have not succeeded in eliminating biased expert testimony. Recommends creation of an organization to assist courts in obtaining reliable expert witness testimony. Quotes Principle III and Opinion 6.01. Cites Principles I, II, and V and Opinions 1.02 and 9.07. Murphy, *Expert Witnesses at Trial: Where are the Ethics?* 14 Geo. J. Legal Ethics 217, 231-32 (2000).

Journal 2000 Discusses traditional medical ethics and the physician's duty to benefit patients. Concludes that in the twenty-first century, physicians will no longer be expected to determine on their own what will benefit their patients. Quotes Principle II and Opinion 8.08. Veatch, *Doctor Does Not Know Best: Why in the New Century Physicians Must Stop Trying to Benefit Patients*, 25 J. Med. & Phil. 701, 710, 711 (2000).

Journal 1999 Provides examples in which psychiatrists might use deception in their practice. Explains the motivations for such conduct and raises questions about possible blameworthiness for such conduct. Quotes Principles II and III. Haroun & Morris, *Weaving a Tangled Web: The Deceptions of Psychiatrists*, 10 J. Contemp. Leg. Issues 227, 235 (1999).

Journal 1999 Examines fraud and abuse throughout government health care programs, with emphasis on enforcement and available sanctions. Concludes that consideration of strategies for revising enforcement protocols is advisable. Quotes Principle II. Jost & Davies, *The Empire Strikes Back: A Critique of the Backlash Against Fraud and Abuse Enforcement*, 51 Ala. L. Rev. 239, 240 (1999).

Journal 1999 Describes historical and present views regarding medical diagnosis. Discusses pressures physicians face that may affect the diagnostic process. Suggests that legal institutions can reduce these pressures, which will enhance the physician-patient therapeutic relationship. Quotes Principle II and Opinion 9.07. Noah, *Pigeonholing Illness: Medical Diagnosis as a Legal Construct*, 50 Hastings L. J. 241, 301, 302 (1999).

Journal 1999 Analyzes the federal rules of evidence from a feminist perspective. Proposes a new "apology" evidence rule to serve as an exception to the general rule that statements by party-opponents are admissible during trial. Suggests that physicians who commit medical errors may ease patients' anger by apologizing. The new evidence rule would permit physicians to be more forthcoming in this regard. Quotes Principles I and II. Orenstein, *Apology Excepted: Incorporating a Feminist Analysis into Evidence Policy Where You Would Least Expect It*, 28 S.W. U. L. Rev. 221, 264 (1999).

Journal 1999 Evaluates changes in direct-to-consumer advertising of prescription pharmaceuticals. Discusses FDA regulation of this type of advertising. Recognizes the important role of the FDA in this context. Quotes Principles II and III. Terzian, *Direct-to-Consumer Prescription Drug Advertising*, 25 Am. J. Law & Med. 149, 165 (1999).

Journal 1998 Discusses gag provisions in physicians' contracts with managed care organizations. Examines effects of gag rules on physicians. Explores state legislation and proposed federal legislation pertaining to gag provisions. Cites Principle II. Munoz, Nichols, Okata, Pitt, & Seager, *The Two Faces of Gag Provisions: Patients and Physicians in a Bind*, 17 Yale L. & Pol'y Rev. 249, 258 (1998).

Journal 1997 Reports on a study of physician attitudes regarding expert witnesses. Notes that a majority of physicians believe that medical expert testimony should be subject to peer review and, when appropriate, medical licensing board discipline. Quotes Principles II and VI, and Opinion 9.07. Eitel, Hegeman, & Evans, *Medicine on Trial: Physicians' Attitudes about Expert Medical Witnesses*, 18 J. Legal Med. 345, 355, 358 (1997).

Journal 1997 Discusses physician frustration with managed care plans caused by gag clauses and cost-containment mechanisms. Reviews the development of managed care organizations and federal attempts at limiting the use of gag clauses. Concludes that gag clauses are inherently flawed and compromise quality health care. Quotes Principles II and V, Fundamental Elements (1), and Opinion 8.13. Note, *Physicians, Bound and Gagged: Federal Attempts to Combat Managed Care's Use of Gag Clauses*, 21 Seton Hall Legis. J. 567, 601-02 (1997).

Journal 1997 Discusses the need for balance between business ethics and medical ethics in the context of managed care. Explores two models for integrating ethics and managed care. Proposes the adoption of a collective responsibility model to improve quality of care. Quotes Principles I, II, III, IV, and V. Cites Preamble. References Opinion 8.13. Regan, *Regulating the Business of Medicine: Models for Integrating Ethics and Managed Care*, 30 Colum. J.L. & Soc. Probs. 635, 651, 656, 657 (1997).

Journal 1996 Discusses the trend toward conserving resources expended on health care by withholding services absent a showing of necessity. Claims that the high standard of care physicians owe patients is jeopardized by medical treatment decisions based on coverage concerns. Concludes that the legal structure regarding health care plans should be changed. Quotes Preamble, Principles I, II, III, IV, V, VI, and VII and Opinion 2.03. Hirshfeld & Thomason, *Medical Necessity Determinations: The Need for a New Legal Structure*, 6 Health Matrix 3, 8-9 (1996).

Journal 1996 Considers the impact of gag clauses on the physician-patient relationship. Undertakes an extensive legal, ethical, and policy analysis. Concludes that gag clauses are violative of legal and ethical principles. Quotes Principles II, V, and VI, and Fundamental Elements (1). Cites Preamble. Martin & Bjerknes, *The Legal and Ethical Implications of Gag Clauses in Physician Contracts*, XXII Am. J. Law & Med. 433, 465-66 (1996).

Journal 1996 Examines the issue of attorney-client sexual relationships and the ethical problems inherent in such conduct. Recommends promulgation of a rule regulating such relationships. Quotes Principle II. Myers, Sonenshein, & Hofstein, *To Regulate or Not To Regulate Attorney-Client Sex? The Ethical Question in Pennsylvania*, 69 Temp. L. Rev. 741, 780 (1996).

Journal 1996 Discusses the ethical implications of sexual misconduct in the medical field. Examines the current civil and criminal tools used to curb physician-patient misconduct. Notes the inadequacy of physician reporting. Proposes a statutory approach to discipline physicians who abuse their fiduciary duties. Quotes Principle II. References Opinion 8.14. Note, *Sexual Conduct Within the Physician-Patient Relationship: A Statutory Framework for Disciplining this Breach of Fiduciary Duty*, 1 Widener L. Symp. J. 501, 507 (1996).

Journal 1994 Compares Texas law with Illinois law on the issue of ex parte communications between defense counsel and the patient/plaintiff's physician in civil litigation. Argues that preservation of the physician-patient relationship requires prohibition of such contact. Quotes Principles II and IV and Opinion 5.05. Comment, *From the Land of Lincoln a Healing Rule: Proposed Texas Rule of Civil Procedure Prohibiting Ex Parte Contact Between Defense Counsel and a Plaintiff's Treating Physician*, 25 Tex. Tech L. Rev. 1081, 1081, 1082 (1994).

Journal 1994 Reviews the evolution of the physician-patient relationship, with attention to patient autonomy. Examines the changing health care delivery environment. Quotes Preamble, Principles I, II, III, IV, V, and VI, Fundamental Elements (1) and (2), and Opinions 1.02 and 8.07 (1981) [now Opinion 8.08]. Cites Opinion 1.01. Szczygiel, *Beyond Informed Consent*, 21 Ohio N.U.L. Rev. 171, 217, 218, 220, 225, 226, 256 (1994).

Journal 1993 Discusses physicians' duty to disclose to patients medical treatment alternatives that are not readily available. Proposes that based on the historical development and legal requirements of the informed consent doctrine, physicians should be required to inform patients of nonreadily available alternatives or face liability for breach of such obligation. Quotes Principles I, II, III, IV, and V and Opinion 8.08. Note, *Informed Choice: Physicians' Duty to Disclose Nonreadily Available Alternatives*, 43 Case W. Res. L. Rev. 491, 491, 498-99, 508, 509 (1993).

Journal 1993 Discusses the problems physicians may encounter by exposing an errant colleague, such as harm to the reporting physician's reputation and the fear of litigation. States that problems involving physician competency and unethical behavior should be investigated, and that physicians should take personal responsibility for reporting problems they observe. References Principle II and Opinions 8.14 and 9.031. Morreim, *Am I My Brother's Warden? Responding to the Unethical or Incompetent Colleague*, 23 Hastings Center Rep. 19, 23 (May/June 1993).

Journal 1993 Explores problems associated with parental requests to withhold diagnoses from children. Discusses the physician's conflict between a duty to respect parents' wishes and a duty to tell children the truth. Quotes Principle II. Sigman, Kraut, & La Puma, *Disclosure of a Diagnosis to Children and Adolescents When Parents Object*, 147 Am. J. Diseases Children 764, 766 (1993).

Journal 1991 Examines the issues surrounding judicial use of professional ethics codes in private litigation. Concludes that judges should more extensively use professional ethics codes to define public policy, standards of care, and legal causes of action. Quotes Principle II and Opinion 2.19. Note, *Professional Ethics Codes in Court: Redefining the Social Contract Between the Public and the Professions*, 25 Georgia L. Rev. 1327, 1335, 1351 (1991).

Journal 1990 Examines the extent to which forensic psychiatrists are consulted in medical malpractice cases. Considers the appropriate standard of care, particularly for psychiatric malpractice cases, and the problems associated with its determination. References Principles II and IV. Modlin, *Forensic Psychiatry and Malpractice*, 18 Bull. Am. Acad. Psychiatry Law 153, 161 (1990).

Journal 1990 Discusses the moral dilemma in deciding whether to withdraw artificial nutrition and hydration from a patient and the appropriate role of the judiciary. Concludes that judicial decisions do not represent the moral viewpoint of society and that moral pronouncements should not be made in the courtroom. Quotes Preamble, Principles I, II, III, IV, V, VI, and VII, and Opinion 2.20. Peccarelli, *A Moral Dilemma: The Role of Judicial Intervention in Withholding or Withdrawing Nutrition and Hydration*, 23 John Marshall L. Rev. 537, 539, 540, 541 (1990).

Journal 1989 Discusses the history of the physician-patient privilege up through changes implemented under the Ohio Tort Reform Act of 1987. Aspects of the physician-patient privilege that are most significantly affected by this Tort Reform Act are highlighted, with recommendations for further refinement of the privilege in Ohio. Quotes Principles II, IV and Opinion 5.05. Note, *The Ohio Physician-Patient Privilege: Modified, Revised, and Defined*, 49 Ohio St. L. J. 1147, 1167 (1989).

Journal 1985 Initially describes how existing doctrines protect the value of autonomy in the context of the physician patient relationship, then examines various problems in the current protective scheme. Concludes by recommending the creation of an independent articulable protected interest in patient autonomy. Quotes Principles II and IV. Cites Opinions 4.04 (1984) [now Opinion 8.03 and 8.032] and 6.03 (1984) [now Opinion 6.02]. Shultz, *From Informed Consent to Patient Choice: A New Protected Interest*, 95 Yale L. J. 219, 275 (1985).

III.   A physician shall respect the law and also recognize a responsibility to seek changes in those requirements which are contrary to the best interests of the patient.

Ariz. 1965 Physician appealed denial of medical license which was based on alleged violations of local medical society rules and Principles 3, 5, and 10 (1957) [now Principles III and VII, and Opinions 3.01, 8.11, and 9.06]. Alleged violations included treating a patient without first obtaining a prior treating physician's permission, inadequate patient care, performing operations without hospital privileges, and signing the medical record of a deceased patient who had been treated by interns. The court held that the evidence failed to show any clear violation of the Principles and that a local medical society had no right to prescribe a code of ethics for state licensing purposes. *Arizona State Bd. of Medical Examiners v. Clark*, 97 Ariz. 205, 398 P.2d 908, 914-15, 915 n.3.

Ky. App. 1978 Plaintiff-physician attempted to enjoin defendant medical society from expelling him for actions contrary to a variety of Principles, the most relevant to his alleged unethical behavior being Principle 4 (1957) [now Principles II and III]. After reviewing the procedures followed by the medical society in considering the evidence pertaining to the charges, the court affirmed judgment dismissing the action, concluding that plaintiff was not deprived of due process. *Kirk v. Jefferson County Medical Soc'y*, 577 S.W.2d 419, 421.

Ohio 1980 A physician, charged with violating the state medical licensing statute by distributing controlled substances without a proper license and writing prescriptions for narcotics in the name of one person when they were intended for another, challenged the state medical board's decision to suspend his license and place him on two years probation. Under the statute, a physician could be disciplined for various activities including violation of any provision of a code of ethics of a national professional organization such as the American Medical Association. The board found in part that the physician's actions violated Principles 4 and 7 (1957) [now Principles II and III and Opinions 8.06 and 9.04]. The trial court reversed, holding that the board had insufficient evidence for its decision, and the court of appeals affirmed. On appeal, the supreme court held that expert testimony was not required at a hearing before a medical licensing board because they were experts and could determine for themselves whether the Principles had been violated. *Arlen v. State*, 61 Ohio St. 2d 168, 399 N.E.2d 1251, 1252, 1253-54.

Journal 2003 Uses public policy arguments to support a preponderance standard for medical license revocations in situations involving false testimony by a medical expert witness. Concludes that medical licensing boards can more effectively protect the public by using a preponderance standard. Quotes Principles II, III, and IV, and Opinions 1.02 and 9.07. Widmer, *South Dakota Should Follow Public Policy and Switch to the Preponderance Standard for Medical License Revocation After In Re the Medical License of Dr. Reuben Setliff, M.D.*, 48 S.D. L. Rev. 388, 396-97, 402 (2003).

Journal 2002 Explores the implications of withholding medical treatment when abortion results in a live birth. Concludes that, in these situations, abortive parents and physicians should not solely decide the child's best interest. Quotes Preamble, Principles I and III, and Opinions 2.035, 2.20, and 2.215. Casagrande, *Children Not Meant to Be: Protecting the Interests of the Child When Abortion Results in Live Birth*, 6 Quinnipiac Health L.J. 19, 44, 45, 47-48 (2002).

Journal 2002 Advocates in favor of disclosure of information regarding a physician's clinical experience when obtaining informed consent. Concludes that the physician's experience is material and patients who inquire should be given this information. Quotes Principle Ch. I, Art. I, Sec. 4 (1847) [now Principle II and Opinion 8.12]. Iheukwumere, *Doctor, are You Experienced? The Relevance of Disclosure of Physician Experience to a Valid Informed Consent*, 18 J. Contemp. Health L. & Pol'y 373, 376-77 (2002).

Journal 2002 Considers the dilemma of informed consent in the context of prescribing psychotropic medication to patients with mental illness and mental retardation. Recognizes the need for substituted decisionmaking in certain situations. Concludes that legislation would help address this issue. Quotes Preamble, Principles I, III, IV, VIII, and IX, and Opinion 8.08. O'Sullivan & Borcherding, *Informed Consent for Medication in Persons with Mental Retardation and Mental Illness*, 12 Health Matrix 63, 75, 86, 87, 88 (2002).

Journal 2001 Considers whether or not it is ethical for physicians to prescribe, and pharmacists to dispense, syringes for use by injection drug users. Concludes that ethical considerations suggest such actions are permissible but not obligatory. Quotes Principle III and Opinion 1.02. References Opinion 5.05. Lazzarini, *An Analysis of Ethical Issues in Prescribing and Dispensing Syringes to Injection Drug Users*, 11 Health Matrix 85, 107, 119 (2001).

Journal 2000 Considers the rules governing expert testimony. Explores professional ethical standards affecting expert witnesses and concludes that codes of ethics have not succeeded in eliminating biased expert testimony. Recommends creation of an organization to assist courts in obtaining reliable expert witness testimony. Quotes Principle III and Opinion 6.01. Cites Principles I, II, and V and Opinions 1.02 and 9.07. Murphy, *Expert Witnesses at Trial: Where are the Ethics?* 14 Geo. J. Legal Ethics 217, 231-32 (2000).

Journal 1999 States that current First Amendment opinions do not give clear guidelines on professional speech. Describes the United States Supreme Court's approach to commercial speech. Examines Supreme Court opinions and points out similarities between the Court's stance on commercial and professional speech. Cites Principle III. Halberstam, *Commercial Speech, Professional Speech, and the Constitutional Status of Social Institutions*, 147 U. Pa. L. Rev. 771, 857 (1999).

Journal 1999 Provides examples in which psychiatrists might use deception in their practice. Explains the motivations for such conduct and raises questions about possible blameworthiness for such conduct. Quotes Principles II and III. Haroun & Morris, *Weaving a Tangled Web: The Deceptions of Psychiatrists*, 10 J. Contemp. Leg. Issues 227, 235 (1999).

Journal 1999 Evaluates changes in direct-to-consumer advertising of prescription pharmaceuticals. Discusses FDA regulation of this type of advertising. Recognizes the important role of the FDA in this context. Quotes Principles II and III. Terzian, *Direct-to-Consumer Prescription Drug Advertising*, 25 Am. J. Law & Med. 149, 165 (1999).

Journal 1998 Examines the United States Supreme Court's decision in *Zinermon v. Burch* in relation to other Supreme Court decisions regarding the role of the courts in mental health treatment determinations. Argues that the government must strike a balance between the duty to care for the mentally ill and the duty to respect individual liberty. Provides approaches legislatures could adopt regarding mental health issues. References Principles I and III. Nidich, *Zinermon v. Burch and Voluntary Admissions to Public Hospitals: A Common Sense Proposal for Compromise*, 25 N. Ky. L. Rev. 699, 710 (1998).

Journal 1997 Discusses the practice of physician deselection by managed care organizations. Suggests that deselection harms the physician-patient relationship and creates a conflict of interest. Argues that solutions to deselection should consider effects on the patient rather than on the physician. Quotes Principle III. Cites Principle I and Opinions 8.05 and 8.13. Liner, *Physician Deselection: The Dynamics of a New Threat to the Physician-Patient Relationship*, 23 Am. J. Law & Med. 511, 513, 527 (1997).

Journal 1997 Discusses the need for balance between business ethics and medical ethics in the context of managed care. Explores two models for integrating ethics and managed care. Proposes the adoption of a collective responsibility model to improve quality of care. Quotes Principles I, II, III, IV, and V. Cites Preamble. References Opinion 8.13. Regan, *Regulating the Business of Medicine: Models for Integrating Ethics and Managed Care*, 30 Colum. J.L. & Soc. Probs. 635, 651, 656, 657 (1997).

Journal 1996 Discusses the trend toward conserving resources expended on health care by withholding services absent a showing of necessity. Claims that the high standard of care physicians owe patients is jeopardized by medical treatment decisions based on coverage concerns. Concludes that the legal structure regarding health care plans should be changed. Quotes Preamble, Principles I, II, III, IV, V, VI, and VII and Opinion 2.03. Hirshfeld & Thomason, *Medical Necessity Determinations: The Need for a New Legal Structure*, 6 Health Matrix 3, 8-9 (1996).

Journal 1995 Offers relevant historical perspectives and provides comprehensive ethical and legal discussion of physician-assisted suicide and euthanasia. Highlights important legislative developments, including the Oregon Death with Dignity Act, and analyzes significant judicial opinions. Quotes Principles III, IV, and VI and Opinions 2.21 and 9.12. Cites Opinions 2.20 and 8.11. Stone & Winslade, *Physician-Assisted Suicide and Euthanasia in the United States: Legal and Ethical Observations*, 16 J. Legal Med. 481, 483, 490, 497, 498, 499 (1995).

Journal 1994 Explores the ethical issues involved in a multidisciplinary team working with children in legal proceedings. Focuses on the relationships between professionals and the conflicts that arise regarding disclosure of confidential information and forced disclosure of non-privileged information. Quotes Principles III, IV, Fundamental Elements (4) and Opinions 1.02 (1992) and 5.07 (1992) [now Opinion 5.05]. Cites Opinion 2.02. Glynn, *Multidisciplinary Representation of Children: Conflicts Over Disclosures of Client Communications*, 27 J. Marshall L. Rev. 617, 625, 626, 630-32, 637, 639, 643 (1994).

Journal 1994 Argues that physician aid-in-dying should be protected by the US Constitution and that patients should have a federal cause of action to challenge prohibitive state statutes. Considers how such a cause of action might affect public policy. Quotes Principles I and III. References Opinion 2.06. Note, *Toward a More Perfect Union: A Federal Cause of Action for Physician Aid-In-Dying*, 27 U. Mich. J.L. Ref. 521, 538 (1994).

Journal 1994 Reviews the evolution of the physician-patient relationship, with attention to patient autonomy. Examines the changing health care delivery environment. Quotes Preamble, Principles I, II, III, IV, V, and VI, Fundamental Elements (1) and (2), and Opinions 1.02 and 8.07 (1981) [now Opinion 8.08]. Cites Opinion 1.01. Szczygiel, *Beyond Informed Consent*, 21 Ohio N.U.L. Rev. 171, 217, 218, 220, 225, 226, 256 (1994).

Journal 1993 Discusses physicians' duty to disclose to patients medical treatment alternatives that are not readily available. Proposes that based on the historical development and legal requirements of the informed consent doctrine, physicians should be required to inform patients of nonreadily available alternatives or face liability for breach of such obligation. Quotes Principles I, II, III, IV, and V and Opinion 8.08. Note, *Informed Choice: Physicians' Duty to Disclose Nonreadily Available Alternatives*, 43 Case W. Res. L. Rev. 491, 491, 498-99, 508, 509 (1993).

Journal 1991 Examines the wisdom and likely results of medicalizing psychoactive drugs of abuse. Concludes that although many physicians would consider prescribing psychoactive drugs of abuse for drug abusers in order to end dependence, few would be willing to prescribe such drugs for recreational purposes. Quotes Principle III. Levine, *Medicalization of Psychoactive Substance Use and the Doctor-Patient Relationship*, 69 Milbank Quarterly 623, 624 (1991).

Journal 1990 Discusses the moral dilemma in deciding whether to withdraw artificial nutrition and hydration from a patient and the appropriate role of the judiciary. Concludes that judicial decisions do not represent the moral viewpoint of society and that moral pronouncements should not be made in the courtroom. Quotes Preamble, Principles I, II, III, IV, V, VI, and VII and Opinion 2.20. Peccarelli, *A Moral Dilemma: The Role of Judicial Intervention in Withholding or Withdrawing Nutrition and Hydration*, 23 John Marshall L. Rev. 537, 539, 540, 541 (1990).

IV. A physician shall respect the rights of patients, colleagues, and other health professionals, and shall safeguard patient confidences and privacy within the constraints of the law.

10th Cir. 2001 Plaintiffs, former employees of a public medical center, brought suit against medical director under 42 USC. § 1983, based upon medical director's racially and sexually harassing actions and statements. The district court awarded compensatory and punitive damages against the medical director. Affirming the award of damages, the court quoted Principles I and IV and concluded that the medical director's behavior impacted not only plaintiffs, but the overall public health. *Nieto v. Kapoor*, 268 F.3d 1208, 1223 n. 12.

D. Kan. 1991 With apparent reliance on Principle IV and Opinion 5.05, plaintiff claimed that other than in discovery or judicial proceedings, the physician-patient privilege is absolute and precludes ex parte communications with defense counsel. While recognizing the confidential nature of the physician-patient relationship, the court held that the ethical standards promulgated by the AMA are not binding law and that, where a litigant-patient has placed his or her medical status in issue, the physician is released from the constraints imposed by the physician-patient relationship for the purposes of the litigation. *Bryant v. Hilst*, 136 F.R.D. 487, 490.

N.D. Ohio 1965 Plaintiff-patient alleged that the defendant-malpractice insurer induced physician to reveal confidential information about plaintiff on pretext that plaintiff filed a malpractice suit. In denying defendant's motion for reconsideration of the court's earlier opinion, the court confirmed its holding that actions of a third party inducing a physician to divulge confidential information may result in liability to the patient. In so holding, the court quoted (with incorrect citation to Ch. II, Sec.1) Principles Ch. I, Sec.2 (1912), [now Principle IV and Opinion 5.08], to emphasize the medical profession's established views regarding confidentiality. *Hammonds v. Aetna Casualty & Sur. Co.*, 243 F. Supp. 793, 803.

M.D. Pa. 1987 Plaintiff in a medical malpractice action sought to preclude his treating physicians from serving as defendant's expert witnesses at trial. The court held that defense counsel's failure to provide prior notice of ex parte communication with plaintiff's treating physicians barred their use as defense experts. Referring to *Petrillo v. Syntex Laboratories, Inc.*, 148 Ill. App. 3d 581, 499 N.E.2d 952 (1986), the court noted that the court there favorably cited Principle IV and Opinions 5.05, 5.06, and 5.07 (1984) in support of a public policy protecting confidentiality between physician and patient and against ex parte discussion. *Manion v. N.P.W. Medical Ctr. of N.E. Pa., Inc.*, 676 F.Supp. 585, 591.

Ala. 1973 Physician revealed patient information to the patient's employer, contrary to instructions of patient. Patient sued for breach of fiduciary duty. Citing Principle 9 (1957) [now Principle IV and Opinion 5.05] as well as cases from other states, the court held that even in the absence of a testimonial privilege statute, as a matter of public policy, a physician has a fiduciary duty not to make extrajudicial disclosures of patient information acquired in the course of treatment unless the public interest or the private interest of the patient demands otherwise. In holding that the physician had breached his contract with patient, the court found the Principles together with state licensing requirements sufficient to establish the public policy of confidentiality. *Horne v. Patton*, 291 Ala. 701, 287 So. 2d 824, 829, 832.

Alaska 1977 Physician-school board member failed to fully comply with state's conflict of interest law by refusing to reveal the names of patients from whom he had received over $100 in income. The physician claimed a legal privilege or ethical duty not to disclose the information under Principle 9 (1957) [now Principle IV and Opinion 5.05] and, alternatively, that the conflict of interest law unconstitutionally invaded a patient's right to privacy. The court held that disclosure was not barred by a legal privilege or ethical mandate, but that the conflict of interest law unconstitutionally invaded patient privacy due to the absence of protective regulations. In ruling on the ethical duty issue, the court noted that under Alaska law, a physician's license may be revoked for violating the Principles. However, the court found this licensing provision irrelevant to the privileged relationship exception in the conflict of interest law. The court found that otherwise the privilege exception in the statute could be changed by the American Medical Association, a private organization, simply by amending the Principles. *Falcon v. Alaska Pub. Offices Comm'n*, 570 P.2d 469, 474 n.13.

Ariz. App. 1992 Employer argued that workers' compensation statute abrogated the physician-patient privilege statute, permitting ex parte communications with employee's treating physician. Recognizing that a physician is ethically bound to protect the confidentiality of privileged information pursuant to Principle IV, yet lacks the legal training to distinguish between privileged and unprivileged information, the court held that a claimant has the right to insist that his attorney be present when his employer interviews the employee's physician. *Salt River Project v. Industrial Comm'n*, 1992 Ariz. App. LEXIS 323, 129 Ariz. Adv. Rep. 39.

Ariz. App. 1989 In a medical malpractice action, defense counsel interviewed several of plaintiff's treating physicians ex parte and notified plaintiff of this in preparation for a medical liability review panel hearing. Plaintiff moved to bar all testimony by those physicians and to disqualify defense counsel from representing defendants. The appellate court noted a physician's obligation of confidentiality pursuant to Principle IV and Opinion 5.05 and held that defense counsel in a medical malpractice action may not engage in non-consensual ex parte communications with plaintiff's treating physicians. *Duquette v. Superior Court*, 161 Ariz. 269, 778 P.2d 634, 641.

Cal. 1976 Parents sued psychotherapists to recover for murder of daughter by psychiatric patient, alleging that failure to warn victim of patient's violent threat was a proximate cause of her death. In considering whether such a revelation would have been a violation of professional ethics, the Court noted that Principle 9 (1957) [now Principle IV and Opinion 5.05] recognized that the confidential nature of a physician-patient communication must yield when disclosure is necessary to protect an individual or community as a whole. The court concluded that, in the circumstances of this case, disclosure would not have violated medical ethics and held that psychotherapists are under a duty to warn when they determine or should determine that a patient poses a serious danger of violence to someone else. *Tarasoff v. Regents of Univ. of Cal.*, 17 Cal.3d 425, 551 P.2d 334, 347, 131 Cal. Rptr. 14, 27.

Cal. 1970 Psychiatrist-witness in civil assault case applied for writ of habeas corpus after being held in contempt of court for refusing to produce patient's psychiatric records. Patient, plaintiff in the assault action, neither expressly claimed nor waived the statutory psychotherapist-patient privilege. The court held that the litigant-patient exception to the statutory psychotherapist-patient privilege does not unconstitutionally infringe rights of privacy of either psychotherapists or their patients. The court noted that in such a context a psychiatrist does not violate Principle 9 (1957) [now Principle IV and Opinion 5.05] since the Principle allows for legally compelled disclosure. *In re Lifschutz*, 2 Cal. 3d 415, 467 P.2d 557, 565-66 n.9, 85 Cal. Rptr. 829, 837-38 n.9.

Cal. App. 1982 Defendant was convicted of lewd act with a child and child molestation or annoyance, after licensed clinical psychologist reported defendant's admission of sexual conduct to authorities. The court held that the psychologist's testimony was properly admitted since a statute requiring the reporting of actual or suspected child abuse expressly made the psychotherapist-patient privilege inapplicable. The court quoted Principle 9 (1957) [now Principle IV and Opinions 2.02 and 5.05] in concluding the disclosure was not a breach of professional ethics. *People v. Stritzinger*, 137 Cal. App. 3d 126, 186 Cal. Rptr. 750, 752 rev'd, 34 Cal.3d 505, 668 P.2d 738, 194 Cal. Rptr. 431 (1983).

Colo. 1989 Spouse of police officer killed by released psychiatric patient sued state mental hospital and psychiatrist for negligence. Patient had blamed police for his misfortunes during repeated involuntary commitments for paranoid schizophrenia, and psychiatrist knew that patient would have access to a gun after release. The court held that a psychiatrist owed a duty of care in determining whether patient had propensity for violence and posed unreasonable risk of serious bodily harm to others. In so holding, the court cited Principle 9 (1957) [now Principle IV and Opinion 5.05], in support of the view that there are situations in which the need to protect an individual or the community from the threat of harm from a patient may outweigh the strong policy in favor of non-disclosure of patient confidences. *Perreira v. State*, 768 P.2d 1198, 1210 n.7.

Del. Super. 1993 Plaintiff-patient brought action for invasion of privacy, breach of confidentiality, and breach of implied contract against defendants, a physician and nurse. Plaintiff alleged that defendant-nurse, without plaintiff's consent, informed plaintiff's mother and grandmother that she was pregnant. Plaintiff also alleged that defendant-physician was liable for the nurse's conduct based on respondeat superior. The defendants questioned whether plaintiff had stated a cause of action and, if so, whether the cause should be treated as a medical malpractice action. Quoting Principle IV and noting that the legislature and the courts had recognized the duty of confidentiality, the court held that plaintiff had a cause of action for breach of confidentiality. *Martin v. Baehler*, 1993 Del. Super. LEXIS 199.

D.C. App. 1985 Patient sued plastic surgeon for breach of confidential physician-patient relationship following surgeon's use of before and after photographs of her plastic surgery in a department store presentation. In considering whether such a breach was an actionable tort, the court made reference to an earlier case quoting Principles Ch. II, Sec. 2 (1947) [erroneously cited in the earlier case as Ch. II, Sec. 1 (1943) [now Principle IV and Opinion 5.05], as evidence of the strong public policy which exists in favor of maintaining a patient's confidences. *Vassiliades v. Garfinckel's, Brooks Bros.*, 492 A.2d 580, 590, 591.

Fla. App. 1995 The court considered the issue of the effect of § 455.241(2) of the Florida Statutes on right of defense in a medical malpractice action to engage in ex parte communications with plaintiff's non-party treating physician. The court held that a 1988 amendment to § 455.241(2) negated the applicability of the statute to medical malpractice cases. The dissent, citing *Petrillo v. Syntex Laboratories, Inc.*, 148 Ill. App. 3d 581, 499 N.E.2d 952 (1986), quoted Principles II and IV and Opinions 5.05, 5.06, and 5.08 as strong public policy support for its position that ex parte communications should be barred altogether. *Castillo-Plaza v. Green*, 655 So. 2d 197, 206 n.4.

Ill. 1997 Trial court held various statutory sections, including those permitting unlimited disclosure of a patient's medical records, unconstitutional. On appeal, state supreme court affirmed. Regarding provisions mandating consent to the disclosure of medical records, the court noted, with reference to Principle IV and Opinion 5.05, the crucial importance of confidentiality in the physician-patient relationship. *Best v. Taylor Machine Works*, 179 Ill. 2d 367, 689 N.E. 2d 1057, 1099.

Ill. 1997 Plaintiffs brought action for medical malpractice and loss of consortium against physicians. Defendants sought the release of medical information according to a statute providing for unlimited access to a plaintiff's medical records. The trial court found this provision unconstitutional as a violation of separation of powers and of patients' privacy rights. On appeal, the court agreed that the statute violated separation of powers. Further, with apparent reference to Principle IV, the court noted the ethical duty of physicians to maintain patient confidentiality. The court, in turn, held that the statute violated the right to privacy, as patients hold confidentiality of personal medical information to be an integral part of privacy interests. *Kunkel v. Walton*, 179 Ill. 2d 519, 689 N.E. 2d 1047, 1055.

Ill. App. 1987 In appeal of malpractice action, an issue was whether expert testimony of plaintiff's treating physician, based upon discussions with the defense counsel without patient's consent, was admissible. The court held that ex parte communications between a plaintiff's treating physician and legal adversary violated public policy. In determining the existence of such a policy favoring the sanctity of the doctor-patient relationship, the court noted *Petrillo v. Syntex Laboratories Inc.*, 148 Ill. App. 3d 581, 499 N.E.2d 952 (1st Dist. 1986) and its reference to the Principles and Opinions, namely Principle IV and Opinion 5.05 (1984), which establish an ethical obligation to keep physician-patient communications confidential, generally requiring a patient's consent before information is released. *Yates v. El-Deiry*, 160 Ill. App. 3d 198, 513 N.E.2d 519, 522.

Ill. App. 1986 Defense attorney in product liability suit was held in contempt of court for conducting ex parte discussions with plaintiff-patient's treating physician without patient's consent and contrary to authorized methods of discovery. The court held that the strong public policy favoring physician-patient confidentiality articulated in Principles II and IV and Opinions 5.05, 5.06, 5.07, and 5.08 (1984) justified a rule against such ex parte discussions. Further, the court held that the public has the right to rely on physicians to faithfully execute their ethical obligations. *Petrillo v. Syntex Laboratories, Inc.*, 148 Ill. App. 3d 581, 499 N.E.2d 952, 957, 958, 959 cert. denied, 483 US 1007 (1987).

Ill. App. 1979 Patient filed suit against physician for breach of contract and breach of confidential relationship after physician's employee disclosed patient's name to police. Patient alleged that implied contract arose out of a statutory physician-patient privilege, and provisions of the Canons of Medical Ethics, with apparent reference to Principle 9 (1957) [now Principle IV and Opinion 5.05]. The court held that disclosure of patient's name alone by a physician or the physician's agents is insufficient to state a cause of action in contract and does not violate the physician-patient privilege. *Geisberger v. Willuhn*, 72 Ill. App. 3d 435, 390 N.E.2d 945, 946, 948.

Ind. App. 1996 A patient filed suit against a mental health counseling center for disclosing to a third party death threats made by the patient during therapy. The patient claimed this was a breach of the standard of care owed to her. The trial court found that the counseling center was not statutorily prohibited from disclosing death threats the patient made. On appeal, the court affirmed the decision. It noted, with apparent reference to Principle IV and Opinion 5.05, that physicians may disclose confidential information to ensure the safety of the public or of individuals. In clarifying its holding, the court observed that while free and frank communication should be promoted to aid proper diagnosis and treatment, public policy supports disclosure of confidential information when appropriate. *Rocca v. Southern Hills Counseling Center, Inc.*, 671 N.E. 2d 913, 916.

Me. 1999 Physician appealed decision of the Board of Licensure in Medicine imposing a civil penalty for his failure to release medical records to patient's physicians. Physician argued that the Board did not specify the ethical standards that his conduct violated. The court vacated the Board's decision on the grounds that the physician was denied the opportunity to refute evidence of a violation of professional standards or to develop a defense predicated on those standards. The Board, in defense of its decision, presented Opinions 7.01 and 7.02 to the court. The court, in vacating the decision, pointed out that the hearing record did not demonstrate which Opinions the Board applied. Furthermore, the court, quoting Principle IV, stated that the physician had a responsibility to protect the patient's medical records. *Balian v. Board of Licensure in Medicine*, 722 A.2d 364, 368.

Md. Att'y Gen. 1989 Except as required by statute, physicians are not legally obligated to report that an adult has been sexually assaulted. Quoting Principle IV regarding the safeguarding of patient confidences within the constraints of the law, the opinion concludes that a physician must consider the confidential nature of the physician-patient relationship when deciding whether to report that a patient has been sexually assaulted. *Maryland Att'y Gen. Op. No. 89-022.*

Md. Att'y Gen. 1986 State attorney general opined that statute authorized physicians to report to the Motor Vehicle Administration patients with certain disorders that would impair their ability to drive. The opinion cites Principle IV in support of the conclusion that, where required by law, a physician's disclosure of patient information is proper. *Maryland Att'y Gen. Op. No. 86-030 71 Op. Att'y. Gen. 407, 410.*

Md. Att'y Gen. 1977 Opinion addresses the obligation of a psychiatrist to report child abuse information obtained from a parent-patient. Referring to state statutes and to Principle 9 (1957) [now Principle IV and Opinions 2.02 and 5.05], the opinion concludes that the question of whether to disclose suspected child abuse is a matter left to the individual psychiatrist's professional and moral judgment. *Maryland Att'y. Gen. Opinion, 62 Op. Att'y Gen. 157, 160.*

Mass. 1989 Physician appealed after being disciplined for discussing anticipated deposition testimony with malpractice defendant's attorney one day prior to scheduled deposition. The court, referring to Principle IV, noted that the American Medical Association's ethical standards did not specifically address situation presented. After weighing the fact that physician had specifically asked attorney whether discussion was appropriate, the court held that the physician's behavior did not constitute gross misconduct and thus he could not be disciplined under licensing statute. *Hellman v. Board of Registration in Medicine, 404 Mass. 800, 537 N.E.2d 150, 153 n.4.*

Mass. 1984 Employee sued employer for libel and invasion of privacy following disclosure of medical facts about employee to other employees. In part, claim involved disclosure of opinion about employee's mental state to his supervisor by physician retained by employer. Citing Principle 9 (1957) [now Principle IV and Opinions 5.05 and 5.09], the court held that a physician retained by an employer may disclose to the employer information concerning an employee if receipt of the information is reasonably necessary to serve a substantial and valid business interest of the employer. *Bratt v. Intn'l Business Mach. Corp., 392 Mass. 508, 467 N.E.2d 126, 137 n.23.*

Minn. 1976 Plaintiff-patient in malpractice action appealed trial court's order to provide authorization for private, informal interview between defense counsel and patient's treating physician. In holding that formal pretrial discovery provided the exclusive procedure by which defendant could obtain medical testimony, the court noted, without deciding the issue, that a physician who discloses confidential patient information in a private interview may be subject to tort liability for breach of patient's right to privacy or professional discipline for unprofessional conduct, citing Principle 9 (1957) [now Principle IV and Opinion 5.05]. *Wenninger v. Muesing, 240 N.W.2d 333, 337 n.3.*

Mo. 1998 Defendant convicted of first degree murder claimed that a physician's testimony at trial violated Principle IV and the statutory physician-patient privilege because the physician contacted the press, provided interviews about his examination of defendant, and testified for the prosecution to rebut defendant's posttraumatic stress disorder defense. The court stated that the defendent waived any privilege and that it was not its place to enforce professional ethical standards. *State v. Johnson, 968 S.W.2d 123, 131.*

Mo. 1993 Patient sued physicians alleging a breach of fiduciary duty of confidentiality for participating in an unauthorized ex parte discussion with defendant's attorney. While recognizing this duty, the court held that, where the plaintiff's medical condition is in issue, this constitutes a waiver of both the testimonial privilege and the physician's fiduciary duty in so far as the information is related to the medical issues. Quoting Opinion 5.05 and citing Principle IV, the court stated that courts may apply ethical principles to frame the specific limits of the legal duty of confidentiality. *Brandt v. Medical Defense Assoc., 856 S.W.2d 667, 671 n.1.*

Mo. 1989 In a personal injury suit, plaintiff challenged trial court's authority to compel plaintiff to authorize ex parte meetings between defendant insurance company and plaintiff's treating physician. Applying a balancing test between preserving the physician-patient confidential and fiduciary relationship, the physician-patient testimonal privilege, and the quest for truth in civil litigation, the court held that such information could be obtained through the methods of formal discovery. The court quoted Principle IV and Opinion 5.05 (1984) as statements of the policy underlying medical confidentiality and a basis for a patient's affirmative right to rely on the confidential nature of disclosures to a treating physician. *State ex. rel. Woytus v. Ryan, 776 S.W.2d 389, 392-93.*

Mo. App. 1985 In a prohibition proceeding arising from a medical malpractice action, defense attorneys sought order compelling plaintiff to authorize a private interview between defense attorneys and physician who treated plaintiff for injuries allegedly caused by defendant-physician. The appellate court, after discussing Principle IV and Opinion 5.05 (1984), held that the defense attorneys had the right to seek an ex parte interview with the treating physician, subject to the willingness of the physician to grant the interview. Furthermore, the court noted that Opinion 5.05 prevents a physician from revealing a patient's confidences only where there is a lack of consent from the patient and found that consent did exist here in the form of a medical authorization executed by plaintiff during pendency of the malpractice action. *State ex rel. Stufflebam v. Appelquist, 694 S.W.2d 882, 886, 888 n.7, overruled by State ex. rel. Woytus v. Ryan, 776 S.W.2d 389 (Mo. 1989).*

N.J. 1985 Plaintiff provided authorization for release of decedent's medical records from former treating physicians but refused to consent to depositions or interviews between defense counsel and physicians. The court noted physicians' ethical duty to avoid unauthorized disclosure, as stated in Principle 9 (1957) [now Principle IV and Opinion 5.05], but recognized that a patient's right to confidentiality was not absolute. After balancing the competing interests involved, the court held that defense counsel had a right to seek ex parte interviews of decedent's other treating physicians regarding litigation matters, provided procedural safeguards were met including clear statements that participation in such an interview is voluntary on the part of a physician. *Stempler v. Speidell, 100 N.J. 368, 495 A.2d 857, 860, cert. denied, 483 US 1007 (1987).*

N.J. 1979 In wrongful death action against a psychiatrist whose patient murdered plaintiff's decedent, the court concluded, in accord with Principle 9 (1957) [now Principle IV], that a psychiatrist may owe a duty to warn potential victims of possible danger from psychiatrist's patient despite the general emphasis on confidentiality. The court also noted the Preamble and Principles 1 and 3 (1957) [now revised Preamble, Principle I, and Opinion 5.05] in discussing the psychiatrist-patient relationship. *McIntosh v. Milano, 168 N.J. Super. 466, 403 A.2d 500, 510, 512-13.*

N.J. 1962 Parents sued pediatrician for unauthorized disclosure to life insurer of deceased infant's congenital heart defect. The court quoted Principle 9 (1957) [now Principle IV and Opinion 5.05] as an articulation of a physician's legal duty to his or her patient subject to exceptions of compelling social or patient interests. The court held that the parents had lost their limited right to nondisclosure by filing an insurance claim. *Hague v. Williams, 37 N.J. 328, 181 A.2d 345, 347.*

N.J. Super. 2002 Patient brought suit against physician for releasing her medical records to opposing counsel in a divorce action without her authorization or consent. The lower court dismissed the complaint for failure to state a claim and ruled the records were discoverable. The New Jersey Superior Court reversed holding that the patient had a cause of action against both the physician and opposing counsel. Quotes Principle IV. *Crescenzo v. Crane, 350 N.J. Super. 531, 796 A.2d 283, 290.*

N.J. Super. 1991 Physician's estate sued hospital alleging that it violated state law against discrimination by restricting the physician's surgery privileges and requiring him to inform patients of his HIV-infected status before performing invasive procedures. The defendant hospital was also alleged to have breached its duty to maintain confidentiality of his seropositive diagnosis. The court held that the hospital had not discriminated against the physician since the hospital had relied on ethical and professional standards, including a report of the Council on Ethical and Judicial Affairs of the AMA dealing with the issue of AIDS [now Opinions 9.13 and 9.131]. However, the hospital was held to have breached its fiduciary duty to maintain the confidentiality of the physician's medical records. Referring to *McIntosh v. Milano, 168 N.J. Super. 466, 403 A.2d 500 (1979)* which had quoted AMA Principles of Medical Ethics sec. 9 (1957) [now Principle IV and Opinion 5.05] in applying the "duty to warn" exception, the court noted that the disclosure in this case went far beyond the medical personnel directly involved in the treatment of the physician and those patients entitled to informed consent. *Estate of Behringer v. Medical Ctr., 249 N.J. Super. 597, 614, 633, 592 A.2d 1251, 1259, 1268.*

N.J. Super. 1988 Several portions of state Department of Corrections regulations concerning exceptions to privileged communications between psychologist and inmates were invalidated by appellate court because they permitted disclosure of confidences that did not present clear and imminent danger to the inmate or others, or failed to identify any intended victim. Court made general reference (with erroneous quotation) to Principle 9 (1957) [now Principle IV and Opinion 5.05]. *In re Rules Adoption, 224 N.J. Super. 252, 540 A.2d 212, 215.*

N.J. Super. 1987 Defendant in a personal injury suit sought to offer testimony from plaintiff's treating physician regarding plaintiff's prognosis. The court denied plaintiff's motion to exclude that evidence, despite the ethical obligation of physicians to uphold patients' communications as confidential under Principle 9 (1957) [now Principle IV and Opinion 5.05]. The court's decision was based on New Jersey case law permitting disclosure of a patient's medical condition to someone having a legitimate interest where the physical condition of the patient is made an element of a claim. *Kurdek v. West Orange Bd. of Educ.*, 222 N.J. Super. 218, 536 A.2d 332, 335.

N.J. Super. 1967 In a suit for separate maintenance, communications between plaintiff-wife and her psychiatrist were not protected from disclosure during depositions, despite Principle 9 (1957) [now Principle IV and Opinion 5.05] which prohibited physicians from disclosing patient confidences except where necessary to protect the welfare of the individual or of the community. The court concluded that the patient had only a limited right of nondisclosure, subject to exceptions created by supervening interest of society and that the institution of litigation by the patient constituted a vitiation of that right. *Ritt v. Ritt*, 98 N.J. Super. 590, 238 A.2d 196, 199 rev'd, 52 N.J. 177, 244 A.2d 497 (1968).

N.Y. Sup. 2000 Physician brought wrongful discharge claim against corporate employer. The physician alleged she was discharged because she refused to reveal confidential medical information regarding employees. With apparent reference to Principle IV and Opinions 5.05 and 5.09, the affidavit filed by the physician claimed she had an ethical and legal duty to protect patient confidentiality. The court found termination of an employee at will based upon such grounds is sufficient to state a cause of action for breach of contract. The court ruled that obligations of good faith and fair dealing may be implied in a contract for the employment of a physician and that no physician should be placed in the position of choosing between retaining employment or violating ethical standards. *Horn v. New York Times*, 186 Misc. 2d 469, 719 N.Y.S. 2d 471, 474.

N.Y. Sup. 1977 Plaintiff, a psychiatric patient, sued her psychiatrist and the psychiatrist's spouse for violating several state statutes and her privacy rights by publishing a book about the intimate details of plaintiff's psychotherapy. The court found for plaintiff, basing its decision in part upon Principle 9 (1957) [now Principle IV and Opinion 5.05] which requires a physician to uphold the confidences of a patient. *Doe v. Roe*, 93 Misc. 2d 201, 400 N.Y.S.2d 668, 674.

N.Y. Surr. 1977 In a discovery proceeding, respondent-psychiatrist, who had treated some patients of deceased psychiatrist subsequent to his death, allegedly misappropriated decedent's patient records. Estate petitioned court for return of records and damages for injury to value of decedent's practice. Respondent sought dismissal of claim arguing that estate could not sell patient records. The court rejected respondent's request. In so ruling, the court noted that under Principle 9 (1957) [now Principle IV and Opinion 5.05] prohibiting physicians from revealing patient confidences, various guidelines had been issued regarding sale of a medical practice [now Opinion 7.04]. Whether respondent's actions had interfered with the estate's efforts to dispose of decedent's practice in keeping with these guidelines presented the court with factual issues for later resolution. *Estate of Finkle*, 90 Misc. 2d 550, 395 N.Y.S.2d 343, 346.

N.C. 1990 Plaintiff in a malpractice case was granted an order prohibiting ex parte conferences between defendant's attorney and non-party treating physicians. The court noted that both the Principles of Medical Ethics and Current Opinions affirm the physician's duty to protect patient confidentiality, in apparent reference to Principle IV and Opinion 5.05. In consideration of (1) the patient's right to privacy, (2) physician-patient confidentiality, (3) the adequacy of formal discovery procedures, and (4) the dilemma in which non-party treating physicians are placed by ex parte conferences, the court held that an attorney may not interview a patient's non-party treating physicians privately without express authorization. *Crist v. Moffatt*, 326 N.C. 326, 333, 389 S.E.2d 41, 46.

Ohio 1999 Patients brought a class action suit against hospital on grounds that the hospital disclosed patients' confidential medical information to the hospital's law firm, in order to determine whether the patients were eligible for government benefits to pay for unpaid hospital bills. The trial court granted defendants' motion for summary judgment. On appeal, the court held that a physician or a hospital can be held liable for unauthorized out-of-court disclosure of patients' confidential information. Additionally, the court found that an independent tort exists for unauthorized, unprivileged disclosure of patients' private medical information to a third party. The court cited Principle 9 (1957) [now Principle IV and Opinion 5.05], noting that courts have looked to such sources in providing a cause of action for breach of patient confidentiality. *Biddle v. Warren General Hospital*, 86 Ohio St. 3d 395, 715 N.E.2d 518, 523.

Ohio 1997 Estates of victims who were killed by their mentally ill son brought suit against son's psychotherapist for failing to disclose potential for violence. Son had been institutionalized and treated for schizophrenia. After release, he continued to take medication and see a psychotherapist. Despite parents' objections and attempts to have him involuntarily recommitted, psychotherapist reduced his medication and continued to recommend outpatient treatment. The court held that the psychotherapist had a duty to exercise reasonable care to control the son so as to prevent him from causing harm to his family. The court expressed concern for safeguarding the confidentiality of psychotherapeutic communications but noted that Principle 9 (1957) [now Principle IV and Opinion 5.05] has long allowed breaches of confidence when it becomes necessary to protect the welfare of the individual or the community. *Estates of Morgan v. Fairfield Family Counseling Center, 77 Ohio St. 3d 284, 303, 673 N.E.2d 1311, 1326.*

Ohio 1991 State medical board revoked license of physician who had consensual sexual relations with his patient. The court upheld the board's ruling that this violated Principles I, II, and IV. Dissenting judge, citing AMA Council on Ethical and Judicial Affairs, Sexual Misconduct in the Practice of Medicine, 266 JAMA 2741 [now Opinion 8.14], argued that until 1991, the AMA did not clearly deem sexual contact with a patient unethical. *Pons v. Ohio State Medical Bd., 66 Ohio St. 3d 619, 623, 625, 614 N.E.2d 748, 752, 753.*

Ohio 1988 Administrator sued psychiatrist for wrongful death after recently discharged patient killed her infant daughter. In determining whether a professional judgment rule should be adopted in the malpractice standard of care where the prediction of violent behavior is involved, the court referred favorably to Principle 9 (1957) [now Principle IV and Opinion 5.05] which allows breaches of patient confidences when necessary to protect potential victims. *Littleton v. Good Samaritan Hosp., 39 Ohio St. 3d 86, 529 N.E.2d 449, 459 n.19.*

Ohio App. 1999 Physician appealed trial court's affirmation of state medical board's decision to suspend his medical license because the physician engaged in sexual relationships with mothers of his pediatric patients. On appeal, the physician claimed that he was denied due process because physicians were not adequately notified that having sexual relations with parents of pediatric patients was unethical. The physician also claimed that the board had not presented adequate evidence that AMA Principles I and IV, extend to the parents of pediatric patients. The court quoted Principles I and IV, and stated that medical experts who testified were of the opinion that having sexual relationships with parents of pediatric patients constituted ethical violations. *Gladieux v. Ohio State Medical Board, 1999 WL 770959, *2, *4.*

Okla. 1988 In response to a police request, physician reported patient treated for a penile bite. Patient sued physician for negligence after information furnished by physician led to patient's arrest and conviction for rape. Patient alleged a tortious breach of the physician-patient confidential relationship, breach of contract, violation of licensing statute, and breach of Principle 9 (1957) [now Principle IV and Opinion 5.05]. The court reasoned that the benefit of the divulgence inured to the public at large and thus fell within the public policy exception to the testimonial privilege, created no liability in tort or contract, and was not a breach of medical ethics under the licensing statute or the Principles. *Bryson v. Tillinghast, 749 P.2d 110, 113, 114.*

Pa. 1973 Plaintiff in personal injury suit resulting from auto accident claimed that trial court should have allowed showing on cross-examination that defendant's expert medical witness, who had treated plaintiff, violated Principle 9 (1957) [now Principle IV and Opinion 5.05] by ex parte communications with defense counsel, in order to impeach his medical testimony. The court held that any connection between an alleged breach of medical ethics and the credibility of a physician on the witness stand was tenuous. Therefore, the trial court's decision barring further inquiry in this regard was proper. *Downey v. Weston, 451 Pa. 259, 301 A.2d 635, 638.*

Pa. Super. 1988 Plaintiff-patient sued her physician for breach of confidentiality when physician conferred with defense counsel in plaintiff's malpractice suit against the hospital (physician's employer). In its majority opinion, the court cited Principle IV, commenting that it gave very little guidance to physicians but nonetheless was not violated by the physician. The court also noted Opinion 5.07 (1986) finding that the plaintiff's suit minimized her expectations of confidentiality. The dissent, however, interpreted these same provisions, along with Opinion 5.05 (1986), as protecting plaintiff's expectations of confidentiality. *Moses v. McWilliams, 379 Pa. Super. 150, 549 A.2d 950, 956, 962 (dissent), appeal denied, 521 Pa. 630, 558 A.2d 532 (1989).*

S.C. 2003 Worker's Compensation Commission ordered injured employee's attorney to stop obstructing *ex parte* contacts between rehabilitative nurse hired by employer and treating physicians regarding employee's medical condition. The South Carolina Supreme Court reversed and held that the Worker's Compensation Act did not authorize such *ex parte* communication. Quotes Principle IV. *Brown v. Bi-Lo, Inc, 354 S.C. 436, 581 S.E.2d 836, 840, n. 5.*

S.C. App. 1997 Patient sued physician for breaching duty of confidentiality after physician divulged patient's emotional health status in a letter which was introduced during patient's divorce proceeding. The trial court dismissed the action for failure to state a cause of action, finding state law did not support a duty of confidentiality. The appeals court reversed. In part, it found a basis for such an action in medical and ethical principles, with apparent reference to Principle IV. Absent a compelling public interest in disclosure, confidences must be preserved. The court remanded to consider whether the disclosure was essential to the best interests of the patient or others. *McCormick v. England*, 328 S.C. 627, 494 S.E. 2d 431, 435.

Tenn. App. 1994 Plaintiff sought damages for wrongful death from defendant-surgeon. Defendant requested that the court require plaintiff to sign a form authorizing release of medical records and information to defense counsel. Trial court denied defendant's motion noting, with apparent reference to Principle IV and Opinion 5.05, that confidential relationship exists between physician and patient. Appellate court affirmed although it did not reach the ethical issue of the propriety of disclosures by a physician. *Wright v. Wasudev*, 1994 Tenn. App. LEXIS 657.

Utah Att'y Gen. 1978 A physician who, acting in good faith, discloses confidential information to proper authorities concerning a patient's unfitness to drive is not liable for doing so. Reference is made to Principle 9 (1957) [now Principle IV and Opinion 5.05] to support propriety of such disclosure where the public interest is involved. *Utah Att'y Gen. Op. No. 77-294.*

Wash. 1988 Personal representative brought wrongful death action against decedent's physicians. At issue was whether defense counsel in a personal injury action may communicate ex parte with plaintiff's treating physician where plaintiff has waived the physician-patient relationship. In holding that defense counsel may not engage in ex parte communication, and is limited to formal discovery methods, the court cited Principle IV and Opinion 5.05 (1986) with approval, reasoning that the mere threat of disclosure of private conversations between a physician and defense counsel would chill the physician-patient relationship and hinder further treatment. *Loudon v. Mhyre*, 110 Wash. 2d 675, 756 P.2d 138, 141, 141 n.3.

Wash. App. 2000 Patient sued a physician under medical malpractice statute, seeking damages for emotional distress resulting from the physician's disclosure of confidential information to the patient's ex-husband. Trial court granted the defendant's motion for summary judgment. On appeal, the court held that a tort action did exist under the statute for damages resulting from the unauthorized disclosure of confidential information related to health care obtained within the physician-patient relationship. The court quoted Principle IV, stating that the accepted standard of care includes a duty to maintain confidentiality with respect to patient information. *Berger v. Sonneland*, 101 Wash. App. 141, 1 P.3d 1187, 1192.

W. Va. 1993 Plaintiff, in a malpractice action, sought a writ of prohibition to prevent the enforcement of a trial court order allowing ex parte interviews. The court, in granting the writ, held that any benefit from ex parte interviews that occurs is minimal compared to the danger that they will undermine the confidential nature of the physician-patient relationship. Quoting Principles of Medical Ethics Ch. II, sec. 1 (1943) [now Principle IV and Opinion 5.05], the court noted that the medical profession is well aware of the importance of patient confidentiality. *State ex. rel. Kitzmiller v. Henning*, 437 S.E.2d 452, 454.

W. Va. 1988 Patient-wife sued psychiatrist who disclosed subpoenaed confidential information to her husband's attorney in divorce proceedings. The court held that a tort action lies when confidential communications regarding mental health patients are released, except under limited circumstances such as a binding court order. The court, however, declined to recognize an enforceable contractual right to confidentiality, although it noted that some states have recognized such a right based upon Principle IV. *Allen v. Smith*, 368 S.E.2d 924, 928.

Wis. 1995 In medical malpractice suit, the court held that (1) subject to restrictions, defense counsel may engage in ex parte communications with plaintiff's treating physician if the communications do not involve disclosure of confidential information; (2) outside a judicial proceeding, defendant-physician may communicate ex parte with plaintiff's treating physician subject to a physician's duty of confidentiality; and (3) if defense counsel elicits confidential information from a treating physician during ex parte communications, the appropriate sanction is within the discretion of the court. The court expressly overruled *State ex rel. Klieger v. Alby*, 125 Wis. 2d 468, 373 N.W.2d 57 (Ct. App. 1985) and the cases applying it. The majority and concurring opinions referred to Principle IV and Opinion 5.05. *Steinberg v. Jensen*, 194 Wis. 2d 440, 534 N.W.2d 361, 370, 377.

Wis. App. 1994 In medical malpractice suit, defense counsel engaged in ex parte communications with plaintiff's consulting physicians. Plaintiff amended her complaint seeking punitive damages for breach of confidentiality. The court concluded that the rule of *State ex rel. Klieger v. Alby*, 125

Wis. 2d 468, 373 N.W.2d 57 (Ct. App. 1985), which prohibits ex parte communications that have the potential to breach physician-patient confidentiality, was violated and sanctions were required. The court referred to *Petrillo v. Syntax Labs., Inc.*, 148 Ill. App. 3d 581, 499 N.E.2d 952 (1986) and its use of Principle IV and Opinion 5.05. *Steinberg v. Jensen, 186 Wis. 2d 237, 519 N.W.2d 753, 761 n.9, rev'd, 194 Wis. 2d 440, 534 N.W.2d 361 (1995).*

Wis. Att'y Gen. 1987 Physicians may report cases of suspected child abuse or neglect when a patient discloses that he or she has abused a child in some manner. Where report is made in good faith, physicians are immune from any civil or criminal liability. Passing reference is made to Principle 9 (1957) [now Principle IV and Opinions 2.02 and 5.05] in support of this position. *Wisconsin Att'y Gen. Op. 10-87 (Mar. 16, 1987) (LEXIS, States library, Wis. file).*

Journal 2003 Considers the legal, medical, and ethical issues of physician-patient confidentiality in disclosure of paternity. Concludes that a balancing test should be applied to making determinations regarding disclosure of paternity. Quotes Principles I, IV, and V, and Opinions 1.02, 5.055, and 10.01. Cites Principle II and Opinion 5.05. Richards & Wolf, *Medical Confidentiality and Disclosure of Paternity, 48 S.D. L. Rev. 409, 411, 412, 413 (2003).*

Journal 2003 Uses public policy arguments to support a preponderance standard for medical license revocations in situations involving false testimony by a medical expert witness. Concludes that medical licensing boards can more effectively protect the public by using a preponderance standard. Quotes Principles II, III, and IV, and Opinions 1.02 and 9.07. Widmer, *South Dakota Should Follow Public Policy and Switch to the Preponderance Standard for Medical License Revocation After In Re the Medical License of Dr. Reuben Setliff, M.D., 48 S.D. L. Rev. 388, 396-97, 402 (2003).*

Journal 2002 Analyzes the expanded use of the Civil False Claims Act in prosecuting health care fraud. Concludes that, in enforcing the law, government must balance its promises to beneficiaries, health care providers, and the public. Quotes Principles I, II, and IV. Krause, *"Promises to Keep": Health Care Providers and the Civil False Claims Act, 23 Cardozo L. Rev. 1363, 1365 (2002).*

Journal 2002 Considers the dilemma of informed consent in the context of prescribing psychotropic medication to patients with mental illness and mental retardation. Recognizes the need for substituted decisionmaking in certain situations. Concludes that legislation would help address this issue. Quotes Preamble, Principles I, III, IV, VIII, and IX, and Opinion 8.08. O'Sullivan & Borcherding, *Informed Consent for Medication in Persons with Mental Retardation and Mental Illness, 12 Health Matrix 63, 75, 86, 87, 88 (2002).*

Journal 2002 Considers the ethical and legal issues regarding breach of confidentiality in situations where a patient is pregnant and uses teratogenic substances. Concludes that a breach of confidentiality causes damage to the physician-patient relationship. Quotes Principle IV and Opinion 10.01. Plambeck, *Divided Loyalties: Legal and Bioethical Considerations of Physician-Pregnant Patient Confidentiality and Prenatal Drug Abuse, 23 J. Legal Med. 1, 8, 25 (2002).*

Journal 2002 Analyzes the role of prognostication in physician-patient communication. Concludes that the patient-physician model of shared decision-making offers the best hope for reestablishing prognostication. Quotes Principles Ch. I, Art. I, Sec. 2 and 4 (1846) [now Principle IV and Opinions 8.12 and 10.01]. Cites Opinion 8.08. Rich, *Prognostication in Clinical Medicine: Prophecy or Professional Responsibility? 23 J. Legal Med. 297, 299, 318, 327 (2002).*

Journal 2002 Considers the case of Ferguson v. City of Charleston. Concludes that the Supreme Court's rationale in that case reflects insights from feminist legal theory. Quotes Opinion 10.01. Cites Principles II and IV. Taslitz, *A Feminist Fourth Amendment?: Consent, Care, Privacy, and Social Meaning in Ferguson v. City of Charleston, 9 Duke J. Gender L. & Pol'y 1, 18, 19 (2002).*

Journal 2001 Discusses issues surrounding the privacy of genetic information. Considers the social, ethical, and legal responses to problems that arise in this context. Concludes with a unique view of privacy that would protect the right of individuals not to know genetic information about themselves. Quotes Principle IV and Opinion 10.01. Laurie, *Challenging Medical-Legal Norms: The Role of Autonomy, Confidentiality, and Privacy in Protecting Individual and Familial Group Rights in Genetic Information, 22 J. Legal Med. 1, 24 (2001).*

Journal 2001 Considers ethical aspects of physician conflicts of interest in the context of human subjects research. Focuses on conflicts that are associated with clinical trials of new drugs and devices. Concludes by discussing the impact of these conflicts of interest on trust in the physician-patient relationship. References Principle IV and Opinion 8.032. Miller, *Trusting Doctors: Tricky Business When It Comes to Clinical Research, 81 B.U.L. Rev. 423, 427-28 (2001).*

Journal 2001 Considers conflicts of interest in clinical research and other types of medical practice. Compares the way in which doctors and lawyers address conflicts of interest in professional practice. Concludes that physicians are unaware of the need to create a meaningful conflict-of-interest doctrine for medical practice. Quotes Preamble, Principle IV, and Opinions 2.07, 8.03, 8.031, and 10.01. Moore, *What Doctors Can Learn from Lawyers about Conflicts of Interest*, 81 B.U.L. Rev. 445, 447, 449-50 (2001).

Journal 2001 Discusses linkages between governmental regulation of medical privacy and reduced medical error. Concludes that protection of patient privacy and the reduction of medical error will be important aspects of health care reform and will spur structural changes in health care delivery that will positively affect evolution of medical malpractice law. Quotes Principle IV. Terry, *An eHealth Diptych: The Impact of Privacy Regulation on Medical Error and Malpractice Litigation*, 27 Am. J.L. & Med. 361, 402 (2001).

Journal 2000 Discusses the development and history of the ethical doctrine of informed consent. Examines the current state of the law in Pennsylvania and concludes it does not adequately fulfill the goals of ethical and legal doctrines. Quotes Principle IV and Opinion 10.01. References Opinion 8.08. Warren, *Pennsylvania Medical Informed Consent Law: A Call to Protect Patient Autonomy Rights By Abandoning the Battery Approach*, 38 Duq. L. Rev. 917, 925 (2000).

Journal 1999 Examines reporting of AIDS and HIV under Texas law. Discusses limitations on a physician's ability to warn potentially at-risk third parties. Concludes that Texas law should be changed to place a duty upon physicians to notify at-risk third parties of a patient's HIV-positive status. Quotes Principle IV and Opinion 10.01. Acosta, *The Texas Communicable Disease Prevention and Control Act: Are We Offering Enough Protection to Those Who Need It Most?* 36 Hous. L. Rev. 1819, 1822, 1830, 1831 (1999).

Journal 1999 Discusses whether a physician has the duty to disclose cancer-related gene mutations to a patient's children. Reviews current legislation regarding disclosure of genetic information. Argues that the potential for harm outweighs imposition of a duty to disclose. Quotes Principle IV. Brownrigg, *Mother Still Knows Best: Cancer-Related Gene Mutations, Familial Privacy, and a Physician's Duty to Warn*, 26 Fordham Urb. L. J. 247 (1999).

Journal 1999 Discusses the use of expert witnesses. Points out that, although some professions have a code of ethics, there is not a single source that defines professional ethics for expert witnesses. Argues that ethical and professional standards for expert witnesses must be defined. Cites Principle IV. Lubet, *Expert Witnesses: Ethics and Professionalism*, 12 Geo. J. Legal Ethics 465, 466 (1999).

Journal 1999 Discusses the practice of male circumcision in the United States. Examines situations where the state may intervene in parental decision-making affecting minor children. Argues that males should be afforded the same protection as females in statutes prohibiting the mutilation of genital organs. Quotes Principle IV. Povenmire, *Do Parents Have the Legal Authority to Consent to the Surgical Amputation of Normal, Healthy Tissue from their Infant Children?: The Practice of Circumcision in the United States*, 7 Am. U. J. Gender Soc. Pol. & L. 87, 96 (1999).

Journal 1999 Discusses the need for physicians to advocate on behalf of patients' rights in the context of health care delivery. Evaluates the nature and scope of the physician's role as advocate, noting that physicians cannot be expected to engage in attorney-like advocacy. Quotes Principles IV and VI, Fundamental Elements (2), (4), and (6) [now Opinion 10.01], Patient Responsibilities 5 [now Opinion 10.02], and Opinions 2.03, 2.07, 2.09, 2.16, 2.19, 3.06, 4.01, 4.04, 6.01, 7.02, 8.02, 8.03, 8.13, 8.132, 9.06, 9.07, and 9.131. Cites Opinions 5.05, 5.09, 7.01, 8.135, and 9.02. Sage, *Physicians as Advocates*, 35 Hous. L. Rev. 1529, 1537, 1541, 1542, 1552-53, 1554, 1556, 1557, 1559, 1561-62, 1564, 1571, 1574, 1576, 1580 (1999).

Journal 1999 Discusses the Department of Health and Human Services recommendations for federal legislation regarding confidentiality of health information. Points out that the recommendations include an exception for law enforcement access to medical records. Argues that such an exception must be narrow and clearly defined. Quotes Principle IV. Van Der Goes, *Opportunity Lost: Why and How to Improve the HHS-Proposed Legislation Governing Law Enforcement Access to Medical Records*, 147 U. Pa. L. Rev. 1009, 1063 (1999).

Journal 1999 Explores Model Rules of Professional Conduct focusing on the attorney-client relationship. Compares confidentiality provisions in the Model Rules with the rules of confidentiality governing the medical profession. Observes that existing confidentiality rules are incomplete and ambiguous. Concludes that one remedy is to embrace a discretionary confidentiality rule. Quotes Opinion 5.05. Cites Principle IV and Opinion 5.07. Zer-Gutman, *Revising the Ethical Rules of*

Attorney-Client Confidentiality: Towards a New Discretionary Rule, 45 Loy. L. Rev. 669, 683-84, 699, 709, 718 (1999).

Journal 1998 Discusses issues of privacy arising out of collection and dissemination of genetic information about specific individuals. Emphasizes the need for privacy and confidentiality in this context. Suggests that future public policy should accommodate this need. Quotes Principle IV. Balint, *Issues of Privacy and Confidentiality in the New Genetics*, 9 Alb. L. J. Sci. & Tech. 27, 32 (1998).

Journal 1998 Recommends the passage of Ohio's proposed bill that would recognize an accountant-client privilege. Describes current recognized privileges, including the physician-patient privilege. Quotes Principle IV. Canning, *Privileged Communications in Ohio and What's New on the Horizon: Ohio House Bill 52 Accountant-Client Privilege*, 31 Akron L. Rev. 505, 550 (1998).

Journal 1998 Suggests that professional ethics correspond well to many governmental areas. Argues that the professional rules are more difficult for politically appointed attorneys. Indicates that ethical questions for government-appointed attorneys are often resolved through personal ethics rather than professional codes. Cites Principle IV. Lund, *The President as Client and the Ethics of the President's Lawyers*, 61 L. & Contemp. Probs. 65, 68 (1998).

Journal 1998 Discusses issues of patient consent regarding disclosure of medical information. Points out that recent changes in the health care system have presented medical record privacy concerns. Discloses findings of a study regarding hospital consent forms and calls for more research to be conducted. Cites Principle IV and Opinion 5.05. Merz, Sankar, & Yoo, *Hospital Consent for Disclosure of Medical Records*, 26 J. Law, Med. & Ethics 241, 248 (1998).

Journal 1998 Examines the transition from paper medical records to electronic medical records. Identifies issues of confidentiality and privacy that arise as a result of the move to electronic medical records. Concludes that federal protection is needed to safeguard personal medical information. Quotes Principle IV and Opinions 5.07 and 5.075. Cites Opinion 8.061. Tsai, *Cheaper and Better: The Congressional Administrative Simplification Mandate Facilitates the Transition to Electronic Medical Records*, 19 J. Legal Med. 549, 570, 581 (1998).

Journal 1998 Explores the increased use and benefits of telemedicine. Points out that there is inadequate protection of privacy rights regarding electronic medical information. Concludes that federal law does not uniformly address medical record privacy and that Missouri law lacks adequate specificity. Quotes Principle IV. References Opinion 5.05. Young, *Telemedicine: Patient Privacy Rights of Electronic Medical Records*, 66 UMKC L. Rev. 921, 926 (1998).

Journal 1997 Discusses the Massachusetts statute that prohibits disclosure of a person's HIV status without obtaining informed consent. Suggests that legislation should be enacted mandating reporting of HIV to the department of public health. Quotes Principle IV. Agnello, *Advocating for a Change in the Massachusetts HIV Statute: Putting an End to Physician Uncertainty*, 2 J. Trial App. Advoc. 105, 107 (1997).

Journal 1997 Discusses the need for health care providers to have accurate medical information to treat patients effectively. Explains the benefits of computerized patient medical records and the privacy and confidentiality concerns raised. Concludes that patient privacy needs to be assured to improve service. Quotes Principle IV. Cuzmanes & Orlando, *Automation of Medical Records: The Electronic Superhighway and Its Ramifications for Health Care Providers*, 6 J. Pharmacy & L. 19, 27 (1997).

Journal 1997 Discusses principles of autonomy in the physician-patient relationship. Notes that rights to privacy and confidentiality are grounded in patient autonomy. Concludes that patients may be harmed when privacy rights are breached. Quotes Principle IV. Doyal, *Human Need and the Right of Patients to Privacy*, 14 J. Contemp. Health L. & Pol'y 1, 3 (1997).

Journal 1997 Considers principles of confidentiality in the physician-patient relationship. Notes the current trend emphasizing public reporting obligations of physicians to protect members of society. Emphasizes need for balance between patient rights and societal interests. Quotes Principle IV and Opinion 5.05. References Preamble. Jozefowicz, *The Case Against Having Professional Privilege in the Physician-Patient Relationship*, 16 Med. & L. 385, 386-87, 391 (1997).

Journal 1997 Suggests that ex parte conferences between treating physicians and opposing counsel undermine the physician-patient relationship. Notes that there are no significant benefits within the fact-finding process that justify the conflicts of interest created. Concludes that ex parte conferences are unnecessary. Quotes Principle IV and Opinion 5.05. Kassel, *Counterpoint . . . Defense Counsel's Ex Parte Communication with Plaintiff's Doctors: A Bad One-Sided Deal*, 9 S.C. Law. 42, 43 (Sept./Oct. 1997).

Journal 1997 Discusses the need for balance between business ethics and medical ethics in the context of managed care. Explores two models for integrating ethics and managed care. Proposes the adoption of a collective responsibility model to improve quality of care. Quotes Principles I, II, III, IV, and V. Cites Preamble. References Opinion 8.13. Regan, *Regulating the Business of Medicine: Models for Integrating Ethics and Managed Care*, 30 Colum. J.L. & Soc. Probs. 635, 651, 656, 657 (1997).

Journal 1997 Explores confidentiality problems that arise as a result of new health information systems. Examines legal aspects of medical records confidentiality. Advocates legislation at the national level to protect privacy of personal health information. Cites Principles of Medical Ethics § 9 (1957) [now Principle IV]. Turkington, *Medical Record Confidentiality Law, Scientific Research, and Data Collection in the Information Age*, 25 J. Law, Med. & Ethics 113, 126 (1997).

Journal 1996 Explores whether patients have a duty to disclose their HIV status to treating physicians. Suggests that recognizing such a duty may subject patients to a lower standard of care and provide a disincentive to be tested. Concludes that courts should not impose a duty to disclose on patients. Quotes Principle 9 (1957) [now Principle IV] and Opinion 9.131. DeNatale & Parrish, *Health Care Workers' Ability to Recover in Tort for Transmission or Fear of Transmission of HIV from a Patient*, 36 Santa Clara L. Rev. 751, 782-83, 787 (1996).

Journal 1996 Discusses the trend toward conserving resources expended on health care by withholding services absent a showing of necessity. Claims that the high standard of care physicians owe patients is jeopardized by medical treatment decisions based on coverage concerns. Concludes that the legal structure regarding health care plans should be changed. Quotes Preamble, Principles I, II, III, IV, V, VI, and VII and Opinion 2.03. Hirshfeld & Thomason, *Medical Necessity Determinations: The Need for a New Legal Structure*, 6 Health Matrix 3, 8-9 (1996).

Journal 1996 Discusses sexual abuse litigation in which accusers have recovered memories of molestation in psychotherapy sessions. Observes that to successfully defend against such claims, it is necessary for the accused to have access to the clinical record. Posits that confidentiality problems can be eliminated with *in camera* record inspections. References Principle IV and Opinion 5.05. Loftus, Paddock, & Guernsey, *Patient-Psychotherapist Privilege: Access to Clinical Records in the Tangled Web of Repressed Memory Litigation*, 30 U. Rich L. Rev. 109, 127 (1996).

Journal 1996 Reviews two Washington state supreme court decisions in which subsequent treating physicians testified against their patients and on behalf of defendant physicians in malpractice litigation. Observes that these decisions erode the physician-patient privilege. Posits that the decisions are inconsistent with current medical ethics and proposes a statutory enactment as a solution. Quotes Opinion 5.05. Cites Principle 9 (1957) [now Principle IV]. Oppenheim, *Physicians as Experts Against Their Own Patients? What Happened to the Privilege?*, 63 Def. Couns. J. 254, 257, 261 (1996).

Journal 1996 Considers prearraignment forensic evaluations. Notes the prohibition against use of such evaluations. Examines underlying ethical precepts. Observes that principles of beneficence are misapplied to forensic psychiatry in this context. Advocates a new ethical framework. Quotes Preamble. References Principle IV and Opinion 5.05. Ornish, Mills, & Ornish, *Prearraignment Forensic Evaluations: Toward a New Policy*, 24 Bull. Am. Acad. Psychiatry Law 453, 454, 469 (1996).

Journal 1996 Examines the psychiatrist-patient duty of confidentiality. Notes that Principles of Medical Ethics prohibit the disclosure of patient confidences and medical records. Observes that exceptions to this prohibition exist when required by law or to protect the community. Quotes Principle 9 (1957) [now Principle IV and Opinion 5.05]. Sadoff, *Ethical Obligations for the Psychiatrist: Confidentiality, Privilege, and Privacy in Psychiatric Treatment*, 29 Loy. L.A. L. Rev. 1709, 1710, 1711 (1996).

Journal 1996 Examines the theories courts have used when evaluating claims for emotional distress damages arising from HIV misdiagnosis. Observes that the physical injury requirement is outdated but notes that alternatives may give rise to potentially unlimited liability. Concludes that physicians should be afforded good faith immunity from suits. Quotes Principle 9 (1957) [now Principle IV]. Schmid, *Protecting the Physician in HIV Misdiagnosis Cases*, 46 Duke L. J. 431, 458 (1996).

Journal 1995 Discusses the belief of health care providers that they have an ethical obligation to warn the partners of HIV-positive patients. Examines both the scope of a Massachusetts statute that prevents providers from releasing HIV test results of patients and possible defenses that providers may assert. Quotes Principle IV and Opinion 5.05. Friedland, *HIV Confidentiality and the Right to Warn—The Health Care Provider's Dilemma*, 80 Mass. L. Rev. 3, 4 (March 1995).

Journal 1995 Examines federal legislative proposals intended to protect confidentiality of computerized medical records. Concludes that proposed legislation will significantly undermine confidentiality. Cites Opinion 5.07. References Principle IV. Hoge, *Proposed Federal Legislation Jeopardizes Patient Privacy,* 23 Bull. Am. Acad. Psychiatry Law 495, 498, 500 (1995).

Journal 1995 Offers relevant historical perspectives and provides comprehensive ethical and legal discussion of physician-assisted suicide and euthanasia. Highlights important legislative developments, including the Oregon Death with Dignity Act, and analyzes significant judicial opinions. Quotes Principles III, IV, and VI and Opinions 2.21 and 9.12. Cites Opinions 2.20 and 8.11. Stone & Winslade, *Physician-Assisted Suicide and Euthanasia in the United States: Legal and Ethical Observations,* 16 J. Legal Med. 481, 483, 490, 497, 498, 499 (1995).

Journal 1994 Compares Texas law with Illinois law on the issue of ex parte communications between defense counsel and the patient/plaintiff's physician in civil litigation. Argues that preservation of the physician-patient relationship requires prohibition of such contact. Quotes Principles II and IV and Opinion 5.05. Comment, *From the Land of Lincoln a Healing Rule: Proposed Texas Rule of Civil Procedure Prohibiting Ex Parte Contact Between Defense Counsel and a Plaintiff's Treating Physician,* 25 Tex. Tech L. Rev. 1081, 1081, 1082 (1994).

Journal 1994 Considers whether an exception should be made to physician-patient confidentiality that would allow a physician to reveal parental medical history to a child. Concludes that such an exception would not completely erode physician-patient confidentiality. Quotes Principles IV, Fundamental Elements (4), and Opinion 5.05. Cites Principle I and Fundamental Elements (1). Friedland, *Physician-Patient Confidentiality: Time to Re-Examine a Venerable Concept in Light of Contemporary Society and Advances in Medicine,* 15 J. Legal Med. 249, 257, 264, 276 (1994).

Journal 1994 Explores the ethical issues involved in a multidisciplinary team working with children in legal proceedings. Focuses on the relationships between professionals and the conflicts that arise regarding disclosure of confidential information and forced disclosure of non-privileged information. Quotes Principles III and IV, Fundamental Elements (4), and Opinions 1.02 (1992) and 5.07 (1992) [now Opinion 5.05]. Cites Opinion 2.02. Glynn, *Multidisciplinary Representation of Children: Conflicts Over Disclosures of Client Communications,* 27 J. Marshall L. Rev. 617, 625, 626, 630-32, 637, 639, 643 (1994).

Journal 1994 Discusses physician-patient confidentiality and the exception that permits breach of a patient's confidence if required by law. Argues that this is always a legitimate exception to the confidentiality rule. Quotes Principle IV and Fundamental Elements (4). McConnell, *Confidentiality and the Law,* 20 J. Med. Ethics 47, 47 (1994).

Journal 1994 Reviews the evolution of the physician-patient relationship, with attention to patient autonomy. Examines the changing health care delivery environment. Quotes Preamble, Principles I, II, III, IV, V, and VI, Fundamental Elements (1) and (2), and Opinions 1.02 and 8.07 (1981) [now Opinion 8.08]. Cites Opinion 1.01. Szczygiel, *Beyond Informed Consent,* 21 Ohio N.U.L. Rev. 171, 217, 218, 220, 225, 226, 256 (1994).

Journal 1994 Discusses the importance of confidentiality in the physician-patient relationship and under what circumstances patient information may be released. Examines unique considerations that apply when a physician provides medical care to a minor or an HIV-infected individual. Quotes Principle IV and Fundamental Elements (4). Weiner & Wettstein, *Confidentiality of Patient-Related Information,* 112 Arch. Ophthalmology 1032, 1033 (1994).

Journal 1993 Discusses family privacy rights and considers the meaning of justice, self respect, and the fundamental principles of physician ethics. Concludes that physicians have an ethical duty to intervene in domestic violence so long as such intervention does not breach confidentiality or violate patient autonomy. Quotes Principle IV and Opinion 5.05. References Opinions 8.14 and 9.131. Jecker, *Privacy Beliefs and the Violent Family: Extending the Ethical Argument for Physician Intervention,* 269 JAMA 776, 778, 779 (1993).

Journal 1993 Discusses physicians' duty to disclose to patients medical treatment alternatives that are not readily available. Proposes that based on the historical development and legal requirements of the informed consent doctrine, physicians should be required to inform patients of nonreadily available alternatives or face liability for breach of such obligation. Quotes Principles I, II, III, IV, and V and Opinion 8.08. Note, *Informed Choice: Physicians' Duty to Disclose Nonreadily Available Alternatives,* 43 Case W. Res. L. Rev. 491, 491, 498-99, 508, 509 (1993).

Journal 1993 Explores the idea of reverse informed consent, which would impose a duty on patients to inform health care professionals of their infectious status. Concludes that such a duty is justified. Quotes Principles IV and VI and Opinions 8.11 and 9.131. Oddi, *Reverse Informed Consent: The Unreasonably Dangerous Patient*, 46 Vand. L. Rev. 1417, 1449, 1463, 1465, 1479 (1993).

Journal 1993 Discusses the issues surrounding the confidentiality of electronic and computerized medical records. Concludes that any legal standard addressing this problem should balance the need to protect patient confidentiality with the practical constraints, such as cost and accessibility limiting ideal security. References Principle IV and Opinion 5.07. Waller & Fulton, *The Electronic Chart; Keeping it Confidential and Secure*, 26 J. Health & Hosp. L. 104, 105 (April 1993).

Journal 1992 Discusses legal issues in the context of disclosing health information in adoptions. Presents the arguments for and against disclosure, including the traditional view favoring nondisclosure. References Principle IV. Blair, *Lifting the Genealogical Veil: The Blueprint for Legislative Reform of the Disclosure of Health-Related Information in Adoption*, 70 No. Carolina L. Rev. 681, 692 (1992).

Journal 1991 Discusses the case of *Crist v. Moffat*, which prohibits ex parte communications with a plaintiff's treating physician in North Carolina. Examines the physician-patient privilege and looks at various jurisdictions that permit and forbid ex parte communications. Quotes Principle IV and Opinion 5.06. Comment, *Shielding the Plaintiff and Physician: The Prohibition of Ex Parte Contacts With a Plaintiff's Treating Physician*, 13 Campbell L. Rev. 233, 243, 248 (1991).

Journal 1990 Examines the relationship between professional ethics and professional autonomy, perceived problems of health care rationing under a prospective payment vs a fee-for-service system, and the relationship between professional ethics and the problem of rationing. Concludes that rationing is inevitable, forcing important ethical questions to be addressed. Quotes Principles IV and VI. Agich, *Rationing and Professional Autonomy*, 18 Law, Med. & Health Care 77, 79, 82 (1990).

Journal 1990 Examines the extent to which forensic psychiatrists are consulted in medical malpractice cases. Considers the appropriate standard of care, particularly for psychiatric malpractice cases, and the problems associated with its determination. References Principles II and IV. Modlin, *Forensic Psychiatry and Malpractice*, 18 Bull. Am. Acad. Psychiatry Law 153, 161 (1990).

Journal 1990 Discusses the moral dilemma in deciding whether to withdraw artificial nutrition and hydration from a patient and the appropriate role of the judiciary. Concludes that judicial decisions do not represent the moral viewpoint of society and that moral pronouncements should not be made in the courtroom. Quotes Preamble, Principles I, II, III, IV, V, VI, and VII, and Opinion 2.20. Peccarelli, *A Moral Dilemma: The Role of Judicial Intervention in Withholding or Withdrawing Nutrition and Hydration*, 23 John Marshall L. Rev. 537, 539, 540, 541 (1990).

Journal 1990 Presents current issues, policies, legislation, and judicial decisions regarding impaired physicians. Concludes by proposing enhanced confidentiality requirements in disciplinary proceedings and nationwide adoption of a uniform law in this area. Quotes Opinion 4.07. References Principle IV. Walzer, *Impaired Physicians: An Overview and Update of the Legal Issues*, 11 J. Legal Med. 131, 174, 192 (1990).

Journal 1989 Discusses the history of the physician-patient privilege up through changes implemented under the Ohio Tort Reform Act of 1987. Aspects of the physician-patient privilege that are most significantly affected by this Tort Reform Act are highlighted, with recommendations for further refinement of the privilege in Ohio. Quotes Principles II and IV and Opinion 5.05. Note, *The Ohio Physician-Patient Privilege: Modified, Revised, and Defined*, 49 Ohio St. L. J. 1147, 1167 (1989).

Journal 1985 Initially describes how existing doctrines protect the value of autonomy in the context of the physician-patient relationship, then examines various problems in the current protective scheme. Concludes by recommending the creation of an independent articulable protected interest in patient autonomy. Quotes Principles II and IV. Cites Opinions 4.04 (1984) [now Opinion 8.03 and 8.032] and 6.03 (1984) [now Opinion 6.02]. Shultz, *From Informed Consent to Patient Choice: A New Protected Interest*, 95 Yale L. J. 219, 275 (1985).

Journal 1983 Examines the evolution and impact of decisions in *Tarasoff v. Regents of the University of California*, 131 Cal. Rptr. 14 (Cal. 1976) and *McIntosh v. Milano*, 403 A.2d 500 (N.J. Super. 1979) which established a duty on the part of a physician or psychotherapist to warn third parties foreseeably endangered by a patient. In establishing such a duty, the courts endeavored to balance the physician's duty to warn endangered third parties with the duty to maintain confidentiality within the physician-patient relationship. Quotes Principle IV. Roth & Levin, *Dilemma* *of Tarasoff: Must Physicians Protect the Public or Their Patients? 11 Law, Med. & Health Care 104, 106 (1983).*

Journal 1981 Observes that a reevaluation of medicine and the medical profession is occurring on at least three levels: theoretical, educational, and professional. Notes that physicians are facing various challenges to the exercise of many of their societal functions and emphasizes that physicians view law and the medical profession as the source most responsible for these challenges. Quotes Principle IV. Schwartz & Gibson, *Defining the Role of the Physician: Medical Education, Tradition, and the Legal Process, 18 Houston L. Rev. 779, 791 (1981).*

V.   A physician shall continue to study, apply, and advance scientific knowledge, maintain a commitment to medical education, make relevant information available to patients, colleagues, and the public, obtain consultation, and use the talents of other health professionals when indicated.

S.D. Ind. 1992 Drug manufacturer sought protective order to prevent disclosure of patients' and physicians' names from adverse drug reaction reports. Plaintiff, quoting Principle V which requires that physicians "make relevant information available to . . . the public," argued that requiring the disclosure of physicians' names would not deter physicians from reporting adverse drug reactions. The court held that the Principle notwithstanding, disclosure of physicians' names would seriously undermine the FDA's voluntary reporting system. *In re Eli Lilly & Co., 142 F.R.D. 454, 458.*

D.S.C. 1968 Military dependent sued government physicians under Federal Tort Claims Act where child with acute abdominal pain was twice referred to naval hospital with diagnosis of possible appendicitis and twice sent home without treatment, eventually suffering ruptured appendix and serious complications. In finding for the plaintiff, the court quoted Principle 8 (1957) [now Principle V and Opinion 8.04] in considering whether the physicians had a duty to seek consultation in such a situation. *Steeves v. United States, 294 F. Supp. 446, 454.*

Minn. 1999 Plaintiffs sought declaratory relief against hospital for its refusal to grant plaintiffs access to peer review materials. The trial court granted the defendant's motion for summary judgment. On appeal the Minnesota Supreme Court held that physicians' private right to access a hospital's peer review materials did not outweigh public interest in quality health care. The court stated that quality care could be jeopardized if physicians had access to peer review material. The court also cited Principle V, stating that physicians have an ethical duty to participate in the peer review process. *Amaral v. Saint Cloud Hospital, 598 N.W.2d 379, 388.*

Tex. 1993 Estate of man who committed suicide after taking drug filed suit against manufacturer and sought adverse reaction or drug experience reports submitted to the FDA. These reports are voluntarily submitted by physicians and other health care providers and, according to 21 C.F.R. § 314.430(e)(4)(ii), the FDA must keep the identity of the reporters and the patients confidential. Noting the public interest in the voluntary reporting system and that the trial court had ordered disclosure of confidential information without applying the standard of relevance and need, the court denied disclosure of the reporters' identities. Quoting Principle V, the dissent declared that the decision adversely affected public health and safety by leaving drug manufacturers free to conceal important information. *Eli Lilly & Co. v. Marshall, 850 S.W.2d 155, 163.*

Journal 2003 Examines policy options for integration of traditional and modern medicine. Concludes that solid cross-sectoral linkages between different traditions can stabilize an integrated health care system. Quotes Preamble and Opinion V. Holliday, *Traditional Medicines in Modern Societies: An Exploration of Integrationist Options through East Asian Experience, 28 J. Med. & Phil. 373, 387 (2003).*

Journal 2003 Considers the legal, medical, and ethical issues of physician-patient confidentiality in disclosure of paternity. Concludes that a balancing test should be applied to making determinations regarding disclosure of paternity. Quotes Principles I, IV, and V, and Opinions 1.02, 5.055, and 10.01. Cites Principle II and Opinion 5.05. Richards & Wolf, *Medical Confidentiality and Disclosure of Paternity, 48 S.D. L. Rev. 409, 411, 412, 413 (2003).*

Journal 2002 Reviews how changes in the health care delivery system underscore the importance of information in patient empowerment. Concludes that patients should use information to take charge of their health care. Quotes Principle V and Opinion 10.02. Cites Opinion 10.01. Kane,

Information is the Key to Patient Empowerment, 11 Annals Health L. 25, 29-30, 44 (2002).

Journal 2002 Evaluates pain management treatment for prisoners. Concludes that withholding treatment for, or failing to adequately treat, pain violates the Eighth Amendment. Quotes Principle V and Opinion 2.20. McGrath, *Raising the "Civilized Minimum" of Pain Amelioration for Prisoners to Avoid Cruel and Unusual Punishment, 54 Rutgers L. Rev. 649, 657, 660 (2002).*

Journal 2002 Evaluates the application of biomedical knowledge in clinical practice. Concludes that serious inadequacies exist in the current practice of evidence-based medicine. Quotes Principle V and Opinion 9.08. References Opinion 9.095. Noah, *Medicine's Epistemology: Mapping the Haphazard Diffusion of Knowledge in the Biomedical Community, 44 Ariz. L. Rev. 373, 404, 447, 448 (2002).*

Journal 2000 Discusses patent law and policy. Examines whether or not those who practice medicine should be excused from patent laws because of the conflict that medical procedure patents create with respect to the practice of medicine. Concludes that Congress should repeal section 287(c) of the Patent Act. Quotes Principle V and Opinions 9.08 and 9.09. Cites Opinion 8.03. References Opinion 10.01. Ho, *Patents, Patients, and Public Policy: An Incomplete Intersection at 35 U.S.C. § 287(c), 33 U.C. Davis L. Rev. 601, 603, 623, 624, 625, 631 (2000).*

Journal 2000 Considers the rules governing expert testimony. Explores professional ethical standards affecting expert witnesses and concludes that codes of ethics have not succeeded in eliminating biased expert testimony. Recommends creation of an organization to assist courts in obtaining reliable expert witness testimony. Quotes Principle III and Opinion 6.01. Cites Principles I, II, and V and Opinions 1.02 and 9.07. Murphy, *Expert Witnesses at Trial: Where are the Ethics? 14 Geo. J. Legal Ethics 217, 231-32 (2000).*

Journal 2000 Describes possible solutions designed to improve post-approval regulation of prescription drugs so that fewer patients will suffer from adverse drug reactions. Concludes that the FDA along with physicians and clinical researchers should rethink the existing approach to monitoring of unexpected side effects. Quotes Principle V and Opinion 9.032. Cites Opinion 5.05. Noah, *Adverse Drug Reactions: Harnessing Experimental Data to Promote Patient Welfare, 49 Cath. U. L. Rev. 449, 477, 497-98 (2000).*

Journal 2000 Evaluates the regulatory framework governing prescription drugs. Considers problems faced by elderly patients when taking FDA-approved medications. Concludes that in order to optimize patient safety, the existing regulatory system must undergo important structural changes. Quotes Principle V and Opinion 9.032. Noah & Brushwood, *Adverse Drug Reactions in Elderly Patients: Alternative Approaches to Postmarket Surveillance, 33 J. Health L. 383, 400, 445 (2000).*

Journal 1997 Discusses physician frustration with managed care plans caused by gag clauses and cost-containment mechanisms. Reviews the development of managed care organizations and federal attempts at limiting the use of gag clauses. Concludes that gag clauses are inherently flawed and compromise quality health care. Quotes Principles II and V, Fundamental Elements (1), and Opinion 8.13. Note, *Physicians, Bound and Gagged: Federal Attempts to Combat Managed Care's Use of Gag Clauses, 21 Seton Hall Legis. J. 567, 601-02 (1997).*

Journal 1997 Discusses the need for balance between business ethics and medical ethics in the context of managed care. Explores two models for integrating ethics and managed care. Proposes the adoption of a collective responsibility model to improve quality of care. Quotes Principles I, II, III, IV, and V. Cites Preamble. References Opinion 8.13. Regan, *Regulating the Business of Medicine: Models for Integrating Ethics and Managed Care, 30 Colum. J.L. & Soc. Probs. 635, 651, 656, 657 (1997).*

Journal 1996 Discusses the trend toward conserving resources expended on health care by withholding services absent a showing of necessity. Claims that the high standard of care physicians owe patients is jeopardized by medical treatment decisions based on coverage concerns. Concludes that the legal structure regarding health care plans should be changed. Quotes Preamble, Principles I, II, III, IV, V, VI, and VII, and Opinion 2.03. Hirshfeld & Thomason, *Medical Necessity Determinations: The Need for a New Legal Structure, 6 Health Matrix 3, 8-9 (1996).*

Journal 1996 Considers the impact of gag clauses on the physician-patient relationship. Undertakes an extensive legal, ethical, and policy analysis. Concludes that gag clauses are violative of legal and ethical principles. Quotes Principles II, V, and VI, and Fundamental Elements (1). Cites Preamble. Martin & Bjerknes, *The Legal and Ethical Implications of Gag Clauses in Physician Contracts, XXII Am. J. Law & Med. 433, 465-66 (1996).*

Journal 1994 Reviews the evolution of the physician-patient relationship, with attention to patient autonomy. Examines the changing health care delivery environment. Quotes Preamble, Principles I, II, III, IV, V, and VI, Fundamental Elements (1) and (2), and Opinions 1.02 and 8.07 (1981) [now Opinion 8.08]. Cites Opinion 1.01. Szczygiel, *Beyond Informed Consent, 21 Ohio N.U.L. Rev. 171, 217, 218, 220, 225, 226, 256 (1994)*.

Journal 1993 Discusses physicians' duty to disclose to patients medical treatment alternatives that are not readily available. Proposes that based on the historical development and legal requirements of the informed consent doctrine, physicians should be required to inform patients of nonreadily available alternatives or face liability for breach of such obligation. Quotes Principles I, II, III, IV, and V and Opinion 8.08. Note, *Informed Choice: Physicians' Duty to Disclose Nonreadily Available Alternatives, 43 Case W. Res. L. Rev. 491, 491, 498-99, 508, 509 (1993)*.

Journal 1990 Discusses the moral dilemma in deciding whether to withdraw artificial nutrition and hydration from a patient and the appropriate role of the judiciary. Concludes that judicial decisions do not represent the moral viewpoint of society and that moral pronouncements should not be made in the courtroom. Quotes Preamble, Principles I, II, III, IV, V, VI, and VII, and Opinion 2.20. Peccarelli, *A Moral Dilemma: The Role of Judicial Intervention in Withholding or Withdrawing Nutrition and Hydration, 23 John Marshall L. Rev. 537, 539, 540, 541 (1990)*.

VI.   A physician shall, in the provision of appropriate patient care, except in emergencies, be free to choose whom to serve, with whom to associate, and the environment in which to provide medical care.

2d Cir. 1980 Appeal by hospital of National Labor Relations Board order to employ two part-time staff physicians on a full-time basis and to consider their applications for permanent admitting privileges. Physicians had joined picket line in sympathy with striking union employees without giving advance notice and were allegedly denied full-time positions in retaliation. The court held that support of the strike was activity protected by the National Labor Relations Act but that the physicians lost protection when they told patients the facility was unable to provide adequate care, in careless disregard of the truth. Further, the court noted that the failure to give notice before striking raised ethical questions under Principle 5 (1957) [now Principle VI]. *Montefiore Hosp. & Medical Ctr. v. NLRB, 621 F.2d 510, 516*.

4th Cir. 1984 Prisoner sued private physician under 42 U.S.C. Sec. 1983 for failure to provide medical treatment in violation of his eighth amendment rights. The court held that the exercise of the physician's medical judgment did not constitute action under color of state law. While not specifically referring to Principle VI (1980), the court cited the Principles for the general proposition that the physician-patient relationship is independent of state administrative supervision. This concept is apparently embodied in Principle VI. *Calvert v. Sharp, 748 F.2d 861, 863, cert. denied, 471 US 1132 (1975)*.

6th Cir. 1989 Plaintiff, a chiropractic association, alleged that the American Medical Association and several other professional associations violated antitrust law by conspiring to contain and ultimately eliminate the practice of chiropractic. The court provided a historical overview of the Association's gradual, but incomplete, recognition of chiropractors and limited licensed practitioners referring specifically to Principle 3 (1957) as well as to the Opinions and Reports of the Judicial Council Sec. 3, Para. 8 (1969) and to the Opinions and Reports 3.60 and 3.70 (1977) [now Principles VI and Opinions 3.01 and 3.04]. Based on its reading of these Principles and Opinions, the court reversed the trial court's grant of summary judgment to the Association because there remained a material issue of fact of whether it had continued to illegally boycott chiropractic. *Chiropractic Coop. Ass'n v. AMA, 867 F.2d 270, 272-75*.

W.D. Ark. 1989 Physician sued hospital alleging that it had acted in bad faith when it terminated his employment for failure to accept responsibility for "medical" as opposed to "surgical" patients. Plaintiff argued that the incorporation of the AMA's Principles of Medical Ethics into the hospital's by-laws gave him the right to choose which patients to serve, in apparent reference to Principle VI. While recognizing this right, the court held that the hospital had a corresponding right to consider such a refusal in its employment decisions. *Maxey v. United States, 1989 US Dist. LEXIS 5827*.

N.D. Ga. 1981 Decedent's widow brought wrongful death action against hospital, treating physician, and physician supervising a group of emergency room physicians who had independent contracts with the hospital. Plaintiff claimed the supervising physician was vicariously liable in damages to her under the doctrine of respondeat superior. The court noted that the traditional control test used to identify agency relationships is ineffective in the context of physician-hospital relationships because physicians are bound by Principle 6 (1957) [now most closely embodied by the independent judgment aspects of Principle VI] which requires physicians to practice medicine according to their independent professional judgment. *Stewart v. Midani, 525 F. Supp. 843, 848-49.*

E.D. Mich. 1986 Plaintiff-chiropractors claimed violation of the Sherman Antitrust Act alleging that the American Medical Association conspired with others to injure them professionally and financially. In support of their claim, plaintiffs cited Principle 3 (1957) and the Opinions and Reports of the Judicial Council Sec.3, Para. 8 (1969) [now Principles VI and Opinions 3.01 and 3.04]. The court, noting the 1977 change in the Association's position regarding chiropractic reflected in the Opinions and Reports of the Judicial Council 3.60 and 3.70 (1977) [now Opinion 3.04], held that plaintiffs failed to demonstrate evidence of an overt act by the Association within the statutory limitations period. Summary judgment entered for Association. *Chiropractic Coop. Ass'n v. AMA, 1986-2 Trade Cas. (CCH) & 67,294, aff'd in part and rev'd in part, 867 F.2d 270 (6th Cir. 1989).*

E.D. Mich. 1985 In an antitrust case brought by plaintiff-chiropractic association against the American Medical Association, plaintiffs presented the court with a motion in limine asking that the court strike defendant's affirmative defense of a good faith concern with public health and patient care. Plaintiffs argued that the defense was unprecedented, in conflict with existing law, and dramatically wrong. Plaintiffs referred to Principle 3 (1957) [now Principle VI and Opinions 3.01 and 3.04] as the source of the AMA's antitrust violations. The court denied plaintiffs' motion to strike, stating that under the rule of reason test, the Association had the right to present evidence that its actions furthered the public interest and patient care. *Chiropractic Coop. Ass'n v. AMA, 617 F. Supp. 264, 266, aff'd in part and rev'd in part, 867 F.2d 270 (6th Cir. 1989).*

D.N.M. 1987 In an antitrust action against major health insurance provider and state medical society, group of chiropractors alleged that a conspiracy existed in which the insurer refused to provide health cost reimbursement coverage for chiropractic services. Plaintiffs urged court to apply a per se analysis, rather than the rule of reason analysis, to determine the legality of defendants' restrictive practices. The court declined to apply the per se test. In part, court's conclusion was based on view that concerns of defendant-physicians about relationship with chiropractors because of ethical restrictions imposed by Principle 3 (1957) [now Principle VI and Opinions 3.01 and 3.04] deserved more consideration than the per se test would afford. *Johnson v. Blue Cross/Blue Shield, 677 F. Supp. 1112, 1118.*

D. Vt. 1986 Prisoner sued prison officials and private physician under section 42 U.S.C. Sec. 1983, claiming cruel and unusual punishment in violation of his constitutional rights after physician allegedly frightened the prisoner while he was physically restrained, performed a colonoscopy with the examining room door open to a main hallway, and allowed guards to participate in the exam. The court held that although state law required the provision of medical care to inmates, the ethical canons upon which the physician patient relationship was based were not derived from state law and the physician's actions did not constitute state action. In so holding, the court relied on *Calvert v. Sharpe, 748 F.2d 861 (4th cir. 1984)* which cites generally to the Principles for the proposition that the physician-patient relationship is independent of state supervision. Principle VI reflects this concept. *Nash v. Wennar, 645 F.Supp. 238, 242.*

Ariz. 1984 Mother sued hospital and physicians after minor son was transferred to another facility for solely financial reasons although emergency surgical care was medically indicated. In holding that the hospital's transfer policy pre-empted further care by the physicians and that the record revealed no physician negligence, the court stated that generally the standard of care for physicians is determined by what is usually done by members of the profession. The court then cited Principle VI, apparently for the proposition that in emergency situations there may be an ethical, rather than legal, obligation to provide care. *Thompson v. Sun City Community Hosp., Inc., 141 Ariz. 597, 688 P.2d 605, 612 n.7.*

Ariz. App. 1980 Malpractice suit against a paid on-call physician for refusal to treat decedent resulting in delay in treatment. The court quoted Principle 5 (1957) [now Principle VI and Opinion 8.11] as establishing an ethical duty to provide emergency care. However, court distinguished any such ethical obligation from its holding that physician had a contractual duty to treat emergency patients to the best of his ability. *Hiser v. Randolph, 126 Ariz. 608, 617 P.2d 774, 776 n.1, 777, 778.*

Cal. App. 2003 Patient and her husband sued medical clinic for terminating care after the patient filed malpractice claims against two clinic physicians. Clinic's policy required termination of all medical care for patients and their families in such a situation. Appeals court upheld summary judgment for the clinic on several claims, but denied summary judgment on claims for interference with contractual relations, negligent infliction of emotional distress, and breach of fiduciary duty. Quotes Principles VI and VIII. *Scripps Clinic v. Superior Court, 108 Cal. App.4th 917, 134 Cal. Rptr. 2d 101, 117.*

Cal. App. 1978 Surviving spouse sued physicians who were on emergency surgical call panel for malpractice where patient died during surgery. Although defendants claimed immunity under state Good Samaritan statute, the court held the statute inapplicable since the legislative purpose was to encourage physicians to render care on an irregular basis to unattended persons discovered by chance at the scene of an emergency. In so holding, the court noted that Principle 5 (1957) [now Principle VI and Opinions 8.11 and 9.06] imposed an ethical duty to render emergency medical care. *Colby v. Schwartz, 78 Cal. App. 3d 885, 144 Cal. Rptr. 624, 627 n.2.*

Ky. App. 1989 Malpractice suit was initiated against physician for failure to treat plaintiff's brother where defendant had repeatedly rebuffed plaintiff's request for emergency assistance and told him to get in line or sign in. Plaintiff removed his brother to another hospital where he subsequently died of heart attack. Plaintiff argued that defendant was under a duty to treat based upon, inter alia, the AMA Code of Ethics [apparently Principle VI and Opinion 8.11]. The court rejected the argument, finding that a breach of ethical standards may establish grounds for professional discipline, but not a civil cause of action, and held that defendant was under no legal duty to treat. *Noble v. Sartori, 1989 Ky. App. LEXIS 67.*

N.J. Super. 1994 Plaintiff-physician alleged that nursing home violated public policy when it terminated his at-will employment in retaliation for his refusal to see and treat patients in excess of his original work load. With apparent reference to Principle VI, physician argued that caring for excessive numbers of patients violated his ethical responsibilities and public policy. The court held that even though physician's objections to nursing home's practices may have supported a reasonable belief that public policy was violated, there was insufficient evidence that objections contributed to termination. *Fineman v. New Jersey Dept. of Human Servs., 272 N.J. Super. 606, 640 A.2d 1161, 1163, 1166, 1169-70, cert. denied, 138 N.J. 267, 649 A.2d 1287 (1994).*

N.J. Super. 1960 Plaintiff, a graduate of a school of osteopathy and licensed to practice medicine and surgery in New Jersey, sought to compel the defendant medical society to admit him to full membership. Defendant claimed as an affirmative defense that to admit plaintiff would violate Principle 3 (1957) [now Principle VI and Opinion 3.01] because plaintiff possessed a degree in osteopathy rather than an M.D. The court noted that the defendant society had virtually monopolistic control of medical practice in the state and that exclusion from membership caused substantial injury. In view of this, the court ordered the defendant society to admit plaintiff to its membership. To bar membership of a licensed graduate of an approved school of osteopathy would, the court held, violate public policy. *Falcone v. Middlesex County Medical Soc'y, 62 N.J. Super. 184, 162 A.2d 324, 328-29, aff'd, 34 N.J. 582, 170 A.2d 791 (1961).*

N.Y. Sup. 1993 Defendant was charged with violating state statute imposing criminal sanction on a physician who refuses to treat a person seeking emergency medical care. Defendant sought dismissal of the charge challenging the constitutionality of the statute and arguing that [it requires mens rea.] The court denied defendant's motion for dismissal, concluding that the statute was constitutional and that the legislature clearly imposed strict liability. The court quoted Principle VI in support of its strict liability conclusion. *People v. Anyakora, 162 Misc. 2d 47, 616 N.Y.S.2d 149, 155.*

Ohio App. 1991 Medical corporation sought an injunction to enforce a covenant not to compete against defendant-physician. The lower court granted summary judgment based on a referee's report which concluded that under Principle VI and Opinions 6.11, 9.02, and 9.06 (1989), restrictive covenants were *per se* unenforceable as a matter of public policy. While recognizing a strong public interest in allowing open access to health care, the appellate court in reversing held that Opinion 9.02, which applied specifically to restrictive covenants, only "discouraged" such covenants. *Ohio Urology, Inc. v. Poll, 72 Ohio. App. 446, 450, 451, 594 N.E.2d 1027, 1030, 1031.*

Wash. 1951 Plaintiff, a charitable, not-for-profit medical corporation, offered prepaid health care services to members and their families. Suit was filed against county medical society and others for damages and injunction for defendants' alleged efforts to monopolize prepaid medical care in area and unlawfully restrain competition by plaintiff and its physicians. Defendants alleged as affirmative defense that their efforts were designed to curb unethical prepaid contract practice by plaintiff. Court examined at length American Medical Association's position regarding contract practice including Principles Ch. III, Art. VI, Secs. 3 and 4 (1947) [now Principle VI and Opinions 8.05 and 9.06] concluding nothing in plaintiff's practice violated the Association's ethical guidelines. Further, quoting Principles Ch. III, Art. III, Sec.1 (1947) [now Opinion 8.04] dealing with consultations, court noted that defendants' efforts impeded plaintiff's physicians from obtaining consultations. Court concluded that defendants' actions constituted unlawful, monopolistic behavior and issued an injunction, although it declined to award damages. *Group Health Coop. v. King County Medical Soc'y,* 39 Wash. 2d 586, 237 P.2d 737, 744, 750-51, 759-60.

Wash. App. 1984 Plaintiff-pathologist sued his corporate employer and one of its subsidiaries for breach of his employment contract; defendants counterclaimed, alleging that plaintiff had tortiously interfered with defendants' business relationships. Plaintiff had discouraged the transfer of laboratory specimens for analysis at a distant lab because he allegedly believed that to do so would be a violation of medical ethics, particularly Principle 6 (1957) [now Principle VII]. In finding for plaintiff, the court acknowledged that a physician was bound to uphold duly prescribed medical ethical principles despite his employment status, especially where such a principle coincided with a public policy favoring acts that tend to prevent a deterioration of the quality of medical care. *Wood v. Upjohn Co.,* No. 6093-1-II (Sept. 4, 1984) (LEXIS, States library, Wash. file).

Journal 2001 Discusses the prohibition on non-lawyer ownership of legal service providers. Considers how ethical rules and standards governing physicians have been directed toward preserving independent judgment. Concludes that ethical conflicts created by abandoning the prohibition on non-lawyer ownership of legal service providers may be managed by following the medical ethics model. Quotes Principle VI and Opinions 2.03, 2.09, 8.02, 8.021, 8.03, 8.05, 8.051, 8.054, 8.13, and 8.132. Harris & Foran, *The Ethics of Middle-Class Access to Legal Services and What We Can Learn from the Medical Profession's Shift to a Corporate Paradigm,* 70 Fordham L. Rev. 775, 817, 821, 822, 823, 824 (2001).

Journal 2000 Examines the ethical, social, and moral dilemmas faced by gays and lesbians who desire to have genetically related children. Discusses assisted reproductive technologies most commonly used by gays and lesbians. Explores the barriers associated with access to reproductive technologies by these individuals. Quotes Principle VI. DeLair, *Ethical, Moral, Economic and Legal Barriers to Assisted Reproductive Technologies Employed by Gay Men and Lesbian Women,* 4 DePaul J. Health Care L. 147, 150 (2000).

Journal 2000 Discusses and evaluates different systems for addressing consumer concerns about managed health care. Asserts that current legal systems for identifying and resolving consumer concerns are not understood by most consumers and are not accessible by many, especially the uninsured. Concludes that several immediate steps are realistic for moving toward reform. Cites Principle VI. References Opinions 8.13 and 9.065. Kinney, *Tapping and Resolving Consumer Concerns About Health Care,* 26 Am. J. Law & Med. 335, 337, 375 (2000).

Journal 2000 Discusses managed care in terms of problems, responses, and accomplishments. Demonstrates how a physician union's collective bargaining process can benefit patients and physicians in addressing problems with managed care. Concludes that barriers preventing such unions should be removed. Quotes Principles VI and VII and Opinion 10.01. Rugg, *An Old Solution to a New Problem: Physician Unions Take the Edge Off Managed Care,* 34 Colum. J. L. & Soc. Probs. 1, 41 (2000).

Journal 2000 Examines current laws prohibiting discrimination in the context of access to health care, placing emphasis on people with HIV/AIDS. Considers the implications of *Bragdon v. Abbott.* Concludes that everyone should be entitled to health care in the absence of an acceptable justification for its denial. Quotes Preamble, Principle VI, and Opinion 9.131. Shepherd, *HIV, the ADA, and the Duty to Treat,* 37 Hous. L. Rev. 1055, 1061, 1083-84 (2000).

Journal 1999 Discusses potential conflicts between a criminal defense attorney's religious beliefs and representation of the client. Explores theories that would allow an attorney to put religious beliefs over the client's interest. Offers analogies within the physician-patient relationship. Concludes that a defense attorney is bound by duty and must set aside conflicting religious beliefs. Quotes Principle VI and Opinions 8.11, 9.06, and 9.12. Reza, *Religion and the Public Defender,* 26 Fordham Urb. L. J. 1051, 1062, 1063 (1999).

Journal 1999 Discusses the need for physicians to advocate on behalf of patients' rights in the context of health care delivery. Evaluates the nature and scope of the physician's role as advocate, noting that physicians cannot be expected to engage in attorney-like advocacy. Quotes Principles IV and VI, Fundamental Elements (2), (4), and (6) [now Opinion 10.01], Patient Responsibilities 5 [now Opinion 10.02], and Opinions 2.03, 2.07, 2.09, 2.16, 2.19, 3.06, 4.01, 4.04, 6.01, 7.02,

8.02, 8.03, 8.13, 8.132, 9.06, 9.07, and 9.131. Cites Opinions 5.05, 5.09, 7.01, 8.135, and 9.02. Sage, *Physicians as Advocates*, 35 Hous. L. Rev. 1529, 1537, 1541, 1542, 1552-53, 1554, 1556, 1557, 1559, 1561-62, 1564, 1571, 1574, 1576, 1580 (1999).

Journal 1999 Discusses whether health care professionals have the right to refuse to treat patients under common law and federal statutes and regulations. Explores the impact of the Americans with Disabilities Act and the United States Supreme Court decision in *Bragdon v. Abbott* on the duties of health care professionals in the context of providing treatment to HIV-positive patients. Quotes Principle VI and Opinions 2.23 and 9.131. White, *Health Care Professionals and Treatment of HIV-Positive Patients*, 20 J. Legal Med. 67, 86 (1999).

Journal 1998 Discusses the development and existence of the corporate practice of medicine doctrine. Points out that the doctrine is inconsistent with recent changes in the health care system. Suggests that the ban on corporate practice should be eliminated. Cites Principle VI. Freiman, *The Abandonment of the Antiquated Corporate Practice of Medicine Doctrine: Injecting a Dose of Efficiency into the Modern Health Care Environment*, 47 Emory L. J. 697, 712 (1998).

Journal 1998 Focuses on conflicts of interest and pressures physicians face when treating professional athletes. Discusses case law regarding team physician liability. Concludes that team physicians and their attorneys need to be aware of conflicts of interest that may arise from treatment of professional athletes. Quotes Principle VI (1957) [now most closely embodied by the independent judgment aspects of Principle VI]. Polsky, *Winning Medicine: Professional Sports Team Doctors' Conflicts of Interest*, 14 J. Contemp. Health L. & Pol'y 503, 505 (1998).

Journal 1997 Reports on a study of physician attitudes regarding expert witnesses. Notes that a majority of physicians believe that medical expert testimony should be subject to peer review and, when appropriate, medical licensing board discipline. Quotes Principles II and VI, and Opinion 9.07. Eitel, Hegeman, & Evans, *Medicine on Trial: Physicians' Attitudes about Expert Medical Witnesses*, 18 J. Legal Med. 345, 355, 358 (1997).

Journal 1997 Analyzes the prohibition against employment agreements between corporations and licensed physicians. Discusses the origins and development of the corporate practice of medicine doctrine. Proposes that state legislatures should adopt doctrinal modifications to aid in the movement toward managed care. Quotes Principle VI. Mars, *The Corporate Practice of Medicine: A Call for Action*, 7 Heath Matrix 241, 267 (1997).

Journal 1996 Discusses the trend toward conserving resources expended on health care by withholding services absent a showing of necessity. Claims that the high standard of care physicians owe patients is jeopardized by medical treatment decisions based on coverage concerns. Concludes that the legal structure regarding health care plans should be changed. Quotes Preamble, Principles I, II, III, IV, V, VI, and VII and Opinion 2.03. Hirshfeld & Thomason, *Medical Necessity Determinations: The Need for a New Legal Structure*, 6 Health Matrix 3, 8-9 (1996).

Journal 1996 Considers the impact of gag clauses on the physician-patient relationship. Undertakes an extensive legal, ethical, and policy analysis. Concludes that gag clauses are violative of legal and ethical principles. Quotes Principles II, V, and VI, and Fundamental Elements (1). Cites Preamble. Martin & Bjerknes, *The Legal and Ethical Implications of Gag Clauses in Physician Contracts*, XXII Am. J. Law & Med. 433, 465-66 (1996).

Journal 1996 Discusses commercialization of the medical industry. Addresses ethical and policy considerations that form the basis for the corporate practice of medicine doctrine. Observes that the doctrine is now outdated. Quotes Principle VI. Parker, *Corporate Practice of Medicine: Last Stand or Final Downfall?*, 29 J. Health & Hosp. L. 160, 167, 173 (1996).

Journal 1996 Examines the recent trend in health care laws and ethics to focus on the alleviation of suffering. Expresses concern that such a focus may result in the valuation of one life over another. Emphasizes the need to evaluate multiple, diverse responses to suffering. Quotes Principle VI. References Opinion 2.162. Shepherd, *Sophie's Choices: Medical and Legal Responses to Suffering*, 72 Notre Dame L. Rev. 103, 106, 133 (1996).

Journal 1995 Examines the rights of health care professionals to refuse to participate in patient care on the basis of conscientious objection. Suggests steps that health care facilities may take when dealing with health care professionals who object to participating in patient care. Quotes Principles I and VI and Opinions 1.02, 2.035, and 9.055. Dellinger & Vickery, *When Staff Object to Participating In Care*, 28 J. Health & Hospital Law 269, 272, 276 (1995).

Journal 1995 Offers relevant historical perspectives and provides comprehensive ethical and legal discussion of physician-assisted suicide and euthanasia. Highlights important legislative developments, including the Oregon Death with Dignity Act, and analyzes significant judicial opinions. Quotes Principles III, IV, and VI and Opinions 2.21 and 9.12. Cites Opinions 2.20 and 8.11. Stone & Winslade, *Physician-Assisted Suicide and Euthanasia in the United States: Legal and Ethical Observations*, 16 J. Legal Med. 481, 483, 490, 497, 498, 499 (1995).

Journal 1995 Examines the history of Medicaid physician reimbursement and physician participation. Concludes that states should facilitate tie-ins among Medicaid patients and privately insured patients rather than raising physician fees. Cites Principle VI. Watson, *Medicaid Physician Participation: Patients, Poverty, and Physician Self-Interest*, XXI Am. J. Law & Med. 191, 218 (1995).

Journal 1994 Analyzes the corporate practice of medicine doctrine. Asserts that viability of the doctrine is questionable in the modern health care industry. Quotes Principle VI. Dowell, *The Corporate Practice of Medicine Prohibition: A Dinosaur Awaiting Extinction*, 27 J. Health & Hospital Law 369, 370 (1994).

Journal 1994 Explores how the Americans with Disabilities Act has created, through federal civil rights mechanisms, a legal duty to treat HIV-infected patients. Discusses previous attempts to create a professional obligation to treat patients with AIDS. Quotes Principle VI and Opinion 9.131. Cites Opinion 9.12. Halevy & Brody, *Acquired Immunodeficiency Syndrome and the Americans with Disabilities Act: A Legal Duty to Treat*, 96 Am. J. Med. 282, 283, 284 (1994).

Journal 1994 Reviews the evolution of the physician-patient relationship, with attention to patient autonomy. Examines the changing health care delivery environment. Quotes Preamble, Principles I, II, III, IV, V, and VI, Fundamental Elements (1) and (2), and Opinions 1.02 and 8.07 (1981) [now Opinion 8.08]. Cites Opinion 1.01. Szczygiel, *Beyond Informed Consent*, 21 Ohio N.U.L. Rev. 171, 217, 218, 220, 225, 226, 256 (1994).

Journal 1993 Explores the traditional view that lawyers have unfettered discretion to select clients and New York's antidiscrimination disciplinary rule, statutes, and case law. Concludes that the legal profession should prohibit invidious or improper discrimination. Quotes Principle VI and Opinions 9.12 and 9.131. Begg, *Revoking the Lawyers' License to Discriminate in New York: The Demise of a Traditional Professional Prerogative*, 7 Geo. J. Legal Ethics 275, 298, 299 (1993).

Journal 1993 Addresses both patient rights under California consent and confidentiality laws relating to AIDS and prohibitions on unreasonable searches and seizures under the US Constitution. Concludes that any health care worker who can document an exposure to blood or body fluids should have the option of compelling a nonconsenting patient to be tested for HIV. Quotes Principle VI and Opinion 9.131. Comment, *Nonconsensual HIV Testing in the Health Care Setting: The Case for Extending the Occupational Protections of California Proposition 96 to Health Care Workers*, 26 Loy. L.A. L. Rev. 1251, 1269 (1993).

Journal 1993 Discusses physicians' duty to disclose to patients medical treatment alternatives that are not readily available. Proposes that based on the historical development and legal requirements of the informed consent doctrine, physicians should be required to inform patients of nonreadily available alternatives or face liability for breach of such obligation. Quotes Principles I, II, III, IV, and V and Opinion 8.08. Note, *Informed Choice: Physicians' Duty to Disclose Nonreadily Available Alternatives*, 43 Case W. Res. L. Rev. 491, 491, 498-99, 508, 509 (1993).

Journal 1993 Explores the idea of reverse informed consent, which would impose a duty on patients to inform health care professionals of their infectious status. Concludes that such a duty is justified. Quotes Principles IV and VI and Opinions 8.11 and 9.131. Oddi, *Reverse Informed Consent: The Unreasonably Dangerous Patient*, 46 Vand. L. Rev. 1417, 1449, 1463, 1465, 1479 (1993).

Journal 1992 Discusses the plight of undocumented aliens and their need for access to medical care. Considers existing systems for providing such care, as well as barriers to the receipt of medical attention. Cites Principles VI and VII. Loue, *Access to Health Care and the Undocumented Alien*, 13 J. Legal Med. 271, 291 (1992).

Journal 1991 Considers whether physicians have an obligation to provide medical care to HIV-infected patients. Examines various sources for such a duty, including a moral obligation not to discriminate and a social responsibility to provide access to health care. Quotes Opinion 9.131. Cites Principle VI. Daniels, *Duty to Treat or Right to Refuse?*, 21 Hastings Center Rep. 36, 37, 42 (March/April 1991).

Journal 1991 Discusses the problem of noncompliant patients and whether a physician may deny treatment to these individuals. Concludes that physicians are not relieved of their duty to treat noncompliant patients, especially because these patients may not be able to adequately control their behavior. Cites Principle VI and Opinion 9.12. Orentlicher, *Denying Treatment to the Noncompliant Patient*, 265 JAMA 1579, 1581 (1991).

Journal 1990 Examines the relationship between professional ethics and professional autonomy, perceived problems of health care rationing under a prospective payment vs a fee-for-service system, and the relationship between professional ethics and the problem of rationing. Concludes that rationing is inevitable, forcing important ethical questions to be addressed. Quotes Principles IV and VI. Agich, *Rationing and Professional Autonomy*, 18 Law, Med. & Health Care 77, 79, 82 (1990).

Journal 1990 Considers the propriety of HIV testing for hospital patients prior to nonemergency surgery. Concludes that testing of patients should be permitted so long as it is not done with the intent, nor the effect, of discriminating against individual patients. Quotes Principle VI and Opinion 9.131. Naccasha, *The Permissibility of Routine AIDS Testing in the Health Care Context*, 5 Notre Dame J.L. Ethics & Pub. Pol'y, 223, 241 (1990).

Journal 1990 Discusses a physician's duty to treat AIDS patients. Concludes that there is a weak basis for imposing an ethical duty to treat, but suggests that a legal duty may be fashioned. Quotes Principle V (1980) [now Principle VI]. Note, *Ethics and AIDS: A Summary of the Law and a Critical Analysis of the Individual Physician's Ethical Duty to Treat*, XVI Am. J. Law & Med. 249, 262 (1990).

Journal 1990 Discusses the moral dilemma in deciding whether to withdraw artificial nutrition and hydration from a patient and the appropriate role of the judiciary. Concludes that judicial decisions do not represent the moral viewpoint of society and that moral pronouncements should not be made in the courtroom. Quotes Preamble, Principles I, II, III, IV, V, VI, and VII, and Opinion 2.20. Peccarelli, *A Moral Dilemma: The Role of Judicial Intervention in Withholding or Withdrawing Nutrition and Hydration*, 23 John Marshall L. Rev. 537, 539, 540, 541 (1990).

Journal 1989 Discusses the legal and ethical challenges that AIDS poses for health care providers. Proposes that health care providers actively participate in preventing HIV infection, providing care for HIV-infected individuals, and fighting AIDS and its associated stigma. Quotes Principle VI and Opinion 9.131. Forrester, *AIDS: The Responsibility to Care*, 34 Vill. L. Rev. 799, 811 (1989).

Journal 1989 Discusses common law developments in the 1960s and 1970s that established a duty to provide emergency care and treatment. Observes that the common law met with only limited success in this regard and concludes that the Consolidated Omnibus Budget Reconciliation Act of 1985 offers the greatest likelihood for creating a nationally enforceable legal duty to provide emergency care. Quotes Principle VI. Rothenberg, *Who Cares? The Evolution of the Legal Duty to Provide Emergency Care*, 26 Houston L. Rev. 21, 22 (1989).

Journal 1988 Noting that safety precautions have been recommended by CDC and OSHA, observes that, despite these measures, if health care providers believe that a risk of contagion exists when caring for HIV seropositive patients, they may take steps to limit exposure by reducing care. Against this background, it is suggested that policies be developed to help ensure that the threat of AIDS does not limit access to care for such patients. Quotes Principle 5 (1980) [sic] [now Principle VI]. Brennan, *Ensuring Adequate Health Care for the Sick: The Challenge of the Acquired Immunodeficiency Syndrome as an Occupational Disease*, 1988 Duke L. J. 29, 47.

Journal 1988 Discusses the question of whether health professionals are obligated to subject themselves to the risks that attend treating patients with communicable diseases, particularly AIDS. Examines the ethical pronouncements and codes of the nursing and medical professions in this respect, noting that the most recent statements of professional values imply the existence of an obligation to treat HIV-infectious patients. Quotes Opinion 8.10 (1986) [now Opinion 8.11] and Principle VI. Cites Opinion 9.11 (1986) [now Opinion 9.12]. Freedman, *Health Professions, Codes, and the Right to Refuse to Treat HIV-Infectious Patients*, 18 Hastings Center Rep. 20 (Supp.), 23, 24 (April/May 1988).

Journal 1986 Examines common law and statutory law applicable to patient dumping, and emphasizes the antidumping provisions of COBRA. Weaknesses in this federal legislative scheme are highlighted and recommendations for strengthening the statute and maximizing access to emergency medical care are offered. Quotes Principle VI and Opinion 8.10 (1986) [now Opinion 8.11]. Note, *Preventing Patient Dumping: Sharpening the COBRA's Fangs*, 61 N. Y. U. L. Rev. 1186, 1189-90 (1986).

VII. A physician shall recognize a responsibility to participate in activities contributing to the improvement of the community and the betterment of public health.

Ariz. 1965 Physician appealed denial of medical license which was based on alleged violations of local medical society rules and Principles 3, 5, and 10 (1957) [now Principles III and VII, and Opinions 3.01, 8.11, and 9.06]. Alleged violations included treating a patient without first obtaining a prior treating physician's permission, inadequate patient care, performing operations without hospital privileges, and signing the medical record of a deceased patient who had been treated by interns. The court held that the evidence failed to show any clear violation of the Principles and that a local medical society had no right to prescribe a code of ethics for state licensing purposes. *Arizona State Bd. of Medical Examiners v. Clark*, 97 Ariz. 205, 398 P.2d 908, 914-15, 915 n.3.

Journal 2003 Discusses conflicts of interest caused when managed care organizations provide financial incentives to physicians. Concludes that the focus of managed care is not well-suited for the doctor-patient relationship. Quotes Opinion 8.03. Cites Principle VII. References Opinion 8.051. Hall, *Bargaining with Hippocrates: Managed Care and the Doctor-Patient Relationship*, 54 S.C. L. Rev. 689, 696, 735 (2003).

Journal 2003 Considers a legislative plan allowing voluntary, consensual organ donation by condemned prisoners. Concludes that, in view of the current organ shortage, the benefits of such a plan outweigh the concerns. Quotes Principle VII and Opinion 2.06. Perales, *Rethinking the Prohibition of Death Row Prisoners as Organ Donors: A Possible Lifeline to Those on Organ Donor Waiting Lists*, 34 St. Mary's L. J. 687, 721, 725 (2003).

Journal 2001 Examines international ethical guidelines for psychiatrists. Observes that many psychiatrists are unaware of the relevant guidelines. Concludes that information about these guidelines should be more widely disseminated with a goal of increased compliance. Quotes Principle VII. Martens, *Necessity of Adapting Psychiatric Treatment to Relevant Ethical Guidelines*, 20 Med. Law 393, 394 (2001).

Journal 2000 Discusses managed care in terms of problems, responses, and accomplishments. Demonstrates how a physician union's collective bargaining process can benefit patients and physicians in addressing problems with managed care. Concludes that barriers preventing such unions should be removed. Quotes Principles VI and VII and Opinion 10.01. Rugg, *An Old Solution to a New Problem: Physician Unions Take the Edge Off Managed Care*, 34 Colum. J. L. & Soc. Probs. 1, 41 (2000).

Journal 1996 Discusses the trend toward conserving resources expended on health care by withholding services absent a showing of necessity. Claims that the high standard of care physicians owe patients is jeopardized by medical treatment decisions based on coverage concerns. Concludes that the legal structure regarding health care plans should be changed. Quotes Preamble, Principles I, II, III, IV, V, VI, and VII and Opinion 2.03. Hirshfeld & Thomason, *Medical Necessity Determinations: The Need for a New Legal Structure*, 6 Health Matrix 3, 8-9 (1996).

Journal 1996 Proposes an alternative method of capital punishment to allow for organ donation by executed prisoners. Provides justifications for this proposal. Concludes that physicians should be able to ethically participate in this process. Quotes Principle VII. Cites Opinion 2.06. References Opinion 2.162 (1994) [subsequently amended]. Patton, *A Call for Common Sense: Organ Donation and the Executed Prisoner*, 3 Va. J. Soc. Pol'y & L. 387, 404, 405, 407-10 (1996).

Journal 1995 Explores the debates and commentaries regarding patenting medical instruments and processes. Concludes that current patent law fails to address the ethical concerns of physicians and their patients. Quotes Principles of Medical Ethics §10 (1971) [now Principle VII] and Principle §2 (1971) [now Opinion 9.095] and Opinions 9.08 and 9.09. Reisman, *Physicians and Surgeons as Inventors: Reconciling Medical Process Patents and Medical Ethics*, 10 High Tech. L. J. 355, 356, 368-70, 385 (1995).

Journal 1992 Discusses the problem of discrimination based on HIV status, particularly among women and children. Examines medical and public health issues involving HIV. Cites Principle VII. References Opinion 9.131. Gittler & Rennart, *HIV Infection Among Women and Children and Antidiscrimination Laws: An Overview*, 77 Iowa L. Rev. 1313, 1363 (1992).

Journal 1992 Discusses the plight of undocumented aliens and their need for access to medical care. Considers existing systems for providing such care, as well as barriers to the receipt of medical attention. Cites Principles VI and VII. Loue, *Access to Health Care and the Undocumented Alien, 13 J. Legal Med. 271, 291 (1992).*

Journal 1990 Discusses the moral dilemma in deciding whether to withdraw artificial nutrition and hydration from a patient and the appropriate role of the judiciary. Concludes that judicial decisions do not represent the moral viewpoint of society and that moral pronouncements should not be made in the courtroom. Quotes Preamble, Principles I, II, III, IV, V, VI, and VII, and Opinion 2.20. Peccarelli, *A Moral Dilemma: The Role of Judicial Intervention in Withholding or Withdrawing Nutrition and Hydration, 23 John Marshall L. Rev. 537, 539, 540, 541 (1990).*

VIII. A physician shall, while caring for a patient, regard responsibility to the patient as paramount.

Cal. App. 2003 Patient and her husband sued medical clinic for terminating care after the patient filed malpractice claims against two clinic physicians. Clinic's policy required termination of all medical care for patients and their families in such a situation. Appeals court upheld summary judgment for the clinic on several claims, but denied summary judgment on claims for interference with contractual relations, negligent infliction of emotional distress, and breach of fiduciary duty. Quotes Principles VI and VIII. *Scripps Clinic v. Superior Court, 108 Cal. App.4th 917, 134 Cal. Rptr. 2d 101, 117.*

Journal 2002 Examines how managed care has adversely affected information disclosure in the physician-patient relationship. Concludes that, unless courts expand applicability of principles of informed consent, patient self-determination and autonomy will continue to be undermined. Quotes Principle VIII and Opinions 8.03, 8.053, 8.054, and 8.08. Morris, *Dissing Disclosure: Just What the Doctor Ordered, 44 Ariz. L. Rev. 313, 344, 349, 362, 363, 366 (2002).*

Journal 2002 Considers the dilemma of informed consent in the context of prescribing psychotropic medication to patients with mental illness and mental retardation. Recognizes the need for substituted decisionmaking in certain situations. Concludes that legislation would help address this issue. Quotes Preamble, Principles I, III, IV, VIII, and IX, and Opinion 8.08. O'Sullivan & Borcherding, *Informed Consent for Medication in Persons with Mental Retardation and Mental Illness, 12 Health Matrix 63, 75, 86, 87, 88 (2002)*

Journal 2002 Discusses legal and medical policies that protect confidentiality in the physician-patient relationship. Concludes that reducing the current level of privacy protection would jeopardize health care. Quotes Preamble and Opinions 2.136, 5.05, and 10.01. References Principles VIII and IX. Sciarrino, *Ferguson v. City of Charleston: "The Doctor Will See You Now, Be Sure to Bring Your Privacy Rights in With You!" 12 Temp. Pol. & Civ. Rts. L. Rev. 197, 213, 215, 220, 221, 222 (2002).*

IX. A physician shall support access to medical care for all people.

Journal 2002 Considers the dilemma of informed consent in the context of prescribing psychotropic medication to patients with mental illness and mental retardation. Recognizes the need for substituted decisionmaking in certain situations. Concludes that legislation would help address this issue. Quotes Preamble, Principles I, III, IV, VIII, and IX, and Opinion 8.08. O'Sullivan & Borcherding, *Informed Consent for Medication in Persons with Mental Retardation and Mental Illness, 12 Health Matrix 63, 75, 86, 87, 88 (2002).*

Journal 2002 Discusses legal and medical policies that protect confidentiality in the physician-patient relationship. Concludes that reducing the current level of privacy protection would jeopardize health care. Quotes Preamble and Opinions 2.136, 5.05, and 10.01. References Principles VIII and IX. Sciarrino, *Ferguson v. City of Charleston: "The Doctor Will See You Now, Be Sure to Bring Your Privacy Rights in With You!" 12 Temp. Pol. & Civ. Rts. L. Rev. 197, 213, 215, 220, 221, 222 (2002).*

Adopted June 1957; revised June 1980; revised June 2001.

1.00 Introduction

1.01 Terminology

The term "ethical" is used in opinions of the Council on Ethical and Judicial Affairs to refer to matters involving (1) moral principles or practices and (?) matters of social policy involving issues of morality in the practice of medicine. The term "unethical" is used to refer to professional conduct which fails to conform to these moral standards or policies.

Many of the Council's opinions lay out specific duties and obligations for physicians. Violation of these principles and opinions represents unethical conduct and may justify disciplinary action such as censure, suspension, or expulsion from medical society membership. (II)

Issued prior to April 1977.

Updated June 1994 and June 1996.

Journal 1994 Discusses the role of professional societies in establishing ethical guidelines for physicians in the context of using medical innovations and new technologies. Observes that these standards must be supplemented by additional external measures or incentives in order to be most effective. Cites Opinions 1.01, 1.02, 8.061, 9.04, and 9.131. Orentlicher, *The Influence of a Professional Organization on Physician Behavior*, 57 Alb. L. Rev. 583, 592, 593, 594, 595, 596 (1994).

Journal 1994 Reviews the evolution of the physician-patient relationship, with attention to patient autonomy. Examines the changing health care delivery environment. Quotes Preamble, Principles I, II, III, IV, V, and VI, Fundamental Elements (1) and (2), and Opinions 1.02 and 8.07 (1981) [now Opinion 8.08]. Cites Opinion 1.01. Szczygiel, *Beyond Informed Consent*, 21 Ohio N.U.L. Rev. 171, 217, 218, 220, 225, 226, 256 (1994).

1.02 The Relation of Law and Ethics

The following statements are intended to clarify the relationship between law and ethics.

Ethical values and legal principles are usually closely related, but ethical obligations typically exceed legal duties. In some cases, the law mandates unethical conduct. In general, when physicians believe a law is unjust, they should work to change the law. In exceptional circumstances of unjust laws, ethical responsibilities should supersede legal obligations.

The fact that a physician charged with allegedly illegal conduct is acquitted or exonerated in civil or criminal proceedings does not necessarily mean that the physician acted ethically. (III)

Issued prior to April 1977.

Updated June 1994.

Journal 2003 Considers the legal, medical, and ethical issues of physician-patient confidentiality in disclosure of paternity. Concludes that a balancing test should be applied to making determinations regarding disclosure of paternity. Quotes Principles I, IV, and V, and Opinions 1.02, 5.055, and 10.01. Cites Principle II and Opinion 5.05. Richards & Wolf, *Medical Confidentiality and Disclosure of Paternity*, 48 S.D. L. Rev. 409, 411, 412, 413 (2003).

Journal 2003 Uses public policy arguments to support a preponderance standard for medical license revocations in situations involving false testimony by a medical expert witness. Concludes that medical licensing boards can more effectively protect the public by using a preponderance standard. Quotes Principles II, III, and IV, and Opinions 1.02 and 9.07. Widmer, *South Dakota Should Follow Public Policy and Switch to the Preponderance Standard for Medical License Revocation After In Re the Medical License of Dr. Reuben Setliff, M.D.*, 48 S.D. L. Rev. 388, 396-97, 402 (2003).

Journal 2002 Discusses issues regarding regulation of elderly drivers. Concludes that mandating physicians to report unfit elderly patients will protect the public and help resolve ethical and legal dilemmas. Quotes Opinions 1.02, 2.24, 5.05, and 10.01. Kane, *Driving into the Sunset: A Proposal for Mandatory Reporting to the DMV by Physicians Treating Unsafe Elderly Drivers*, 25 U. Haw. L. Rev. 59, 59, 61, 62, 67, 69, 82, 83 (2002).

Journal 2001 Considers whether or not it is ethical for physicians to prescribe, and pharmacists to dispense, syringes for use by injection drug users. Concludes that ethical considerations suggest such actions are permissible but not obligatory. Quotes Principle III and Opinion 1.02. References Opinion 5.05. Lazzarini, *An Analysis of Ethical Issues in Prescribing and Dispensing Syringes to Injection Drug Users*, 11 Health Matrix 85, 107, 119 (2001).

Journal 2001 Explores utilization of the Gannett Principles to develop uniform ethical and legal standards in journalism. Concludes that these principles are an inevitable and useful response to legal realities. Quotes Opinion 1.02. Storey, *Does Ethics Make Good Law? A Case Study*, 19 Cardozo Arts & Ent. L.J. 467, 470 (2001).

Journal 2000 Considers the rules governing expert testimony. Explores professional ethical standards affecting expert witnesses and concludes that codes of ethics have not succeeded in eliminating biased expert testimony. Recommends creation of an organization to assist courts in obtaining reliable expert witness testimony. Quotes Principle III and Opinion 6.01. Cites Principles I, II, and V and Opinions 1.02 and 9.07. Murphy, *Expert Witnesses at Trial: Where are the Ethics?* 14 Geo. J. Legal Ethics 217, 231-32 (2000).

Journal 1995 Examines the rights of health care professionals to refuse to participate in patient care on the basis of conscientious objection. Suggests steps that health care facilities may take when dealing with health care professionals who object to participating in patient care. Quotes Principles I and VI and Opinions 1.02, 2.035, and 9.055. Dellinger & Vickery, *When Staff Object to Participating In Care*, 28 J. Health & Hospital Law 269, 272, 276 (1995).

Journal 1994 Explores the ethical issues involved in a multidisciplinary team working with children in legal proceedings. Focuses on the relationships between professionals and the conflicts that arise regarding disclosure of confidential information and forced disclosure of non-privileged information. Quotes Principles III, IV, Fundamental Elements (4) and Opinions 1.02 (1992) and 5.07 (1992) [now Opinion 5.05]. Cites Opinions 2.02. Glynn, *Multidisciplinary Representation of Children: Conflicts Over Disclosures of Client Communications*, 27 J. Marshall L. Rev. 617, 625, 626, 630-32, 637, 639, 643 (1994).

Journal 1994 Discusses the role of professional societies in establishing ethical guidelines for physicians in the context of using medical innovations and new technologies. Observes that these standards must be supplemented by additional external measures or incentives in order to be most effective. Cites Opinions 1.01, 1.02, 8.061, 9.04, and 9.131. Orentlicher, *The Influence of a Professional Organization on Physician Behavior*, 57 Alb. L. Rev. 583, 592, 593, 594, 595, 596 (1994).

Journal 1994 Reviews the evolution of the physician-patient relationship, with attention to patient autonomy. Examines the changing health care delivery environment. Quotes Preamble, Principles I, II, III, IV, V, and VI, Fundamental Elements (1) and (2), and Opinions 1.02 and 8.07 (1981) [now Opinion 8.08]. Cites Opinion 1.01. Szczygiel, *Beyond Informed Consent*, 21 Ohio N.U.L. Rev. 171, 217, 218, 220, 225, 226, 256 (1994).

Journal 1992 Argues that legal ethics and state laws governing attorney conduct are in conflict. Concludes that legal ethics continue to play a prominent role because states are "weakly committed" to regulation of the profession. Cites Opinion 1.02. Koniak, *The Law Between the Bar and the State*, 70 No. Carolina L. Rev. 1389, 1396 (1992).

Journal 1991 Explores ethical problems unique to the field of forensic psychiatry. Presents the results of a survey of members of the American Academy of Psychiatry and the Law (AAPL), asking their opinions regarding proposed ethical guidelines. Quotes Opinions 1.02 and 5.09. Weinstock, Leong, & Silva, *Opinions by AAPL Forensic Psychiatrists on Controversial Ethical Guidelines: A Survey*, 19 Bull. Am. Acad. Psychiatry Law 237, 238 (1991).

Opinions on Social Policy Issues

2.01 Abortion

The Principles of Medical Ethics of the AMA do not prohibit a physician from performing an abortion in accordance with good medical practice and under circumstances that do not violate the law. (III, IV)

Issued prior to April 1977.

U.S. 1973 Pregnant woman and physician sought declaratory relief and injunction against Texas criminal abortion statute. In holding that the constitutional right of privacy includes a woman's decision whether to terminate a pregnancy prior to viability, the Court reviewed the medical and legal history of abortion, including the AMA's lobbying efforts in support of criminal abortion statutes (1859, 1871), its opposition to induced abortion except when threat to life or health of mother exists (1967), its statement that lobbying efforts were consistent with the Principles of Medical Ethics (1957), and the Preamble, Sec. 10 (1971) [now Opinion 2.01], which stated that a physician was not prohibited from performing an abortion in accordance with good medical practice and consistent with local law. *Roe v. Wade, 410 U.S. 113, 144 n.39.*

Journal 2000 Examines physician value neutrality (PVN). Defines PVN as providing a foundation to suggest physicians must keep their values—religious, political, or otherwise—out of the patient-physician relationship. Concludes it is not clear how values can be removed from the patient-physician relationship without removing the very thing PVN supporters are trying to protect, the intrinsic value of persons. References Opinions 2.01, 2.02, 8.032, 8.05, 8.08, and 8.132. Beckwith & Peppin, *Physician Value Neutrality: A Critique, 28 J. L. Med. & Ethics 67, 72-73 (2000).*

Journal 1995 Examines four essential principles of bioethics—patient autonomy, nonmaleficence, beneficence, and justice—describes their application in clinical settings according to bioethical norms and AMA opinions. Concludes that such an approach promotes compassionate medical caregiving and that laws should reflect these values. Quotes Opinions 2.01 and 8.18. References Opinion 2.211. Cohen, *Toward a Bioethics of Compassion, 28 Ind. L. Rev. 667, 673, 681-82, 683 (1995).*

2.015 Mandatory Parental Consent to Abortion

Physicians should ascertain the law in their state on parental involvement to ensure that their procedures are consistent with their legal obligations.

Physicians should strongly encourage minors to discuss their pregnancy with their parents. Physicians should explain how parental involvement can be helpful and that parents are generally very understanding and supportive. If a minor expresses concerns about parental involvement, the physician should ensure that the minor's reluctance is not based on any misperceptions about the likely consequences of parental involvement.

Physicians should not feel or be compelled to require minors to involve their parents before deciding whether to undergo an abortion. The patient, even an adolescent, generally must decide whether, on balance, parental involvement is advisable. Accordingly, minors should ultimately be allowed to decide whether parental involvement is appropriate. Physicians should explain under what circumstances (eg, life-threatening emergency) the minor's confidentiality will need to be abrogated.

Physicians should try to ensure that minor patients have made an informed decision after giving careful consideration to the issues involved. They should encourage their minor patients to consult alternative sources if parents are not going to be involved in the abortion decision. Minors should be urged to seek the advice and counsel of those adults in whom they have confidence, including professional counselors, relatives, friends, teachers, or the clergy. (III, IV)

Issued June 1994 based on the report "Mandatory Parental Consent to Abortion," adopted June 1992 (JAMA. 1993; 269: 82-86).

6th Cir. 1999 Plaintiff challenged state law requiring minors to appeal, within 24 hours, a denied petition to bypass parental consent to obtain an abortion. The court stated that the 24-hour appeal requirement did not unduly burden the minor's ability to obtain an abortion. The dissent cited Opinion 2.015, to support its view that the 24-hour appeal requirement imposed an undue burden by jeopardizing the minor's ability to obtain an abortion. *Memphis Planned Parenthood v. Sundquist, 175 F.3d 456, 473.*

8th Cir. 1995 Court held several provisions of the South Dakota abortion law unconstitutional, including parental notice provision. In ruling that parental notice requirement, which lacked a bypass provision, unduly burdened liberty interests of some minors, the court cited AMA Council on Ethical and Judicial Affairs, Mandatory Parental Consent to Abortion, 269 JAMA 82 (1993) [now Opinion 2.015]. *Planned Parenthood v. Miller, 63 F.3d 1452, 1462.*

Mass. 1997 Plaintiffs brought suit seeking a declaration that statute prohibiting, with certain exceptions, a pregnant unmarried minor from obtaining an abortion unless either both parents consent or a judge authorizes the procedure, is unconstitutional. The court concluded that the statute did not facially violate due process or equal protection and was thus constitutional. However, the court struck down the provision requiring both parents' consent as lacking sufficient justification to overcome the minor's constitutional right to choose. The court cited AMA Council on Ethical and Judicial Affairs, Mandatory Parental Consent to Abortion, 269 JAMA 82 (1993) [now Opinion 2.015]. *Planned Parenthood League of Massachusetts, Inc. v. Attorney General, 424 Mass. 586, 596, 608, 677 N.E.2d 101, 107, 114.*

N.J. 2000 Prior to the effective date of the Parental Notification for Abortion Act, the plaintiffs sought a declaratory judgment and preliminary injunction precluding the enforcement of the Act. The trial court dismissed the challenge, but the state supreme court struck down the statute. The state, in support of the Act, argued that it was passed to facilitate and foster familial communications. The court rejected this as a legitimate governmental interest, noting that the Act applies to many young women who are justified in not telling there parents about their abortion decisions. The court quoted AMA Council on Ethics and Judicial Affairs, Mandatory Parental Consent to Abortion, 269 JAMA 82 (1983) [now Opinion 2.015] in support of this argument. *Planned Parenthood of Central New Jersey v. Farmer, 165 N.J. 609, 762 A.2d 620, 640.*

Journal 2003 Uses the medical self-consent rights of minors to challenge the legal assumption that teens lack decisional capacity for abortions. Concludes with discussion of an empirical study that supports this challenge. References Opinion 2.015. Ehrlich, *Grounded in the Reality of Their Lives: Listening to Teens Who Make the Abortion Decision without Involving Their Parents, 18 Berkeley Women's L. J. 61, 72, 84-85, 175-76 (2003).*

Journal 2003 Explores conflict in the legal treatment of minors in situations involving reproductive decision-making and the commission of crimes. Concludes that different approaches are justified. References Opinion 2.015. Ehrlich, *Shifting Boundaries: Abortion, Criminal Culpability and the Indeterminate Legal Status of Adolescents, 18 Wis. Women's L.J. 77, 105 (2003).*

Journal 2002 Argues attorneys should be appointed to represent minors in judicial bypass proceedings. Concludes that appointing a guardian ad litem raises ethical and constitutional problems. References Opinion 2.015. Graybill, *Assisting Minors Seeking Abortions in Judicial Bypass*

Proceedings: A Guardian ad Litem is No Substitute for an Attorney, 55 Vand. L. Rev. 581, 583 (2002).

Journal 2002 Examines how Alabama juvenile courts are handling petitions for waiver of parental consent for abortion. Concludes the courts are not correctly handling these matters, thus adversely affecting the rights of pregnant minors. References Opinion 2.015. Silverstein & Speitel, *"Honey, I Have No Idea": Court Readiness to Handle Petitions to Waive Parental Consent for Abortion,* 88 Iowa L. Rev. 75, 116, 117 (2002).

Journal 2001 Considers proposed state legislation requiring a minor to notify a parent when she intends to obtain an abortion. Concludes that notification serves the minor's best interests. References Opinion 2.015. Collett, *Protecting Our Daughters: The Need for the Vermont Parental Notification Law,* 26 Vt. L. Rev. 101, 106-07 (2001).

Journal 2000 Explores issues associated with mandatory parental consent to abortion laws. Examines the failure of the United States Supreme Court to consider medical decision-making by minors when evaluating the constitutionality of such laws. References Opinion 2.015. Ehrlich, *Minors as Medical Decision Makers: The Pretextual Reasoning of the Court in the Abortion Cases,* 7 Mich. J. Gender & L. 65, 91 (2000).

Journal 1999 Discusses minors' rights to an abortion. Examines parental notification requirements and procedures to bypass parental notification laws. Argues that minors should be afforded the same rights in seeking an abortion as adult women. References Opinion 2.015. Katz, *The Pregnant Child's Right to Self-Determination,* 62 Alb. L. Rev. 1119, 1142 (1999).

Journal 1998 Discusses parental consent laws pertaining to minors seeking abortions. Examines *Roe v. Wade* and the federal constitutional challenge to the Massachusetts parental consent law. States that the purpose of parental involvement laws is to limit abortion rights, rather than to promote family discourse. References Opinion 2.015. Ehrlich, *Journey Through the Courts: Minors, Abortion and the Quest for Reproductive Fairness,* 10 Yale J. L. & Feminism 1, 19 (1998).

Journal 1997 Addresses the issue of teenage pregnancy. Examines governmental actions that have made it more difficult for teenagers to receive abortions. Suggests that parental consent and judicial bypass provisions are an infringement on their reproductive freedom. Advocates lawyer participation in abortion reform. References Opinion 2.015. Schiff, *The Lawyer's Role in Restoring Adolescents' Abortion Rights,* 44 Fed. Law. 60, 62 (May 1997).

Journal 1996 Reviews Supreme Court decisions that address parental involvement in the abortion decisions of mature minors. Suggests that the Court's position on parental involvement should be reevaluated. Posits that many young women are mature enough to make their own pregnancy decisions. References Opinion 2.015. O'Shaughnessy, *The Worst of Both Worlds?: Parental Involvement Requirements and the Privacy Rights of Mature Minors,* 57 Ohio St. L. J. 1731, 1764-65 (1996).

2.02   Abuse of Spouses, Children, Elderly Persons, and Others at Risk

The following are guidelines for detecting and treating family violence:

Due to the prevalence and medical consequences of family violence, physicians should routinely inquire about physical, sexual, and psychological abuse as part of the medical history. Physicians must also consider abuse in the differential diagnosis for a number of medical complaints, particularly when treating women.

Physicians who are likely to have the opportunity to detect abuse in the course of their work have an obligation to familiarize themselves with protocols for diagnosing and treating abuse and with community resources for battered women, children, and elderly persons.

Physicians also have a duty to be aware of societal misconceptions about abuse and prevent these from affecting the diagnosis and management of abuse. Such misconceptions include the belief that abuse is a rare occurrence; that abuse does not occur in "normal" families; that abuse is a private problem best resolved without outside interference; and that victims are responsible for the abuse.

In order to improve physician knowledge of family violence, physicians must be better trained to identify signs of abuse and to work cooperatively with the range of community services currently involved. Hospitals should require additional training for those physicians who are likely to see victims of abuse. Comprehensive training on family violence should be required in medical school curricula and in residency programs for specialties in which family violence is likely to be encountered.

The following are guidelines for the reporting of abuse:

Laws that require the reporting of cases of suspected abuse of children and elderly persons often create a difficult dilemma for the physician. The parties involved, both the suspected offenders and the victims, will often plead with the physician that the matter be kept confidential and not be disclosed or reported for investigation by public authorities.

Children who have been seriously injured, apparently by their parents, may nevertheless try to protect their parents by saying that the injuries were caused by an accident, such as a fall. The reason may stem from the natural parent-child relationship or fear of further punishment. Even institutionalized elderly patients who have been physically maltreated may be concerned that disclosure of what has occurred might lead to further and more drastic maltreatment by those responsible.

The physician should comply with the laws requiring reporting of suspected cases of abuse of spouses, children, elderly persons, and others.

Public officials concerned with the welfare of children and elderly persons have expressed the opinion that the incidence of physical violence to these persons is rapidly increasing and that a very substantial percentage of such cases is unreported by hospital personnel and physicians. A child or elderly person brought to a physician with a suspicious injury is the patient whose interests require the protection of law in a particular situation, even though the physician may also provide services from time to time to parents or other members of the family.

The obligation to comply with statutory requirements is clearly stated in the Principles of Medical Ethics. Absent such legal requirement, for mentally competent, adult victims of abuse, physicians should not report to state authorities without the consent of the patient. Physicians, however, do have an ethical obligation to intervene. Actions should include, but would not be limited to: suggesting the possibility of abuse with the adult patient, discussing the safety mechanisms available to the adult patient (eg, reporting to the police or appropriate state authority), making available to the adult patient a list of community and legal resources, providing ongoing support, and documenting the situation for future reference. Physicians must discuss possible interventions and the problem of family violence with adult patients in privacy and safety. (I, III)

Issued December 1982.

Updated June 1994 based on the report "Physicians and Family Violence: Ethical

Considerations," adopted December 1991 (*JAMA*. 1992; 267: 3190-93); updated June 1996; and updated June 2000 based on the report "Domestic Violence Intervention," adopted June 1998.

Cal. App. 1982 Defendant was convicted of lewd act with a child and child molestation or annoyance, after licensed clinical psychologist reported defendant's admission of sexual conduct to authorities. The court held that the psychologist's testimony was properly admitted since a statute requiring the reporting of actual or suspected child abuse expressly made the psychotherapist-patient privilege inapplicable. The court quoted Principle 9 (1957) [now Principle IV and Opinions 2.02 and 5.05] in concluding the disclosure was not a breach of professional ethics. *People v. Stritzinger, 137 Cal. App. 3d 126, 186 Cal. Rptr. 750, 752 rev'd 34 Cal. 3d 505, 668 p.2d 738, 194 Cal. Rptr. 431 (1983).*

Md. Att'y Gen. 1977 Opinion addresses the obligation of a psychiatrist to report child abuse information obtained from a parent-patient. Referring to state statutes and to Principle 9 (1957) [now Principle IV and Opinions 2.02 and 5.05] the opinion concludes that the question of whether to disclose suspected child abuse is a matter left to the individual psychiatrist's professional and moral judgment. *Maryland Att'y. Gen. Opinion, 62 Op. Att'y Gen. Md. 157, 160.*

Wis. Att'y Gen. 1987 Physicians may report cases of suspected child abuse or neglect when a patient discloses that he or she has abused a child in some manner. Where report is made in good faith, physicians are immune from any civil or criminal liability. Passing reference is made to Principle 9 (1957) [now Principle IV and Opinions 2.02 and 5.05] in support of this position. *Wisconsin Att'y Gen. Op. 10-87 (March 16, 1987) (LEXIS, States library, Wis. file).*

Journal 2000 Examines physician value neutrality (PVN). Defines PVN as providing a foundation to suggest physicians must keep their values—religious, political, or otherwise—out of the patient-physician relationship. Concludes it is not clear how values can be removed from the patient-physician relationship without removing the very thing PVN supporters are trying to protect, the intrinsic value of persons. References Opinions 2.01, 2.02, 8.032, 8.05, 8.08, and 8.132. Beckwith & Peppin, *Physician Value Neutrality: A Critique, 28 J. L. Med. & Ethics 67, 72-73 (2000).*

Journal 2000 Examines public policies and medical practices intended to protect victims of domestic violence. Explores the possibility of liability for failure to act by health care professionals. Concludes that states need to develop public policy initiatives to address this and other related issues. References Opinion 2.02. Brown-Cranstoun, *Kringen v. Boslough and Saint Vincent Hospital: A New Trend for Healthcare Professionals Who Treat Victims of Domestic Violence? 33 J. Health L. 629, 649, 650 (2000).*

Journal 2000 Discusses the physical health consequences of psychological intimate partner violence (IPV). Concludes that clinicians should screen for psychological, physical, and sexual IPV in order to minimize physical health consequences. References Opinion 2.02. Coker, Smith, Bethea, King, & McKeown, *Physical Health Consequences of Physical and Psychological Intimate Partner Violence, 9 Arch. Fam. Med. 451, 456, 457 (2000).*

Journal 2000 Describes the epidemiology of intimate partner violence. Explores medical, legal, and law enforcement responses to intimate partner violence. Urges further research relating to medical and legal issues associated with intimate partner violence as well as additional training of attorneys, health care providers, judges, and law enforcement personnel. References Opinion 2.02. Loue, *Intimate Partner Violence: Bridging the Gap Between Law and Science, 21 J. Legal Med. 1, 18 (2000).*

Journal 2000 Examines public reporting statutes and introduces the provisions of the Violence Against Women Act (VAWA). Compares VAWA and public reporting laws. Concludes that VAWA is superior legislation because it requires women to initiate their own claims against abusers. References Opinion 2.02. Vital, *Mandatory Reporting Statutes and the Violence Against Women Act: An Analytical Comparison, 10 Geo. Mason U. Civ. Rts. L. J. 171, 189 (2000).*

Journal 1999 Discusses the basis for holding professionals liable for failing to report abuse. Explains reasons why professionals should be held liable in tort when they fail to report abuse. Argues that imposing such liability will increase early detection and deter future abuse. References Opinion 2.02. Jones, *Kentucky Tort Liability for Failure to Report Family Violence, 26 N. Ky. L. Rev. 43, 58 (1999).*

Journal 1998 Emphasizes that physicians need to be aware of the signs of domestic violence. Points out that, because many victims seek medical treatment, physicians are in a key position to identify domestic violence. Argues that Florida should follow other states' examples and adopt a mandatory reporting act. References Opinion 2.02. Makar, *Domestic Violence: Why the Florida Legislature Must Do More to Protect the "Silent" Victims*, 72 Fla. Bar J. 10, 16 (Nov. 1998).

Journal 1998 Discusses proposed legislation in New York that would mandate physician reporting of domestic violence. Argues that mandatory reporting harms patients by threatening the physician-patient relationship. Suggests that victims of domestic violence may be less likely to seek treatment or will be hesitant to speak freely with their physicians if reporting is mandatory. Cites Opinion 2.02. McFarlane, *Mandatory Reporting of Domestic Violence: An Inappropriate Response for New York Health Care Professionals*, 17 Buff. Pub. Int. L. J. 1, 29 (1998).

Journal 1998 Points out that most victims of elder abuse are socially isolated and thus few incidents of elder abuse are reported to authorities. Argues that current protections against elder abuse are inadequate. Suggests that the legal system and health professionals can make a difference in reducing elder abuse. Quotes Opinion 5.05. References Opinion 2.02. Moskowitz, *Saving Granny from the Wolf: Elder Abuse and Neglect—The Legal Framework*, 31 Conn. L. Rev. 77, 116, 120, 121, 122 (1998).

Journal 1997 Considers the best interests of children who are victims of domestic abuse. Advocates a rebuttable presumption against granting custody to a perpetrator. Concludes that courts should be educated about domestic violence. References Opinion 2.02. Comment, *Protecting Children Exposed to Domestic Violence in Contested Custody and Visitation Litigation*, 6 B.U. Pub. Int. L. J. 501, 502, 505 (1997).

Journal 1997 Reviews the historical treatment of domestic violence in tort law. Explores the difficulties victims of domestic violence suffer in pursuing traditional forms of relief. Considers this issue in the context of divorce proceedings. Offers practical guidance for achieving justice. References Opinion 2.02. Dalton, *Domestic Violence, Domestic Torts and Divorce: Constraints and Possibilities*, 31 New. Eng. L. Rev. 319, 354 (1997).

Journal 1996 Considers means of combating spousal abuse problems. Suggests various schemes of liability to increase aid to victims and reporting of problems. Observes that physicians may play an important role in eliminating spousal abuse. Concludes that imposition of civil liability on physicians for failure to report abuse will help remedy problems. References Opinion 2.02. Jones, *Battered Spouses' Damage Actions Against Non-Reporting Physicians*, 45 DePaul L. Rev. 191 (1996).

Journal 1994 Explores the ethical issues involved in a multidisciplinary team working with children in legal proceedings. Focuses on the relationships between professionals and the conflicts that arise regarding disclosure of confidential information and forced disclosure of non-privileged information. Quotes Principles III, IV, Fundamental Elements (4) and Opinions 1.02 (1992) and 5.07 (1992) [now Opinion 5.05]. Cites Opinions 2.02. Glynn, *Multidisciplinary Representation of Children: Conflicts Over Disclosures of Client Communications*, 27 J. Marshall L. Rev. 617, 625, 626, 630-32, 637, 639, 643 (1994).

2.03   Allocation of Limited Medical Resources

A physician has a duty to do all that he or she can for the benefit of the individual patient. Policies for allocating limited resources have the potential to limit the ability of physicians to fulfill this obligation to patients. Physicians have a responsibility to participate and to contribute their professional expertise in order to safeguard the interests of patients in decisions made at the societal level regarding the allocation or rationing of health resources.

Decisions regarding the allocation of limited medical resources among patients should consider only ethically appropriate criteria relating to medical need. These criteria include likelihood of benefit, urgency of need, change in quality of life, duration of benefit, and, in some cases, the amount of resources required for successful treatment. In general, only very substantial differences among patients are ethically relevant; the greater the disparities, the more justified the use of these criteria becomes. In making quality of life judgments, patients should first be prioritized so that death or extremely poor outcomes are avoided; then, patients should be prioritized according to change in quality of life, but only when there are very substantial differences among patients. Non-medical criteria, such as ability to pay, age, social worth, perceived obstacles to treatment, patient contribution to illness, or past use of resources should not be considered.

Allocation decisions should respect the individuality of patients and the particulars of individual cases as much as possible. When very substantial differences do not exist among potential recipients of treatment on the basis of the appropriate criteria defined above, a "first-come-first-served" approach or some other equal opportunity mechanism should be employed to make final allocation decisions. Though there are several ethically acceptable strategies for implementing these criteria, no single strategy is ethically mandated. Acceptable approaches include a three-tiered system, a minimal threshold approach, and a weighted formula. Decision-making mechanisms should be objective, flexible, and consistent to ensure that all patients are treated equally.

The treating physician must remain a patient advocate and therefore should not make allocation decisions. Patients denied access to resources have the right to be informed of the reasoning behind the decision. The allocation procedures of institutions controlling scarce resources should be disclosed to the public as well as subject to regular peer review from the medical profession. (I,VII)

Issued March 1981.

Updated June 1994 based on the report "Ethical Considerations in the Allocation of Organs and Other Scarce Medical Resources Among Patients," adopted June 1993 (*Arch Intern Med.* 1995; 155: 29-40).

Journal 2002 Examines whether managed care organizations should be obligated to disclose physician financial incentives that may limit patient care. Concludes that mandatory disclosure is in the best interest of patients and physicians. Quotes Opinions 2.03 and 8.13. Talesh, *Breaking the Learned Helplessness of Patients: Why MCOs Should be Required to Disclose Financial Incentives*, 26 *Law & Psychol. Rev.* 49, 60-61, 63 (2002).

Journal 2001 Examines issues relating to health care cost containment. Concludes that, if physicians are to meet the goals assigned to them in a cost-constrained health care system, then professional standards must be reevaluated and modified to afford meaningful guidance for clinical decision-making in the face of health care spending controls. Quotes Opinions 2.03, 2.09, 2.095, 8.032, and 9.04. Cites Opinions 8.02, 8.021, 8.051, and 8.13. Agrawal, *Resuscitating Professionalism: Self-Regulation in the Medical Marketplace*, 66 Mo. L. Rev. 341, 354, 355, 360, 361, 378, 388 (2001).

Journal 2001 Discusses the prohibition on non-lawyer ownership of legal service providers. Considers how ethical rules and standards governing physicians have been directed toward preserving independent judgment. Concludes that ethical conflicts created by abandoning the prohibition on non-lawyer ownership of legal service providers may be managed by following the medical ethics model. Quotes Principle VI and Opinions 2.03, 2.09, 8.02, 8.021, 8.03, 8.05, 8.051, 8.054, 8.13, and 8.132. Harris & Foran, *The Ethics of Middle-Class Access to Legal Services and What We Can Learn from the Medical Profession's Shift to a Corporate Paradigm*, 70 Fordham L. Rev. 775, 817, 821, 822, 823, 824 (2001).

Journal 2000 Considers how social and political values shape normative understandings of health and disease. Concludes that the challenge for developing universal canonical accounts of health and disease arises out of moral diversity. Quotes Opinion 2.03. Cherry, *Polymorphic Medical Ontologies: Fashioning Concepts of Disease*, 25 J. Med. & Phil. 519, 532 (2000).

Journal 1999 Analyzes federal regulations regarding allocation of organs for transplantation. Explores the political background and controversy surrounding allocation of human organs. Cites

Opinion 2.03. McMullen, *Equitable Allocation of Human Organs: An Examination of the New Federal Regulation*, 20 J. Legal Med. 405, 412 (1999).

Journal 1999 Points out that several states do not allow patients to designate their physicians as health care proxies. Observes that such restrictions inhibit patient autonomy. Provides justification in support of permitting appointments of physicians as proxies. Cites Opinion 2.03. Rai, Siegler, & Lantos, *The Physician as a Health Care Proxy*, 29 Hastings Center Rep. 14, 19 (Sep./Oct. 1999).

Journal 1999 Discusses the need for physicians to advocate on behalf of patients' rights in the context of health care delivery. Evaluates the nature and scope of the physician's role as advocate, noting that physicians cannot be expected to engage in attorney-like advocacy. Quotes Principles IV and VI, Fundamental Elements (2), (4), and (6) [now Opinion 10.01], Patient Responsibilities 5 [now Opinion 10.02], and Opinions 2.03, 2.07, 2.09, 2.16, 2.19, 3.06, 4.01, 4.04, 6.01, 7.02, 8.02, 8.03, 8.13, 8.132, 9.06, 9.07, and 9.131. Cites Opinions 5.05, 5.09, 7.01, 8.135, and 9.02. Sage, *Physicians as Advocates*, 35 Hous. L. Rev. 1529, 1537, 1541, 1542, 1552-53, 1554, 1556, 1557, 1559, 1561-62, 1564, 1571, 1574, 1576, 1580 (1999).

Journal 1999 Explores the impact managed care organizations have had on health care. Explains that patients may not understand restrictions and incentives imposed by their managed care organizations when entering the program. Argues that such information should be disclosed at various times during the period of plan coverage. Cites Opinions 2.03, 8.03, 8.032, 8.051, 8.13 and 8.132. Wolf, *Toward a Systemic Theory of Informed Consent in Managed Care*, 35 Hous. L. Rev. 1631, 1641, 1658, 1661, 1662, 1679 (1999).

Journal 1998 Discusses the physician's fiduciary duty to the patient. Explores the expansion of the "honest services" mail fraud statute to prosecute undisclosed fiduciary breaches. Concludes that the mail fraud statute may be used to prosecute physicians who fail to disclose financial incentives to their patients. Quotes Opinion 8.03. Cites Opinions 2.03 and 8.07 [now Opinion 8.06]. Jones, *Primum Non Nocere: The Expanding "Honest Services" Mail Fraud Statute and the Physician-Patient Fiduciary Relationship*, 51 Vand. L. Rev. 139, 161, 164 (1998).

Journal 1997 Posits that cost-containment schemes in managed care systems have eroded the fiduciary duty physicians owe patients. Notes that MCOs are prohibiting patients from trusting and relying on physicians. Concludes that patients must seek quality assurance from sources other than their physicians. Quotes Opinions 2.03, 2.09, and 8.13. Jacobi, *Patients at a Loss: Protecting Health Care Consumers through Data Driven Quality Assurance*, 45 U. Kan. L. Rev. 705, 720, 721, 759 (1997).

Journal 1996 Examines the role of physicians in managed health care. Posits that the new system of managed care is beneficial because it combines high performance with affordable outcomes. Concludes that outcome-based payment systems, with tort reform, will maximize results. Quotes Opinion 2.03 (1984) [subsequently amended]. Furrow, *Incentivizing Medical Practice: What (If Anything) Happens to Professionalism?*, 1 Widener L. Symp. J. 1, 9 (1996).

Journal 1996 Discusses the trend toward conserving resources expended on health care by withholding services absent a showing of necessity. Claims that the high standard of care physicians owe patients is jeopardized by medical treatment decisions based on coverage concerns. Concludes that the legal structure regarding health care plans should be changed. Quotes Preamble, Principles I, II, III, IV, V, VI, and VII and Opinion 2.03. Hirshfeld & Thomason, *Medical Necessity Determinations: The Need for a New Legal Structure*, 6 Health Matrix 3, 8-9 (1996).

Journal 1996 Considers whether the Oregon Health Plan discriminates on the basis of race by excluding coverage for obesity which disproportionately affects African-American women. Discusses discrimination in federally funded health care programs and the purpose of Title VI. Quotes Opinion 2.03. Jurevic, *Disparate Impact Under Title VI: Discrimination, By Any Other Name, Will Still Have the Same Impact*, 15 St. Louis U. Pub. L. Rev. 237, 253 (1996).

Journal 1996 Discusses conflicts of interest between health care professionals and patients created by managed health care and the drive toward reduction of costs. Suggests that a multi-disciplinary group of health professionals could act as patient advocates to help protect their interests. Quotes Opinion 2.03. Mehlman, *Medical Advocates: A Call for a New Profession*, 1 Widener L. Symp. J. 299, 314 (1996).

Journal 1996 Considers the change from traditional medical care systems to managed care, noting the conflicts of interest this creates between physicians' ethical obligations and financial concerns. Discusses these issues in the context of managed behavioral health care. Suggests community-based care and social supports as a solution. Quotes Opinion 2.03 and 4.04. Petrila, *Ethics, Money, and the Problem of Coercion in Managed Behavioral Health Care*, 40 St. Louis U. L. J. 359, 377 (1996).

Journal 1994 Considers how greater patient autonomy has led to situations in which medical care may be viewed as futile. Suggests that the law has intruded too far into this area of medicine. Quotes Opinion 2.035. Cites Opinions 2.03, 2.095, 2.17, 2.19, 2.20, and 2.22. Cultice, *Medical Futility: When Is Enough, Enough?*, 27 J. Health & Hosp. Law 225, 230, 256 (1994).

Journal 1994 Discusses the practice of physician rationing and how the principles of beneficence and autonomy are consistent with the practice. Explores the objection to using financial incentives, commonly adopted by HMOs, to promote rationing and concludes that rationing should be allowed in some circumstances. Quotes Opinion 2.03. Hall, *Rationing Health Care at the Bedside*, 69 N.Y.U. L. Rev. 693, 704 (1994).

Journal 1994 Observes that health care reform proposals present significant challenges to the role and ethics of attending physicians. Emphasizes that reform proposals must set forth the role envisioned for physicians and must articulate an acceptable ethical framework within which physicians may fulfill that role. Quotes Opinions 4.04, 9.121, and 9.122. Cites Opinions 2.03, 2.09, 5.01, and 8.03. Wolf, *Health Care Reform and the Future of Physician Ethics*, 24 Hastings Center Rep. 28, 32, 40 (March/April 1994).

Journal 1992 Discusses two California cases focusing on the liability of physicians and third-party payors when medically necessary care is denied. Concludes that physicians also may be obligated to advocate patient interests in attempting to secure payment from third parties when appropriate. Quotes Opinion 2.03. Comment, *Who's in Charge: The Doctor or the Dollar? Assessing the Relative Liability of Third Party Payors and Doctors After Wickline and Wilson*, 18 J. Contemp. L. 285, 301, 302 (1992).

Journal 1992 Examines the major health care rationing issues facing the United States including increasing costs and decreasing access. Concludes that the standard of care should not be changed and that rationing should be a separate enterprise undertaken pursuant to explicit criteria. Quotes Opinions 2.03, 2.09, and 4.04. Hirshfeld, *Should Ethical and Legal Standards for Physicians Be Changed to Accommodate New Models for Rationing Health Care?*, 140 Univ. Pa. L. Rev. 1809, 1816 (1992).

Journal 1991 Focuses on the denial of insurance benefits for experimental medical procedures, and explains the *de novo* review process under ERISA. Concludes that there is need for a structure that will permit greater objectivity in the context of data collection as well as judicial determination. Cites Opinions 2.03 and 2.09. Note, *Denial of Coverage for "Experimental" Medical Procedures: The Problem of De Novo Review Under ERISA*, 79 Kentucky L.J. 801, 824 (1990-91).

Journal 1990 Discusses economic considerations in clinical decisionmaking, with emphasis on the standard of care. Concludes that organized medicine has made valuable contributions through development of practice parameters that offer guidance in the exercise of clinical judgment. Cites Opinions 2.03 and 2.09. Hirshfeld, *Economic Considerations in Treatment Decisions and the Standard of Care in Medical Malpractice Litigation*, 264 JAMA 2004, 2007 (1990).

Journal 1990 Discusses efforts of third-party payors to control health care expenditures for beneficiaries. Concludes that financial incentives to limit care and other cost control techniques should be disclosed and that the rationale for such disclosure is compelling. Quotes Opinions 2.03, 2.09, and 8.03. Cites Opinions 2.19, 4.04, and 4.06. Hirshfeld, *Should Third Party Payors of Health Care Services Disclose Cost Control Mechanisms to Potential Beneficiaries?*, 14 Seton Hall Legis. J. 115, 130, 131, 144, 145, 146 (1990).

Journal 1988 Discusses various circumstances that have led to proposals for the rationing of health care by hospitals and other providers in order to contain health care costs. Because of the impact such proposals may have on older persons, focus is placed on the Age Discrimination Act of 1975 and its likely effect on the use of age as a criterion for rationing in the context of heart transplantation. Quotes Opinion 2.02 (1982) [now Opinion 2.03]. Silver, *From Baby Doe to Grandpa Doe: The Impact of the Federal Age Discrimination Act on the Hidden Rationing of Medical Care*, 37 Catholic Univ. L. Rev. 993, 1013 (1988).

Journal 1985 Notes that considerations of cost and availability of advanced medical technology raise troublesome ethical and legal issues. In addressing these issues, examines potential mechanisms for rationing expensive lifesaving medical treatment, concluding that the cost of rationing probably exceeds the benefits. Quotes Opinion 2.02 (1982) [now Opinion 2.03]. Mehlman, *Rationing Expensive Lifesaving Medical Treatments, 1985 Wisconsin L. Rev. 239, 250, 260 (1985).*

2.035 Futile Care

Physicians are not ethically obligated to deliver care that, in their best professional judgment, will not have a reasonable chance of benefiting their patients. Patients should not be given treatments simply because they demand them. Denial of treatment should be justified by reliance on openly stated ethical principles and acceptable standards of care, as defined in Opinion 2.03, "Allocation of Limited Medical Resources," and Opinion 2.095, "The Provision of Adequate Health Care," not on the concept of "futility," which cannot be meaningfully defined. (I, IV)

Issued June 1994.

Journal 2002 Explores the implications of withholding medical treatment when abortion results in a live birth. Concludes that, in these situations, abortive parents and physicians should not solely decide the child's best interest. Quotes Preamble, Principles I and III, and Opinions 2.035, 2.20, and 2.215. Casagrande, *Children Not Meant to Be: Protecting the Interests of the Child When Abortion Results in Live Birth, 6 Quinnipiac Health L.J. 19, 44, 45, 47-48 (2002).*

Journal 2002 Discusses the precautions lawyers must take when advising clients about living wills. Concludes clients must be reminded that medical advances or changes in circumstances may affect their living wills. Quotes Opinion 2.035. Kruse, *A Call for New Perspectives for Living Wills (You Might Like It Here), 37 Real Prop., Prob. & Tr. J. 545, 550 (2002).*

Journal 2001 Observes that many aspects of managed care have increased the tensions between patients and their health care providers. Notes that patient dissatisfaction is on the rise for other reasons as well. Concludes that Congress should take a comprehensive legislative approach in addressing these issues. Quotes Opinion 2.17. Cites Opinion 2.035. References Opinions 2.037 and 2.22. Sanematsu, *Taking a Broader View of Treatment Disputes Beyond Managed Care: Are Recent Legislative Efforts the Cure? 48 UCLA L. Rev. 1245, 1258, 1284 (2001).*

Journal 2000 Considers whether or not age is a sufficient justification to limit or deny access to health care. Concludes that the use of advance care directives, further research, and educational programs can help physicians address this ethical challenge. Quotes Opinion 2.035. Tadd & Bayer, *Commentary: Medical Decision Making Based on Chronological Age—Cause for Concern, 11 J. Clinical Ethics 328, 330 (2000).*

Journal 1998 Explains when a surrogate is required to make health care decisions. Discusses limitations of a surrogate's authority. Emphasizes that the health care provider must recognize that ultimate decision-making regarding care first belongs to the patient, and then to the surrogate. Quotes Opinion 2.035. Cites Opinion 8.11. References Opinion 2.22. O'Neill, *Surrogate Health Care Decisions for Adults in Illinois—Answers to the Legal Questions That Health Care Providers Face on a Daily Basis, 29 Loy. Univ. Chi. L. J. 411, 445, 448 (1998).*

Journal 1997 Examines case law pertaining to medical futility disputes. Reviews hospital policies regarding futility and notes a variety of definitions and guidelines. Concludes that, absent a clear consensus, physicians should not act solely to decide questions of futility. References Opinions 2.035 and 2.22. Johnson, Gibbons, Goldner, Wiener, & Eton, *Legal and Institutional Policy Responses to Medical Futility, 30 J. Health & Hosp. L. 21, 26, 31, 35, 36 (1997).*

Journal 1995 Considers how the judiciary, legislatures, and provider institutions balance the values of patients and their physicians. Recommends that physicians and hospitals promulgate written policies outlining their preferred treatment parameters in any given circumstance. Quotes Opinion 2.035. Daar, *Medical Futility and Implications for Physician Autonomy, XXI Am. J. Law & Med. 221, 234 (1995).*

Journal 1995 Examines the rights of health care professionals to refuse to participate in patient care on the basis of conscientious objection. Suggests steps that health care facilities may take when dealing with health care professionals who object to participating in patient care. Quotes Principles I and VI and Opinions 1.02, 2.035, and 9.055. Dellinger & Vickery, *When Staff Object to Participating In Care*, 28 J. Health & Hospital Law 269, 272, 276 (1995).

Journal 1994 Considers how greater patient autonomy has led to situations in which medical care may be viewed as futile. Suggests that the law has intruded too far into this area of medicine. Quotes Opinion 2.035. Cites Opinions 2.03, 2.095, 2.17, 2.19, 2.20, and 2.22. Cultice, *Medical Futility: When Is Enough, Enough?*, 27 J. Health & Hosp. Law 225, 230, 256 (1994).

2.037   Medical Futility in End-of-Life Care

When further intervention to prolong the life of a patient becomes futile, physicians have an obligation to shift the intent of care toward comfort and closure. However, there are necessary value judgments involved in coming to the assessment of futility. These judgments must give consideration to patient or proxy assessments of worthwhile outcome. They should also take into account the physician or other provider's perception of intent in treatment, which should not be to prolong the dying process without benefit to the patient or to others with legitimate interests. They may also take into account community and institutional standards, which in turn may have used physiological or functional outcome measures.

Nevertheless, conflicts between the parties may persist in determining what is futility in the particular instance. This may interrupt satisfactory decision-making and adversely affect patient care, family satisfaction, and physician-clinical team functioning. To assist in fair and satisfactory decision-making about what constitutes futile intervention:

(1) All health care institutions, whether large or small, should adopt a policy on medical futility; and

(2) Policies on medical futility should follow a due process approach. The following seven steps should be included in such a due process approach to declaring futility in specific cases.

(a) Earnest attempts should be made in advance to deliberate over and negotiate prior understandings between patient, proxy, and physician on what constitutes futile care for the patient, and what falls within acceptable limits for the physician, family, and possibly also the institution.

(b) Joint decision-making should occur between patient or proxy and physician to the maximum extent possible.

(c) Attempts should be made to negotiate disagreements if they arise, and to reach resolution within all parties' acceptable limits, with the assistance of consultants as appropriate.

(d) Involvement of an institutional committee such as the ethics committee should be requested if disagreements are irresolvable.

(e) If the institutional review supports the patient's position and the physician remains unpersuaded, transfer of care to another physician within the institution may be arranged.

(f) If the process supports the physician's position and the patient/proxy remains unpersuaded, transfer to another institution may be sought and, if done, should be supported by the transferring and receiving institution.

14

(g) If transfer is not possible, the intervention need not be offered. (I, V)

Issued June 1997 based on the report "Medical Futility in End-of-Life Care," adopted December 1996 (JAMA. 1999; 281: 937-41).

Journal 2002 Critiques Daniel Callahan's theory of rationing health resources according to age. Concludes age should not be a controlling factor in end-of-life decisionmaking. References Opinion 2.037. Cohen-Almagor, *A Critique of Callahan's Utilitarian Approach to Resource Allocation in Health Care, 17 Issues L. & Med. 247, 261 (2002)*.

Journal 2002 Analyzes ethical positions on futility in light of the California Uniform Health Care Decisions Act. Concludes the Act provides only a preliminary framework and considers AMA guidelines on medical futility in offering suggestions for change. Quotes Opinion 2.037. Ferguson, *Ethical Postures of Futility and California's Uniform Health Care Decisions Act, 75 S. Cal. L. Rev. 1217, 1252-53 (2002)*.

Journal 2001 Observes that many aspects of managed care have increased the tensions between patients and their health care providers. Notes that patient dissatisfaction is on the rise for other reasons as well. Concludes that Congress should take a comprehensive legislative approach in addressing these issues. Quotes Opinion 2.17. Cites Opinion 2.035. References Opinions 2.037 and 2.22. Sanematsu, *Taking a Broader View of Treatment Disputes Beyond Managed Care: Are Recent Legislative Efforts the Cure? 48 UCLA L. Rev. 1245, 1258, 1284 (2001)*.

Journal 2000 Discusses the rise and fall of the futility movement. Focuses on attempts to define and develop a process for resolving futility disputes. Concludes that the decision-making dilemma surrounding treatments of minimal benefit still exists and that talking to patients and families should be viewed as the primary method by which physicians may address this problem. References Opinion 2.037. Helft, Siegler, & Lantos, *The Rise and Fall of the Futility Movement, 343 New Eng. J. Med. 293, 294 (2000)*.

Journal 2000 Evaluates documentation of decision-making in the treatment of hospitalized elderly trauma patients who died. Considers the frequency of withdrawal of therapy and who made the decisions. Concludes that further research is needed regarding methods to resolve disputes involving futility and withdrawal of therapy. References Opinion 2.037. Trunkey, Cahn, Lenfesty, & Mullins, *Management of the Geriatric Trauma Patient at Risk of Death: Therapy Withdrawal Decision Making, 135 Arch. Surg. 34, 35 (2000)*.

Journal 2000 Discusses medical futility and offers a case-based assessment of circumstances under which continued use of treatment may exceed the boundaries of reasonableness. Suggests a procedural approach for making decisions on a case-by-case basis. References Opinion 2.037. Truog, *Futility in Pediatrics: From Case to Policy, 11 J. Clinical Ethics 136, 139, 141 (2000)*.

2.04   The previous Opinion 2.04, "Artificial Insemination by Known Donor," issued prior to April 1977, was replaced by the current Opinion 2.04, "Artificial Insemination by Known Donor."

2.04   Artificial Insemination by Known Donor

Any individual or couple contemplating artificial insemination by husband, partner, or other known donor should be counseled about the full range of infectious and genetic diseases for which the donor or recipient can be screened, including HIV infection. Full medical history disclosure and appropriate diagnostic screening should be recommended to the donor and recipient but are not required.

Informed consent for artificial insemination should include disclosure of risks, benefits, and likely success rate of the method proposed and potential alternative methods. Individuals should receive information about screening, costs, and procedures for confidentiality, when applicable. The prospective parents or parent should be informed of the laws regarding the rights of children conceived by artificial insemination, as well as the laws regarding parental rights and obligations. If the donor is married to the recipient, resultant children will have all the rights of a child conceived naturally.

If the donor and recipient are not married, an appropriate legal rule would treat the situation as if the donor were anonymous: the recipient would be considered the sole parent of the child except in cases where both donor and recipient agree to recognize a paternity right.

Sex selection of sperm for the purposes of avoiding a sex-linked inheritable disease is appropriate. However, physicians should not participate in sex selection for reasons of gender preference. Physicians should encourage a prospective parent or parents to consider the value of both sexes.

If semen is frozen and the donor dies before it is used, the frozen semen should not be used or donated for purposes other than those originally intended by the donor. If the donor left no instructions, it is reasonable to allow the remaining partner to use the semen for artificial insemination but not to donate it to someone else. However, the donor should be advised of such a policy at the time of donation and be given an opportunity to override it. (I, V)

Issued June 1993.

Colo. 1989 State statute prohibiting a sperm donor from asserting his parental status was held to be inapplicable where known donor and unmarried recipient agreed that the donor would have parental rights. Concurring opinion argued that the statute bars any non-husband donor, regardless of relationship to the recipient, from asserting parental rights. However, the concurring opinion found the statute inapplicable because its provision requiring "supervision" by a physician had not been met. In apparent reference to the standards set out under Opinions 2.04 and 2.05, the concurring opinion said that "supervision" should at the least require an examination to determine whether there are any health risks to the recipient as a result of the procedure and to protect the child from hereditary disease. *In re R.C., 775 P.2d 27, 37 n.3.*

Journal 1987 Examines various ethical issues surrounding surrogate motherhood, artificial insemination, in vitro fertilization and embryonic/fetal research. Reports on the positions of four ethics groups: the Warnock Committee of Inquiry into Human Fertilization and Embryology; the AMA's Council on Ethical and Judicial Affairs; the Ethics Committee of the American Fertility Society; and the Ethics Committee of the American College of Obstetricians and Gynecologists. References Opinions 2.04, 2.05, and 2.13 (1986) [now Opinion 2.14]. Quotes Opinion 2.18. Rosner, Cassell, Friedland, Landolt, Loeb, Numann, Ora, Risemberg, & Sordillo, *Ethical Considerations of Reproductive Technologies, 87 N.Y. State J. Med. 398, 399-400 (1987).*

2.05   The previous Opinion 2.05, "Artificial Insemination by Donor," issued 1983, was replaced by the current Opinion 2.05, "Artificial Insemination by Anonymous Donor."

2.05   Artificial Insemination by Anonymous Donor

Thorough medical histories must be taken of all candidates for anonymous semen donation. All potential donors must also be screened for infectious or inheritable diseases which could adversely affect the recipient or the resultant child. Frozen semen should be used for artificial insemination because it enables the donor to be tested for HIV infection at the time of donation, and again after an interval before the original semen is used, thus increasing the likelihood that the semen is free of HIV infection. Physicians should rely on the guidelines formulated by relevant professional organizations, such as the American Society of Reproductive Medicine, the Centers for Disease Control and Prevention, and the Food and Drug Administration, in determining the interval between the initial and final HIV test, which disorders to screen for, and which procedures to use in screening.

Physicians should maintain a permanent record which includes both identifying and non-identifying health and genetic screening information. Other than exceptional situations where identifying information may be required, physicians should release only non-identifying health-related information in order to preserve the confidentiality of the semen donor. Physicians should maintain permanent records of donors to fulfill the following obligations: (1) to exclude individuals from the donor pool who test positive for infectious or inheritable diseases, (2) to limit the number of pregnancies resulting from a single donor source so as to avoid future consanguineous marriages or reproduction, (3) to notify donors of screening results which indicate the presence of an infectious or inheritable disease, and (4) to notify donors if a child born through artificial insemination has a disorder which may have been transmitted by the donor.

Informed consent for artificial insemination should include disclosure of risks, benefits, likely success rate of the method proposed and potential alternative methods, and costs. Both recipients and donors should be informed of the reasons for screening and confidentiality. They should also know the extent of access to non-identifying and identifying information about the donor. Participants should be advised to consider the legal ramifications, if any, of artificial insemination by anonymous donor.

The consent of the husband is ethically appropriate if he is to become the legal father of the resultant child from artificial insemination by anonymous donor. Anonymous donors cannot assume the rights or responsibilities of parenthood for children born through therapeutic donor insemination, nor should they be required to assume them.

In the case of single women or women who are part of a homosexual couple, it is not unethical to provide artificial insemination as a reproductive option.

Sex selection of sperm for the purposes of avoiding a sex-linked inheritable disease is appropriate. However, physicians should not participate in sex selection of sperm for reasons of gender preference. Physicians should encourage a prospective parent or parents to consider the value of both sexes.

In general, it is inappropriate to offer compensation to donors to encourage donation over and above reimbursement for time and actual expenses. (I, V)

Issued June 1993.

Colo. 1989 State statute prohibiting a sperm donor from asserting his parental status was held to be inapplicable where known donor and unmarried recipient agreed that the donor would have parental rights. Concurring opinion argued that the statute bars any non-husband donor, regardless of relationship to the recipient, from asserting parental rights. However, the concurring opinion found the statute inapplicable because its provision requiring "supervision" by a physician had not been met. In apparent reference to the standards set out under Opinions 2.04 and 2.05, the concurring opinion said that "supervision" should at the least require an examination to determine whether there are any health risks to the recipient as a result of the procedure and to protect the child from hereditary disease. *In re R.C., 775 P.2d 27, 37 n.3.*

Journal 1987 Examines various ethical issues surrounding surrogate motherhood, artificial insemination, in vitro fertilization and embryonic/fetal research. Reports on the positions of four ethics groups: the Warnock Committee of Inquiry into Human Fertilization and Embryology; the AMA's Council on Ethical and Judicial Affairs; the Ethics Committee of the American Fertility Society; and the Ethics Committee of the American College of Obstetricians and Gynecologists. References Opinions 2.04, 2.05, and 2.13 (1986) [now Opinion 2.14]. Quotes Opinion 2.18. Rosner, Cassell, Friedland, Landolt, Loeb, Numann, Ora, Risemberg, & Sordillo, *Ethical Considerations of Reproductive Technologies*, 87 N.Y. State J. Med. 398, 399-400 (1987).

2.055 Ethical Conduct in Assisted Reproductive Technology

The following guidelines are intended to emphasize the value of existing standards to ensure ethical practices in assisted reproductive technology (ART):

(1) The medical profession's development of technical and ethical guidelines for ART should continue. Education of the profession and patients should be pursued through widely disseminated information. Such material should include information on clinic-specific success rates.

(2) Fertility laboratories not currently participating in a credible professional accreditation program are encouraged to do so. Professional self-regulation is also encouraged through signed pledges to meet established ethical standards and to comply with laboratory accreditation efforts. Physicians who become aware of unethical practices must report such conduct to the appropriate body. Physicians also should be willing to provide expert testimony when needed. Specialty societies should discuss the development of mechanisms for disciplinary action, such as revocation of membership, for members who fail to comply with ethical standards.

(3) Patients should be fully informed about all aspects of ART applicable to their particular clinical profile. A well-researched, validated informed consent instrument would be useful for the benefit of patients and professionals. Payment based on clinical outcome is unacceptable.

(4) Physicians and clinicians practicing ART should use accurate descriptors of available services, success rates, and fee structure and payment obligations in promotional materials.

If legislation on regulation of ART laboratories, advertising practices, or related issues is adopted, it should include adequate financial resources to ensure the intended action can be implemented. Improved legislative protection may be needed to protect physicians and their professional organizations when they provide testimony on unethical conduct of colleagues. (I, V)

Issued December 1998 based on the report "Issues of Ethical Conduct in Assisted Reproductive Technology," adopted June 1996.

2.06 Capital Punishment

An individual's opinion on capital punishment is the personal moral decision of the individual. A physician, as a member of a profession dedicated to preserving life when there is hope of doing so, should not be a participant in a legally authorized execution. Physician participation in execution is defined generally as actions which would fall into one or more of the following categories: (1) an action which would directly cause the death of the condemned; (2) an action which would assist, supervise, or contribute to the ability of another individual to directly cause the death of the condemned; (3) an action which could automatically cause an execution to be carried out on a condemned prisoner.

Physician participation in an execution includes, but is not limited to, the following actions: prescribing or administering tranquilizers and other psychotropic agents and medications that are part of the execution procedure; monitoring vital signs on site or remotely (including monitoring electrocardiograms); attending or observing an execution as a physician; and rendering of technical advice regarding execution.

In the case where the method of execution is lethal injection, the following actions by the physician would also constitute physician participation in execution: selecting injection sites; starting intravenous lines as a port for a lethal injection device; prescribing, preparing, administering, or supervising injection drugs or their doses or types; inspecting, testing, or maintaining lethal injection devices; and consulting with or supervising lethal injection personnel.

The following actions do not constitute physician participation in execution: (1) testifying as to medical history and diagnoses or mental state as they relate to competence to stand trial, testifying as to relevant medical evidence during trial, testifying as to medical aspects of aggravating or mitigating circumstances during the penalty phase of a capital case, or testifying as to medical diagnoses as they relate to the legal assessment of competence for execution; (2) certifying death, provided that the condemned has been declared dead by another person; (3) witnessing an execution in a totally nonprofessional capacity; (4) witnessing an execution at the specific voluntary request of the condemned person, provided that the physician observes the execution in a nonprofessional capacity; and (5) relieving the acute suffering of a condemned person while awaiting execution, including providing tranquilizers at the specific voluntary request of the condemned person to help relieve pain or anxiety in anticipation of the execution.

Physicians should not determine legal competence to be executed. A physician's medical opinion should be merely one aspect of the information taken into account by a legal decision maker such as a judge or hearing officer. When a condemned prisoner has been declared incompetent to be executed, physicians should not treat the prisoner for the purpose of restoring competence unless a commutation order is issued before treatment begins. The task of re-evaluating the prisoner should be performed by an independent physician examiner. If the incompetent prisoner is undergoing extreme suffering as a result of psychosis or any other illness, medical intervention intended to mitigate the level of suffering is ethically permissible. No physician should be compelled to participate in the process of establishing a prisoner's competence or be involved with treatment of an incompetent, condemned prisoner if such activity is contrary to the physician's personal beliefs. Under those circumstances, physicians should be permitted to transfer care of the prisoner to another physician.

Organ donation by condemned prisoners is permissible only if (1) the decision to donate was made before the prisoner's conviction, (2) the donated tissue is harvested after the prisoner has been pronounced dead and the body removed from the death chamber, and (3) physicians do not provide advice on modifying the method of execution for any individual to facilitate donation. (I)

Issued July 1980.

Updated June 1994 based on the report "Physician Participation in Capital Punishment," adopted December 1992 (JAMA. 1993; 270: 365-68); updated June 1996 based on the report "Physician Participation in Capital Punishment: Evaluations of Prisoner Competence to be Executed; Treatment to Restore Competence to be Executed," adopted in June 1995; updated December 1999; and updated June 2000 based on the report "Defining Physician Participation in State Executions," adopted June 1998.

8th Cir. 2003 Prisoner convicted of capital felony murder was involuntarily medicated after a review panel held he was a danger to himself and others. Thereafter, the state set an execution date for prisoner because he was competent due to the medication. The Court of Appeals, *en banc*, affirmed lower court's denial of the prisoner's habeus corpus petition. Court found state had a duty to medicate the prisoner and that Eighth Amendment is not violated when a prisoner on death row regains competency as a result of involuntary medication. Dissenting judges, with apparent reference to Opinion 2.06, noted that the ethical standards of the AMA prohibit physicians from assisting in executions. *Singleton v. Norris, 319 F.3d 1018, 1036.*

D.D.C. 2001 District court found that the government was permitted to treat the defendant involuntarily with antipsychotic medication in order to render him non-dangerous and mentally competent to stand trial. The court in making its decision that a pretrial detainee is not afforded the same prohibition against involuntary medication as a convicted defendant waiting to be executed apparently relied on Opinion 2.06. *United States v. Weston, 134 F. Supp. 2d 115, 126-27.*

La. 1992 State's attempt to circumvent prohibition against execution of insane prisoners by forcibly medicating prisoner was held to be a violation of the prisoner's right to privacy and constituted cruel and unusual punishment. Noting that a physician's administration of medication in order to facilitate the prisoner's execution is contrary to the AMA's ethical code, in apparent reference to Opinion 2.06, the court held that involuntary administration of medication is not medical treatment but constitutes a part of capital punishment. *State v. Perry, 610 So. 2d 746, 753.*

S.C. 1993 State sought to reverse order vacating death sentence and imposing life imprisonment. The court stated that the critical issue inherent in the state's contention of error was whether the state could forcibly medicate a prisoner solely to make prisoner competent enough to execute. Citing Opinion 2.06, the court held that the AMA's position reinforces the prohibition against the state's use of medication solely to facilitate an insane prisoner's execution. *Singleton v. State, 437 S.E. 2d 53, 61.*

Va. Att'y Gen. 1994 Attorney General responded in the negative when asked whether a physician employed by the Department of Corrections may be disciplined by the Board of Medicine for participating in the execution of a prisoner where "participating" was defined as "attending or observing an execution, for making a determination that death has occurred, for issuing a certificate of death, or for performing any other function that applicable state statutes lawfully require to be performed by a physician in connection with an execution." Citing Opinion 2.06, the Attorney General noted that such ethical opinions are not legally conclusive and that if they conflict with a state statute, the statute controls. *Va. Att'y Gen. Op., 1994 Va. AG LEXIS 12.*

Journal 2003 Considers a legislative plan allowing voluntary, consensual organ donation by condemned prisoners. Concludes that, in view of the current organ shortage, the benefits of such a plan outweigh the concerns. Quotes Principle VII and Opinion 2.06. Perales, *Rethinking the Prohibition of Death Row Prisoners as Organ Donors: A Possible Lifeline to Those on Organ Donor Waiting Lists, 34 St. Mary's L. J. 687, 721, 725 (2003).*

Journal 2003 Discusses history of the death penalty in Colorado. Concludes that the trend is moving toward its abolition. Quotes Opinion 2.06. Radelet, *Capital Punishment in Colorado: 1859-1972, 74 U. Colo. L. Rev. 885, 940 (2003).*

Journal 2002 Addresses the problems arising out of legislative changes in methods of execution. Focuses on the change from electrocution to lethal injection. Concludes that, despite changes, executions are not necessarily more humane. Quotes Opinion 2.06. Denno, *When Legislatures Delegate Death: The Troubling Paradox Behind State Uses of Electrocution and Lethal Injection and*

What it Says About Us, 63 Ohio St. L.J. 63, 112-13 (2002).

Journal 2002 Examines the standard for determining competency to be executed as applied to mentally ill death row inmates. Favors commuting their sentences. Concludes a new standard that comports with the Eighth Amendment should be adopted. Quotes Opinion 2.06. Horstman, *Commuting Death Sentences of the Insane: A Solution for a Better, More Compassionate Society, 36 U.S.F.L. Rev. 823, 848 (2002).*

Journal 2002 Analyzes Arizona case law and other relevant law regarding medical treatment of individuals who are Not Competent to be Executed. Concludes that the law should address this difficult problem in a more uniform manner. Cites Opinion 2.06. Levitt & Ryan, *Not Competent to Be Executed: Dilemmas Faced By Psychiatrists and Attorneys, 23 Am. J. Forensic Psych. 39, 47 (July 2002).*

Journal 2002 Examines medical professionalism. Considers how changes in health care give rise to physician frustration, which has served as an anchor for the Charter on Medical Professionalism. Quotes Opinion 2.06. Miles, *On a New Charter to Defend Medical Professionalism: Whose Profession is it Anyway? 32 Hastings Center Rep. 46, 47 (May/June 2002).*

Journal 2001 Discusses the ethical, legal, and policy arguments affecting physician participation in capital punishment. Examines the tension created by conflicting state death penalty laws and medical practice acts. Concludes that an active role for physicians in lethal injection should be supported in an effort to reduce mishaps that may occur during executions. Quotes Opinion 2.06. Baum, *"To Comfort Always": Physician Participation in Executions, 5 N.Y.U. J. Legis. & Pub. Pol'y 47, 56-57 (2001).*

Journal 2001 Addresses the issue of whether death row prisoners may be compelled to take psychotropic medications to render them mentally competent to be executed. Considers whether physicians should be required to violate principles of medical ethics in order to treat death row inmates for this purpose. Quotes Opinion 2.06. Daugherty, *"Synthetic Sanity": The Ethics and Legality of Using Psychotropic Medications to Render Death Row Inmates Competent for Execution, 17 J. Contemp. H. L. & Pol'y 715, 730 (2001).*

Journal 2001 Discusses policies that consider physician participation in capital punishment to be unethical. Observes that such policies are without merit. Argues that such policies attempt to override the will of the people, their elected representatives, and the administration of justice. Concludes that these policies should be rescinded by state and national medical associations. Quotes Opinion 2.06. Keyes, *The Choice of Participation by Physicians in Capital Punishment, 22 Whittier L. Rev. 809, 810-11, 838 (2001).*

Journal 2000 Explores physicians' views regarding involvement in capital punishment. Concludes that, despite medical society policies, a majority of physicians believe participation in capital punishment is acceptable in certain circumstances. Quotes Opinion 2.06. Farber, Davis, Weiner, Jordan, Boyer, & Ubel, *Physicians' Attitudes About Involvement in Lethal Injection for Capital Punishment, 160 Arch. Intern. Med. 2912, 2912 (2000).*

Journal 2000 Explores issues and concerns associated with capital punishment. Discusses the controversy surrounding ways that physicians participate in capital punishment in this country. Concludes that capital punishment is not needed and cannot be fairly administered. Quotes Opinion 2.06. Martin, *Tessie Hutchinson and the American System of Capital Punishment, 59 Md. L. Rev. 553, 565 (2000).*

Journal 2000 Explores the history and legal rationale behind the prohibition against executing the insane. Considers relevant case law addressing the forced medication issue, especially as it relates to death row inmates. Concludes the ultimate question should focus on what is in the prisoner's best interest. Cites Opinion 2.06. Miller-Rice, *The "Insane" Contradiction of Singleton v. Norris: Forced Medication in a Death Row Inmate's Medical Interest Which Happens to Facilitate His Execution, 22 U. Ark. Little Rock L. Rev. 659, 673 (2000).*

Journal 2000 Explores the debate regarding physician-assisted suicide. Concludes that autonomy should be respected and that an individual's wishes for assisted suicide should be honored, unless the individual is misinformed or legally incompetent. Quotes Opinion 2.211. References Opinion 2.06. Urofsky, *Justifying Assisted Suicide: Comments on the Ongoing Debate, 14 Notre Dame J. L. Ethics & Pub. Pol'y 893, 918, 923 (2000).*

Journal 1999 Discusses the Uniform Declaration of Death Act and the dead-donor rule. Provides ethical justifications for sustaining current policies on non-heart-beating organ donation. Cites

Opinions 2.06 and 2.162. DuBois, *Non-Heart-Beating Organ Donation: A Defense of the Required Determination of Death*, 27 J. Law, Med. & Ethics 126, 128 (1999).

Journal 1998 Describes a survey regarding physician-assisted suicide given to members of the Group for the Advancement of Psychiatry. Discusses the results of the survey, noting that most surveyed psychiatrists oppose assisting patients to die. Cites Opinions 2.06 and 2.20. Kramer, Gruenberg, & Fidler, *Psychiatrists' Attitudes Toward Physician-Assisted Suicide: A Survey*, 19 Am. J. Forensic Psychiatry 81, 87, 90 (1998).

Journal 1998 Explains that a determination of mental capacity to consent must be made when a person requests physician-assisted suicide in a jurisdiction where such practice is legal. Explores the potential for liability in the context of making such a determination. Argues that standards regarding determination of mental capacity must be established by case law or legislation. Cites Opinion 2.211. References Opinion 2.06. Lipschitz, *Psychiatry and Consent for Physician-Assisted Suicide*, 19 Am. J. Forensic Psychiatry 91, 103, 104 (1998).

Journal 1997 Explores the Eighth Amendment prohibition against cruel and unusual punishment in the context of capital punishment. Discusses widely used methods of execution. Suggests that execution methods may be unconstitutionally excessive. Concludes the death penalty should not be imposed until methods are more humane. Quotes Opinion 2.06. Denno, *Getting to Death: Are Executions Constitutional?*, 82 Iowa L. Rev. 319, 385-86 (1997).

Journal 1997 Describes capital punishment in the United States. Considers ethical and moral issues implicated by physician participation. Opines that executions constitute harm and that physician participation contravenes professional ethical obligations. Quotes Opinion 2.06. Michalos, *Medical Ethics and the Executing Process in the United States of America*, 16 Med. & Law 125, 131, 133 (1997).

Journal 1996 Examines how execution practices affect crime deterrence. Explores trend toward private and more humane executions. Discusses similarity between lethal injection and medical procedures. Concludes that deterrence is not served by current execution practices and should not be advanced as support for the death penalty. Cites Opinion 2.06. Abernethy, *The Methodology of Death: Reexamining the Deterrence Rationale*, 27 Colum. Hum. Rts. L. Rev. 379, 410-11 (1996).

Journal 1996 Examines the death penalty statute in New York. Discusses statutory provisions and notes it is unethical for medical personnel to assist with executions. Concludes that the death penalty statute fails to deter crime and may be unconstitutional. Quotes Opinion 2.06. Acker, *When the Cheering Stopped: An Overview and Analysis of New York's Death Penalty Legislation*, 17 Pace L. Rev. 41, 221-22 (1996).

Journal 1996 Discusses the current shortage of available organs for transplant patients. Suggests several new methods for increasing the supply. Includes among these suggestions a proposal that inmates sentenced to death should be allowed to donate organs. Quotes Opinion 2.06. Coleman, *Brother, Can You Spare a Liver? Five Ways to Increase Organ Donation*, 31 Val. U.L. Rev. 1, 30, 31 (1996).

Journal 1996 Discusses the involvement of psychiatrists in capital punishment. Posits that physicians should not aid legal executions. Expresses support for the ethical resolutions of psychiatric and medical associations regarding this issue. Quotes Opinion 2.06. Freedman & Halpern, *The Erosion of Ethics and Morality in Medicine: Physician Participation in Legal Executions in the United States*, 41 N.Y.L. Sch. L. Rev. 169, 174 (1996).

Journal 1996 Proposes an alternative method of capital punishment to allow for organ donation by executed prisoners. Provides justifications for this proposal. Concludes that physicians should be able to ethically participate in this process. Quotes Principle VII. Cites Opinion 2.06. References Opinion 2.162 (1994) [subsequently amended]. Patton, *A Call for Common Sense: Organ Donation and the Executed Prisoner*, 3 Va. J. Soc. Pol'y & L. 387, 404, 405, 407-10 (1996).

Journal 1996 Considers physician participation in execution of capital offenders. Observes that this practice is unethical and contrary to the physician's role as a healer. Concludes that physicians should not participate in any aspect of executions. Quotes Opinion 2.06. Schoenholtz, Freedman, & Halpern, *The Legal Abuse of Physicians in Deaths in the United States: The Erosion of Ethics and Morality in Medicine*, 42 Wayne L. Rev. 1505, 1542 (1996).

Journal 1996 Discusses the role psychiatrists play in capital punishment. Notes that the ethical prohibition against physician participation in the process creates complications for psychiatrists.

References Opinion 2.06. Zwirn, *Professionalism, Mental Disability, and the Death Penalty*, 41 N.Y.L Sch. L. Rev. 163, 165 (1996).

Journal 1995 Summarizes the US Supreme Court's capital punishment jurisprudence. Explores the history and methodology of the New York Court of Appeals' constitutional adjudication of capital punishment issues and examines constitutional challenges to the death penalty in other states. Quotes Opinion 2.06. Falk & Cary, *Death-Defying Feats: State Constitutional Challenges To New York's Death Penalty*, 4 J. L. & Pol'y 161, 233, 234 (1995).

Journal 1995 Explores the relevance of historical account of capital punishment in New York to the contemporary debate regarding televised executions. Concludes that increased publicity may give both the public and the condemned more power over how executions are conducted. Cites Opinion 2.06. Madow, *Forbidden Spectacle: Executions, the Public and the Press in Nineteenth Century New York*, 43 Buff. L. Rev. 461, 475 (1995).

Journal 1994 Argues that assisted suicide is not an implicit right under the fourteenth amendment's liberty guarantee. Suggests that giving physicians the authority to determine the appropriateness of assisted suicide furthers no legitimate state interest. Cites Opinion 2.06. References Opinion 2.211. Marzen, *Out, Out Brief Candle: Constitutionally Prescribed Suicide for the Terminally Ill*, 21 Hastings Const. L.Q. 799, 821 (1994).

Journal 1994 Argues that physician aid-in-dying should be protected by the US Constitution and that patients should have a federal cause of action to challenge prohibitive state statutes. Considers how such a cause of action might affect public policy. Quotes Principles I and III. References Opinion 2.06. Note, *Toward a More Perfect Union: A Federal Cause of Action for Physician Aid-In-Dying*, 27 U. Mich. J.L. Ref. 521, 538 (1994).

Journal 1993 Considers whether criminal penalties should be imposed on a physician who assists in the suicide of a competent, non-terminal patient who requested such assistance. Presents the arguments for and against active euthanasia, with emphasis on the "slippery slope" argument. References Opinions 2.06 and 2.20. Persels, *Forcing the Issue of Physician-Assisted Suicide: Impact of the Kevorkian Case on the Euthanasia Debate*, 14 J. Legal Med. 93, 115 (1993).

Journal 1993 Explores the extent to which physicians may participate in capital punishment. Explains the policy behind prohibiting physicians from taking part in executions. Cites Opinion 2.06. Truog & Brennan, *Participation of Physicians in Capital Punishment*, 329 New Eng. J. Med. 1346 (1993).

Journal 1991 Considers ethical issues raised by the case of *Perry v. Louisiana*, where the state attempted to treat an insane death row inmate in order to render him fit for execution. Explores various ethical questions involving mentally ill defendants/inmates and proposes increased discussion and reform of ethical guidelines. Quotes Opinion 2.06. Note, *Perry v. Louisiana: Medical Ethics on Death Row—Is Judicial Intervention Warranted?*, 4 Georgetown J. Legal Ethics 707, 714 (1991).

Journal 1987 Concludes that a policy or practice of active voluntary euthanasia is not desirable, linking a moral prohibition against active voluntary euthanasia to the moral prohibition against physicians actively participating in capital punishment. In place of any practice of active voluntary euthanasia, recommends increased use of hospices, greater emphasis on training physicians to care for the dying patient, and further research aimed at producing symptomatic relief in dying patients. Cites Opinions 2.06, 8.10 (1986) [now Opinion 8.11], and 9.06. Shewmon, *Active Voluntary Euthanasia: A Needless Pandora's Box*, 3 Issues in Law and Med. 219, 220, 222, 243 (1987).

Journal 1987 Focuses on the decision of the US Supreme Court in *Ford v. Wainwright*, wherein the Court ruled that the Eighth Amendment forbids the execution of a condemned inmate who has become insane. Noting that physicians should not ethically participate in a legally authorized execution, except to make a determination or certification of death, concludes that participation by mental health professionals in assessing competency for execution is incompatible with the general ethics of the profession. Cites Opinion 2.06. Wallace, *Incompetency for Execution: The Supreme Court Challenges the Ethical Standards of the Mental Health Professions*, 8 J. Legal Med. 265, 267 (1987).

Journal 1986 Observes that the AMA policy on capital punishment expressly forbids psychiatrists from making determinations of competency for execution. Compares the psychiatrist's determination of competency for execution to the behavior of Nazi physicians, and condemns as inherently dishonest any therapy not grounded in the patient's best interests. References

Principle I and Opinion 2.06. Sargent, *Treating the Condemned to Death*, 16 Hastings Center Rep. 5, 5 (Dec. 1986).

Journal 1983 Focuses on the medical-ethical dilemma inherent in the application of medical technology to bring about death and observes that medical professional organizations have done little to solve the dilemma. Concludes that there is a need for federal legislation preempting the multiplicity of state-sanctioned methods to reduce the potential of abuse of civil and human rights. References 1980 AMA Policy Statement [now Opinion 2.06]. Finks, *Lethal Injection: An Uneasy Alliance of Law and Medicine*, 4 J. Legal Med. 383, 392, 394 (1983).

2.065 Court-Initiated Medical Treatments in Criminal Cases

Physicians can ethically participate in court-initiated medical treatments only if the procedure being mandated is therapeutically efficacious and is therefore undoubtedly not a form of punishment or solely a mechanism of social control. While a court has the authority to identify criminal behavior, a court does not have the ability to make a medical diagnosis or to determine the type of treatment that will be administered. In accordance with ethical practice, physicians should treat patients based on sound medical diagnoses, not court-defined behaviors. This is particularly important where the treatment involves in-patient therapy, surgical intervention, or pharmacological treatment. In these cases, diagnosis can be made initially by the physician who will do the treatment, but must then be confirmed by an independent physician or a panel of physicians not responsible to the state. A second opinion is not necessary in cases of court-ordered counseling or referrals for psychiatric evaluations.

A recognized, authoritative medical body, such as a national specialty society, should pre-establish scientifically valid treatments for medically determined diagnoses. Such pre-established acceptable treatments should then be applied on a case-by-case basis.

The physician who will perform the treatment must be able to conclude, in good conscience and to the best of his or her professional judgment, that the informed consent was given voluntarily to the extent possible, recognizing the element of coercion that is inevitably present. In cases involving in-patient therapy, surgical intervention, or pharmacological treatment, an independent physician or a panel of physicians not responsible to the state should confirm that the informed consent was given in accordance with these guidelines. (I, III)

Issued December 1998 based on the report "Court-Initiated Medical Treatment in Criminal Cases," adopted June 1998.

2.067 Torture

Torture refers to the deliberate, systematic, or wanton administration of cruel, inhumane, and degrading treatments or punishments during imprisonment or detainment.

Physicians must oppose and must not participate in torture for any reason. Participation in torture includes, but is not limited to, providing or withholding any services, substances, or knowledge to facilitate the practice of torture. Physicians must not be present when torture is used or threatened.

Physicians may treat prisoners or detainees if doing so is in their best interest, but physicians should not treat individuals to verify their health so that torture can begin or continue. Physicians who treat torture victims should not be persecuted. Physicians should help provide support for victims of torture and, whenever possible, strive to change situations in which torture is practiced or the potential for torture is great. (I, III)

Issued December 1999.

2.07 Clinical Investigation

The following guidelines are intended to aid physicians in fulfilling their ethical responsibilities when they engage in the clinical investigation of new drugs and procedures.

(1) A physician may participate in clinical investigation only to the extent that those activities are a part of a systematic program competently designed, under accepted standards of scientific research, to produce data which are scientifically valid and significant.

(2) In conducting clinical investigation, the investigator should demonstrate the same concern and caution for the welfare, safety, and comfort of the person involved as is required of a physician who is furnishing medical care to a patient independent of any clinical investigation.

(3) Minors or mentally incompetent persons may be used as subjects in clinical investigation only if:

(a) The nature of the investigation is such that mentally competent adults would not be suitable subjects.

(b) Consent, in writing, is given by a legally authorized representative of the subject under circumstances in which informed and prudent adults would reasonably be expected to volunteer themselves or their children as subjects.

(4) In clinical investigation primarily for treatment:

(a) The physician must recognize that the patient-physician relationship exists and that professional judgment and skill must be exercised in the best interest of the patient.

(b) Voluntary written consent must be obtained from the patient, or from the patient's legally authorized representative if the patient lacks the capacity to consent, following: (i) disclosure that the physician intends to use an investigational drug or experimental procedure, (ii) a reasonable explanation of the nature of the drug or procedure to be used, risks to be expected, and possible therapeutic benefits, (iii) an offer to answer any inquiries concerning the drug or procedure, and (iv) a disclosure of alternative drugs or procedures that may be available. Physicians should be completely objective in discussing the details of the drug or procedure to be employed, the pain and discomfort that may be anticipated, known risks and possible hazards, the quality of life to be expected, and particularly the alternatives. Especially, physicians should not use persuasion to obtain consent which otherwise might not be forthcoming, nor should expectations be encouraged beyond those which the circumstances reasonably and realistically justify.

(i) In exceptional circumstances, where the experimental treatment is the only potential treatment for the patient and full disclosure of information concerning the nature of the drug or experimental procedure or risks would pose such a serious psychological threat of detriment to the patient as to be medically contraindicated, such information may be withheld from the patient. In these circumstances, such information should be disclosed to a responsible relative or friend of the patient where possible.

(ii) Ordinarily, consent should be in writing, except where the physician deems it necessary to rely upon consent in other than written form because of the physical or emotional state of the patient.

(5) In clinical investigation primarily for the accumulation of scientific knowledge:

(a) Adequate safeguards must be provided for the welfare, safety, and comfort of the subject. It is fundamental social policy that the advancement of scientific knowledge must always be secondary to primary concern for the individual.

(b) Consent, in writing, should be obtained from the subject, or from a legally authorized representative if the subject lacks the capacity to consent, following: (i) disclosure of the fact that an investigational drug or procedure is to be used, (ii) a reasonable explanation of the nature of the procedure to be used and risks to be expected, and (iii) an offer to answer any inquiries concerning the drug or procedure.

(6) No person may be used as a subject in clinical investigation against his or her will.

(7) The overuse of institutionalized persons in research is an unfair distribution of research risks. Participation is coercive and not voluntary if the participant is subjected to powerful incentives and persuasion.

(8) The ultimate responsibility for the ethical conduct of science resides within the institution (academic, industrial, public, or private) which conducts scientific research and with the individual scientist. Research institutions should assure that rigorous scientific standards are upheld by each of their faculty, staff, and students and should extend these standards to all reports, publications, and databases produced by the institution. All medical schools and biomedical research institutions should implement guidelines for a review process for dealing with allegations of fraud. These guidelines should ensure that (a) the process used to resolve allegations of fraud does not damage science, (b) all parties are treated fairly and justly with a sensitivity to reputations and vulnerabilities, (c) the highest degree of confidentiality is maintained, (d) the integrity of the process is maintained by an avoidance of real or apparent conflicts of interest, (e) resolution of charges is expeditious, (f) accurate and detailed documentation is kept throughout the process, and (g) responsibilities to all involved individuals, the public, research sponsors, the scientific literature, and the scientific community is met after resolution of charges. Academic institutions must be capable of, and committed to, implementing effective procedures for examining allegations of scientific fraud. No system of external monitoring should replace the efforts of an institution to set its own standards

which fulfill its responsibility for the proper conduct of science and the training of scientists.

(9) With the approval of the patient or the patient's lawful representative, physicians should cooperate with the press and media to ensure that medical news concerning the progress of clinical investigation or the patient's condition is available more promptly and more accurately than would be possible without their assistance. On the other hand, the Council does not approve of practices designed to create fanfare, sensationalism to attract media attention, and unwarranted expressions of optimism because of short-term progress, even though longer range prognosis is known from the beginning to be precarious. With the approval of the patient or the patient's family, the Council, however, encourages the objective disclosure to the press and media of pertinent information. If at all possible, the identity of the patient should remain confidential if the patient or the patient's family so desires. The situation should not be used for the commercial ends of participating physicians or the institutions involved. (I, III, V)

Issued prior to April 1977.

Updated June 1994 and June 1998.

N.J. 1980 Physician employed to do research sued pharmaceutical company for wrongful discharge claiming that as an employee at will she had a cause of action for termination following her refusal to continue research she viewed as medically unethical. The court held that an employee has a cause of action when discharged contrary to a clearly mandated public policy. However, the court affirmed summary judgment because human testing was not imminent and because plaintiff failed to demonstrate the existence of a clear public policy based upon any statements of medical ethics to support her refusal to continue work on controversial drug. The dissent argued that the Opinions and Reports of the Judicial Council 5.03 and 5.18 (1979) [now Opinion 2.07] and other medical ethical statements did provide a clear expression of public policy and that plaintiff's failure to specifically cite them was merely a technical defect, and not fatal. *Pierce v. Ortho Pharmaceutical Corp., 84 N.J. 58, 417 A.2d 505, 516, 518.*

Wyo. 2000 Physician sought judicial review of Board of Medicine's disciplinary order. Among its holdings, the Board found the physician's participation in a patient case study using testing and treatment procedures of no proven medical efficacy was unprofessional conduct contrary to recognized standards of medical ethics. The Board quoted and relied on Opinion 2.07. The supreme court reversed the Board's decision for failure to provide expert testimony regarding whether the physician's conduct was contrary to the standards set out in Opinion 2.07. *Painter v. Abels, 998 P.2d 931, 935, 939.*

Journal 2002 Challenges the general use of special informed consent disclosure rules in experimental therapy. Discusses the lack of a bright-line distinction between standard and experimental interventions. Concludes that focus should be placed on the distinctiveness of experimentation. Quotes Opinion 2.07. References Opinion 9.032. Noah, *Informed Consent and the Elusive Dichotomy Between Standard and Experimental Therapy, 28 Am. J.L. & Med. 361, 394, 395 (2002).*

Journal 2001 Considers conflicts of interest in clinical research and other types of medical practice. Compares the way in which doctors and lawyers address conflicts of interest in professional practice. Concludes that physicians are unaware of the need to create a meaningful conflict-of-interest doctrine for medical practice. Quotes Preamble, Principle IV, and Opinions 2.07, 8.03, 8.031, and 10.01. Moore, *What Doctors Can Learn from Lawyers about Conflicts of Interest, 81 B.U.L. Rev. 445, 447, 449-50 (2001).*

Journal 1999 Explores the duty to disclose genetic test results in research and clinical settings. Characterizes the legal duty to disclose. Concludes with guidelines regarding ways that medical researchers can reduce the potential for liability in this context. Quotes Opinion 2.07. Furman, *Genetic Test Results and the Duty to Disclose: Can Medical Researchers Control Liability? 23 Seattle Univ. L. R. 391, 408-09 (1999).*

Journal 1999 Discusses the need for physicians to advocate on behalf of patients' rights in the context of health care delivery. Evaluates the nature and scope of the physician's role as advocate, noting that physicians cannot be expected to engage in attorney-like advocacy. Quotes Principles IV and VI, Fundamental Elements (2), (4), and (6) [now Opinion 10.01], Patient Responsibilities 5 [now Opinion 10.02], and Opinions 2.03, 2.07, 2.09, 2.16, 2.19, 3.06, 4.01, 4.04, 6.01, 7.02, 8.02, 8.03, 8.13, 8.132, 9.06, 9.07, and 9.131. Cites Opinions 5.05, 5.09, 7.01, 8.135, and 9.02. Sage, *Physicians as Advocates*, 35 Hous. L. Rev. 1529, 1537, 1541, 1542, 1552-53, 1554, 1556, 1557, 1559, 1561-62, 1564, 1571, 1574, 1576, 1580 (1999).

Journal 1998 Discusses conflicts of interest in the physician-patient relationship arising out of use of financial incentives by managed care organizations. Considers how such conflicts are dealt with in the attorney-client relationship. Suggests that a financial incentive should be legally denounced if it unreasonably interferes with a physician's duty to properly care for and treat patients. Quotes Preamble, Fundamental Elements (1) [now Opinion 10.01] and Opinions 4.04, 5.01, 8.03, 8.13, and 9.06. Cites Fundamental Elements (4) [now Opinion 10.01] and Opinions 2.07, 2.08, and 2.132. Hall, *Third-Party Payor Conflicts of Interest in Managed Care: A Proposal for Regulation Based on the Model Rules of Professional Conduct*, 29 Seton Hall L. Rev. 95, 96, 107, 108, 109, 110, 111, 112, 134, 135, 136 (1998).

Journal 1998 Discusses the use of mentally impaired individuals as research subjects. Argues that a common set of rules needs to be promulgated to protect the decisionally impaired from certain risks of human research. Quotes Opinion 2.07. Sundram, *In Harm's Way: Research Subjects Who are Decisionally Impaired*, 1 J. Health Care L. & Pol'y 36, 43-44 (1998).

Journal 1997 Considers emergency room research informed consent standards. Reviews new federal regulations and related moral and ethical concerns. Concludes that regulations will require a case-by-case approach to balancing competing interests between research and ethics. References Opinion 2.07. Brody, *New Perspectives on Emergency Room Research*, 27 Hastings Center Rep. 7, 9 (Jan./Feb. 1997).

Journal 1997 Considers informed consent and the principle of self-determination. Analyzes the tradition of informed consent in medical research, with emphasis on international considerations. Concludes that research subjects need better protection. Cites Opinion 2.07. Note, *The Informed-Consent Policy of the International Conference on Harmonization of Technical Requirements for Registrations of Pharmaceuticals for Human Use: Knowledge is the Best Medicine*, 30 Cornell Int'l L. J. 203, 209 (1997).

Journal 1993 Considers the legitimacy of neonatal HIV screening studies conducted without parental notice or consent. Asserts that such testing is morally and legally questionable. Quotes Opinion 2.07. Isaacman & Miller, *Neonatal HIV Seroprevalence Studies*, 14 J. Legal Med. 413, 428 (1993).

Journal 1989 Discusses various social control mechanisms that have an impact upon biomedical research. Emphasis is placed upon a comparison of the effectiveness of intra- and extraprofessional methods of control. References Opinion 2.07. Benson, *The Social Control of Human Biomedical Research: An Overview and Review of the Literature*, 29 Soc. Sci. Med. 1, 3 (1989).

2.071 Subject Selection for Clinical Trials

Ethical considerations in clinical research have traditionally focused on protecting research subjects. These protections may be especially important for those from socioeconomically diasdavantaged populations who may be more vulnerable to coercive pressures. The benefits from altruism that result from participation in research, particularly for severely chronically ill persons, may justify equitable consideration of historically disadvantaged populations such as the poor. With these considerations in mind, the following guidelines are offered:

(1) Although the burdens of research should not fall disproportionately on socioeconomically disadvantaged populations, neither should such populations be categorically excluded, or discouraged, from research protocols.

(2) Inclusion and exclusion criteria for a clinical study should be based on

sound scientific principles. Conversely, participants in a clinical trial should be drawn from the qualifying population in the general geographic area of the trial without regard to race, ethnicity, economic status, or gender.

If a subject's primary care physician determines that the subject received a clear medical benefit from the experimental intervention which is now moving towards marketing approval and chooses to seek authorization from the Food and Drug Administration (FDA) for continued use of the investigational therapy during the time period between the end of the protocol and the availability of the drug on the market, the investigator should work with the primary care physician, the product sponsor, and the FDA to allow continued availability of the product. (I, V, VII)

Issued June 1998 based on the report "Subject Selection for Clinical Trials," adopted December 1997 (*IRB*. 1998; 20(2-3): 12-15).

2.075 The Use of Placebo Controls in Clinical Trials

Placebo controls are an important part of medicine's commitment to ensuring that the safety and efficacy of new drugs are sufficiently established. Used appropriately, placebo controls can safely provide valuable data and should continue to be considered in the design of clinical trials. The existence of an accepted therapy does not necessarily preclude the use of such controls; however, physician-investigators should adhere to the following guidelines to ensure that the interests of patients who participate in clinical trials are protected.

(1) Investigators must be extremely thorough in obtaining informed consent from patients. To the extent that research is dependent upon the willingness of patients to accept a level of risk, their understanding of the potential harms involved must be a top priority of any clinical investigation. The possibility presented in some studies that patients often do not fully understand the research protocol and therefore truly cannot give informed consent demonstrates a need to heighten the efforts of researchers to impress upon their subjects the nature of clinical research and the risks involved. Patients are capable of making decisions when presented with sufficient information, and it is the responsibility of the institutional review board (IRB) and the individual investigators involved to ensure that each subject has been adequately informed and has given voluntary consent. Each patient must also be made aware that they can terminate their participation in a study at any time.

(2) Informed consent cannot be invoked to justify an inappropriate trial design. IRBs as well as investigators have an obligation to evaluate each study protocol to determine whether a placebo control is necessary and whether an alternative study design with another type of control would be sufficient for the purposes of research. Protocols that involve conditions causing death or irreversible damage cannot ethically employ a placebo control if alternative treatment would prevent or slow the illness progres-

sion. When studying illnesses characterized by severe or painful symptoms, investigators should thoroughly explore alternatives to the use of placebo controls. In general, the more severe the consequences and symptoms of the illness under study, the more difficult it will be to justify the use of a placebo control when alternative therapy exists. Consequently, there will almost certainly be conditions for which placebo controls cannot be justified. Similarly, the use of a placebo control will more easily be justified as the severity and number of negative side effects of standard therapy increase.

(3) Researchers and IRBs should continue to minimize the amount of time patients are given placebo. The rationale provided by investigators for the length of study will give IRBs the opportunity to ensure that patients are given placebo therapy for as short a time as possible to provide verifiable results. Additionally, the interim data analysis and monitoring currently in practice will allow researchers to terminate the study because of either positive or negative results, thus protecting patients from remaining on placebo unnecessarily. (I, V)

Issued June 1997 based on the report "Ethical Use of Placebo Controls in Clinical Trials," adopted June 1996.

Journal 2003 Provides an update on the Declaration of Helsinki and the FDA's position on placebo-controlled medical research. Concludes that the FDA should reconsider its position in light of the principles articulated in the Declaration. Quotes Opinion 2.075. Michels & Rothman, *Update on Unethical Use of Placebos in Randomised Trials*, 17 Bioethics 188, 200 (2003)

Journal 2001 Reviews federal regulations and discusses challenges associated with developing guidelines relating to the use of placebos. Concludes that the use of placebo controls in human subjects research must be carefully regulated. Quotes Opinion 2.075. Hoffman, *The Use of Placebos in Clinical Trials: Responsible Research or Unethical Practice?* 33 Conn. L. Rev. 449, 454-55, 496 (2001).

2.076 Surgical "Placebo" Controls

The term surgical "placebo" controls refers to the control arm of a research study where subjects undergo surgical procedures that have the appearance of therapeutic interventions, but during which the essential therapeutic maneuver is omitted.

The appropriateness of a surgical "placebo" control should be evaluated on the basis of guidelines provided in Opinion 2.07, "Clinical Investigation," as well as the following requirements:

(1) Surgical "placebo" controls should be used only when no other trial design will yield the requisite data.

(2) Particular attention must be paid to the informed consent process when enrolling subjects in trials that use surgical "placebo" controls. Careful explanation of the risks of the operations must be disclosed, along with a description of the differences between the trial arms emphasizing the essential procedure that will or will not be performed. Additional safeguards around the informed consent process may be appropriate such as using a neutral third party to provide information and get consent, or using consent monitors to oversee the consent process.

(3) The use of surgical "placebo" controls may be justified when an existing, accepted surgical procedure is being tested for efficacy. It is not justified when testing the effectiveness of an innovative surgical technique that represents only a minor modification of an existing, accepted surgical procedure.

(4) When a new surgical procedure is developed with the prospect of treating a condition for which no known surgical therapy exists, using surgical "placebo" controls may be justified, but must be evaluated in light of whether the current standard of care includes a non-surgical treatment and the benefits, risks, and side effects of that treatment.

    (a) If foregoing standard treatment would result in significant injury and the standard treatment is efficacious and acceptable to the patient (in terms of side effects, personal beliefs, etc), then it must be offered as part of the study design.

    (b) When the standard treatment is not fully efficacious, or not acceptable to the patient, surgical "placebo" controls may be used and the standard treatment foregone, but additional safeguards must be put in place around the informed consent process. (I, V)

Issued December 2000 based on the report "Surgical Placebo Controls," adopted June 2000 (*Ann Surg.* 2002; 235: 303-07).

Updated June 2003.

2.077   Ethical Considerations in International Research

Physicians, either in their role as investigators or as decision-makers involved in the deliberations related to the funding or the review of research, hold an ethical obligation to ensure the protection of research participants. When the research is to be conducted in countries with differing cultural traditions, health care systems, and ethical standards, and in particular in countries with developing economies and with limited health care resources, US physicians should respect the following guidelines:

(1) First and foremost, physicians involved in clinical research that will be carried out internationally should be satisfied that a proposed research design has been developed according to a sound scientific design. Therefore, investigators must ascertain that there is genuine uncertainty within the clinical community about the comparative merits of the experimental treatment and the one to be offered as a control in the population among which the study is to be undertaken. In some instances, a three-pronged protocol, which offers the standard treatment in use in the US, a treatment that meets a level of care that is attainable and sustainable by the host country, and a placebo (see Opinion 2.075, "Surgical 'Placebo' Controls"), may be the best method to evaluate the safety and efficacy of a treatment in a given population. When US investigators participate in international research they must obtain approval for such protocols from U.S. Institutional Review Boards (IRBs).

(2) IRBs, which are responsible for ensuring the protection of research participants, must determine that risks have been minimized and that the proto-

col's ratio of risks to benefits is favorable to participants. In evaluating the risks and benefits that a protocol presents to a population, IRBs should obtain relevant input from representatives from the host country and from the research population. It is also appropriate for IRBs to consider the harm that is likely to result from forgoing the research.

(3) Also, IRBs are required to protect the welfare of individual participants. This can best be achieved by assuring that a suitable informed consent process is in place. Therefore, IRBs should ensure that individual potential participants will be informed of the nature of the research endeavor and that their voluntary consent will be sought. IRBs should recognize that, in some instances, information will be meaningful only if it is communicated in ways that are consistent with local customs.

(4) Overall, to ensure that the research does not exploit the population from which participants are recruited, IRBs should ensure that the research corresponds to a medical need in the region where it is undertaken. Furthermore, they should foster research with the potential for lasting benefits, especially when it is undertaken among populations that are severely deficient in health care resources. This can be achieved by facilitating the development of a health care infrastructure that will be of use during and beyond the conduct of the research. Additionally, physicians conducting studies must encourage research sponsors to continue to provide beneficial study interventions to all study participants at the conclusion of the study. (I, IV, VII, VIII, IX)

Issued December 2001 based on the report "Ethical Considerations in International Research," adopted June 2001.

2.079 Safeguards in the Use of DNA Databanks in Genomic Research

The following safeguards should be applied to the use of databases for the purpose of population-based genomic research:

(1) Physicians who participate as investigators in genomic research should have adequate training in genomic research and related ethical issues so as to be able to discuss these issues with patients and/or potential research subjects.

(2) If research is to be conducted within a defined subset of the general population, that is, an identifiable community, then investigators should consult with the community to design a study that will minimize harm not only for individual subjects, but also for the community. When substantial opposition to the research is expressed within the community, investigators should not conduct the study. When the community supports a proposal, investigators nevertheless should obtain individual consent in the usual manner. The same procedure should be followed whether the investigators intend to collect new samples and data or whether they wish to use previously archived data sets.

(3) When obtaining the informed consent of individuals to participate in genomic research, standard informed consent requirements apply (see Opinion 2.07, "Clinical Investigation"). In addition:

(a) Special emphasis should be placed on disclosing the specific standards of privacy contained in the study: whether the material will be coded (ie: encrypted so that only the investigator can trace materials back to specific individuals) or be completely de-identified (ie: stripped of identifiers).

(b) If data are to be coded, subjects should be told whether they can expect to be contacted in the future to share in findings or to consider participating in additional research, which may relate to the current protocol or extend to other research purposes.

(c) Individuals should always be free to refuse the use of their biological materials in research, without penalty.

(d) Disclosure should include information about whether investigators or subjects stand to gain financially from research findings (see Opinion 2.08, "Commercial Use of Human Tissue"). Such disclosure should refer to the possible conflicts of interest of the investigators (see Opinion 8.0315, "Managing Conflicts of Interest in the Conduct of Clinical Trials").

(e) Subjects should be informed of when, if ever, and how archived information and samples will be discarded.

(4) To strengthen the protection of confidentiality, genomic research should not be conducted using information and samples that identify the individuals from whom they were obtained (ie: by name or social security number). Furthermore, to protect subsets of the population from such harms as stigmatization and discrimination, demographic information not required for the study's purposes should be coded. (I, IV, V, VII)

Issued June 2002 based on the report "The Use of DNA Databanks in Genomic Research: The Imperative of Informed Consent," adopted December 2001.

2.08   The previous Opinion 2.08, "Clinical Investigation: Replacement of Vital Humans Organs," issued July 1986, was deleted in 1994 and combined with Opinion 2.07, "Clinical Investigation."

2.08   Commercial Use of Human Tissue

The rapid growth of the biotechnology industry has resulted in the commercial availability of numerous therapeutic and other products developed from human tissue. Physicians contemplating the commercial use of human tissue should abide by the following guidelines:

(1) Informed consent must be obtained from patients for the use of organs or tissues in clinical research.

(2) Potential commercial applications must be disclosed to the patient before a profit is realized on products developed from biological materials.

(3) Human tissue and its products may not be used for commercial purposes without the informed consent of the patient who provided the original cellular material.

(4) Profits from the commercial use of human tissue and its products may be shared with patients, in accordance with lawful contractual agreements.

(5) The diagnostic and therapeutic alternatives offered to patients by their physicians should conform to standards of good medical practice and should not be influenced in any way by the commercial potential of the patient's tissue. (II, V)

Issued June 1994 based on the report "Who Should Profit from the Economic Value of Human Tissue? An Ethical Analysis," adopted June 1990.

S.D. Fla. 2003 Donors of tissue samples sought equitable and injunctive relief against a physician-researcher and affiliated hospitals doing research on Canavan disease. The researcher used the donations to obtain a gene patent and the hospitals restricted any activity related to the patent. District court dismissed all counts except the unjust enrichment claim. Court quoted Opinion 2.08 with respect to disclosure to patients of possible commercial application of research. *Greenberg v. Miami Children's Hospital Research Institute, Inc., 264 F. Supp. 2d 1064, 1070-71, n. 2.*

Journal 2002 Examines various concerns regarding gene patents and discusses other policy alternatives. Concludes that policymakers are exploring alternatives to ensure that gene patents will benefit society. Quotes Opinion 2.08. Cites Opinion 9.095. Andrews, *The Gene Patent Dilemma: Balancing Commercial Incentives with Health Needs, 2 Hous. J. Health L. & Pol'y 65, 74, 104 (2002).*

Journal 1998 Discusses conflicts of interest in the physician-patient relationship arising out of use of financial incentives by managed care organizations. Considers how such conflicts are dealt with in the attorney-client relationship. Suggests that a financial incentive should be legally denounced if it unreasonably interferes with a physician's duty to properly care for and treat patients. Quotes Preamble, Fundamental Elements (1) [now Opinion 10.01] and Opinions 4.04, 5.01, 8.03, 8.13, and 9.06. Cites Fundamental Elements (4) [now Opinion 10.01] and Opinions 2.07, 2.08, and 2.132. Hall, *Third-Party Payor Conflicts of Interest in Managed Care: A Proposal for Regulation Based on the Model Rules of Professional Conduct, 29 Seton Hall L. Rev. 95, 96, 107, 108, 109, 110, 111, 112, 134, 135, 136 (1998).*

2.09 Costs

While physicians should be conscious of costs and not provide or prescribe unnecessary medical services, concern for the quality of care the patient receives should be the physician's first consideration. This does not preclude the physician, individually or through medical or other organizations, from participating in policy-making with respect to social and economic issues affecting health care. (I, VII)

Issued March 1981.

Updated June 1994 and June 1998; Updated December 2003.

Journal 2001 Examines issues relating to health care cost containment. Concludes that, if physicians are to meet the goals assigned to them in a cost-constrained health care system, then professional standards must be reevaluated and modified to afford meaningful guidance for clinical decision-making in the face of health care spending controls. Quotes Opinions 2.03, 2.09, 2.095, 8.032, and 9.04. Cites Opinions 8.02, 8.021, 8.051, and 8.13. Agrawal, *Resuscitating Professionalism: Self-Regulation in the Medical Marketplace, 66 Mo. L. Rev. 341, 354, 355, 360, 361, 378, 388 (2001).*

Journal 2001 Discusses the prohibition on non-lawyer ownership of legal service providers. Considers how ethical rules and standards governing physicians have been directed toward preserving independent judgment. Concludes that ethical conflicts created by abandoning the prohibition on non-lawyer ownership of legal service providers may be managed by following the medical ethics model. Quotes Principle VI and Opinions 2.03, 2.09, 8.02, 8.021, 8.03, 8.05, 8.051, 8.054, 8.13, and 8.132. Harris & Foran, *The Ethics of Middle-Class Access to Legal Services and What We Can Learn from the Medical Profession's Shift to a Corporate Paradigm, 70 Fordham L. Rev. 775, 817, 821, 822, 823, 824 (2001).*

Journal 1999 Discusses the need for physicians to advocate on behalf of patients' rights in the context of health care delivery. Evaluates the nature and scope of the physician's role as advocate, noting that physicians cannot be expected to engage in attorney-like advocacy. Quotes Principles IV and VI, Fundamental Elements (2), (4), and (6) [now Opinion 10.01], Patient Responsibilities 5 [now Opinion 10.02], and Opinions 2.03, 2.07, 2.09, 2.16, 2.19, 3.06, 4.01, 4.04, 6.01, 7.02, 8.02, 8.03, 8.13, 8.132, 9.06, 9.07, and 9.131. Cites Opinions 5.05, 5.09, 7.01, 8.135, and 9.02. Sage, *Physicians as Advocates*, 35 *Hous. L. Rev.* 1529, 1537, 1541, 1542, 1552-53, 1554, 1556, 1557, 1559, 1561-62, 1564, 1571, 1574, 1576, 1580 (1999).

Journal 1997 Posits that cost-containment schemes in managed care systems have eroded the fiduciary duty physicians owe patients. Notes that MCOs are prohibiting patients from trusting and relying on physicians. Concludes that patients must seek quality assurance from sources other than their physicians. Quotes Opinions 2.03, 2.09, and 8.13. Jacobi, *Patients at a Loss: Protecting Health Care Consumers through Data Driven Quality Assurance*, 45 *U. Kan. L. Rev.* 705, 720, 721, 759 (1997).

Journal 1996 Explores changing health care delivery environment and proposes a new approach to medical ethics. Suggests ways to improve the roles of care managers in capitated systems. Advocates disclosure of information to patients regarding coverage limitations and cost-containment policies. Quotes Opinion 2.09. Malinowski, *Capitation, Advances in Medical Technology, and the Advent of a New Era in Medical Ethics*, XXII *Am. J. Law & Med.* 331, 337 (1996).

Journal 1996 Discusses the health care system as it pertains to the elderly. Observes that age-based rationing decisions create significant value conflicts. Suggests that, in developing national health policy, decisions regarding resource allocation for the elderly must incorporate principles of ethical and moral reasoning. Quotes Opinion 2.09. Smith, *Our Hearts Were Once Young and Gay: Health Care Rationing and the Elderly*, 8 *U. Fla. J.L. & Pub. Pol'y* 1, 21 (1996).

Journal 1994 Considers how patients with insufficient financial resources place physicians in a conflict of interest situation with respect to patient needs and the financial interests of the physician, other patients, and society. Suggests that rules of contract and malpractice law do not provide satisfactory guidelines to resolve these conflicts. Cites Opinions 2.09 and 2.095. Mehlman & Massey, *The Patient-Physician Relationship and the Allocation of Scarce Resources: A Law and Economics Approach*, 4 *Kennedy Inst. Ethics J.* 291, 292 (1994).

Journal 1994 Observes that health care reform proposals present significant challenges to the role and ethics of attending physicians. Emphasizes that reform proposals must set forth the role envisioned for physicians and must articulate an acceptable ethical framework within which physicians may fulfill that role. Quotes Opinions 4.04, 9.121, and 9.122. Cites Opinions 2.03, 2.09, 5.01, and 8.03. Wolf, *Health Care Reform and the Future of Physician Ethics*, 24 *Hastings Center Rep.* 28, 32, 40 (March/April 1994).

Journal 1993 Discusses the problem of physicians withholding needed medical treatment from HIV-infected infants. Concludes that current law should be expanded to eliminate this discrimination. Quotes Opinions 2.09, 2.17, 2.20, 2.22, 4.04, and 8.03. Crossley, *Of Diagnoses and Discrimination: Discriminatory Nontreatment of Infants With HIV Infection*, 93 *Columbia L. Rev.* 1581, 1620, 1621 (1993).

Journal 1993 Defines the physician-patient relationship within the framework of contract, tort, and fiduciary law. Concludes that the law does not require a physician to provide care for the nonpaying patient. Quotes Opinion 2.09. Mehlman, *The Patient-Physician Relationship in an Era of Scarce Resources: Is There a Duty to Treat?* 25 *Conn. L. Rev.* 349 (1993).

Journal 1992 Examines the major health care rationing issues facing the United States including increasing costs and decreasing access. Concludes that the standard of care should not be changed and that rationing should be a separate enterprise undertaken pursuant to explicit criteria. Quotes Opinions 2.03, 2.09, and 4.04. Hirshfeld, *Should Ethical and Legal Standards for Physicians Be Changed to Accommodate New Models for Rationing Health Care?*, 140 *Univ. Pa. L. Rev.* 1809, 1816 (1992).

Journal 1991 Focuses on the denial of insurance benefits for experimental medical procedures. Explains the de novo review process under ERISA. Concludes that there is need for a structure that will permit greater objectivity in the context of data collection as well as judicial determination. Cites Opinions 2.03 and 2.09. Note, *Denial of Coverage for "Experimental" Medical Procedures: The Problem of De Novo Review Under ERISA*, 79 *Kentucky L.J.* 801, 824 (1990-91).

Journal 1990 Discusses economic considerations in clinical decisionmaking, with emphasis on the standard of care. Concludes that organized medicine has made valuable contributions through development of practice parameters that offer guidance in the exercise of clinical judgment. Cites Opinions 2.03 and 2.09. Hirshfeld, *Economic Considerations in Treatment Decisions and the Standard of Care in Medical Malpractice Litigation*, 264 JAMA 2004, 2007 (1990).

Journal 1990 Discusses efforts of third-party payors to control health care expenditures for beneficiaries. Concludes that financial incentives to limit care and other cost control techniques should be disclosed and that the rationale for such disclosure is compelling. Quotes Opinions 2.03, 2.09, and 8.03. Cites Opinions 2.19, 4.04, and 4.06. Hirshfeld, *Should Third Party Payors of Health Care Services Disclose Cost Control Mechanisms to Potential Beneficiaries?*, 14 Seton Hall Legis. J. 115, 130, 131, 144, 145, 146 (1990).

2.095 The Provision of Adequate Health Care

Because society has an obligation to make access to an adequate level of health care available to all of its members regardless of ability to pay, physicians should contribute their expertise at a policy-making level to help achieve this goal. In determining whether particular procedures or treatments should be included in the adequate level of health care, the following ethical principles should be considered: (1) degree of benefit (the difference in outcome between treatment and no treatment), (2) likelihood of benefit, (3) duration of benefit, (4) cost, and (5) number of people who will benefit (referring to the fact that a treatment may benefit the patient and others who come into contact with the patient, as with a vaccination or antimicrobial drug).

Ethical principles require that a just process be used to determine the adequate level of health care. To ensure justice, the process for determining the adequate level of health care should include the following considerations: (1) democratic decision making with broad public input at both the developmental and final approval stages, (2) monitoring for variations in care that cannot be explained on medical grounds with special attention to evidence of discriminatory impact on historically disadvantaged groups, and (3) adjustment of the adequate level over time to ensure continued and broad public acceptance.

Because of the risk that inappropriate biases will influence the content of the basic benefits package, it may be desirable to avoid rigid or precise formulas to define the specific components of the basic benefits package. After applying the five ethical values listed above, it will be possible to designate some kinds of care as either clearly basic or clearly discretionary. However, for care that is not clearly basic or discretionary, seemingly objective formulas may result in choices that are inappropriately biased. For that care, therefore, it may be desirable to give equal consideration (eg, through a process of random selection) to the different kinds of care when deciding which will be included in the basic benefits package. The mechanism for providing an adequate level of health care should ensure that the health care benefits for the poor will not be eroded over time. (VII)

Issued June 1994 based on the report "Ethical Issues in Health System Reform: The Provision of Adequate Health Care," adopted December 1993 (JAMA. 1994; 272: 1056-62).

Journal 2001 Examines issues relating to health care cost containment. Concludes that, if physicians are to meet the goals assigned to them in a cost-constrained health care system, then professional standards must be reevaluated and modified to afford meaningful guidance for clinical decision-making in the face of health care spending controls. Quotes Opinions 2.03, 2.09, 2.095, 8.032, and 9.04. Cites Opinions 8.02, 8.021, 8.051, and 8.13. Agrawal, *Resuscitating*

Professionalism: Self-Regulation in the Medical Marketplace, 66 Mo. L. Rev. 341, 354, 355, 360, 361, 378, 388 (2001).

Journal 1996 Considers challenges to the psychiatrist-patient relationship that are triggered by managed care cost-containment methodologies. Offers guidance to psychiatrists for addressing these challenges. References Opinions 2.095, 8.13, and 8.132. Hoge, *APA Resource Document: I. The Professional Responsibilities of Psychiatrists in Evolving Health Care Systems*, 24 Bull. Am. Acad. Psychiatry Law 393, 405 (1996).

Journal 1994 Considers how greater patient autonomy has led to situations in which medical care may be viewed as futile. Suggests that the law has intruded too far into this area of medicine. Quotes Opinion 2.035. Cites Opinions 2.03, 2.095, 2.17, 2.19, 2.20, and 2.22. Cultice, *Medical Futility: When Is Enough, Enough?*, 27 J. Health & Hosp. Law 225, 230, 256 (1994).

Journal 1994 Considers how patients with insufficient financial resources place physicians in a conflict of interest situation with respect to patient needs and the financial interests of the physician, other patients, and society. Suggests that rules of contract and malpractice law do not provide satisfactory guidelines to resolve these conflicts. Cites Opinions 2.09 and 2.095. Mehlman & Massey, *The Patient-Physician Relationship and the Allocation of Scarce Resources: A Law and Economics Approach*, 4 Kennedy Inst. Ethics J. 291, 292 (1994).

2.10   Fetal Research Guidelines

The following guidelines are offered as aids to physicians when they are engaged in fetal research:

(1) Physicians may participate in fetal research when their activities are part of a competently designed program, under accepted standards of scientific research, to produce data which are scientifically valid and significant.

(2) If appropriate, properly performed clinical studies on animals and non-gravid humans should precede any particular fetal research project.

(3) In fetal research projects, the investigator should demonstrate the same care and concern for the fetus as a physician providing fetal care or treatment in a non-research setting.

(4) All valid federal or state legal requirements should be followed.

(5) There should be no monetary payment to obtain any fetal material for fetal research projects.

(6) Competent peer review committees, review boards, or advisory boards should be available, when appropriate, to protect against the possible abuses that could arise in such research.

(7) Research on the so-called dead fetus, macerated fetal material, fetal cells, fetal tissue, or fetal organs should be in accord with state laws on autopsy and state laws on organ transplantation or anatomical gifts.

(8) In fetal research primarily for treatment of the fetus:
   (a) Voluntary and informed consent, in writing, should be given by the gravid woman, acting in the best interest of the fetus.
   (b) Alternative treatment or methods of care, if any, should be carefully evaluated and fully explained. If simpler and safer treatment is available, it should be pursued.

(9) In research primarily for treatment of the gravid female:
   (a) Voluntary and informed consent, in writing, should be given by the patient.
   (b) Alternative treatment or methods of care should be carefully evaluated and fully explained to the patient. If simpler and safer treatment is available, it should be pursued.

(c) If possible, the risk to the fetus should be the least possible, consistent with the gravid female's need for treatment.

(10) In fetal research involving a fetus in utero, primarily for the accumulation of scientific knowledge:

(a) Voluntary and informed consent, in writing, should be given by the gravid woman under circumstances in which a prudent and informed adult would reasonably be expected to give such consent.

(b) The risk to the fetus imposed by the research should be the least possible.

(c) The purpose of research is the production of data and knowledge which are scientifically significant and which cannot otherwise be obtained.

(d) In this area of research, it is especially important to emphasize that care and concern for the fetus should be demonstrated. (I, III, V)

Issued March 1980.

Updated June 1994.

Journal 1991 Explores arguments for and against fetal tissue transplantation research, including arguments for and against the use of federal funds to support such research. Considers whether the donation model is appropriate for the transfer of fetal tissue, and whether a woman who chooses elective abortion is an appropriate donor. References Opinion 2.10. Childress, *Ethics, Public Policy, and Human Fetal Tissue Transplantation Research, Vol 1 Kennedy Inst. Ethics J.* 93, 116 (*June 1991*).

Journal 1991 Considers how the use of in vitro fertilization (IVF) has blurred the distinction between medical practice and research. Argues that medical-professional responsibility standards should be used to curtail the creation of life in vitro. Quotes Opinions 2.10 and 2.14. Comment, *Dangerous Relations: Doctors and Extracorporeal Embryos, The Need For New Limits To Medical Inquiry,* 7 J. Contemp. Health L. & Pol'y 307, 309 (1991).

2.105 Patenting Human Genes

A patent grants the holder the right, for a limited amount of time, to prevent others from commercializing his or her inventions. At the same time, the patent system is designed to foster information sharing. Full disclosure of the invention—enabling another trained in the art to replicate it—is necessary to obtain a patent. Patenting is also thought to encourage private investment into research. Arguments have been made that the patenting of human genomic material sets a troubling precedent for the ownership or commodification of human life. DNA sequences, however, are not tantamount to human life, and it is unclear where and whether qualities uniquely human are found in genetic material.

Genetic research holds great potential for achieving new medical therapies. It remains unclear what role patenting will play in ensuring such development. At this time the Council concludes that granting patent protection should not hinder the goal of developing new beneficial technology and offers the following guidelines:

(1) Patents on processes—for example, processes used to isolate and purify gene sequences, genes and proteins, or vehicles of gene therapy—do not raise the same ethical problems as patents on the substances themselves and are thus preferable.

(2) Substance patents on purified proteins present fewer ethical problems than patents on genes or DNA sequences and are thus preferable.

(3) Patent descriptions should be carefully constructed to ensure that the patent holder does not limit the use of a naturally occurring form of the substance in question. This includes patents on proteins, genes, and genetic sequences.

One of the goals of genetic research is to achieve better medical treatments and technologies. Granting patent protection should not hinder this goal. Individuals or entities holding patents on genetic material should not allow patents to languish and should negotiate and structure licensing agreements in such a way as to encourage the development of better medical technology. (V, VII)

Issued June 1998 based on the report "Patenting the Human Genome," adopted December 1997.

Journal 2001 Examines whether or not DNA patents violate or threaten human dignity. Supports legislation banning patents on the whole human genome. Concludes that only patents that comprise complete commodification of human beings violate human dignity. References Opinion 2.105. Resnik, *DNA Patents and Human Dignity, 29 J. L. Med. & Ethics 152, 158, 159 (2001)*.

2.11 Gene Therapy

Gene therapy involves the replacement or modification of a genetic variant to restore or enhance cellular function or to improve the reaction of non-genetic therapies.

Two types of gene therapy have been identified: (1) somatic cell therapy, in which human cells other than germ cells are genetically altered, and (2) germ line therapy, in which a replacement gene is integrated into the genome of human gametes or their precursors, resulting in expression of the new gene in the patient's offspring and subsequent generations. The fundamental difference between germ line therapy and somatic cell therapy is that germ line therapy affects the welfare of subsequent generations and may be associated with increased risk and the potential for unpredictable and irreversible results. Because of the far-reaching implications of germ line therapy, it is appropriate to limit genetic intervention to somatic cells at this time.

The goal of both somatic cell and germ line therapy is to alleviate human suffering and disease by remedying disorders for which available therapies are not satisfactory. This goal should be pursued only within the ethical tradition of medicine, which gives primacy to the welfare of the patient whose safety and well-being must be vigorously protected. To the extent possible, experience with animal studies must be sufficient to assure the effectiveness and safety of the techniques used, and the predictability of the results.

Moreover, genetic manipulation generally should be utilized only for therapeutic purposes. Efforts to enhance "desirable" characteristics through the insertion of a modified or additional gene, or efforts to "improve" complex human traits—the eugenic development of offspring—are contrary not only to the ethical tradition of medicine, but also to the egalitarian values of our society. Because of the potential for abuse, genetic manipulation to affect non-disease traits may never be acceptable and perhaps should never be pursued. If it is ever allowed, at least three conditions would have to be met before it could be deemed ethically acceptable: (1) there would have to be a clear and meaningful benefit to the person, (2) there would have to be no trade-off with other characteristics or traits, and (3) all citizens would have to have equal access to the genetic technology, irrespective of income or other socioeconomic characteristics. These criteria should be viewed as a minimal, not an exhaustive, test of the ethical propriety of non-disease-related genetic intervention. As genetic technology and knowledge of the human genome develop further, additional guidelines may be required.

As gene therapy becomes feasible for a variety of human disorders, there are several practical factors to consider to ensure safe application of this technology in society. First, any gene therapy research should meet the Council's guidelines on clinical investigation (Opinion 2.07, "Clinical Investigation") and investigators must adhere to the standards of medical practice and professional responsibility. The proposed procedure must be fully discussed with the patient and the written informed consent of the patient or the patient's legal representative must be voluntary. Investigators must be thorough in their attempts to eliminate any unwanted viral agents from the viral vector containing the corrective gene. The potential for adverse effects of the viral delivery system must be disclosed to the patient. The effectiveness of gene therapy must be evaluated fully, including the determination of the natural history of the disease and follow-up examination of subsequent generations. Gene therapy should be pursued only after the availability or effectiveness of other possible therapies is found to be insufficient. These considerations should be reviewed, as appropriate, as procedures and scientific information develop. (I, V)

Issued December 1988.

Updated June 1994 based on the report "Prenatal Genetic Screening," adopted December 1992 (*Arch Fam Med.* 1994; 3: 633-42), and updated June 1996.

Journal 2000 Defines and describes human genetic enhancement. Explores the legal implications of this emerging technology as well as related societal concerns. Quotes Opinion 2.11. References Opinion 2.12. Mehlman, *The Law of Above Averages: Leveling the New Genetic Enhancement Playing Field*, 85 Iowa L. Rev. 517, 527-28, 559 (2000).

Journal 1999 Discusses regulatory concerns regarding genetic technology. Provides ideas on how society might regulate genetic enhancements. Argues that a variety of means of regulation need to be utilized to govern genetic technology. Quotes Opinion 2.11. Cites Opinion 9.065. References Opinion 2.138. Mehlman, *How Will We Regulate Genetic Enhancement?*, 34 Wake Forest L. Rev. 671, 693-94, 695 (1999).

2.12 Genetic Counseling

Three primary areas of prenatal genetic testing are (1) screening or evaluating prospective parents for genetic disease before conception to predict the likelihood of conceiving an affected child; (2) analysis of a pre-embryo at the preimplantation stage of artificial reproductive techniques; and (3) in utero testing after conception, such as ultrasonography, amniocentesis, fetoscopy, and chorionic villus sampling, to determine the condition of the fetus. Physicians engaged in genetic counseling are ethically obligated to provide prospective parents with the basis for an informed decision for childbearing. Counseling should include reasons for and against testing as well as discussion of inappropriate uses of genetic testing. Prenatal genetic testing is most appropriate for women or couples whose medical histories or family backgrounds indicate an elevated risk of fetal genetic disorders. Women or couples without an elevated risk of genetic disease may legitimately request prenatal diagnosis, provided they understand and accept the risks involved. When counseling prospective parents, physicians should avoid the imposition of their personal moral values and the substitution of their own moral judgment for that of the prospective parents.

The physician should be aware that where a genetic defect is found in the fetus, prospective parents may request or refuse an abortion. Physicians who consider the legal and ethical requirements applicable to genetic counseling to be in conflict with their moral values and conscience may choose to limit their services to preconception diagnosis and advice or not provide any genetic services. However, the physician who is so disposed is nevertheless obligated to alert prospective parents when a potential genetic problem does exist, so that the patient may decide whether to seek further genetic counseling from another qualified specialist.

Genetic selection refers to the abortion or discard of a fetus or pre-embryo with a genetic abnormality. In general, it is ethically permissible for physicians to participate in genetic selection to prevent, cure, or treat genetic disease. However, selection to avoid a genetic disease may not always be appropriate, depending on factors such as the severity of the disease, the probability of its occurrence, the age at onset, and the time of gestation at which selection would occur. It would not be ethical to engage in selection on the basis of non-disease-related characteristics or traits. (II, IV, V, VI)

Issued June 1983.

Updated June 1994 based on the report "Prenatal Genetic Screening," adopted December 1992 (*Arch Fam Med* 1994; 3: 633-42).

Journal 2003 Applies professional standards to determine the technology that practitioners should utilize in prenatal diagnosis. Concludes that appropriate uses of prenatal diagnostic methodologies must be articulated by society. Quotes Opinion 2.12. Botkin, *Prenatal Diagnosis and the Selection of Children*, 30 Fla. St. U. L. Rev. 265, 289 (2003).

Journal 2003 Proposes a method to distinguish between good and bad eugenics. Concludes that prenatal testing for Down syndrome, followed by termination of pregnancy, characterizes bad eugenics. References Opinion 2.12. Mahowald, *Aren't We All Eugenicists? Commentary on Paul Lombardo's "Taking Eugenics Seriously"* 30 Fla. St. U. L. Rev. 219, 234 (2003).

Journal 2000 Defines and describes human genetic enhancement. Explores the legal implications of this emerging technology as well as related societal concerns. Quotes Opinion 2.11. References Opinion 2.12. Mehlman, *The Law of Above Averages: Leveling the New Genetic Enhancement Playing Field*, 85 Iowa L. Rev. 517, 527-28, 559 (2000).

Journal 1998 Discusses genetic testing to determine hereditary hearing impairment. Explains ways in which genetic counselors can assist people. Points out how presymptomatic diagnosis can help parents and children. References Opinion 2.12. Chen, Mueller, Prasad, Greinwald, Manaligod, Muilenburg, Verhoeven, Van Camp, & Smith, *Presymptomatic Diagnosis of Nonsyndromic Hearing Loss by Genotyping*, 124 Arch. Otolaryngol. Head Neck Surg. 20, 23 (1998).

Journal 1997 Discusses techniques and possibilities for genetic testing. Presents a series of problems designed as a starting point for understanding the conflicts surrounding genetic testing. Reviews the applications of state-of-the-art genetic research. Suggests potential difficulties that testing may cause in society. References Opinion 2.12. Underwood & Cadle, *Genetics, Genetic Testing, and the Specter of Discrimination: A Discussion Using Hypothetical Cases*, 85 Ky. L. J. 665, 684 (1996-97).

2.13   Genetic Engineering

The Federal Recombinant DNA Advisors Committee and the Food and Drug Administration oversee and regulate gene splicing, recombinant DNA research, chemical synthesis of DNA molecules, and other genetic engineering research. However, for genetic engineering technologies that represent a significant departure from familiar practices there should be independent input from the scientific community, organized medicine, industry, the public, and others, in addition to the federal government, to prevent abuse from any sector of society, private or public. Such departures include the use of novel vectors, gene transfer in utero, potential germ line modification, and gene transfer to normal volunteers.

    If and when gene replacement with normal DNA becomes a practical reality for the treatment of human disorders, the following factors should be considered:

(1) If procedures are performed in a research setting, reference should be made to the Council's guidelines on clinical investigation.

(2) If procedures are performed in a non-research setting, adherence to usual and customary standards of medical practice and professional responsibility would be required.

(3) Full discussion of the proposed procedure with the patient would be required. The consent of the patient or the patient's legal representative should be informed, voluntary and written.

(4) There must be no hazardous or other unwanted virus on the viral DNA containing the replacement or corrective gene.

(5) The inserted DNA must function under normal control within the recipient cell to prevent metabolic damage that could damage tissue and the patient.

(6) The effectiveness of the gene therapy should be evaluated as well as possible. This will include determination of the natural history of the disease and follow-up examination of subsequent generations.

(7) Such procedures should be undertaken in the future only after careful evaluation of the availability and effectiveness of other possible therapy. If simpler and safer treatment is available, it should be pursued.

(8) These considerations should be reviewed, as appropriate, as procedures and scientific information are developed in the future. (I, V, VII)

Issued March 1980.

Updated June 1996.

2.131   Disclosure of Familial Risk in Genetic Testing

(1) Physicians have a professional duty to protect the confidentiality of their patients' information, including genetic information.

(2) Pre- and post-test counseling must include implications of genetic information for patients' biological relatives. At the time patients are considering undergoing genetic testing, physicians should discuss with them

whether to invite family members to participate in the testing process. Physicians also should identify circumstances under which they would expect patients to notify biological relatives of the availability of information related to risk of disease. In this regard, physicians should make themselves available to assist patients in communicating with relatives to discuss opportunities for counseling and testing, as appropriate.

(3) Physicians who order genetic tests should have adequate knowledge to interpret information for patients. In the absence of adequate expertise in pre-test and post-test counseling, a physician should refer the patient to an appropriate specialist.

(4) Physicians should encourage genetic education throughout a medical career. (I, IV, V, VIII)

Issued December 2003 based on the report "Disclosure of Familial Risk in Genetic Testing," adopted June 2003.

2.132   Genetic Testing by Employers

As a result of the human genome project, physicians will be able to identify a greater number of genetic risks of disease. Among the potential uses of the tests that detect these risks will be screening of potential workers by employers. Employers may want to exclude workers with certain genetic risks from the workplace because these workers may become disabled prematurely, impose higher health care costs, or pose a risk to public safety. In addition, exposure to certain substances in the workplace may increase the likelihood that a disease will develop in the worker with a genetic risk for the disease.

(1) It would generally be inappropriate to exclude workers with genetic risks of disease from the workplace because of their risk. Genetic tests alone do not have sufficient predictive value to be relied upon as a basis for excluding workers. Consequently, use of the tests would result in unfair discrimination against individuals who have positive test results. In addition, there are other ways for employers to serve their legitimate interests. Tests of a worker's actual capacity to meet the demands of the job can be used to ensure future employability and protect the public's safety. Routine monitoring of a worker's exposure can be used to protect workers who have a genetic susceptibility to injury from a substance in the workplace. In addition, employees should be advised of the risks of injury to which they are being exposed.

(2) There may be a role for genetic testing in the exclusion from the workplace of workers who have a genetic susceptibility to injury. At a minimum, several conditions would have to be met:

(a) The disease develops so rapidly that serious and irreversible injury would occur before monitoring of either the worker's exposure to the toxic substance or the worker's health status could be effective in preventing the harm.

(b) The genetic testing is highly accurate, with sufficient sensitivity and specificity to minimize the risk of false negative and false positive test results.

(c) Empirical data demonstrate that the genetic abnormality results in an unusually elevated susceptibility to occupational injury.

(d) It would require undue cost to protect susceptible employees by lowering the level of the toxic substance in the workplace. The costs of lowering the level of the substance must be extraordinary relative to the employer's other costs of making the product for which the toxic substance is used. Since genetic testing with exclusion of susceptible employees is the alternative to cleaning up the workplace, the cost of lowering the level of the substance must also be extraordinary relative to the costs of using genetic testing.

(e) Testing must not be performed without the informed consent of the employee or applicant for employment. (IV)

Issued June 1991 based on the report "Genetic Testing by Employers," adopted June 1991 (JAMA. 1991; 266: 1827-30).

Journal 2003 Focuses on the controversial use of genetic information in employment and insurance. Concludes that reformers must reexamine the ethical and legal duties of professionals regarding protection of genetic information. References Opinion 2.132. Partlett, *Misuse of Genetic Information: The Common Law and Professionals' Liability, 42 Washburn L.J. 489, 503 (2003).*

Journal 2001 Discusses same-sex marriages in the transgender community. Explores Defense of Marriage Act statutes. Considers whether same-sex transgender marriages can prevail against attacks brought under such statutes. Cites Opinions 2.132, 2.135, 2.137, 5.08, and 5.09. Frye & Meiselman, *Same-Sex Marriages Have Existed Legally in the United States for a Long Time Now, 64 Alb. L. Rev. 1031, 1053 (2001).*

Journal 2001 Examines the distinction between preplacement and postplacement examinations in the workplace. Analyzes the possible dangers that might result if preplacement medical testing is not restricted. Concludes that any such testing must relate to the potential employee's ability to perform assigned job duties. References Opinions 2.132 and 2.139. Hoffman, *Preplacement Examinations and Job-Relatedness: How to Enhance Privacy and Diminish Discrimination in the Workplace, 49 U. Kan. L. Rev. 517, 534, 535, 556, 565 (2001).*

Journal 2000 Explores the benefits and harms of the new era of genomic medicine. Discusses the needs of tissue donors, noting they should be carefully balanced with the needs of the medical research community. Concludes that a multifaceted effort is essential to ensuring trust in the medical community as the benefits of genomic medicine are realized. References Opinion 2.132. Ashburn, Wilson, & Eisenstein, *Human Tissue Research in the Genomic Era of Medicine, 160 Arch. Intern. Med. 3377, 3378 (2000).*

Journal 2000 Examines the effects of genetic information on medical care. Concludes that the existing rules and regulations, which try to protect a patient's absolute control over personal genetic data, should be modified. Suggests that a statutory board might better decide when personal genetic information may be divulged to others. References Opinion 2.132. Bruns & Wolman, *Morality of the Privacy of Genetic Information: Possible Improvements of Procedures, 19 Med. Law 127, 129 (2000).*

Journal 2000 Evaluates transgender legal and political activity in the United States. Discusses the International Bill of Gender Rights against the background of the Texas case, *Littleton v. Prange.* Cites Opinions 2.132, 2.135, 2.137, 5.08, and 5.09. Frye, *The International Bill of Gender Rights vs. the Cider House Rules: Transgenders Struggle with the Courts Over What Clothing They Are Allowed to Wear on the Job, Which Restroom They are Allowed to Use on the Job, Their Right to Marry, and the Very Definition of Their Sex, 7 Wm. & Mary J. Women & L. 133, 149 (2000).*

Journal 2000 Explores the legal, ethical, social, and economic considerations associated with use of new genetic techniques in the prediction and diagnosis of Alzheimer Disease. Outlines the potential responsibilities and liabilities of physicians in connection with use of these techniques. References Opinions 2.132, 2.139, and 8.032. Kapp, *Physicians' Legal Duties Regarding the Use of Genetic Tests to Predict and Diagnose Alzheimer Disease, 21 J. Legal Med. 445, 456-57, 465-66 (2000).*

Journal 2000 Discusses the adverse effects of predisposition genetic testing on personal and familial relationships as well as insurability and employment opportunities. Concludes that health care providers and policy makers must ensure that individuals who undergo genetic testing have access to proper counseling, appropriate medical resources, and protection from genetic discrimination. References Opinion 2.132. Schneider, *Adverse Impact of Predisposition Testing on Major Life Activities: Lessons from BRCA1/2 Testing, 3 J. Health Care L. & Pol'y 365, 380 (2000)*.

Journal 1999 Explains physicians' potential liability as corporate professionals and how that reinforces professional standards. Discusses physicians' pursuit of preventive health and its impact on reducing company liability. References Opinion 2.132. Draper, *Preventive Law by Corporate Professional Team Players: Liability and Responsibility in the Work of Company Doctors, 15 J. Contemp. Health L. & Pol'y. 525, 564 (1999)*.

Journal 1999 Argues that current Fourth Amendment jurisprudence needs to be changed. Describes two different theories—an anti-discrimination model and an individual rights model—and applies them to different situations. States that the Fourth Amendment needs to protect personal sovereignty for the sake of the individual and society. References Opinion 2.132. Luna, *Sovereignty and Suspicion, 48 Duke L. J. 787, 884 (1999)*.

Journal 1998 Discusses conflicts of interest in the physician-patient relationship arising out of use of financial incentives by managed care organizations. Considers how such conflicts are dealt with in the attorney-client relationship. Suggests that a financial incentive should be legally denounced if it unreasonably interferes with a physician's duty to properly care for and treat patients. Quotes Preamble, Fundamental Elements (1) [now Opinion 10.01] and Opinions 4.04, 5.01, 8.03, 8.13, and 9.06. Cites Fundamental Elements (4) [now Opinion 10.01] and Opinions 2.07, 2.08, and 2.132. Hall, *Third-Party Payor Conflicts of Interest in Managed Care: A Proposal for Regulation Based on the Model Rules of Professional Conduct, 29 Seton Hall L. Rev. 95, 96, 107, 108, 109, 110, 111, 112, 134, 135, 136 (1998)*.

Journal 1998 Discusses the use of genetic information by employers. Argues that people may forego genetic testing for fear that the results will be used by their employers in a discriminatory manner. Concludes that the Minnesota statute prohibiting employers from performing medical tests or obtaining medical information, which is not job related, is better than other approaches. References Opinion 2.132. Rothstein, Gelb, & Craig, *Protecting Genetic Privacy by Permitting Employer Access Only to Job-Related Employee Medical Information: Analysis of a Unique Minnesota Law, 24 Am. J. Law & Med. 399, 400 (1998)*.

Journal 1997 Explores the legality of pre-employment screening techniques. Considers legal reforms that would balance the interests of employers and job applicants. Offers suggestions that would enhance fairness and consistency in this screening process. References Opinion 2.132. Befort, *Pre-Employment Screening and Investigation: Navigating Between a Rock and a Hard Place, 14 Hofstra Lab. L. J. 365, 391 (1997)*.

Journal 1997 Explores parents' legal rights to subject their children to genetic testing for untreatable, late-onset disorders or for carrier status. Examines potential negative aspects of genetic testing. Proposes that parents should not have the right to subject their children to such testing. References Opinion 2.132. Holland, *Should Parents Be Permitted to Authorize Genetic Testing for Their Children?, 31 Fam. L. Q. 321, 346-47 (1997)*.

Journal 1997 Discusses the collection and storage of human tissues. Notes the use of genetic testing by employers. Examines whether those with biomedical experience perceive genetic research as dangerous. Considers problems of privacy and confidentiality raised by genetic technology and the storage of tissues. References Opinion 2.132. Merz, *Psychosocial Risks of Storing and Using Human Tissues in Research, 8 Risk: Health Safety & Env't 235, 236 (1997)*.

Journal 1993 Examines how genetic tests to diagnose disease may be useful to private insurance companies in identifying persons for whom coverage will be provided. Concludes that this issue should be considered as part of the national health care reform debate. References Opinion 2.132. Jecker, *Genetic Testing and the Social Responsibility of Private Health Insurance Companies, 21 J. Law, Med. & Ethics 109, 112 (1993)*.

2.135   Insurance Companies and Genetic Information

Physicians should not participate in genetic testing by health insurance companies to predict a person's predisposition for disease. As a corollary, it may be necessary for physicians to maintain separate files for genetic testing results to ensure that the results are not sent to health insurance companies when requests for copies of patient medical records are fulfilled. Physicians who withhold testing results should inform insurance companies that, when medical records are sent, genetic testing results are not included. This disclosure should occur with all patients, not just those who have undergone genetic testing. (IV)

Issued June 1994 based on the report "Physician Participation in Genetic Testing by Health Insurance Companies," adopted June 1993.

Updated June 1996.

Journal 2001 Discusses same-sex marriages in the transgender community. Explores Defense of Marriage Act statutes. Considers whether same-sex transgender marriages can prevail against attacks brought under such statutes. Cites Opinions 2.132, 2.135, 2.137, 5.08, and 5.09. Frye & Meiselman, *Same-Sex Marriages Have Existed Legally in the United States for a Long Time Now*, 64 *Alb. L. Rev. 1031, 1053 (2001)*.

Journal 2000 Evaluates transgender legal and political activity in the United States. Discusses the International Bill of Gender Rights against the background of the Texas case, *Littleton v. Prange*. Cites Opinions 2.132, 2.135, 2.137, 5.08, and 5.09. Frye, *The International Bill of Gender Rights vs. the Cider House Rules: Transgenders Struggle with the Courts Over What Clothing They Are Allowed to Wear on the Job, Which Restroom They are Allowed to Use on the Job, Their Right to Marry, and the Very Definition of Their Sex*, 7 *Wm. & Mary J. Women & L. 133, 149 (2000)*.

2.136 Genetic Information and the Criminal Justice System

The release of genetic information from a physician's records without the consent of the patient constitutes a breach of confidentiality. Opinion 5.05, "Confidentiality," acknowledges that law and overriding social considerations may permit physicians to disclose confidential information in limited circumstances. However, such circumstances present ethical challenges. The following guidelines are intended to aid physicians in considering the ethical basis for the release of genetic information to the criminal justice system:

(1) Physicians should release a patient's genetic information only with the patient's consent or in compliance with a warrant or other order of a court of law. The circumstances in which law enforcement may seek a suspect's genetic information from the suspect's physician depend on whether any specific suspect has been identified, and if the suspect is in custody.

   (a) If law enforcement personnel have identified a suspect and the suspect cannot be located to provide a genetic sample, physicians should release clinical genetic information only when a warrant or court order mandates such a release.

   (b) When law enforcement personnel have identified a suspect, and the suspect has been located but refuses to provide a sample or is deceased (but his or her body is available), physicians should not be required to release genetic information as in these circumstances a court can authorize collection of a sample from the suspect or from postmortem tissue.

   (c) Searching clinical and research databases of genetic information, or extracting and analyzing DNA from clinical or research tissue repositories, should not be conducted for the mere possibility that there is a match to a suspect's DNA unless there is a warrant or court order to do so.

(2) When genetic information is provided to the judicial system, physicians should provide the minimum amount of information necessary for the

explicit identification procedure being performed. Other elements of the medical record or the results of any genetic testing or genetic diagnosis should not be released without the patient's consent or further warrant or order of the court.

(3) It is unethical for any genetic information obtained from a physician for identification purposes to be used subsequently for other purposes, such as research, unless appropriate ethical guidelines are followed and the informed consent of the individual is obtained (or the legally appropriate surrogate if the individual is incompetent or deceased, in compliance with Opinion 5.051, "Confidentiality of Medical Information Postmortem").

(4) Databases that contain only the genetic identifiers from the specific loci that are typically used for identification purposes do not present the same ethical concerns that are presented by databases which contain genotypic or phenotypic information. Physicians participating in the creation of genetic databases for the exclusive use of the criminal justice system should ensure that the database is not used inappropriately for purposes other than identification.

(5) In general, requiring that the genetic sample be destroyed or returned after the analysis necessary for identification is performed affords protection against inappropriate uses.

(6) When the criminal justice system seeks genetic information for the purposes of identifying a deceased victim, the above relevant guidelines also apply. (III, IV)

Issued June 2001 based on the report "Genetic Information and the Criminal Justice System," adopted June 2000. (J. Law, Med. & Ethics. 2002: 30; 88-94).

Journal 2002 Discusses legal and medical policies that protect confidentiality in the physician-patient relationship. Concludes that reducing the current level of privacy protection would jeopardize health care. Quotes Preamble and Opinions 2.136, 5.05, and 10.01. References Principles VIII and IX. Sciarrino, *Ferguson v. City of Charleston: "The Doctor Will See You Now, Be Sure to Bring Your Privacy Rights in With You!" 12 Temp. Pol. & Civ. Rts. L. Rev. 197, 213, 215, 220, 221, 222 (2002)*

2.137 Ethical Issues in Carrier Screening of Genetic Disorders

All carrier testing must be voluntary, and informed consent from screened individuals is required. Confidentiality of results is to be maintained. Results of testing should not be disclosed to third parties without the explicit informed consent of the screened individual. Patients should be informed as to potential uses for the genetic information by third parties, and whether other ways of obtaining the information are available when appropriate.

Carrier testing should be available uniformly among the at-risk population being screened. One legitimate exception to this principle is the limitation of carrier testing to individuals of childbearing age. In pursuit of uniform access, physicians should not limit testing only to patients specifically requesting testing. If testing is offered to some patients, it should be offered to all patients within the same risk category.

The direction of future genetic screening tests should be determined by well-thought-out and well-coordinated social policy. Third parties, including insurance companies or employers, should not be permitted to discriminate against carriers of genetic disorders through policies which have the ultimate effect of influencing decisions about testing and reproduction. (IV, V)

Issued June 1994 based on the report "Ethical Issues in Carrier Screening for Cystic Fibrosis and Other Genetic Disorders," adopted June 1991.

Journal 2001 Discusses same-sex marriages in the transgender community. Explores Defense of Marriage Act statutes. Considers whether same-sex transgender marriages can prevail against attacks brought under such statutes. Cites Opinions 2.132, 2.135, 2.137, 5.08, and 5.09. Frye & Meiselman, *Same-Sex Marriages Have Existed Legally in the United States for a Long Time Now*, 64 Alb. L. Rev. 1031, 1053 (2001).

Journal 2000 Evaluates transgender legal and political activity in the United States. Discusses the International Bill of Gender Rights against the background of the Texas case, *Littleton v. Prange*. Cites Opinions 2.132, 2.135, 2.137, 5.08, and 5.09. Frye, *The International Bill of Gender Rights vs. the Cider House Rules: Transgenders Struggle with the Courts Over What Clothing They Are Allowed to Wear on the Job, Which Restroom They are Allowed to Use on the Job, Their Right to Marry, and the Very Definition of Their Sex*, 7 Wm. & Mary J. Women & L. 133, 149 (2000).

2.138 Genetic Testing of Children

Genetic testing of children implicates important concerns about individual autonomy and the interest of the patients. Before testing of children can be performed, there must be some potential benefit from the testing that can reasonably be viewed as outweighing the disadvantages of testing, particularly the harm from abrogating the children's future choice in knowing their genetic status. When there is such a potential benefit, parents should decide whether their children will undergo testing. If parents unreasonably request or refuse testing of their child, the physician should take steps to change or, if necessary, use legal means to override the parents' choice. Applying these principles to specific circumstances yields the following conclusions:

(1) When a child is at risk for a genetic condition for which preventive or other therapeutic measures are available, genetic testing should be offered or, in some cases, required.

(2) When a child is at risk for a genetic condition with pediatric onset for which preventive or other therapeutic measures are not available, parents generally should have discretion to decide about genetic testing.

(3) When a child is at risk for a genetic condition with adult onset for which preventive or other therapeutic measures are not available, genetic testing of children generally should not be undertaken. Families should still be informed of the existence of tests and given the opportunity to discuss the reasons why the tests are generally not offered for children.

(4) Genetic testing for carrier status should be deferred until either the child reaches maturity, the child needs to make reproductive decisions, or, in the case of children too immature to make their own reproductive decisions, reproductive decisions need to be made for the child.

(5) Genetic testing of children for the benefit of a family member should not be performed unless the testing is necessary to prevent substantial harm to the family member.

When a child's genetic status is determined incidentally, the information should be retained by the physician and entered into the patient record.

Discussion of the existence of this finding should then be taken up when the child reaches maturity or needs to make reproductive decisions, so that the individual can decide whether to request disclosure of the information. It is important that physicians be consistent in disclosing both positive and negative results in the same way since if physicians raise the existence of the testing results only when the results are positive, individuals will know what the results must be. This information should not be disclosed to third parties. Genetic information should be maintained in a separate portion of the medical record to prevent mistaken disclosure.

When a child is being considered for adoption, the guidelines for genetic testing should be the same as for other children. (IV)

Issued June 1996 based on the report "Testing Children for Genetic Status," adopted June 1995.

Journal 1999 Discusses regulatory concerns regarding genetic technology. Provides ideas on how society might regulate genetic enhancements. Argues that a variety of means of regulation need to be utilized to govern genetic technology. Quotes Opinion 2.11. Cites Opinion 9.065. References Opinion 2.138. Mehlman, *How Will We Regulate Genetic Enhancement?*, 34 Wake Forest L. Rev. 671, 693-94, 695 (1999).

Journal 1998 Discusses ramifications of genetic research. Points out that genetic information affects not only the tested individual, but the person's family as well. Suggests that a greater awareness of potential risk will reduce possible hazards stemming from genetic research. Cites Opinion 2.138. Green & Thomas, *DNA: Five Distinguishing Features for Policy Analysis*, 11 Harv. J. L. & Tech. 571, 582-83 (1998).

Journal 1997 Discusses the National Human Genome Research Institute and the activities of the Office of Genome Ethics. Offers an overview and evaluation, with emphasis on bioethical education and counsel that was provided to genetic researchers. References Opinion 2.138. Green, *NHGRI's Intramural Ethics Experiment*, 7 Kennedy Inst. of Ethics J. 181, 185, 188 (1997).

2.139 Multiplex Genetic Testing

Multiplex testing—where tests are offered for several different medical conditions in a single session—presents a series of challenges to adequate communication between the patient and the physician. It increases the total number of marginally indicated or non-indicated tests, thereby bolstering the rate of false results. These results may lead to psychological stress and misinformed life-altering decisions, and may also impact the ability of a physician to obtain informed consent. Multiplex testing and its resultant information may also have widespread societal implications that include discriminatory practices against not only individuals but specific ethnic groups that have been designated "at risk" populations.

Before such tests reach health care providers, clinics, and drugstores, the ethical and social implications of these tests must be well-understood, and careful restrictions and regulations must be established. The following guidelines are offered on the future possibilities of multiplex genetic testing:

(1) Physicians should not routinely order tests for multiple genetic conditions.

(2) Tests for more than one genetic condition should be ordered only when clinically relevant and after the patient has had full counseling and has given informed consent for each test.

(3) Efforts should be made to educate clinicians and society about the uncertainty surrounding genetic testing. (IV, V)

Issued June 1998 based on the report "Multiplex Genetic Testing," adopted December 1996 (*Hastings Center Report*. 1998; 28(4): 15-21).

Journal 2001 Examines the distinction between preplacement and postplacement examinations in the workplace. Analyzes the possible dangers that might result if preplacement medical testing is not restricted. Concludes that any such testing must relate to the potential employee's ability to perform assigned job duties. References Opinions 2.132 and 2.139. Hoffman, *Preplacement Examinations and Job-Relatedness: How to Enhance Privacy and Diminish Discrimination in the Workplace*, 49 U. Kan. L. Rev. 517, 534, 535, 556, 565 (2001).

Journal 2000 Explores issues relating to genetic privacy and considers how the law should evolve in this context. Identifies contrasting ideological viewpoints regarding the role government should play in regulating public use of personal genetic data. Concludes that because of unregulated information markets, people may be afraid to use genetic technologies. References Opinion 2.139. Fedder, *To Know or Not to Know: Legal Perspectives on Genetic Privacy and Disclosure of an Individual's Genetic Profile*, 21 J. Legal Med. 557, 563 (2000).

Journal 2000 Explores the legal, ethical, social, and economic considerations associated with use of new genetic techniques in the prediction and diagnosis of Alzheimer Disease. Outlines the potential responsibilities and liabilities of physicians in connection with use of these techniques. References Opinions 2.132, 2.139, and 8.032. Kapp, *Physicians' Legal Duties Regarding the Use of Genetic Tests to Predict and Diagnose Alzheimer Disease*, 21 J. Legal Med. 445, 456-57, 465-66 (2000).

2.14 In Vitro Fertilization

The technique of in vitro fertilization and embryo transplantation enables certain couples previously incapable of conception to bear a child. It is also useful in the field of research directed toward an understanding of how genetic defects arise and are transmitted and how they might be prevented or treated. Because of serious ethical and moral concerns, however, any fertilized egg that has the potential for human life and that will be implanted in the uterus of a woman should not be subjected to laboratory research.

All fertilized ova not utilized for implantation and that are maintained for research purposes shall be handled with the strictest adherence to the Principles of Medical Ethics, to the guidelines for research and medical practice expressed in the Council's opinion on fetal research, and to the highest standards of medical practice. (I, V, VII)

Issued June 1983.

Journal 1991 Considers how the use of in vitro fertilization (IVF) has blurred the distinction between medical practice and research. Argues that medical-professional responsibility standards should be used to curtail the creation of life in vitro. Quotes Opinions 2.10 and 2.14. Comment, *Dangerous Relations: Doctors and Extracorporeal Embryos, The Need For New Limits To Medical Inquiry*, 7 J. Contemp. Health L. & Pol'y 307, 309 (1991).

Journal 1987 Examines various ethical issues surrounding surrogate motherhood, artificial insemination, in vitro fertilization and embryonic/fetal research. Reports on the positions of four ethics groups: the Warnock Committee of Inquiry into Human Fertilization and Embryology; the AMA's Council on Ethical and Judicial Affairs; the Ethics Committee of the American Fertility Society; and the Ethics Committee of the American College of Obstetricians and Gynecologists. References Opinions 2.04, 2.05, and 2.13 (1986) [now Opinion 2.14]. Quotes Opinion 2.18. Rosner, Cassell, Friedland, Landolt, Loeb, Numann, Ora, Risemberg, & Sordillo, *Ethical Considerations of Reproductive Technologies*, 87 N.Y. State J. Med. 398, 399-400 (1987).

Frozen Pre-embryos

The practice of freezing extra pre-embryos harvested during the in vitro fertilization process (IVF) has enhanced the ability of infertile couples to preserve embryos for future implantation. This practice has also posed a number of ethical and legal dilemmas, including questions regarding decision-making authority over the pre-embryos and appropriate uses of pre-embryos.

This country's cultural and legal traditions indicate that the logical persons to exercise control over a frozen pre-embryo are the woman and man who provided the gametes (the ovum and sperm). The gamete providers have a fundamental interest at stake, their potential for procreation. In addition, the gamete providers are the parties most concerned with the interests of a frozen pre-embryo and most likely to protect those interests.

Gamete providers should be able to use the pre-embryos themselves or donate them for use by other parties, but not sell them. In addition, research on pre-embryos should be permitted as long as the pre-embryos are not destined for transfer to a woman for implantation and as long as the research is conducted in accordance with the Council's guidelines on fetal research. Frozen pre-embryos may also be allowed to thaw and deteriorate.

The gamete providers should have an equal say in the use of their pre-embryos and, therefore, the pre-embryos should not be available for use by either provider or changed from their frozen state without the consent of both providers. The man and woman each has contributed half of the pre-embryo's genetic code. In addition, whether a person chooses to become a parent and assume all of the accompanying obligations is a particularly personal and fundamental decision. Even if the individual could be absolved of any parental obligations, he or she may have a strong desire not to have offspring. The absence of a legal duty does not eliminate the moral duty many would feel toward any genetic offspring.

Advance agreements are recommended for deciding the disposition of frozen pre-embryos in the event of divorce or other changes in circumstances. Advance agreements can help ensure that the gamete providers undergo IVF and pre-embryo freezing after a full contemplation of the consequences but should not be mandatory. (I, III, IV, V)

Issued March 1992 based on the report "Frozen Pre-Embryos," adopted December 1989 (JAMA. 1990; 263: 2484-87).

Updated June 1994.

Journal 2003 Reviews legal methods for resolving disputes involving disposition of cryopreserved preembryos. Concludes that federal legislation is needed to address existing problems. Cites Opinion 2.141. Windsor, *Disposition of Cryopreserved Preembryos After Divorce*, 88 Iowa L. Rev. 1001, 1026 (2003).

Journal 2001 Examines the ethical and legal dilemmas associated with stem cell and fetal tissue research. Discusses current federal law. Concludes that Congress should allow researchers to obtain stem cells from discarded human embryos provided by in vitro fertilization clinics. Cites Opinion 2.141. Casell, *Lengthening the Stem: Allowing Federally Funded Researchers to Derive Human Pluripotent Stem Cells From Embryos*, 34 U. Mich. J. L. Ref. 547, 563 (2001).

Journal 1999 Describes cryopreservation and in vitro fertilization (IVF) procedures. Examines statutory and case law regarding the use of IVF and discusses theories about how frozen preembryos should be discarded. Concludes by suggesting that, in legal disputes, the party opposing implantation ordinarily should prevail. Quotes Opinion 2.141. Fiestal, *A Solomonic Decision: What Will be the Fate of Frozen Preembryos?* 6 Cardozo Women's L. J. 103, 110 (1999).

Journal 1999 Describes the approaches various courts have taken toward disposition of cryopreserved embryos after dissolution of marriage. Concludes that, while a prior agreement should be binding, various contract defenses may apply where circumstances have substantially changed. References Opinion 2.141. Haut, *Divorce and the Disposition of Frozen Embryos*, 28 Hofstra L. Rev. 493, 519 (1999).

Journal 1998 Addresses the ethical and legal issues regarding storage and disposition of frozen human embryos. Suggests that courts should seek to honor the donors' wishes. Proposes that future legislation should mandate embryo disposition after a certain length of time. Quotes Opinion 2.141. Forster, *The Legal and Ethical Debate Surrounding the Storage and Destruction of Frozen Human Embryos: A Reaction to the Mass Disposal in Britain and the Lack of Law in the United States*, 76 Wash. U. L. Q. 759, 766-67, 770 (1998).

Journal 1998 Discusses legal issues regarding reproductive biotechnology, with emphasis on freezing of eggs and embryos, research involving frozen embryos, and cloning. Argues that legislation should protect society from unacceptable uses of reproductive technology but, at the same time, ensure advancement of technology for the benefit of society. References Opinion 2.141. Godoy, *Where is Biotechnology Taking the Law? An Overview of Assisted Reproductive Technology, Research on Frozen Embryos and Human Cloning*, 19 J. Juv. L. 357, 363 (1998).

Journal 1990 Considers ways in which the frozen pre-embryo can be legally described and argues that it should not be considered either person or property. Concludes that in vitro fertilization research is valuable to society and proposes research guidelines. References Opinion 2.141. Martin & Lagod, *The Human Preembryo, the Progenitors, and the State: Toward a Dynamic Theory of Status, Rights, and Research Policy*, 5 High Tech. L. J. 257, 304 (1990).

Journal 1990 Considers problems created by frozen pre-embryos that result from in vitro fertilization therapy. Explores problems with disposing of these pre-embryos and how prior agreements between couples have surfaced as a potential solution. References Opinion 2.141. Robertson, *Prior Agreements for Disposition of Frozen Embryos*, 51 Ohio St. L. J. 407, 419 (1990).

2.145 Pre-embryo Splitting

The technique of splitting in vitro fertilized pre-embryos may result in multiple genetically identical siblings.

The procedure of pre-embryo splitting should be available so long as both gamete providers agree. This procedure may greatly increase the chances of conception for an infertile couple or for a couple whose future reproductive capacity will likely be diminished. Pre-embryo splitting also can reduce the number of invasive procedures necessary for egg retrieval and the necessity for hormonal stimulants to generate multiple eggs. The use and disposition of any pre-embryos that are frozen for future use should be consistent with the Council's opinion on frozen pre-embryos (Opinion 2.141, "Frozen Pre-embryos").

The use of frozen pre-embryo identical siblings many years after one child has been born raises new ethical issues. Couples might wait until they can discover the mental and physical characteristics of a child before transferring a genetically identical sibling for implantation, they might sell their frozen pre-embryos based upon the outcome of a genetically identical child, or they might decide to transplant a genetically identical sibling based on the need to harvest the child's tissue.

The Council does not find that these considerations are sufficient to prohibit pre-embryo splitting for the following reasons:

(1) It would take many years to determine the outcome of a child and most families want to complete their childbearing within a shorter time.

(2) The sale of pre-embryos can and should be prohibited.

(3) The small number of couples who might bear identical siblings solely for purposes of harvesting their tissue does not outweigh the benefits which might be derived from pre-embryo splitting. Additionally, it is not evident that a sibling would have negative psychological or emotional consequences from having acted as an organ or tissue donor. Indeed, the child may derive psychological benefits from having saved the life of a sibling.

To the extent possible, discussion of these issues should be had with gamete providers prior to pre-embryo splitting and freezing so as to inform the prospective parents of possible future ethical dilemmas. (I, III, IV, V)

Issued June 1994.

2.146 Cloning-for-Biomedical-Research

Stem cells derived from cloned human embryos resulting from somatic cell nuclear transfer technology are promising as a potential source of treatment in a wide range of diseases. However, much controversy arises from the necessity to destroy embryos in order to extract their stem cells for use in biomedical research. The conflict centers on the moral status of embryos, a question that divides ethical opinion and that cannot be resolved by medical science.

(1) While the pluralism of moral visions that underlie this debate must be respected, physicians collectively must continue to be guided by their paramount obligation to the welfare of their patients. In this light, cloning-for-biomedical-research is consistent with medical ethics. Every physician remains free to decide whether to participate in stem cell research or to use its products.

(2) Cloning-for-biomedical-research requires appropriate oversight and monitoring. At a minimum, not only is the oversight of an institutional review board required, but also that of a regulatory body, such as the Office for Human Research Protections, to monitor progress in the field, assist in developing relevant guidelines, and ensure that the technique of cloning-for-biomedical-research is used only if uniquely promising.

(3) Informed consent by subjects participating in cloning-for-biomedical-research is governed by standard principles: voluntary participation and disclosure of all relevant risks and benefits to subjects. Disclosure to the donor of the oocyte and the donor of the somatic cell also must include:

(a) Description of the procurement procedures specific to the donor

(b) Statement of the intention to create a cloned human embryo through introduction of the somatic cell's nucleus into the enucleated egg for research purposes (and not for transfer to a woman's uterus)

(c) Acknowledgment that the extraction of stem cells will require the cloned embryo's destruction

(d) The intention to derive immortal cell lines from the stem cells to be used in research and possibly in therapeutic contexts; primary and secondary uses should be disclosed and individuals should be free to refuse the use of their biological materials for specified purposes

(e) Potential commercial uses and patent or ownership issues (as described in Opinion E-2.08, "Commercial Use of Human Tissue")

(4) The informed consent process for potential recipients of stem cells derived from cloned embryos should conform with ethical standards outlined in the Council on Ethical and Judicial Affairs' Opinion E-2.07, "Clinical Investigation," and address additional disclosures including provenance of stem cells.

(5) Due to the possibilities of contamination by infectious agents from other species and damage to DNA during growth of new tissues and organs, products of cloning-for-biomedical-research raise ethical concerns similar to those surrounding xenotransplantation. Therefore, the informed consent process for potential recipients of these products also should conform to Opinion E-2.169, "The Ethical Implications of Xenotransplantation." (V)

Issued December 2003 based on the report "Cloning-for-Biomedical-Research," adopted June 2003.

2.147 Cloning-to-Produce-Children

Somatic cell nuclear transfer (SCNT) is the process in which the nucleus of a somatic cell of an organism is transferred into an enucleated oocyte. "Cloning-to-produce-children" is the application of SCNT to the creation of a human being that shares all of its nuclear genes with the donor of the human somatic cell.

To clarify the many existing misconceptions about this use of cloning, physicians should help educate the public about the intrinsic limits of cloning-to-produce-children as well as about the current ethical and legal protections that would prevent certain uses of cloned human embryos. These include the following:

(1) Using cloning-to-produce-children as an approach to replicate a person (the donor of the somatic cell) is a concept based on the mistaken notion that one's genotype largely determines one's individuality. A cloned child created via this process would not be identical to the donor of the somatic cell.

(2) Current ethical and legal standards hold that under no circumstances should any use of cloning occur without informed consent from the somatic cell and the oocyte donor(s).

(3) Current ethical and legal standards hold that a child produced from a clone would be entitled to the same rights, freedoms, and protections as every other individual in society. The fact that a human clone's nuclear genes would derive from a single individual rather than two would not change its moral standing.

Physicians have an ethical obligation to consider the harms and benefits of new medical procedures and technologies. Physicians should not participate in cloning-to-produce-children at this time because further investigation and discussion regarding the harms and benefits of this use of cloning are required. Concerns include:

(1) Unknown physical harms introduced by SCNT technology. SCNT has not yet been refined and its long-term safety has not yet been proven. The risk

of producing individuals with genetic anomalies gives rise to an obligation to seek better understanding of—and potential medical therapies for—the unforeseen medical consequences that could stem from cloning-to-produce-children.

(2) Psychosocial harms introduced by cloning, including violations of privacy and autonomy. Cloning-to-produce children risks limiting, at least psychologically, the seemingly unlimited potential of new human beings and thus creating enormous pressures on the cloned child to live up to expectations based on the life of the somatic cell donor.

(3) The impact of cloning-to-produce-children on familial and societal relations. The family unit may be altered with the introduction of this use of cloning, and more thought is required on a societal level regarding how to construct familial relations.

(4) Potential effects on the gene pool. Like other interventions that can change individuals' reproductive patterns and the resulting genetic characteristics of a population, cloning-to-produce-children has the potential to be used in a eugenic or discriminatory fashion—practices that are incompatible with the ethical norms of medical practice. Moreover, cloning-to-produce-children could alter irreversibly the gene pool and exacerbate genetic problems that arise from deleterious genetic mutations, resulting in harms to future generations.

Two potentially realistic and possibly appropriate medical uses of cloning-to-produce-children are for assisting individuals or couples to reproduce and for generating tissues when the donor is not harmed or sacrificed. Given the unresolved issues regarding cloning identified above, the medical profession should not undertake cloning-to-produce-children at this time and pursue alternative approaches that raise fewer ethical concerns.

Because SCNT technology is not limited to the United States, physicians should help establish international guidelines governing uses. (V)

Issued December 1999 based on the report "The Ethics of Human Cloning," adopted June 1999.

Updated December 2003, based on the report "Cloning-for-Biomedical-Research," adopted June 2003.

Journal 1999 Discusses arguments against cloning. Points out that, as medical knowledge advances, and physicians can safely undertake this procedure, increasing emphasis will be placed on ethical concerns. Concludes that cloning may benefit infertile couples and single people who want to have children without involving a third party in their procreational activities. References Opinion 2.147. Orentlicher, *Cloning and the Preservation of Family Integrity*, 59 La. L. Rev. 1019, 1022 (1999).

2.15   Financial Incentives to Living Donors

The voluntary donation of organs in appropriate circumstances is to be encouraged. It is unethical to participate in a procedure to enable a living donor to receive payment, other than for the reimbursement of expenses necessarily incurred in connection with removal, for any of the donor's solid organs.

Issued June 1984.

Updated June 1994 based on the report "Financial Incentives for Organ Procurement: Ethical Aspects of Future Contracts for Cadaveric Donors," adopted December 1993 (*Arch Intern Med.* 1995; 155: 581-89); updated June 2004 based on the report, "Cadaveric Organ Donation: Encouraging the Study of Motivation," adopted June 2002.

Journal 2003 Proposes a moral, communitarian approach to address organ shortages. Concludes the next step should involve a demonstration that the communitarian approach can succeed. Quotes Opinion 2.155. Cites Opinion 2.15. Etzioni, *Organ Donation: A Communitarian Approach,* 13 Kennedy Inst. Ethics J. 1, 3, 4, 16 (March 2003).

Journal 2003 Examines the benefits of paired organ exchanges and proposes a statutory framework for implementation. Concludes this approach supplements the current U.S. organ procurement system without resorting to use of financial incentives. Quotes Opinion 2.15. Morley, *Increasing the Supply of Organs for Transplantation Through Paired Organ Exchanges, 21 Yale L. & Pol'y Rev. 221, 255 (2003).*

Journal 2003 Suggests that financial incentives for organ procurement should be reconsidered. Concludes that the ban on marketing organs should be lifted. References Opinion 2.15. Veatch, *Why Liberals Should Accept Financial Incentives for Organ Procurement, 13 Kennedy Inst. Ethics J. 19, 34 (March 2003).*

Journal 1995 Examines legal and ethical issues surrounding organ transplant procurement practices, with emphasis on a possible commercial system. Concludes that adequate market safeguards need to be developed to protect vulnerable donors and citizens. References Opinions 2.15 and 2.167. Banks, *Legal and Ethical Safeguards: Protection of Society's Most Vulnerable Participants in a Commercialized Organ Transplantation System, XXI Am. J. Law & Med. 45, 77, 79, 95-96, 103-04 (1995).*

2.151   Cadaveric Organ Donation: Encouraging the Study of Motivation

Physicians have an obligation to hold their patients' interests paramount and to support access to medical care (Principles VIII and IX). To discharge these obligations, physicians should participate in efforts to increase organ donation including promotion of voluntary donation. Beyond educational programs, however, physicians should support innovative approaches to encourage organ donation. Such efforts may include encouragement of and, if appropriate, participation in the conduct of ethically designed research studies of financial incentives.

Because the potential benefits and harms of financial incentives for cadaveric organ donation are unknown, physicians have an obligation to study financial incentives. Whether or not they are ethical depends upon the balance of benefits and harms that result from them. Physicians should encourage and support pilot studies, limited to relatively small populations, that investigate the effects of financial incentives for cadaveric organ donation for the purpose of examining and possibly revising current policies in the light of scientific evidence.

Pilot studies of the effects of financial incentives for cadaveric organ donation should be implemented only after certain considerations have been met, including:

(1) Consultation and advice is sought from the population within which the pilot study is to take place.

(2) Objectives and strategies as well as sound scientific design, measurable outcomes and set time frames are clearly defined in written protocols that

are publicly available and approved by appropriate oversight bodies, such as Institutional Review Boards.

(3) Incentives are of moderate value and at the lowest level that can be reasonably expected to increase organ donation.

(4) Payment for an organ from a living donor is not a part of any study.

(5) Financial incentives apply to cadaveric donation only, and must not lead to the purchase of donated organs; the distribution of organs for transplantation should continue to be governed by United Network for Organ Sharing (UNOS), based on ethically appropriate criteria related to medical need. (I, III, V, VII, VIII, IX)

Issued December 2002 based on the report "Cadaveric Organ Donation: Encouraging the Study of Motivation," adopted June 2002, (*Transplantation* 2003; 76(4): 748-751).

2.155 Mandated Choice and Presumed Consent for Cadaveric Organ Donation

A system of mandated choice for organ donation, in which individuals are required to express their preferences regarding organ donation when renewing their drivers' licenses or performing some other state-mandated task, is an ethically appropriate strategy for encouraging donation and should be pursued. To be effective, information on the importance of organ donation and the success of organ transplantation should be provided when the donation decision is made.

A system of presumed consent for organ donation, in which individuals are assumed to consent to be organ donors after death unless they indicate their refusal to consent, raises serious ethical concerns. For presumed consent to be ethically acceptable, effective mechanisms for documenting and honoring refusals to donate must be in place. In addition, when there is no documented refusal by the individual decedent, the family of the decedent would have to be contacted to verify that they do not know of any objections to donation by the decedent while living. (I, III, V)

Issued June 1994 based on the report "Strategies for Cadaveric Organ Procurement: Mandated Choice and Presumed Consent," adopted December 1993 (*JAMA*. 1994; 272: 809-12).

Journal 2003 Explores the ethical, legal, and clinical implications of non-heart beating organ donation. Concludes that, if ambiguities are clarified, non-heart beating organ donation can achieve an ethical good. References Opinions 2.155 and 2.162. Bell, *Non-heart Beating Organ Donation: Old Procurement Strategy—New Ethical Problems*, 29 J. Med. Ethics 176, 181 (2003).

Journal 2003 Recommends a modified version of mandated choice for organ procurement. Concludes that the modified version recognizes arguments favoring mandated donation while still relying on the importance of individual consent. References Opinion 2.155. Chouhan & Draper, *Modified Mandated Choice for Organ Procurement*, 29 J. Med. Ethics 157, 162 (2003).

Journal 2003 Proposes a moral, communitarian approach to address organ shortages. Concludes the next step should involve a demonstration that the communitarian approach can succeed. Quotes Opinion 2.155. Cites Opinion 2.15. Etzioni, *Organ Donation: A Communitarian Approach*, 13 Kennedy Inst. Ethics J. 1, 3, 4, 16 (March 2003).

Journal 2002 Considers ethical incentives to increase organ donation. Concludes that market-based incentives are unethical. References Opinion 2.155. Delmonico, Arnold, Scheper-Hughes, Siminoff, Kahn & Youngner, *Ethical Incentives—Not Payment—for Organ Donation*, 346 New Eng. J. Med. 2002, 2005 (2002).

Journal 2001 Explores ways to overcome barriers to organ donation. Clarifies ethical constraints affecting societal efforts to increase the supply of organs. Supports the rights of individuals to make organ donation decisions, but emphasizes the importance of doing so as members of communities—particularly small communities of families. Quotes Opinion 2.155. Childress, *The Failure to Give: Reducing Barriers to Organ Donation, 11 Kennedy Inst. Ethics J. 1, 13, 14 (2001).*

Journal 1997 Explores the current policies on cadaveric organ procurement in the United States. Offers improvements to help save lives and end the waste of suitable organs. Discusses pertinent ethical and legal issues. References Opinion 2.155. MacDonald, *Organ Donation: The Time Has Come to Refocus the Ethical Spotlight, 8 Stan. L. & Pol'y Rev. 177, 179, 185 (1997).*

2.157   Organ Procurement Following Cardiac Death

Given the increasing need for donor organs, protocols for procurement following cardiac death have been developed. In some instances, patients or their surrogate decision makers request withdrawal of life support and choose to serve as organ donors. In these cases, the organs can be preserved best by discontinuation of life support in the operating room so that organs can be removed two minutes following cardiac death. In other scenarios, patients who suffer unexpected cardiac death may be cannulated and perfused with cold preserving fluid (in situ preservation) to maintain organs. Both of these methods may be ethically permissible, with attention to certain safeguards.

(1) When securing consent for life support withdrawal and organ retrieval, the health care team must be certain that consent is voluntary. This is particularly true where surrogate decisions about life-sustaining treatment may be influenced by the prospect of organ donation. If there is any reason to suspect undue influence, a full ethics consultation should be required.

(2) In all instances, it is critical that there be no conflict of interest in the health care team. Those health care professionals providing care at the end of life must be separated from providers participating in the transplant team.

(3) Further pilot programs should assess the success and acceptability of organ removal following withdrawal of life-sustaining treatment.

(4) In cases of in situ preservation of cadaveric organs, the prior consent of the decedent or the consent of the decedent's surrogate decision maker makes perfusion ethically permissible. Perfusion without either prior specific consent to perfusion or general consent to organ donation violates requirements for informed consent for medical procedures and should not be permitted.

(5) The recipients of such procured organs should be informed of the source of the organs as well as any potential defects in the quality of the organs, so that they may decide with their physicians whether to accept the organs or wait for more suitable ones.

(6) Clear clinical criteria should be developed to ensure that only appropriate candidates, whose organs are reasonably likely to be suitable for transplantation, are considered eligible to donate organs under these protocols.
(I, III, V)

Issued June 1996 based on the reports "Ethical Issues in the Procurement of Organs Following Cardiac Death: The Pittsburgh Protocol," and "Ethical Issues in Organ Procurement Following Cardiac Death: In Situ Preservation of Cadaveric Organs," adopted December 1994.

2.16　Organ Transplantation Guidelines

The following statement is offered for guidance of physicians as they seek to maintain the highest level of ethical conduct in the transplanting of human organs.

(1) In all professional relationships between a physician and a patient, the physician's primary concern must be the health of the patient. The physician owes the patient primary allegiance. This concern and allegiance must be preserved in all medical procedures, including those which involve the transplantation of an organ from one person to another where both donor and recipient are patients. Care must, therefore, be taken to protect the rights of both the donor and the recipient, and no physician may assume a responsibility in organ transplantation unless the rights of both donor and recipient are equally protected. A prospective organ transplant offers no justification for a relaxation of the usual standard of medical care for the potential donor.

(2) When a vital, single organ is to be transplanted, the death of the donor shall have been determined by at least one physician other than the recipient's physician. Death shall be determined by the clinical judgment of the physician, who should rely on currently accepted and available scientific tests.

(3) Full discussion of the proposed procedure with the donor and the recipient or their responsible relatives or representatives is mandatory. The physician should ensure that consent to the procedure is fully informed and voluntary, in accordance with the Council's guidelines on informed consent. The physician's interest in advancing scientific knowledge must always be secondary to his or her concern for the patient.

(4) Transplant procedures of body organs should be undertaken (a) only by physicians who possess special medical knowledge and technical competence developed through special training, study, and laboratory experience and practice, and (b) in medical institutions with facilities adequate to protect the health and well-being of the parties to the procedure.

(5) Recipients of organs for transplantation should be determined in accordance with the Council's guidelines on the allocation of limited medical resources.

(6) Organs should be considered a national, rather than a local or regional, resource. Geographical priorities in the allocation of organs should be prohibited except when transportation of organs would threaten their suitability for transplantation.

(7) Patients should not be placed on the waiting lists of multiple local transplant centers, but rather on a single waiting list for each type of organ.
(I, III, V)

Issued prior to April 1977.

Updated June 1994 based on the report "Ethical Considerations in the Allocation of Organs and Other Scarce Medical Resources Among Patients," adopted June 1993.

Journal 2003 Considers the cause of persistent shortages of vaccines and other critical drugs. Concludes that government should take specific steps to encourage pharmaceutical manufacturers to supply these essential products. References Opinion 2.16. Noah, *Triage in the Nation's Medicine Cabinet: The Puzzling Scarcity of Vaccines and Other Drugs*, 54 S.C. L. Rev. 741, 755 (2003).

Journal 2003 Provides a moral and legal framework for considering the possibility of progress in managing technology applicable to organ transplantation. Concludes that progress in increasing the supply of organs will require an evolution in moral thinking. Quotes Opinion 2.16. Shapiro, *On the Possibility of "Progress" in Managing Biomedical Technologies: Markets, Lotteries, and Rational Moral Standards in Organ Transplantation*, 31 Cap. U. L. Rev. 13, 29 (2003).

Journal 2002 Provides ethical arguments in favor of transplantation in HIV-patients. Concludes that preventing such transplants is unethical and discriminatory. References Opinions 2.16 and 9.131. Halpern, Ubel, & Caplan, *Solid-Organ Transplantation in HIV-Infected Patients*, 347 New Eng. J. Med. 284, 287 (2002).

Journal 2000 Examines the criteria for organ transplantation. Explores the use of cognitive ability as an exclusion criterion for organ transplantation in children. Concludes that other useful neurologic criteria can be established to inform equitable allocation decisions. References Opinion 2.16. Orr, Johnston, Ashwal, & Bailey, *Should Children with Severe Cognitive Impairment Receive Solid Organ Transplants?* 11 J. Clinical Ethics 219, 222-23, 228 (2000).

Journal 1999 Examines the new federal rule mandating broader organ allocation. Raises various constitutional questions, particularly with respect to state laws regulating allocation of organs. Suggests that Congress needs to develop clearer guidelines in this area. Quotes Opinion 2.16. Chen, *Organ Allocation and the States: Can the States Restrict Broader Organ Sharing?*, 49 Duke L. J. 261, 273 (1999).

Journal 1999 Attributes distrust and dissatisfaction with managed care organizations to individualism and cynicism in society. Argues that proposed reforms will not solve society's problems with managed care organizations. Recommends an alternate health care system that would strike a balance between considerations of patient autonomy and cost containment. References Opinion 2.16. Harris, *The Regulation of Managed Care: Conquering Individualism and Cynicism in America*, 6 Va. J. Soc. Pol'y. & L. 315, 329 (1999).

Journal 1999 Discusses the need for physicians to advocate on behalf of patients' rights in the context of health care delivery. Evaluates the nature and scope of the physician's role as advocate, noting that physicians cannot be expected to engage in attorney-like advocacy. Quotes Principles IV and VI, Fundamental Elements (2), (4), and (6) [now Opinion 10.01], Patient Responsibilities 5 [now Opinion 10.02], and Opinions 2.03, 2.07, 2.09, 2.16, 2.19, 3.06, 4.01, 4.04, 6.01, 7.02, 8.02, 8.03, 8.13, 8.132, 9.06, 9.07, and 9.131. Cites Opinions 5.05, 5.09, 7.01, 8.135, and 9.02. Sage, *Physicians as Advocates*, 35 Hous. L. Rev. 1529, 1537, 1541, 1542, 1552-53, 1554, 1556, 1557, 1559, 1561-62, 1564, 1571, 1574, 1576, 1580 (1999).

Journal 1987 Discusses the issue of the right of the individual to consent to organ removal and then examines the doctrine of informed consent as it is applied in the context of live organ donation. Evaluates the extent to which removal of non-regenerative organs disrupts the basis for application of the traditional informed consent model with special attention to children and incompetent patients. Quotes Opinion 2.15 (1986) [now Opinion 2.16]. Adams, *Live Organ Donors and Informed Consent: A Difficult Minuet*, 8 J. Legal Med. 555, 560-61 (1987).

2.161   Medical Applications of Fetal Tissue Transplantation

The principal ethical concern in the use of human fetal tissue for transplantation is the degree to which the decision to have an abortion might be influenced by the decision to donate the fetal tissue. In the application of fetal tissue transplantation the following safeguards should apply: (1) The Council on Ethical and Judicial Affairs' guidelines on clinical investigation and organ transplantation are followed, as they pertain to the recipient of the fetal tissue transplant (see Opinion 2.07, "Clinical Investigation," and Opinion 2.16, "Organ Transplantation Guidelines"); (2) a final decision regarding abortion is made before initiating a discussion of the transplantation use of fetal tissue; (3) decisions regarding the technique used to induce abortion, as well as the timing of the abortion in relation to the gestational age of the fetus, are based on concern for the safety of the pregnant woman; (4) fetal tissue is not provided in exchange for financial remuneration above that which is necessary to cover reasonable expenses; (5) the recipient of the tissue is not designated by the donor; (6) health care personnel involved in the termination of a particular pregnancy do not participate in or receive any benefit from the transplantation of tissue from the abortus of the same pregnancy; and (7) informed consent on behalf of both the donor and the recipient is obtained in accordance with applicable law. (I, IV, V)

Issued March 1992 based on the report "Medical Applications of Fetal Tissue Transplantation," adopted June 1989 (JAMA. 1990; 263: 565-70).

Updated June 1996.

Journal 2002 Observes that changes in the health professions challenge certain assumptions about professional ethics. Concludes that these long-standing assumptions must be re-examined. Cites Opinion 2.161. References Opinion 8.13. Kelley, *The Meanings of Professional Life: Teaching Across the Health Professions*, 27 J. Med. & Phil. 475, 485, 490, 491 (2002).

Journal 1990 Presents an update on current medical research regarding Parkinson's disease. Discusses the relevance of fetal tissue transplantation to this research. References Opinion 2.161. Joynt, *Neurology*, 263 JAMA 2660 (1990).

2.162 Anencephalic Neonates as Organ Donors

Anencephaly is a congenital absence of major portion of the brain, skull, and scalp. Anencephalic neonates are thought to be unique from other brain-damaged beings because of a lack of past consciousness with no potential for future consciousness.

Physicians may provide anencephalic neonates with ventilator assistance and other medical therapies that are necessary to sustain organ perfusion and viability until such time as a determination of death can be made in accordance with accepted medical standards, relevant law, and regional organ procurement organization policy. Retrieval and transplantation of the organs of anencephalic infants are ethically permissible only after such determination of death is made, and only in accordance with the Council's guidelines for transplantation. (I, III, V)

Issued March 1992 based on the report "Anencephalic Infants as Organ Donors," adopted December 1988.

Updated June 1994; updated December 1994 based on the report "The Use of Anencephalic Neonates as Organ Donors," adopted December 1994; (JAMA. 1995; 273: 1614-18.) and updated June 1996 based on the report "Anencephalic Infants as Organ Donors—Reconsideration," adopted December 1995.

Journal 2003 Explores the ethical, legal, and clinical implications of non-heart beating organ donation. Concludes that, if ambiguities are clarified, non-heart beating organ donation can achieve an ethical good. References Opinions 2.155 and 2.162. Bell, *Non-heart Beating Organ Donation: Old Procurement Strategy—New Ethical Problems*, 29 J. Med. Ethics 176, 181 (2003).

Journal 2003 Discusses how legal norms can be challenged by advances in medical knowledge. Concludes that sources beyond the law should be considered to prevent untoward legal outcomes. References Opinion 2.162. Mayo, *Sex, Marriage, Medicine, and Law: "What Hope of Harmony?"* 42 Washburn L.J. 269, 271 (2003).

Journal 1999 Discusses legal, medical, social, and ethical issues regarding organ donation by anencephalic infants. Points out the dangers surrounding anencephalic organ donation versus parents' needs for good to come out of the lives of their anencephalic children. References Opinion 2.162. Bard, *The Diagnosis is Anencephaly and the Parents Ask About Organ Donation: Now What? A Guide for Hospital Counsel and Ethics Committees*, 21 W. New Eng. L. Rev. 49, 62 (1999).

Journal 1999 Discusses the Uniform Declaration of Death Act and the dead-donor rule. Provides ethical justifications for sustaining current policies on non-heart-beating organ donation. Cites Opinions 2.06 and 2.162. DuBois, *Non-Heart-Beating Organ Donation: A Defense of the Required Determination of Death*, 27 J. Law, Med. & Ethics 126, 128 (1999).

Journal 1999 Explains that shortages in available organs have prompted a movement that favors modifying the dead-donor rule. Discusses different proposals to amend the dead-donor rule. Suggests that even the slightest modification of the rule will prompt strong opposition. References Opinion 2.162. Robertson, *The Dead Donor Rule*, 29 Hastings Center Rep. 6, 13 (Nov./Dec. 1999).

Journal 1999 Discusses national and international legislative proposals addressing human cloning. Considers human cloning for reproductive and nonreproductive reasons. Undertakes legal analysis and concludes that human cloning should not be banned completely. Cites Opinion 2.162. Smith, *Ignorance is Not Bliss: Why a Ban on Human Cloning is Unacceptable*, 9 Health Matrix. 311, 330, 331 (1999).

Journal 1998 Examines American and British views on the brain death test and advance directives. Points out that the brain death test has been criticized in cases where patients woke up after being in a coma for long periods of time. Argues that better utilization of advance directives may dissipate arguments for euthanasia. References Opinion 2.162. Trew, *Regulating Life and Death: The Modification and Commodification of Nature*, 29 U. Tol. L. Rev. 271, 292 (1998).

Journal 1996 Explores courses of treatment for infants born with hypoplastic left heart syndrome. Discusses the various treatment options available to infants, and their frequency. Notes the controversy surrounding the AMA's opinion on anencephalic infants as organ donors. References Opinion 2.162 [subsequently amended]. Caplan, Cooper, Garcia-Prats, & Brody, *Diffusion of Innovative Approaches to Managing Hypoplastic Left Heart Syndrome*, 150 Arch. Pediatr. Adolesc. Med. 487, 490 (1996).

Journal 1996 Describes the impact of federal laws on medical decisions for anencephalic infants. Discusses selective nontreatment of such infants and the debate regarding availability of their organs for transplantation. Quotes Opinions 2.162 (1994) [subsequently amended] and 2.17. Crossley, *Infants with Anencephaly, the ADA, and the Child Abuse Amendments*, 11 Issues in Law & Med. 379, 385, 409 (1996).

Journal 1996 Proposes an alternative method of capital punishment to allow for organ donation by executed prisoners. Provides justifications for this proposal. Concludes that physicians should be able to ethically participate in this process. Quotes Principle VII. Cites Opinion 2.06. References Opinion 2.162 (1994) [subsequently amended]. Patton, *A Call for Common Sense: Organ Donation and the Executed Prisoner*, 3 Va. J. Soc. Pol'y & L. 387, 404, 405, 407-10 (1996).

Journal 1996 Examines the recent trend in health care laws and ethics to focus on the alleviation of suffering. Expresses concern that such a focus may result in the valuation of one life over another. Emphasizes the need to evaluate multiple, diverse responses to suffering. Quotes Principle VI. References Opinion 2.162. Shepherd, *Sophie's Choices: Medical and Legal Responses to Suffering*, 72 Notre Dame L. Rev. 103, 106, 133 (1996).

Journal 1994 Criticizes both the White House's proposed National Bioethics Advisory Commission and certain purely private ethical advisory bodies. Proposes that an appropriately organized new federal advisory body could provide essential guidance in developing public bioethical policies, particularly if the meaningful input of ethics scholars at universities, ethics centers, and other private organizations and public commissions were sought. Cites Opinion 2.162. Capron, *Ethics: Public and Private*, 24 Hastings Center Rep. 26, 27 (November/December 1994).

2.165   Fetal Umbilical Cord Blood

Human umbilical cord blood has been identified as a viable source of hematopoietic stem cells that can be used as an alternative to bone marrow for transplantation. It is obtained by clamping the umbilical cord immediately after delivery.

The use of umbilical cord blood raises two main ethical problems. First, the exact timing of the clamping has a significant impact on the neonate. Studies indicate that early clamping may cause an abrupt surge in arterial pressure, resulting in intraventricular hemorrhage (particularly in premature infants). Second, there is a risk that the infant donor will develop a need for his or her own cord blood later in life. If that child was a donor and this later need arises, he or she might be without blood, when he or she could have had his or her own blood stored.

To avoid health risks, normal clamping protocol should be followed and not altered in such a way that might endanger the infant. Additionally, parents of the infant must be fully informed of the risks of the donation and written consent should be obtained from them.

The second concern, that the child may need the blood later in life, is more complex. The possibility that an infant donor would be in need of his or her own umbilical cord blood is highly speculative. There are a number of reasons why the infant may not need the blood later. The diseases that are treated by bone marrow transplantation are not common, and there may be other treatment alternatives available, particularly in the future when the illness would occur. Additionally, the demand for fetal umbilical cord blood will increase as it becomes medically certain that the blood may be used in persons unrelated to the donor. This situation will reduce the need to store a particular infant's blood since umbilical cord blood from other donors would be available. If the blood is sufficient for use in unrelated individuals, then the donor may obtain the cord blood from another donor later in life, making the need to store his or her own blood unnecessary. These original donors, however, should be given priority in receipt of such blood if they need a donation later in life.

For all of these reasons, it would generally not be unethical to use the cord blood. However, if the child-donor is known to be at risk for an illness that is treated by bone marrow donation, the child should not be used as a donor, and his or her blood should be stored for future use. (I, V)

Issued June 1994.

Updated June 1996.

2.167 The Use of Minors as Organ and Tissue Donors

Minors need not be prohibited from acting as sources of organs, but their participation should be limited. Different procedures pose different degrees of risk and do not all require the same restrictions. In general, minors should not be permitted to serve as a source when there is a very serious risk of complications (eg, partial liver or lung donation, which involve a substantial risk of serious immediate or long-term morbidity). If the safeguards in the remainder of this opinion are followed, minors may be permitted to serve as a source when the risks are low (eg, blood or skin donation, in which the donated tissue can regenerate and spinal or general anesthesia is not required), moderate (eg, bone marrow donation, in which the donated tissue can regenerate but brief general or spinal anesthesia is required), or serious (eg, kidney donation, which involve more extensive anesthesia and major invasive surgery).

If a child is capable of making his or her own medical treatment decisions, he or she should be considered capable of deciding whether to be an organ or tissue donor. However, physicians should not perform organ retrievals of serious risk without first obtaining court authorization. Courts should confirm that the mature minor is acting voluntarily and without coercion.

If a child is not capable of making his or her own medical decisions, all transplantations should have parental approval, and those which pose a serious risk should receive court authorization. In the court authorization process, the evaluation of a child psychiatrist or psychologist must be sought and a guardian ad litem should be assigned to the potential minor donor in order to fully represent the minor's interests.

When deciding on behalf of immature children, parents and courts should ensure that transplantation presents a "clear benefit" to the minor source, which entails meeting the following requirements:

(1) Ideally the minor should be the only possible source. All other available sources of organs, both donor pools and competent adult family members, must be medically inappropriate or significantly inferior. An unwilling potential donor does not qualify him/her as medically inappropriate.

(2) For transplantations of moderate or serious risk, the transplantation must be necessary with some degree of medical certainty to provide a substantial benefit; that is, it both prevents an extremely poor quality of life and ensures a good quality of life for the recipient. A transplant should not be allowed if it merely increases the comfort of the recipient. If a transplant is not presently considered to provide a substantial benefit but is expected to do so within a period of time, the transplant need not be delayed until it meets this criterion, especially if the delay would significantly decrease the benefits derived from the transplant by the recipient.

(3) The organ or tissue transplant must have a reasonable probability of success in order for transplantation to be allowed. What constitutes a reasonable chance of success should be based on medical judgments about the physical condition of the recipient and the likelihood that the transplant will not be rejected, futile, or produce benefits which are very transient. Children should not be used for transplants that are considered experimental or non-standard.

(4) Generally, minors should be allowed to serve as a source only to close family members.

(5) Psychological or emotional benefits to the potential source may be considered, though evidence of future benefit to the minor source should be clear and convincing. Possible benefits to a child include continued emotional bonds between the minor and the recipient, increased self-esteem, and prevention of adverse reaction to death of a sibling. Whether a child will capture these benefits depends upon the child's specific circumstances. A minor's assent or dissent to a procedure is an important piece of evidence that demonstrates whether the transplant will offer psychological benefits to the source. Dissent from incompetent minors should be powerful evi-

dence that the donation will not provide a clear benefit, but may not present an absolute bar. Every effort should be made to identify and address the child's concerns in this case.

(6) It is essential to ensure that the potential source does not have any underlying conditions that create an undue individual risk. (I, V)

Issued June 1994 based on the report "The Use of Minors as Organ and Tissue Donors," adopted December 1993.

2.169 The Ethical Implications of Xenotransplantation

Xenotransplantation includes any procedure that involves the transplantation, implantation, or infusion into a human recipient of either (a) live cells, tissues, or organs from a non-human animal source or (b) human body fluids, cells, tissues or organs that have had ex vivo contact with live non-human animal cells, tissues, or organs. Although xenotransplantation offers a potential source of tissue, and organs for medical procedures, research in this area may uncover physical and psychological conditions that require medical attention. As such, physicians need to be involved in developing and implementing guidelines for continued research. Therefore, the following guidelines are offered for the medical and scientific communities:

(1) Physicians should encourage education and public discussion of xenotransplantation because of the potential unique risks such procedures pose to individual patients and the public.

(2) The medical and scientific communities should support oversight for the development of clinical trial protocols and of ongoing xenotransplantation research.

(3) Given the uncertain risk xenotransplantation poses to society, participants in early clinical trials may have to agree to (a) postoperative measures such as life-long surveillance, disclosure of sexual contacts, autopsy; and (b) a waiver of the traditional right to withdraw from a clinical trial until the risk of late xenozoonoses is reasonably known not to exist. These requirements may continue even if the transplanted tissue is rejected or removed. The informed consent process should include a discussion of the above issues as well as potential risks to third parties and psychological concerns associated with receiving an organ or tissue graft from an animal. Careful attention must be paid to both the content of the consent disclosure and the manner in which consent is obtained.

(4) It would be ethical to include children and incompetent adults in xenotransplantation research protocols only when the patients are terminally ill and alternative treatments are not available.

(5) Allocation protocols must be fair and in accordance with Opinion 2.03, "Allocation of Limited Medical Resources," which recommends that decisions regarding the allocation of medical resources among patients be based only on ethically appropriate criteria relating to medical need. These criteria include, but are not limited to, the likelihood of benefit, the urgency of need, the change in quality of life, the duration of benefit, and, in some cases, the amount of resources required for treatment.

(6) Sponsors of xenotransplantation research should assure that adequate funding exists for life-long surveillance and treatment of complications arising from xenotransplantation procedures on research subjects.

(7) At a minimum, all on-going research should adhere to the Public Health Service Guideline on Infectious Disease Issues in Xenotransplantation, FDA guidelines relating to xenotransplantation, Opinion 2.07 "Clinical Research," and any additional precautionary measures believed to minimize potential risks to the public or to patients. It is inappropriate to participate in xenograft procedures outside federal guidelines.

(8) All xenotransplantation research should continue to promote high standards of care and humane treatment of all animals used in research (H-460.979, "Use of Animals in Research") and to apply these standards to the care and treatment of animals used as sources of transplantation material. (IV, VII)

Issued June 2001 based on the report "The Ethical Implications of Xenotransplantation," adopted December 2000.

2.17 Quality of Life

In the making of decisions for the treatment of seriously disabled newborns or of other persons who are severely disabled by injury or illness, the primary consideration should be what is best for the individual patient and not the avoidance of a burden to the family or to society. Quality of life, as defined by the patient's interests and values, is a factor to be considered in determining what is best for the individual. It is permissible to consider quality of life when deciding about life-sustaining treatment in accordance with Opinions 2.20, "Withholding or Withdrawing Life-Sustaining Medical Treatment," 2.215, "Treatment Decisions for Seriously Ill Newborns," and 2.22, "Do-Not-Resuscitate Orders." (I, III, IV)

Issued March 1981.

Updated June 1994.

N.J. Super. 1983 Guardian of elderly nursing home patient suffering from severe organic brain syndrome sought to remove nasogastric tube from patient. Trial court granted guardian's petition, and patient's guardian ad litem appealed. Appellate court reversed, in part based upon Opinions 2.11 (1981) and 5.17 (1979) [now Opinions 2.17 and 2.20], and held that it is improper and would violate medical ethics to allow dehydration and starvation in a non-comatose, non-brain-dead patient not facing imminent death, not maintained by any life-support machine, and not able to speak for herself. *In re Conroy, 190 N.J. Super. 453, 464 A.2d 303, 313-15, rev'd, 98 N.J. 321, 486 A.2d 1209 (1985).*

Journal 2001 Observes that many aspects of managed care have increased the tensions between patients and their health care providers. Notes that patient dissatisfaction is on the rise for other reasons as well. Concludes that Congress should take a comprehensive legislative approach in addressing these issues. Quotes Opinion 2.17. Cites Opinion 2.035. References Opinions 2.037 and 2.22. Sanematsu, *Taking a Broader View of Treatment Disputes Beyond Managed Care: Are Recent Legislative Efforts the Cure? 48 UCLA L. Rev. 1245, 1258, 1284 (2001).*

Journal 1999 Advocates on behalf of allowing physicians to legally prescribe marijuana in certain medical situations. Discusses use of marijuana to slow the process of severe weight loss among AIDS patients. Argues in favor of reclassifying marijuana from a Schedule I drug to a Schedule II drug, thus allowing lawful prescription use. Cites Opinion 2.17. Wolfson, *A Quality of Mercy: The*

Struggle of the AIDS-Afflicted to Use Marijuana as Medicine, 22 T. Jefferson L. Rev. 1, 24 (1999).

Journal 1999 Discusses the decision in *Conant v. McCaffrey*, which precluded the government from prosecuting physicians who recommended marijuana to patients for medical use. Examines the ramifications of removing physician judgment from medical decisions. Argues that the federal government should retract its restriction on the medical prescription and use of marijuana. Cites Opinion 2.17. Dixon, *Conant v. McCaffrey: Physicians, Marijuana, and the First Amendment, 70 U. Colo. L. Rev. 975, 977 (1999).*

Journal 1997 Considers percutaneous endoscopic gastrostomy tubes and the lack of standards for their placement. Discusses the medical and ethical problems involved, and creates a method for reconciling them. Recommends that patients in a persistent vegetative state not undergo the procedure. References Opinion 2.17. Rabeneck, McCullough, & Wray, *Ethically Justified, Clinically Comprehensive Guidelines for Percutaneous Endoscopic Gastrostomy Tube Placement, 349 Lancet 496, 497, 498 (1997).*

Journal 1996 Explores decision-making standards employed in the removal of medical treatment from incompetent patients. Suggests substituted judgment and best interests standards be replaced by a standard that focuses on patient dignity. Concludes that treatment should be removed when empirical evidence suggests a majority of individuals would want it removed. Cites Opinion 2.16 (1986) [now Opinion 2.17]. Cantor, *Discarding Substituted Judgment and Best Interests: Toward a Constructive Preference Standard for Dying, Previously Competent Patients Without Advance Instructions, 48 Rutgers L. Rev. 1193, 1234, 1247 (1996).*

Journal 1996 Examines the medical use of marijuana in a legal and ethical context. Posits that legal prohibitions against medical use of marijuana infringe upon patient autonomy and the physician-patient relationship. Concludes that societal laws should be modified to allow for regulated medical use of marijuana. Quotes Opinion 2.17. Comment, *Medical Use of Marijuana: Legal and Ethical Conflicts in the Patient-Physician Relationship, 30 U. Rich. L. Rev. 249, 268-69 (1996).*

Journal 1996 Describes the impact of federal laws on medical decisions for anencephalic infants. Discusses selective nontreatment of such infants and the debate regarding availability of their organs for transplantation. Quotes Opinions 2.162 (1994) [subsequently amended] and 2.17. Crossley, *Infants with Anencephaly, the ADA, and the Child Abuse Amendments, 11 Issues in Law & Med. 379, 385, 409 (1996).*

Journal 1994 Considers how greater patient autonomy has led to situations in which medical care may be viewed as futile. Suggests that the law has intruded too far into this area of medicine. Quotes Opinion 2.035. Cites Opinions 2.03, 2.095, 2.17, 2.19, 2.20, and 2.22. Cultice, *Medical Futility: When Is Enough, Enough?, 27 J. Health & Hosp. Law 225, 230, 256 (1994).*

Journal 1993 Discusses the problem of physicians withholding needed medical treatment from HIV-infected infants. Concludes that current law should be expanded to eliminate this discrimination. Quotes Opinions 2.09, 2.17, 2.20, 2.22, 4.04, and 8.03. Crossley, *Of Diagnoses and Discrimination: Discriminatory Nontreatment of Infants With HIV Infection, 93 Columbia L. Rev. 1581, 1620, 1621 (1993).*

Journal 1993 Argues that society should not permit euthanasia because of lack of protection against potential abuses. Recommends that health care providers be taught to treat pain and more effectively care for dying patients, rather than to affirmatively end life. Quotes Opinions 2.17 and 2.20. Dickey, *Euthanasia: A Concept Whose Time Has Come?, 8 Issues in Law & Med. 521, 523, 524 (1993).*

Journal 1992 Suggests that triage and cost-benefit analysis are the most effective means to evaluate issues associated with allocating scarce medical resources to disabled infants. Concludes both that selective treatment can never be considered murder and that governmental intrusion in this area should be minimal. Quotes Opinions 2.10 (1982) [now Opinion 2.17] and 2.18 (1986) [now Opinion 2.20]. Smith, *Murder, She Wrote or Was It Merely Selective Nontreatment?, 8 J. Contemp. Health L. & Pol'y 49, 53 (1992).*

Journal 1990 Questions the value of medical treatment that is futile or may prolong suffering. Proposes that physicians be permitted to write Do-Not-Resuscitate orders, in certain cases, without the consent of the family. Quotes Opinion 2.17. Hackler & Hiller, *Family Consent to Orders Not To Resuscitate: Reconsidering Hospital Policy, 264 JAMA 1281, 1282 (1990).*

Journal 1989 Examines the federal Baby Doe rule, and its implementing regulations, which require treatment of disabled infants in all but the most obviously hopeless cases. Concludes that the rule is insensitive to the complexities of the moral issue, and that state constitutions may prohibit local legislative adoption of the federal requirements. Quotes Opinion 2.14 (1984) [now Opinion 2.17]. Newman, *Baby Doe, Congress and the States: Challenging the Federal Treatment Standard for Impaired Infants,* XV Am. J. Law and Med. 1, 42, 47 (1989).

Journal 1986 Discusses the fact that the legal system has granted substantial professional autonomy to physicians. As a result, medical professionals have exerted dominance over individual health care decisions, particularly in the context of infanticide, or withholding of treatment from severely handicapped infants. Quotes Opinion 2.10 (1982) [now Opinion 2.17]. Malone, *Medical Authority and Infanticide,* 1 J. Law & Health 77, 94, 96 (1985-86).

Journal 1985 Discusses the constitutional rights of newborns with birth defects, noting that they are persons within the meaning of the fourteenth amendment. Observes that the fundamental right to life applies equally to healthy newborns as well as newborns with birth defects and concludes that the newborn's future quality of life with a disability should not be a factor in assessing whether medical treatment is in the child's best interest. Quotes from Opinion 2.10 (1982) [now Opinion 2.17]. Comment, *Withholding Life-saving Treatment From Defective Newborns: An Equal Protection Analysis,* 29 St. Louis Univ. L. J. 853, 854 (1985).

Journal 1982 From a legal viewpoint, focuses on the effect of abortion decisions on nontreatment of defective neonates issues as well as decisions that directly address the nontreatment issue. Also provides general discussion of the wide range of moral attitudes expressed by physicians on withholding treatment, the meaning of the terms ordinary and extraordinary care, and the question of who should bear the responsibility for deciding to treat or not to treat defective neonates. Quotes Opinion 2.10 (1981) [now Opinion 2.17]. Taub, *Withholding Treatment From Defective Newborns,* 10 Law, Med. & Health Care 4, 8 (Feb. 1982).

Journal 1981 Discusses a Danville, Illinois, case in which the Illinois Department of Children and Family Services successfully opposed the decision of the physician and parents not to feed newborn Siamese twins. Focuses on both moral and legal aspects of nontreatment decisions, and discusses the common, yet controversial nature of decisions not to treat, categorization of birth defects for purposes of moral decisionmaking, the importance of medical and social information in nontreatment decisions, the legal duty to treat such children, and substantive and procedural criteria for nontreatment decisions. Quotes Opinion 2.10 (1981) [now Opinion 2.17]. Robertson, *Dilemma in Danville,* 11 Hastings Center Rep. 5, 7 (Oct. 1981).

2.18   Surrogate Mothers

"Surrogate" motherhood involves the artificial insemination of a woman who agrees, usually in return for payment, to give the resulting child to the child's father by surrendering her parental rights. Often, the father's infertile wife becomes the child's adoptive mother. The woman bearing the child is in most cases genetically related to the child, though gestational surrogacy (in which the ovum is provided by the father's infertile wife or other donor) is possible as well.

Ethical, social, and legal problems may arise in surrogacy arrangements. Surrogate motherhood may commodify children and women's reproductive capacities, exploit poor women whose decision to participate may not be wholly voluntary, and improperly discourage or interfere with the formation of a natural maternal-fetal or maternal-child bond. Psychological impairment may occur in a woman who deliberately conceives with the intention of bearing a child which she will give up. In addition, the woman who has contracted to bear the child may decide to have an abortion or to refuse to relinquish her parental rights. Alternatively, if there is a subsequent birth of a disabled child, prospective parents and the birth mother may not want to or will be unable to assume the responsibilities of parenthood.

On the other hand, surrogate motherhood arrangements are often the last hope of prospective parents to have a child that is genetically related to at least one of them. In addition, most surrogacy arrangements are believed by the parties involved to be mutually beneficial, and most are completed without mishap or dispute. In light of the concerns expressed above, however, some safeguards are necessary to protect the welfare of the child and the birth mother. The Council believes that surrogacy contracts, while permissible, should grant the birth mother the right to void the contract within a reasonable period of time after the birth of the child. If the contract is voided, custody of the child should be determined according to the child's best interests.

In gestational surrogacy, in which the surrogate mother has no genetic tie to the fetus, the justification for allowing the surrogate mother to void the contract becomes less clear. Gestational surrogacy contracts should be strictly enforceable (ie, not voidable by either party). (I, II, IV)

Issued December 1983.

Updated June 1994.

Journal 2000 Examines questions regarding the legality of such practices as voluntary stopping of eating and drinking (VSED), use of risky analgesics, and terminal sedation. Explores the distinctions between physician-assisted suicide and other palliative interventions. Concludes VSED, risky analgesics, and certain types of terminal sedation are lawful and should be made available to dying patients who make informed decisions to accept the risks involved. Quotes Opinions 2.21 and 2.211. Cites Opinions 2.18 and 2.20. Cantor & Thomas, *The Legal Bounds of Physician Conduct Hastening Death*, 48 Buff. L. Rev. 83, 110, 131, 158 (2000).

Journal 1990 Argues that gestational surrogacy, because of its inherent medical, ethical, and legal complications, is not an acceptable reproductive alternative. Discusses the California Superior Court case of *Johnson v. Calvert* in which a gestational surrogacy contract was held valid and the genetic parents were found to have exclusive custody and parental rights. Quotes Opinion 2.18 (1988). Rothenberg, *Gestational Surrogacy and the Health Care Provider: Put Part of the IVF Genie Back Into the Bottle*, 18 Law, Med. & Health Care 345, 346 (1990).

Journal 1987 Examines various ethical issues surrounding surrogate motherhood, artificial insemination, in vitro fertilization and embryonic/fetal research. Reports on the positions of four ethics groups: the Warnock Committee of Inquiry into Human Fertilization and Embryology; the AMA's Council on Ethical and Judicial Affairs; the Ethics Committee of the American Fertility Society; and the Ethics Committee of the American College of Obstetricians and Gynecologists. References Opinions 2.04, 2.05, and 2.13 (1986) [now Opinion 2.14]. Quotes Opinion 2.18. Rosner, Cassell, Friedland, Landolt, Loeb, Numann, Ora, Risemberg, & Sordillo, *Ethical Considerations of Reproductive Technologies*, 87 N.Y. State J. Med. 398, 399-400 (1987).

2.19   Unnecessary Medical Services

Physicians should not provide, prescribe, or seek compensation for medical services that they know are unnecessary. (II, VII)

Issued prior to April 1977.

Updated June 1996; Updated December 2003.

Journal 1999 Discusses the need for physicians to advocate on behalf of patients' rights in the context of health care delivery. Evaluates the nature and scope of the physician's role as advocate, noting that physicians cannot be expected to engage in attorney-like advocacy. Quotes Principles IV and VI, Fundamental Elements (2), (4), and (6) [now Opinion 10.01], Patient Responsibilities 5 [now Opinion 10.02], and Opinions 2.03, 2.07, 2.09, 2.16, 2.19, 3.06, 4.01, 4.04, 6.01, 7.02, 8.02, 8.03, 8.13, 8.132, 9.06, 9.07, and 9.131. Cites Opinions 5.05, 5.09, 7.01, 8.135, and 9.02.

Sage, *Physicians as Advocates*, 35 Hous. L. Rev. 1529, 1537, 1541, 1542, 1552-53, 1554, 1556, 1557, 1559, 1561-62, 1564, 1571, 1574, 1576, 1580 (1999).

Journal 1994 Considers how greater patient autonomy has led to situations in which medical care may be viewed as futile. Suggests that the law has intruded too far into this area of medicine. Quotes Opinion 2.035. Cites Opinions 2.03, 2.095, 2.17, 2.19, 2.20, and 2.22. Cultice, *Medical Futility: When Is Enough, Enough?*, 27 J. Health & Hosp. Law 225, 230, 256 (1994).

Journal 1991 Looks at the physician as a fiduciary and the law governing fiduciary relationships. Concludes that fiduciary concepts are a valuable basis for establishing ethical and legal guidelines for physician behavior. Quotes Opinions 2.19, 8.03 (1989) [now Opinion 8.032], and 8.06. Healey & Dowling, *Controlling Conflicts of Interest in the Doctor-Patient Relationship: Lessons From Moore v. Regents of the University of California*, 42 Mercer L. Rev. 989, 997, 998 (1991).

Journal 1991 Examines the issues surrounding judicial use of professional ethics codes in private litigation. Concludes that judges should more extensively use professional ethics codes to define public policy, standards of care, and legal causes of action. Quotes Principle II and Opinion 2.19. Note, *Professional Ethics Codes in Court: Redefining the Social Contract Between the Public and the Professions*, 25 Georgia L. Rev. 1327, 1335, 1351 (1991).

Journal 1990 Discusses efforts of third-party payors to control health care expenditures for beneficiaries. Concludes that financial incentives to limit care and other cost control techniques should be disclosed and that the rationale for such disclosure is compelling. Quotes Opinions 2.03, 2.09, and 8.03. Cites Opinions 2.19, 4.04, and 4.06. Hirshfeld, *Should Third Party Payors of Health Care Services Disclose Cost Control Mechanisms to Potential Beneficiaries?*, 14 Seton Hall Legis. J. 115, 130, 131, 144, 145, 146 (1990).

Journal 1986 Discusses the Missouri living will statute and the Death-Prolonging Procedures Act. Examines the extent to which these laws ensure individuals the right to make choices regarding personal medical treatment in the event of terminal illness, even if they become incompetent. Quotes Opinion 2.12 (1981) [now Opinion 2.19]. Johnson, *The Death-Prolonging Procedures Act and Refusal of Treatment in Missouri*, 30 St. Louis Univ. L. J. 805, 816 (1986).

2.20   Withholding or Withdrawing Life-Sustaining Medical Treatment

The social commitment of the physician is to sustain life and relieve suffering. Where the performance of one duty conflicts with the other, the preferences of the patient should prevail. The principle of patient autonomy requires that physicians respect the decision to forego life-sustaining treatment of a patient who possesses decision-making capacity. Life-sustaining treatment is any treatment that serves to prolong life without reversing the underlying medical condition. Life-sustaining treatment may include, but is not limited to, mechanical ventilation, renal dialysis, chemotherapy, antibiotics, and artificial nutrition and hydration.

There is no ethical distinction between withdrawing and withholding life-sustaining treatment.

A competent, adult patient may, in advance, formulate and provide a valid consent to the withholding or withdrawal of life-support systems in the event that injury or illness renders that individual incompetent to make such a decision. A patient may also appoint a surrogate decision maker in accordance with state law.

If the patient receiving life-sustaining treatment is incompetent, a surrogate decision maker should be identified. Without an advance directive that designates a proxy, the patient's family should become the surrogate decision maker. Family includes persons with whom the patient is closely associated. In the case when there is no person closely associated with the patient, but there are persons who both care about the patient and have sufficient relevant knowledge of the patient, such persons may be appropriate surrogates. Physicians should provide all relevant medical information and explain to surrogate decision makers that decisions regarding withholding or withdrawing life-sustaining treatment should be based on substituted judgment (what the patient would have decided) when there is evidence of the patient's preferences and values. In making a substituted judgment, decision makers may consider the patient's advance directive (if any); the patient's values about life and the way it should be lived; and the patient's attitudes towards sickness, suffering, medical procedures, and death. If there is not adequate evidence of the incompetent patient's preferences and values, the decision should be based on the best interests of the patient (what outcome would most likely promote the patient's well-being).

Though the surrogate's decision for the incompetent patient should almost always be accepted by the physician, there are four situations that may require either institutional or judicial review and/or intervention in the decision-making process: (1) there is no available family member willing to be the patient's surrogate decision maker; (2) there is a dispute among family members and there is no decision maker designated in an advance directive; (3) a health care provider believes that the family's decision is clearly not what the patient would have decided if competent; and (4) a health care provider believes that the decision is not a decision that could reasonably be judged to be in the patient's best interests. When there are disputes among family members or between family and health care providers, the use of ethics committees specifically designed to facilitate sound decision making is recommended before resorting to the courts.

When a permanently unconscious patient was never competent or had not left any evidence of previous preferences or values, since there is no objective way to ascertain the best interests of the patient, the surrogate's decision should not be challenged as long as the decision is based on the decision maker's true concern for what would be best for the patient.

Physicians have an obligation to relieve pain and suffering and to promote the dignity and autonomy of dying patients in their care. This includes providing effective palliative treatment even though it may foreseeably hasten death.

Even if the patient is not terminally ill or permanently unconscious, it is not unethical to discontinue all means of life-sustaining medical treatment in accordance with a proper substituted judgment or best interests analysis.
(I, III, IV, V)

Issued December 1984 as Opinion 2.18, Withholding or Withdrawing Life-Prolonging Medical Treatment, and Opinion 2.19, Withholding or Withdrawing Life-Prolonging Medical Treatment—Patients' Preferences. In 1989, these opinions were renumbered 2.20 and 2.21, respectively.

Updated June 1994 based on the reports "Decisions Near the End of Life" and "Decisions to Forego Life-Sustaining Treatment for Incompetent Patients," both adopted June 1991 (Decisions Near the End of Life. JAMA. 1992; 267: 2229-33), and updated June 1996. [In March, 1981, the Council on Ethical and Judicial Affairs issued Opinion 2.11, *Terminal Illness*. The opinion was renumbered 2.15 in 1984 and was deleted in 1986.]

U.S. 1997 Several physicians and terminally ill patients sued the state seeking a declaration that its prohibition against physician-assisted suicide violates the Fourteenth Amendment's Equal Protection Clause. The trial court disagreed, but the Second Circuit reversed, holding that the state accords different treatment to those terminally ill patients who wish to hasten their death by self-administering prescribed drugs and to those patients who wish to do so by directing the removal of life support systems. The Supreme Court reversed holding that the prohibition against assisting suicide does not violate the Equal Protection Clause. The Court concluded that there is a distinction between assisting suicide and withdrawing treatment quoting reports of the AMA Council on Ethical and Judicial Affairs [now Opinions 2.20 and 2.211]. *Vacco v. Quill, 117 S. Ct. 2293, 2298, 138 L. Ed. 2d 834.*

U.S. 1990 Parents of patient in persistent vegetative state appealed denial of request to discontinue gastrotomy feeding tube. The Supreme Court held that the federal constitution did not forbid the state's requirement of clear and convincing evidence of an incompetent patient's wishes regarding the withdrawal of life-prolonging treatment. The Court acknowledged that a competent person has a liberty interest under the Due Process clause in refusing unwanted medical care; however, the Court assumed the existence of a constitutionally protected right to refuse artificial hydration and nutrition only for purposes of the case. In a concurring opinion, Justice O'Connor cited Opinion 2.20 for the proposition that artificial feeding cannot be distinguished from other forms of medical treatment. In his dissent, Justice Brennan likewise cited Opinion 2.20 for this point. *Cruzan v. Director, Missouri Department of Health, 497 U.S. 261.*

9th Cir. 1996 Suit was brought by several physicians and not-for-profit corporation which provides information, assistance, and counseling to competent terminally ill adult patients contemplating suicide, asserting that a state statute making it a crime to aid anyone in attempting to commit suicide unconstitutionally prevents terminally ill patients from exercising their protected liberty interests. Appeals court, en banc, held that the choice of how and when to die is a liberty interest and that the statute violates the due process rights of competent, terminally ill adults who wish to hasten their deaths by obtaining medication prescribed by their physicians. Stating that physician-assisted suicide runs counter to medical ethics, the dissent cited Opinions 2.20, 2.21, and 2.211 and quoted Opinion 2.211. *Compassion in Dying v. Washington, 79 F.3d 790, 840, 855, replacing 49 F.3d 586 (9th Cir. 1995).*

Ariz. 1987 Guardian of nursing home patient in persistent vegetative state sought removal of nasogastric tube and retention of Do Not Resuscitate and Do Not Hospitalize orders. Patient had not communicated desires regarding life-sustaining procedures while competent. In assessing whether safeguarding the integrity of the medical profession might be a state interest that outweighed the patient's right to refuse medical treatment, the court noted Opinion 2.18 (1986) [now Opinion 2.20] to support the view that the medical profession itself now recognizes that it is no longer obligated to provide medical treatment in all situations. Since the Opinion would allow the disputed orders for a patient suffering from an irreversible coma, the court concluded that the same action would be allowed in a case of irreversible chronic vegetative state and thus concluded that the case did not bring into disrepute the ethical integrity of the medical profession. *Rasmussen v. Fleming, 154 Ariz. 207, 741 P.2d 674, 684, 685.*

Ariz. App. 1986 Guardian of nursing home patient in persistent vegetative state sought removal of nasal gastric tube and retention of Do Not Resuscitate and Do Not Hospitalize orders. Patient had not communicated her desires regarding life-sustaining procedures while competent. The court quoted Opinion 2.18 (1986) [now Opinion 2.20] in holding that competing state interests, including the ethical integrity of the medical profession, did not outweigh patient's constitutional right to privacy and held that rights of incompetent patient could be asserted vicariously. *Rasmussen v. Fleming, 154 Ariz. 200, 741 P.2d 667, 671, 672, 673 n.4, aff'd in part and rev'd in part, 154 Ariz. 207, 741 P.2d 674 (1987).*

Cal. App. 1988 Conservator sought an injunction requiring physician to remove nasogastric feeding tube from a patient who was in a persistent vegetative state. The court held that while a conservator may authorize withdrawal or withholding of medical treatment, he may not force a physician to do so against the physician's personal moral objections if the patient can be transferred to the care of a physician who will follow the directive. Citing Opinion 2.18 (1986) [now Opinion 2.20], the court noted that the physician's compliance with the conservator's decision would not have violated the ethical code of the medical profession. *Morrison v. Abramovice, 206 Cal. App. 3d 304, 309, 253 Cal. Rptr. 530, 533.*

Cal. App. 1988 Conservator of patient in persistent vegetative state sought permission for removal of nasogastric feeding tube claiming such relief would serve the patient's best interests. Patient had expressed a desire never to be kept alive through artificial means. The court held that a conservator is authorized to order that artificial life support be withdrawn after considering medical advice and the patient's best interests. In so holding, the court quoted Opinion 2.18 (1986) [now Opinion 2.20] showing support within the medical community for its analysis. *In re Drabick, 200*

Cal. App. 3d 185, 245 Cal. Rptr. 840, 845 n.8.

Cal. App. 1986 Mentally competent, physically debilitated patient sought authorization to discontinue forced feedings through nasogastric tube. Patient had dictated instructions to her lawyers and signed them with an x by means of a pen held in her mouth. In holding that a competent adult patient has the legal right to refuse medical treatment even though such refusal will hasten her death, the court quoted Opinion 2.18 (1986) [now Opinion 2.20]. *Bouvia v. Superior Court, 179 Cal. App. 3d 1127, 225 Cal. Rptr. 297, 303-04.*

Conn. 1989 Family of comatose, terminal patient in nursing home sought injunction to discontinue life support services. In holding that removal of a gastrostomy tube was authorized by statute and no compelling state interests outweighed the patient's rights, the court cited Opinion 2.18 (1986) [now Opinion 2.20] for its view that the provision of nutrition and hydration is a form of life-prolonging medical treatment. *McConnell v. Beverly Enterprises-Connecticut, Inc., 209 Conn. 692, 553 A.2d 596, 603 n.13.*

Fla. App. 1986 Husband of terminally ill patient in persistent vegetative state sought declaratory judgment to permit removal of nasogastric feeding tube. In recognizing a right to allow the natural consequence of removal of artificial life sustaining measures, the court quoted Opinion 2.18 (1986) [now Opinion 2.20]. *Corbett v. D'Alessandro, 487 So. 2d 368, 371 n.1.*

Ill. 1989 Daughter of permanently unconscious patient petitioned to withdraw life-prolonging gastrotomy feeding tube. The court cited with approval Opinion 2.18 (1986) [now Opinion 2.20] that the American Medical Association considers artificial hydration and nutrition to be medical treatments which may be withdrawn under certain circumstances. The court based the right to refuse life-prolonging procedures upon the state's common law of informed consent, probate law, and power of attorney for health care statute. The court established guidelines for a guardian's exercise of this right. The patient must be terminally ill, in a persistent vegetative state, and the guardian must exercise the substituted judgment of the patient as shown through clear and convincing evidence in a judicial proceeding. *In re Longeway, 133 Ill. 2d 33, 549 N.E.2d 292, 295-96.*

Ill. App. 1988 Guardian of patient in persistent vegetative state petitioned to withdraw artificial feeding tube. Prior to her incompetence, the patient had stated in writing and in conversations with friends that she desired no artificial means of treatment if there was no hope for her recovery, and had completed a living will form, but had failed to obtain the requisite number of witness signatures. The trial court dismissed the case upon the patient's death. On appeal, the court held that the guardian, using the doctrine of substituted judgment, could consent to the removal of a feeding tube from a patient in a persistent vegetative state. In so holding, the court quoted Opinion 2.18 [now Opinion 2.20], noting that it was within a physician's ethical parameters to discontinue such treatment. *In re Prange, 166 Ill. App. 3d 1091, 520 N.E.2d 946, vacated, 121 Ill. 2d 570, 527 N.E.2d 303 (1988).*

Ind. 1991 State statute provided procedures by which parents of an incompetent patient, in consultation with the patient's physician, could withhold or withdraw life-prolonging medical treatment. The court held that barring any challenge from the treating physician or interested parties, the family could make these decisions without a court proceeding. Quoting Opinion 2.20 (1989), the court concluded that medical treatment includes artificial nutrition and hydration. *In re Lawrance, 579 N.E.2d 32, 40.*

Kan. App. 1998 Physician was convicted of attempted murder of a terminally ill patient, and intentional and malicious second-degree murder of another terminally ill patient. The court quoted Opinion 2.22, to exemplify a physician's duty to provide cardiopulmonary resuscitation unless the physician believes that such action would be futile. Additionally, the court referenced Opinion 2.20, in support of a physician's duty to provide a terminally ill patient adequate pain relief. The court reversed the physician's convictions, stating that the jury could not disregard the testimony of several physicians who concurred with the defendant-physician's treatment of the deceased patients. *State v. Naramore, 25 Kan. App. 2d 302, 965 P.2d 211, 214, 216.*

Ky. 1993 In a declaratory judgment action, the court was asked to allow a surrogate to exercise the right to withdraw life-prolonging treatment for a patient who had orally expressed her wishes not to be sustained artificially. Since common law recognizes a patient's right to withdraw or withhold medical treatment, the court held that a surrogate could rely on the patient's statement of choice made before patient became incompetent to exercise "substituted judgment." The court quoted from guidelines for state courts deciding life-sustaining medical treatment cases issued by the National Center for State Courts. Citing Opinion 2.20 and other sources, the Guidelines stated that a consensus had already been reached on the primary ethical issues relating to life-prolonging treatment. *DeGrella v. Elston, 858 S.W.2d 698, 707 n.5.*

Me. 1987 Guardian sought to have nasogastric feeding tube withdrawn from patient in persistent vegetative state. Investigation by a state agency corroborated evidence of patient's prior statements that he desired no life-sustaining procedures if in a persistent vegetative state. The court noted that under state's common law an individual has a personal right to refuse medical treatment, including life-sustaining procedures. The court held that where the patient had clearly and convincingly expressed his desire not to be maintained by life-sustaining procedures if in a persistent vegetative state, health professionals had a duty to respect that decision. The court cited Opinion 2.18 (1986) [now Opinion 2.20] for the concept that artificial hydration and nutrition should be equated with other life-sustaining treatments in delineating the patient's right to reject such treatment. *In re Gardner, 534 A.2d 947, 954.*

Md. Att'y Gen. 1988 Attorney general was asked whether persons with capacity to decide about medical care have a right to instruct that artificially administered sustenance not be provided if they become terminally ill or permanently comatose. An opinion was also requested regarding decisionmaking for incompetent persons who have given no prior instructions about artificial feeding. In response, Opinion 2.18 (1986) [now Opinion 2.20] is cited to support the view that no distinction should be drawn between artificial feeding and other forms of life-prolonging treatment. Further, in delineating procedures for deciding to forego treatment for an incompetent, terminally ill patient who has given no prior instructions, Opinion 2.18 (1986) [now Opinion 2.20] is also cited in terms of the physician's role in advising whether withdrawal is medically proper. Finally, while disallowing family members, without court approval, to terminate tube feeding for a nonterminal, permanently comatose patient, it is recognized that under this Opinion it is not unethical to discontinue life-sustaining treatment for such a patient. *Maryland Att'y Gen. Op. No. 88-046, 73 Op. Att'y Gen. 162.*

Mass. 1992 Request of parents of a patient in a persistent vegetative state to employ "substituted judgment" in order to withdraw medical treatment was granted. Citing Opinion 2.18 (1986) [now Opinion 2.20], the court noted that medical treatment includes artificial hydration and nutrition. *In re Doe, 411 Mass. 512, 517 n.11, 583 N.E.2d 1263, 1267 n.11.*

Mass. 1986 Guardian of patient in persistent vegetative state who, according to trial court, would have declined food and water, sued for declaratory judgment requesting authority to have artificial hydration and nutrition discontinued. The court held that while the hospital had a right to refuse to participate in the removal of the gastrostomy tube, the guardian was authorized to transfer the patient to other physicians who would honor the guardian's request. The court cited Opinion 2.18 (1986) [now Opinion 2.20] in finding that the patient's right to refuse medical treatment did not violate the state's interest in the maintenance of the ethical integrity of the medical profession as long as the hospital was not forced to participate in the removal or clamping of the gastronomy tube. *Brophy v. New England Sinai Hosp., Inc., 398 Mass. 417, 497 N.E.2d 626, 638-39 n.38.*

Mich. App. 2001 State brought criminal action against physician for the murder of a patient by lethal injection. The trial court convicted the physician of second-degree murder and delivering a controlled substance. On appeal, the trial court decision was affirmed. The physician asked the appellate court to conclude that euthanasia is legal and to reverse his conviction on constitutional grounds. The appellate court relied on Washington v. Glucksberg, 521 U.S. 702 (1997) in determining there is no constitutional right to commit euthanasia, so that an individual can be free from intolerable and irremediable suffering. In discussing Glucksberg, the court observed that a state has a legitimate interest in protecting the integrity and ethics of the medical profession. The court noted Glucksberg's reference to Opinions 2.20, 2.21, and 2.211 in this regard. *People v. Kevorkian, 248 Mich. App. 373, 639 N.W.2d 291, 305 n. 42.*

Mo. 1988 Parents-guardians of a nonterminal patient in a persistent vegetative state sought a declaratory judgment after a state hospital refused to terminate artificial hydration and nutrition. The court found that the patient's burden in being fed through gastronomy tube did not outweigh the state's interest in preserving life and that guardians could not order withdrawal of hydration and nutrition. The court, in refusing to classify artificial hydration and nutrition as medical treatment, rejected Opinion 2.18 (1986) [now Opinion 2.20] which expresses a contrary view. *Cruzan v. Harmon, 760 S.W.2d 408, 423 n.18, aff'd, 497 U.S. 261.*

N.J. 1987 Husband applied to court for authorization to discontinue wife's hydration and nutrition after nursing home refused his request to do so. The court held that the right of a patient in an irreversible vegetative state to refuse life-sustaining procedures may be exercised by the patient's family or close friend after two independent neurologists have confirmed the diagnosis and prognosis. The court further stated that the processes of surrogate decision-making should be substantially the same regardless of type of medical facility. In so holding, the court cited Opinion 2.18 (1986) [now Opinion 2.20] with approval. *In re Jobes*, 108 N.J. 394, 529 A.2d 434, 446.

N.J. 1987 Elderly nursing home patient was comatose in a persistent vegetative state. Patient's designee, under power of attorney for health care decisions, sought appointment as guardian and authorization for removal of patient's artificial nutrition and hydration. The court held that where there is clear and convincing proof that patient would refuse such treatment if competent, a surrogate may effect that decision regardless of the patient's life expectancy. The court quoted with approval Opinion 2.18 (1986) [now Opinion 2.20] stating that artificial hydration and nutrition is a form of medical treatment. *In re Peter*, 108 N.J. 365, 529 A.2d 419, 427-28.

N.J. 1987 Husband of competent, terminally ill patient applied to be special medical guardian to effectuate patient's desire to remove respirator. In holding that the right of a competent, terminally ill patient to decline medical treatment outweighed the state's interests in preserving life, preventing suicide, protecting innocent third parties, and safeguarding the integrity of the medical profession, the court cited as reflective of the views of the medical profession the Judicial Council's report at 253 J.A.M.A. 2424 (1985) [now Opinion 2.20]. *In re Farrell*, 108 N.J. 335, 529 A.2d 404, 412.

N.J. Super. 1983 Guardian of elderly nursing home patient suffering from severe organic brain syndrome sought to remove nasogastric tube from patient. Trial court granted guardian's petition, and patient's guardian ad litem appealed. Appellate court reversed, in part based upon Opinions 2.11 (1981) and 5.17 (1979) [now Opinions 2.17 and 2.20], and held that it is improper and would violate medical ethics to allow dehydration and starvation in a non-comatose, non-brain-dead patient not facing imminent death, not maintained by any life-support machine, and not able to speak for herself. *In re Conroy*, 190 N.J. Super. 453, 464 A.2d 303, 313-15, rev'd, 98 N.J. 321, 486 A.2d 1209 (1985).

N.Y. 1990 Jehovah's Witness was given blood transfusion against her express wishes. The court held that the lower court erred in ordering the transfusions without giving the patient or her family notice and a hearing. Barring any superior interest of the state, the patient had a right to determine the course of her own treatment. Concurring opinion argued that the majority rule created an absolute right to refuse treatment. Quoting from Opinion 2.21 (1989) [now Opinion 2.20], the concurring opinion held that a physician had a corresponding ethical duty to render treatment which, in his judgment, benefits the patient. Note that Opinion 2.20 does not retain the specific language of former Opinion 2.21 relied on by concurring judge. *Fosmire v. Nicoleau*, 75 N.Y.2d 218, 236 n.2, 551 N.E.2d 77, 87 n.2, 551 N.Y.S.2d 876, 886 n.2.

N.Y. Sup. 2003 Mother petitioned court to remove her daughter from a respirator. Hospital policy denied mother the authorization to withdraw care. Court granted petition and held parents have a right to refuse medical treatment for their children. Applying the best interest test, the court held that the burdens of prolonging life exceeded the benefits and that, absent extraordinary circumstances or disagreement between parents, judicial intervention is not required to withhold medical treatment from a minor in a vegetative state. Quotes Opinion 2.215. References Opinion 2.20. *In re AB*, 196 Misc. 2d 940, 768 N.Y.S. 2d 256, 268-69.

N.Y. Sup. 1986 Plaintiff petitioned for judicial authorization to remove feeding tube from her 33-year-old husband, a patient in a permanent chronic vegetative state. In denying the petition, the court noted the American Medical Association's position set out in 245 JAMA 819 (1981), later included as Opinion 2.11 (1981) [now Opinion 2.20] that, in such cases, members of the family and physicians should decide whether to continue treatment. However, the court concluded that the legislature must resolve the issue and denied the petition. *Delio v. Westchester County Medical Center*, 134 Misc. 2d 206, 510 N.Y.S.2d 415, 419, rev'd, 129 A.D. 2d 1, 516 N.Y.S. 2d 677 (1987).

Ohio App. 1989 The divorced parents of a patient in a persistent vegetative state each petitioned to be appointed guardian of their son. The mother was initially appointed guardian and testified that it would be in the best interests of her son, and consistent with his wishes, to terminate nutrition and hydration. Over the father's objections, the probate court granted the mother, as guardian, the right to make decisions regarding her son's treatment and care. On appeal, the appellate court modified the lower court's order, pursuant to a state statute enacted after that order was entered. Although recognizing that the lower court's decision was consistent with the position of the American Medical Association as articulated in Opinion 2.20, the appellate court held that to allow termination of nutrition and hydration in this case would violate the public policy as expressed in recent legislation. *Couture v. Couture, 48 Ohio App. 3d 208, 549 N.E.2d 571, 574.*

Pa. Super. 1995 Parent of nursing home patient in persistent vegetative state sought removal of gastrostomy tube. Nursing home refused to comply with request without court order. Trial court, applying best interests test, authorized removal of tube. On appeal, court held that consent of close family member, with approval of two qualified physicians, is sufficient without court order to terminate life sustaining treatment for patient in a long-term persistent vegetative state. Court referred to *In re Grant,* 109 Wash. 2d 545, 747 P.2d 445 (1987) citing Opinion 2.18 [now Opinion 2.20] for proposition that medical ethical principles permit withdrawal of nutrition and hydration for patient in persistent vegetative state. *In re Fiori, 438 Pa. Super. 610, 652 A.2d 1350, 1354, app. granted, 655 A.2d 989 (Pa. 1995).*

Phila. Co. 1987 In a declaratory judgment action, the court held that a patient has a right to withhold or withdraw medical treatment. This right is subject to the state's interest in (1) the preservation of life, (2) protection of innocent third parties, (3) prevention of suicide, and (4) protecting the ethical integrity of the medical profession. The court held that the withholding or withdrawal of life support by a physician or hospital or their agents did not constitute a criminal act or give rise to any civil liability. Citing Opinion 2.18 (1986) [now Opinion 2.20]), the court noted that respect for a patient's autonomy and decision to withdraw life support was consistent with medical ethics. *In re Doe, 16 Phila. 229, 1987 Phila. Cty. Rptr. LEXIS 30 (1987).*

Tenn. App. 2002 Patient was in a vegetative state and had metastasized breast cancer. Her family sought to terminate nutrition and hydration. Trial court found clear and convincing evidence showed patient did not want to live by artificial nutrition. However, court also ruled that state statute required a valid written document in order for an incompetent person to refuse nutrition and hydration. Appellate court reversed, holding that lower court misinterpreted the statute. The court held that patient had an inherent fundamental right to refuse medical treatment. Quotes Opinion 2.18 [now Opinion 2.20]. *San Juan-Torregosa v. Garcia, 80 S.W.3d 539, 543.*

Va. Att'y Gen. 1990 Attorney general answered in the affirmative when asked whether a competent adult could create a document authorizing a surrogate to consent to the withholding or withdrawal of medical treatment if the person later enters a persistent vegetative state but is not terminally ill. Quoting Opinion 2.18 (1986) [now Opinion 2.20], the Attorney General concluded that medical treatment includes artificial hydration and nutrition. *Va. Att'y Gen. Op., 1990 Va. AG LEXIS 63.*

Wash. 1987 Court authorization sought by guardian to withhold mechanical or artificial life-sustaining procedures from incompetent patient with terminal disorder. Trial court denied request as premature because patient was not yet comatose or vegetative, and did not yet need intrusive medical procedures. Supreme court held that an incompetent patient in an advanced stage of a terminal illness has right to have life-sustaining treatment withheld, a right which stems from the constitutional right of privacy and the common law right to be free of bodily invasion. Court quoted Opinion 2.18 (1986) [now Opinion 2.20] in support of the right of a terminally ill, noncomatose patient to have life-sustaining procedures withheld including the right to withhold artificial means of nutrition and hydration. *In re Grant, 109 Wash. 2d 545, 747 P.2d 445, 450, 454.*

Wis. 1992 Guardian may consent to the withholding or withdrawal of life-prolonging medical treatment on behalf of an incompetent patient and/or a patient for whom the guardian cannot reasonably make a "substituted judgment" where (1) the patient is in a persistent vegetative state with no reasonable chance of recovery, and (2) the guardian in good faith determines that it is in the patient's "best interest." The court referred to the concurring opinion in *Cruzan v. Director, Missouri Dept. of Health,* 497 U.S. 261 (1990) which quoted Opinion 2.20 (1989) in holding that medical treatment includes nutrition and hydration. Further, citing Opinion 2.18 (1986) [now Opinion 2.20], the court found the actions here consistent with current medical ethics. Thus, the state's interest in protecting the integrity of the medical profession was not implicated. *L.W. v. L.E. Phillips Career Dev. Ctr., 167 Wis. 2d 53, 71, 72, 91, 482 N.W.2d 60, 66, 74.*

Journal 2003 Discusses whether patients may assert a claim of medical malpractice for inadequate treatment of pain. Concludes courts should find that failure to adequately treat pain constitutes negligence. Quotes Opinion 2.20. Mayer, *Bergman v. Chin: Why an Elder Abuse Case is a Stride in the Direction of Civil Culpability for Physicians Who Undertreat Patients Suffering from Terminal Pain, 37 New Eng. L. Rev. 313, 340 (2003).*

Journal 2002 Suggests a reconceptualization for bioethics that integrates an analysis of the history of moral change. Concludes that bioethical textbooks should include discussion about the history of bioethics and medical ethics. Quotes Opinion 2.20. References Opinions 6.02, 6.03, 6.04 [now Opinion 8.06], and 8.032. Baker, *Bioethics and History*, 27 J. Med. & Phil. 447, 455, 469 (2002).

Journal 2002 Explores the implications of withholding medical treatment when abortion results in a live birth. Concludes that, in these situations, abortive parents and physicians should not solely decide the child's best interest. Quotes Preamble, Principles I and III, and Opinions 2.035, 2.20, and 2.215. Casagrande, *Children Not Meant to Be: Protecting the Interests of the Child When Abortion Results in Live Birth*, 6 Quinnipiac Health L.J. 19, 44, 45, 47-48 (2002).

Journal 2002 Considers a judicial model to evaluate the relationship between law and bioethics. Concludes that, in this regard, ethics may justify court decisions but likely will not break new ground. Quotes Opinion 2.20. Gross, *Wagging the Watchdog: Law and the Emergence of Bioethical Norms*, 21 Med. & L. 687, 702 (2002).

Journal 2002 Considers the use of nonlegal materials in United States Supreme Court decisions. Concludes that law alone cannot answer complex legal questions. Cites Opinions 2.20 and 2.211. Hasko, *Persuasion in the Court: Nonlegal Materials in U.S. Supreme Court Opinions*, 94 Law Libr. J. 427, 444, 453 (2002).

Journal 2002 Examines competing interests regarding genetic testing. Argues that testing of employees should be banned. Concludes that Congress should pass legislation prohibiting genetic testing in the workplace. Quotes Opinion 2.20. Krumm, *Genetic Discrimination: Why Congress Must Ban Genetic Testing in the Workplace*, 23 J. Legal Med. 491, 506 (2002).

Journal 2002 Evaluates pain management treatment for prisoners. Concludes that withholding treatment for, or failing to adequately treat, pain violates the Eighth Amendment. Quotes Principle V and Opinion 2.20. McGrath, *Raising the "Civilized Minimum" of Pain Amelioration for Prisoners to Avoid Cruel and Unusual Punishment*, 54 Rutgers L. Rev. 649, 657, 660 (2002).

Journal 2002 Examines key factors that led to the current palliative care crisis. Analyzes state legislative and judicial efforts to improve palliative care. Concludes with model legislation that holds physicians accountable for inadequate palliative care. Quotes Opinions 2.21 and 2.211. References Opinion 2.20. Oken, *Curing Healthcare Providers' Failure to Administer Opioids in the Treatment of Severe Pain*, 23 Cardozo L. Rev. 1917, 1925-26, 1952, 1954 (2002).

Journal 2001 Explores the similarities and differences between active voluntary euthanasia, terminal sedation, and assisted suicide. Examines the problems with making moral distinctions based on physicians' intentions. Concludes that, with proper safeguards, active voluntary euthanasia and assisted suicide are more protective of patient self determination. Quotes Opinions 2.20 and 2.21. Gauthier, *Active Voluntary Euthanasia, Terminal Sedation, and Assisted Suicide*, 12 J. Clinical Ethics 43, 43-44, 49 (2001).

Journal 2001 Examines the role of telemedicine in end-of-life decision-making. Concludes that telemedicine should not be used as a substitute for face-to-face discussions, but as a method to supplement such discussions with input from other experienced clinicians. Cites Opinion 2.20. Pronovost & Williams, *Telemedicine and End-of-Life Care: What's Wrong with This Picture?* 12 J. Clinical Ethics 64, 68 (2001).

Journal 2001 Discusses the North Carolina case of *In Re Cartrette*, which focuses on a mother's decision to terminate life support for her incompetent daughter, who is neither terminally ill nor PVS. Argues against sole reliance on a quality of life assessment as a predicate for surrogate decision-making for a patient who has never been competent. Urges adoption of best interests standard. Quotes Opinion 2.20. Sabo, *Limiting a Surrogate's Authority to Terminate Life-Support for an Incompetent Adult*, 79 N.C.L. Rev. 1815, 1815 (2001).

Journal 2000 Examines questions regarding the legality of such practices as voluntary stopping of eating and drinking (VSED), use of risky analgesics, and terminal sedation. Explores the distinctions between physician-assisted suicide and other palliative interventions. Concludes VSED, risky analgesics, and certain types of terminal sedation are lawful and should be made available to dying patients who make informed decisions to accept the risks involved. Quotes Opinions 2.21 and 2.211. Cites Opinions 2.18 and 2.20. Cantor & Thomas, *The Legal Bounds of Physician Conduct Hastening Death*, 48 Buff. L. Rev. 83, 110, 131, 158 (2000).

Journal 2000 Examines various laws associated with physician-assisted suicide, including the Oregon Death with Dignity Act, the Legal Drug Abuse and Prevention Act of 1998, and the Pain Relief Promotion Act of 1999 (PRPA). Argues that the Supreme Court should declare the PRPA unconstitutional. References Opinion 2.20. Fallek, *The Pain Relief Promotion Act: Will It*

Spell Death to "Death With Dignity" or Is It Unconstitutional? 27 Fordham Urb. L. J. 1739, 1755 (2000).

Journal 2000 Considers the question of whether physician-assisted suicide and euthanasia should be legalized. Concludes that, under basic moral and common law principles, the intentional taking of human life by a private person is wrong. References Opinions 2.20, 2.21, and 2.211. Gorsuch, *The Right to Assisted Suicide and Euthanasia*, 23 Harv. J. L. & Pub. Pol'y 599, 653, 707 (2000).

Journal 2000 Examines advance directive pregnancy provisions. Discusses the right to refuse medical treatment and the right to terminate pregnancy. Concludes the Minnesota advance directive pregnancy presumption balances the woman's right to terminate a pregnancy and the right to refuse medical treatment with the state interest in potential life. References Opinion 2.20. Jerdee, *Breaking Through the Silence: Minnesota's Pregnancy Presumption and the Right to Refuse Medical Treatment*, 84 Minn. L. Rev. 971, 980 (2000).

Journal 2000 Examines legal and ethical issues bearing upon pain management. Asserts that health care professionals have a legal and ethical duty to relieve pain and suffering of patients whenever possible. Suggests that this duty is legally enforceable. Quotes Principle V and Opinions 2.20 and 9.011. Rich, *A Prescription for the Pain: The Emerging Standard of Care for Pain Management*, 26 Wm. Mitchell L. Rev. 1, 35-36, 85 (2000).

Journal 2000 Examines existing law governing a parent's authority to make health care decisions for a child. Concludes that, consistent with principles of beneficence and autonomy, parents generally should retain their status as primary decision-makers for their children. Cites Opinion 2.20. Rosato, *Using Bioethics Discourse to Determine When Parents Should Make Health Care Decisions for their Children: Is Deference Justified?* 73 Temp. L. Rev. 1, 40, 44 (2000).

Journal 1999 States that a distrust of the medical profession arose from changes in the health care system and federal law. Explains how legislation may help alleviate some of the distrust. Suggests that people need more access to information about their health plans. References Opinions 2.20 and 2.225. Cerminara, *Protecting Participants in and Beneficiaries of ERISA-Governed Managed Health Care Plans*, 29 U. Mem. L. Rev. 317, 324 (1999).

Journal 1999 Discusses use of the hierarchical decision-making model for end-of-life decisions. Proposes that a consensus-based decision-making model, which synthesizes therapeutic jurisprudence and preventive law, should replace the hierarchical decision-making model. Argues that the consensus-based model would decrease court involvement and advance the interests of those affected by the decision. Quotes Opinion 2.20. Hafemeister, *End-of-Life Decision Making, Therapeutic Jurisprudence, and Preventive Law: Hierarchical v. Consensus-Based Decision-Making Model*, 41 Ariz. L. Rev. 329 (1999).

Journal 1999 States that the Patient Self-Determination Act is the medical field's version of the Miranda warning. Suggests that, although the act is followed, many patients do not understand how to exercise their right to medical self-determination. Argues that informed consent should be required in relation to advance directives. Cites Opinion 2.20. Pope, *The Maladaptation of Miranda to Advance Directives: A Critique of the Implementation of the Patient Self-Determination Act*, 9 Health Matrix 139, 178 (1999).

Journal 1999 Examines legal and policy issues regarding physician-assisted suicide. Distinguishes between refusing treatment and assisted suicide. Concludes that there are too many dangers posed by physician-assisted suicide to warrant legalization. Quotes Opinion 2.211. Cites Opinions 2.20 and 2.21. Pratt, *Too Many Physicians: Physician-Assisted Suicide After Glucksberg/Quill*, 9 Alb. L. J. Sci. & Tech. 161, 208 (1999).

Journal 1999 Evaluates liability theories used in cases alleging failure to follow do-not-resuscitate orders and advance directives. Analyzes the impact of legal liability as a means to ensure compliance with such orders and directives. Concludes that there is an increased need for open communication among physicians, patients, and patients' family members. Quotes Opinion 2.20. Rodriguez, *Suing Health Care Providers for Saving Lives: Liability for Providing Unwanted Life-Sustaining Treatment*, 20 J. Legal Med. 1, 62 (1999).

Journal 1999 Explains the rule of double effect. Distinguishes between assisted suicide and pain control for terminally ill patients. Suggests that the rule of double effect needs to be adequately defined so physicians will understand that they can ethically give terminally ill patients drugs that will alleviate their pain, but that also may hasten their death. Cites Opinion 2.20. Sulmasy

& Pellegrino, *The Rule of Double Effect: Clearing Up the Double Talk*, 159 Arch. Intern. Med. 545, 550 (1999).

Journal 1998 Explains that the United States Supreme Court's decisions in *Washington* and *Vacco* left the door open for future constitutional challenges regarding the right to physician-assisted suicide. States that the Court did not explicitly deny the existence of a right to physician-assisted suicide. Quotes Opinion 2.20. Cites Opinion 2.211. Cohen, *The Open Door: Will the Right to Die Survive Washington v. Glucksberg and Vacco v. Quill?*, 16 In Pub. Interest 79, 94 (1998).

Journal 1998 Describes a survey regarding physician-assisted suicide given to members of the Group for the Advancement of Psychiatry. Discusses the results of the survey, noting that most surveyed psychiatrists oppose assisting patients to die. Cites Opinions 2.06 and 2.20. Kramer, Gruenberg, & Fidler, *Psychiatrists' Attitudes Toward Physician-Assisted Suicide: A Survey*, 19 Am. J. Forensic Psychiatry 81, 87, 90 (1998).

Journal 1998 Discusses legal aspects of physician-assisted suicide. Identifies acceptable end-of-life choices and compares them to physician-assisted suicide. Points out that physician-assisted suicide has the potential for abuse and that safeguards have not been implemented to protect people from that risk. Quotes Opinion 2.211. Cites Opinions 2.20 and 8.08. Mitchell, *Physician-Assisted Suicide: A Survey of the Issues Surrounding Legalization*, 74 N. D. L. Rev. 341, 349 (1998).

Journal 1998 Points out that the court in *Vacco v. Quill* did not reject the practice of physician-assisted suicide and left the subject open for state experimentation. Discusses routes some states have taken regarding assisted suicide. Concludes that access to assisted suicide is outweighed by the risk it will be utilized by depressed and mentally ill people. Quotes Opinions 2.20 and 2.211. Moore, *Physician-Assisted Suicide: Does "The End" Justify the Means?*, 40 Ariz. L. Rev. 1471, 1472, 1481-82, 1491 (1998).

Journal 1998 Discusses consequences physician-assisted suicide may have on disabled individuals. Weighs potential benefits and disadvantages stemming from physician-assisted suicide. Concludes that only a small number of people with disabilities would benefit from physician-assisted suicide and that the benefits are outweighed by the risk of abuse. Cites Opinion 2.20. National Council on Disability, *Assisted Suicide: A Disability Perspective*, 14 Issues L. & Med. 273, 292 (1998).

Journal 1998 Observes that the Patient Self-Determination Act does not obligate physicians to discuss advance directives with patients. Explains that physicians may elect not to discuss advance directives with patients because of lack of time and reimbursement for such discussions. Emphasizes that patients, physicians, and health care providers may benefit from advance directives. Quotes Opinion 2.20. Rich, *Advance Directives: The Next Generation*, 19 J. Legal Med. 63, 79 (1998).

Journal 1998 Provides a historical view on parents' rights to make medical decisions for their children. Argues that parents have the right to make medical decisions for their children when the decisions are supported by medical evidence. This right extends to decisions regarding life-sustaining medical treatment. Quotes Opinion 2.20. Walters, *Life-Sustaining Medical Decisions Involving Children: Father Knows Best*, 15 T. M. Cooley L. Rev. 115, 128, 138, 151 (1998).

Journal 1997 Reviews the criminalization of physician-assisted suicide. Discusses informed consent, the double effect, and the right to die. Explains the current state of the law and the position Illinois has taken. Advocates the adoption of a law authorizing physician-assisted suicide in Illinois. References Opinion 2.20. Comment, *An Illinois Physician-Assisted Suicide Act: A Merciful End to a Terminally Ill Criminal Tradition*, 28 Loy. U. Chi. L. J. 763, 775 (1997).

Journal 1997 Discusses Pennsylvania Supreme Court case of *In Re Fiori*. Explains that the court extended the right to refuse medical treatment to patients in permanent vegetative states. Notes that the court now allows family members to exercise this right on behalf of such patients. Quotes Opinion 2.20. Comment, *Surrogate Health Care Decision Making: The Pennsylvania Supreme Court Recognizes the Right of an Individual in a Permanent Vegetative State to Refuse Life-Sustaining Measures through a Surrogate Decision Maker*, 35 Duq. L. Rev. 849, 859-60 (1997).

Journal 1997 Discusses goals of care included in advance directives and whether they can be used to predict specific interventions and results. Offers insights provided by survey of physicians at Massachusetts General Hospital. Cites Opinions 2.20 and 2.21. Fischer, Alpert, Stoeckle, & Emanuel, *Can Goals of Care Be Used to Predict Intervention Preferences in an Advance Directive?*, 157 Arch. Intern. Med. 801, 807 (1997).

Journal 1997 Examines the evolution of the Indiana health care system. Discusses developments in Indiana jurisprudence regarding the physician-patient relationship. Explores various challenges facing the relationship and recognizes the need for legal rules to help address these challenges. Quotes Opinion 8.08. Cites Opinions 2.20, 9.06, and 9.12. Kinney & Selby, *History and Jurisprudence of the Physician-Patient Relationship in Indiana*, 30 Ind. L. Rev. 263, 269, 272, 276 (1997).

Journal 1996 Proposes a model state statute allowing and controlling physician-assisted suicide. Analyzes the constitutionality of the act and offers public policy justifications for the act's provisions. Concludes that proponents of physician-assisted suicide should provide precise, carefully tailored examples of regulations. Quotes Opinion 2.211. Cites Opinion 2.20. Baron, Bergstresser, Brock, Cole, Dorfman, Johnson, Schnipper, Vorenberg, & Wanzer, *A Model State Act to Authorize and Regulate Physician-Assisted Suicide*, 33 Harv. J. Legis. 1, 2, 7 (1996).

Journal 1996 Explores the issue of legalizing physician-assisted suicide. Opines that the current state of technology increases life expectancy but with a concomitant decrease in dignity and autonomy surrounding one's death. Notes that the elderly are committing suicide at an increasing rate. Cites Opinions 2.20, 2.21, and 2.211. Morgan & Sutherland, *Last Rights? Confronting Physician-Assisted Suicide in Law and Society: Legal Liturgies on Physician-Assisted Suicide*, 26 Stetson L. Rev. 481, 484 (1996).

Journal 1996 Considers the right to death with dignity. Suggests that the AMA's position undermines mitigation of suffering and the individuals' right to self-determination. Concludes that restrictions on the right to death with dignity may be constitutionally impermissible. Quotes Opinion 2.211. Cites Opinion 2.20. Note, *Who Decides if There is Triumph in the Ultimate Agony? Constitutional Theory and the Emerging Right to Die With Dignity*, 37 Wm. & Mary L. Rev. 827, 829 (1996).

Journal 1996 Discusses the physician's duty to relieve pain. Considers current attitudes toward pain management. Concludes that, consistent with principles of beneficence, physicians are obligated to provide pain relief and palliation. Quotes Opinion 2.20. Post, Blustein, Gordon, & Dubler, *Pain: Ethics, Culture, and Informed Consent to Relief*, 24 J. Law, Med. & Ethics 348, 349, 356 (1996).

Journal 1996 Discusses children's rights to consent to or refuse life-sustaining medical treatment. Compares the rights of children to those of adults in a medical decision-making context. Proposes reforms to allow minors legal rights to make decisions regarding withdrawal of life-sustaining treatment. Quotes Opinion 2.20. Rosato, *The Ultimate Test of Autonomy: Should Minors Have a Right to Make Decisions Regarding Life-Sustaining Treatment?*, 49 Rutgers L. Rev. 1, 80-81, 82 (1996).

Journal 1995 Explores reluctance of long-term care facilities to allow patients to forgo life-sustaining tube feeding. Concludes that policies must be adopted to ensure that patients' rights to refuse artificial nutrition and hydration are protected. Cites Opinion 2.20. Meisel, *Barriers to Forgoing Nutrition and Hydration in Nursing Homes*, XXI Am. J. Law & Med. 335, 353-54 (1995).

Journal 1995 Examines the problem of determining when a patient has lost decision-making capacity. Compares the authority of the treating physician with that of the patient's designated agent in making such a determination. Cites Opinion 2.20. Schneiderman, Teetzel, & Kalmanson, *Who Decides Who Decides? When Disagreement Occurs Between the Physician and the Patient's Appointed Proxy About the Patient's Decision-Making Capacity*, 155 Arch. Intern. Med. 793, 796 (1995).

Journal 1995 Offers relevant historical perspectives and provides comprehensive ethical and legal discussion of physician-assisted suicide and euthanasia. Highlights important legislative developments, including the Oregon Death with Dignity Act, and analyzes significant judicial opinions. Quotes Principles III, IV, and VI and Opinions 2.21 and 9.12. Cites Opinions 2.20 and 8.11. Stone & Winslade, *Physician-Assisted Suicide and Euthanasia in the United States: Legal and Ethical Observations*, 16 J. Legal Med. 481, 483, 490, 497, 498, 499 (1995).

Journal 1994 Considers how greater patient autonomy has led to situations in which medical care may be viewed as futile. Suggests that the law has intruded too far into this area of medicine. Quotes Opinion 2.035. Cites Opinions 2.03, 2.095, 2.17, 2.19, 2.20, and 2.22. Cultice, *Medical Futility: When Is Enough, Enough?*, 27 J. Health & Hosp. Law 225, 230, 256 (1994).

Journal 1994 Discusses whether a patient's prior expression of treatment choices in an advance directive accurately represents future choices. Concludes that patients are capable of making stable scenario- and treatment-specific advance directives, that their choices become more stable with repeat consideration, and that illness has little effect on stability of choices. Cites Opinion 2.20. Emanuel, Emanuel, Stoeckle, Hummel, & Barry, *Advance Directives: Stability of Patients' Treatment Choices*, 154 Arch. Intern. Med. 209, 217 (1994).

Journal 1994 Analyzes physicians' attitudes about whether to initiate or withhold tube feeding when patients' preferences are unknown. Concludes that patient prognosis and quality of life are the most important influences on physician decisions about tube feeding. Cites Opinion 2.20. Hodges, Tolle, Stocking, & Cassel, *Tube Feeding: Internists' Attitudes Regarding Ethical Obligations*, 154 Arch. Intern. Med. 1013, 1020 (1994).

Journal 1994 Examines the various types of advance health care directives and reviews pertinent Arkansas law. Concludes that directives should conform to each person's values, health status, and medical prognosis. Cites Opinion 2.20. Leflar, *Advance Health Care Directives Under Arkansas Law*, 1994 Ark. L. Notes 37, 42.

Journal 1994 Examines how state laws have accommodated medical developments in the area of treatment decisions and how they serve to resolve and encourage conflict in health care decision-making. Considers the roles of physicians, hospitals, and families and how their wishes may conflict with those of the patient. Cites Opinion 2.20. Tarantino, *Withdrawal of Life Support. Conflict Among Patient Wishes, Family, Physicians, Courts and Statutes, and the Law*, 42 Buff. L. Rev. 623, 638, 639, 646 (1994).

Journal 1994 Determines that physicians are not taking the responsibility for initiating discussions about end-of-life medical treatment and that many patients falsely assume that their physicians would know what kind of treatments they would want. Concludes that physician-patient communication is improved slightly when there is an advance directive, but that there is still a lack of detailed discussion about end-of-life treatments. Cites Opinion 2.20. Virmani, Schneiderman, & Kaplan, *Relationship of Advance Directives to Physician-Patient Communication*, 154 Arch. Intern. Med. 909, 913 (1994).

Journal 1993 Analyzes the implications of giving patients and their families an absolute right to control medical treatment. Argues that courts should refrain from ordering physicians to treat patients when physicians believe that treatment would be ineffective. Quotes Fundamental Elements (5) and Opinions 2.11 (1982) [now Opinion 2.20] and 2.18 (1986) [now Opinion 2.20]. Comment, *Beyond Autonomy: Judicial Restraint and the Legal Limits Necessary to Uphold the Hippocratic Tradition and Preserve the Ethical Integrity of the Medical Profession*, 9 J. Contemp. Health L. & Pol'y 451, 467, 468 (1993).

Journal 1993 Discusses Ohio's living will statute in light of the *Cruzan* decision. Presents the medical implications of the persistent vegetative state patient. Quotes Opinion 2.18 (1986) [now Opinion 2.20]. Comment, *One Step Forward, Two Steps Back: A Constitutional and Critical Look at Ohio's New Living Will Statute*, 54 Ohio St. L. J. 445, 447, 460, 470 (1993).

Journal 1993 Discusses the problem of physicians withholding needed medical treatment from HIV-infected infants. Concludes that current law should be expanded to eliminate this discrimination. Quotes Opinions 2.09, 2.17, 2.20, 2.22, 4.04, and 8.03. Crossley, *Of Diagnoses and Discrimination: Discriminatory Nontreatment of Infants With HIV Infection*, 93 Columbia L. Rev. 1581, 1620, 1621 (1993).

Journal 1993 Discusses the relationship between a physician's professional conscience and end of life decisionmaking. Considers the issue of futile medical treatment. Examines case law concerning a patient's right to demand treatment and a physician's obligation to provide it. References Opinions 2.20 and 2.22. Daar, *A Clash at the Bedside: Patient Autonomy v. A Physician's Professional Conscience*, 44 Hastings L. J. 1241, 1257, 1268, 1286 (1993).

Journal 1993 Argues that society should not permit euthanasia because of lack of protection against potential abuses. Recommends that health care providers be taught to treat pain and more effectively care for dying patients, rather than to affirmatively end life. Quotes Opinions 2.17 and 2.20. Dickey, *Euthanasia: A Concept Whose Time Has Come?*, 8 Issues in Law & Med. 521, 523, 524 (1993).

Journal 1993 Discusses the legal distinction between "the right to die" and physician-assisted suicide. Examines how the law is applied and whether it should be reformed in light of public opinion and changing ethical standards. References Opinion 2.20. Gostin, *Drawing a Line Between Killing and Letting Die: The Law, and Law Reform, on Medically Assisted Dying*, 21 J. Law, Med. & Ethics 94, 98 (1993).

Journal 1993 Considers how life-sustaining treatments have led to prolonged life under unacceptable circumstances. Recommends quality assurance programs that promote discussion between physicians and patients regarding life-sustaining treatment problems. Cites Opinions 2.20 and 2.21. Pearlman, Cain, Patrick, Appelbaum-Maizel, Starks, Jecker, & Uhlmann, *Insights Pertaining* *to Patient Assessments of States Worse than Death, 4 J. Clinical Ethics 33, 40 (1993).*

Journal 1993 Considers whether criminal penalties should be imposed on a physician who assists in the suicide of a competent, non-terminal patient who requested such assistance. Presents the arguments for and against active euthanasia, with emphasis on the "slippery slope" argument. References Opinions 2.06 and 2.20. Persels, *Forcing the Issue of Physician-Assisted Suicide: Impact of the Kevorkian Case on the Euthanasia Debate, 14 J. Legal Med. 93, 115 (1993).*

Journal 1993 Discusses legal and ethical issues raised by physician aid-in-dying. Concludes that passive euthanasia for competent, terminal adults is the accepted norm and physician aid-in-dying is the new frontier. Quotes Opinion 2.18 (1986) [now Opinion 2.20]. Risley, *Ethical and Legal Issues in the Individual's Right to Die, 20 Ohio N.U.L. Rev. 597, 605 (1993).*

Journal 1992 Considers when it is appropriate to withdraw artificial food and nutrition from an incompetent patient under the Indiana "Living Wills" statute. Concludes that, in Indiana, it is appropriate to remove artificial nutrition and hydration that only "prolongs the dying process." Quotes Opinion 2.20. Anderson, *A Medical-Legal Dilemma: When Can "Inappropriate" Nutrition and Hydration Be Removed in Indiana? 67 Ind. L. J. 479, 480 (1992).*

Journal 1992 Analyzes the arguments for and against active euthanasia, including ethical concerns, the slippery slope argument, and the proper role of the physician. Suggests that active euthanasia may be acceptable when its administration is restricted to physicians. References Opinions 2.20 and 2.21. Brock, *Voluntary Active Euthanasia, 22 Hastings Center Rep. 10 (March/April 1992).*

Journal 1992 Examines several issues regarding persistent vegetative state (PVS) patients, including whether PVS patients are really dead, whether nutrition and hydration should be withheld, whether life-sustaining treatments are futile or medically inappropriate, and whether ordinary standards for decisionmaking should be applied to PVS patients. Concludes that life-sustaining therapy may be withheld or continued, but that withdrawal of nutrition and hydration, as well as active euthanasia, present more difficult questions. References Opinions 2.20 and 2.22. Brody, *Special Ethical Issues in the Management of PVS Patients, 20 Law, Med. & Health Care 104, 109 (1992).*

Journal 1992 Examines ethical and legal issues surrounding cardiopulmonary resuscitation and emergency cardiac care. Discusses advance directives and proxy decisionmaking, medical futility, resource allocation, and Do-Not-Resuscitate orders. References Opinions 2.20 and 2.22. Comment, *Ethical Considerations in Resuscitation, 268 JAMA 2282, 2283, 2287 (1992).*

Journal 1992 Defines the right of terminally ill, competent patients to die with the assistance of a physician and argues that it is essentially the same as the right to die by refusing life-sustaining medical treatment. Concludes that courts should balance patients' rights with compelling state interests in assessing the scope of this right. Cites Opinion 2.20. Comment, *Physician Assisted Suicide and the Right to Die With Assistance, 105 Harvard L. Rev. 2021, 2027, 2035 (1992).*

Journal 1992 Discusses the Iowa living will statute, comparing it to similar laws in other states. Proposes a revised statute to address problems arising in light of recent court decisions.. References Opinion 2.20. Goldman, *Revising Iowa's Life-Sustaining Procedures Act: Creating a Practical Guide to Living Wills in Iowa, 76 Iowa L. Rev. 1137, 1149 (1992).*

Journal 1992 Explores various health policy issues addressed by the Indiana state legislature. Considers Indiana lawmakers' responses to the following concerns: health care access; tort reform; the right to die; medicaid reimbursements; and discrimination against AIDS patients. Cites Opinion 2.18 (1986) [now Opinion 2.20]. Kumar & Kinney, *Indiana Lawmakers Face National Health Policy Issues, 25 Indiana L. Rev. 1271, 1275, 1276 (1992).*

Journal 1992 Discusses the need for a policy governing life-sustaining treatment decisions for incompetent adult wards of the state. Provides a basic outline for such a policy and proposes a model policy statement. Quotes Opinion 2.20. McKnight & Bollis, *Foregoing Life-Sustaining Treatment for Adult Developmentally Disabled, Public Wards: A Proposed Statute, XVIII Am. J. Law & Med. 203, 206, 220, 227 (1992).*

Journal 1992 Observes that the fundamental question in *Cruzan* was whether there should be judicial oversight regarding decisions to forego life-sustaining treatment. Concludes that *Cruzan* did not resolve this issue. Cites Opinion 2.18 (1986) [now Opinion 2.20]. Meisel, *A Retrospective on Cruzan, 20 Law, Med. & Health Care 340, 345 (1992).*

Journal 1992 Explores evolution of the legal consensus that terminating life support is legitimate under some circumstances. Suggests that the consensus will continue to spread in the absence of opposition and may extend to mercy killing and futility cases. Quotes Opinion 2.18 (1986) [now Opinion 2.20]. Meisel, *The Legal Consensus About Forgoing Life-Sustaining Treatment: Its Status and Its Prospects*, 2 Kennedy Inst. Ethics J. 309, 325 (1992).

Journal 1992 Considers the debate surrounding medical futility. Observes that this debate is encouraging reexamination of the nature of patient entitlement to medical care as well as the "ends of medicine." References Opinions 2.20, 2.21, and 2.22. Miles, *Medical Futility*, 20 Law, Med. & Health Care 310, 311, 313 (1992).

Journal 1992 Analyzes North Carolina's living will and health care power of attorney statutes in light of the *Cruzan* case. Notes recent changes to both statutes and problems that continue to exist. Quotes Opinion 2.21 (1992) [now Opinion 2.20]. Note, *Exercising the Right to Die: North Carolina's Amended Natural Death Act and the 1991 Health Care Power of Attorney Act*, 70 No. Carolina L. Rev. 2108, 2116 (1992).

Journal 1992 Explains how the "terminal condition" requirement in natural death acts may reduce the number of people who fall within the scope of coverage. Also indicates that omission of nutrition and hydration from the list of treatments that may be withdrawn limits patient choices. Quotes Opinion 2.20. References Opinion 2.22. Note, *State Natural Death Acts: Illusory Protection of Individuals' Life-Sustaining Treatment Decisions*, 29 Harvard J. Legis. 175, 186, 194, 195, 201 (1992).

Journal 1992 Discusses the impact of physicians' values on end-of-life decision making for patients. Examines how and why physician values may become dominant. References Opinions 2.20, 2.22, and 9.121. Orentlicher, *The Illusion of Patient Choice in End-Of-Life Decisions*, 267 JAMA 2101, 2102 (1992).

Journal 1992 Contrasts physician-assisted suicide and voluntary euthanasia. Recommends legalization of physician-assisted suicide and proposes guidelines for implementation. References Opinion 2.20. Quill, Cassel, & Meier, *Care of the Hopelessly Ill: Proposed Clinical Criteria for Physician-Assisted Suicide*, 327 New Eng. J. Med. 1380, 1381 (1992).

Journal 1992 Suggests that triage and cost-benefit analysis are the most effective means to evaluate issues associated with allocating scarce medical resources to disabled infants. Concludes both that selective treatment can never be considered murder and that governmental intrusion in this area should be minimal. Quotes Opinions 2.10 (1982) [now Opinion 2.17] and 2.18 (1986) [now Opinion 2.20]. Smith, *Murder, She Wrote or Was It Merely Selective Nontreatment?*, 8 J. Contemp. Health L. & Pol'y 49, 53 (1992).

Journal 1991 Discusses the manner in which competent and incompetent patients could exercise the right to refuse life-sustaining medical treatment prior to *Cruzan*. Analyzes the effect *Cruzan* had on these rights. Concludes that *Cruzan* had limited far-reaching impact and failed to answer several important questions. Cites Opinion 2.20. Albert, *Cruzan v. Director, Missouri Department of Health: Too Much Ado*, 12 J. Legal Med. 331, 338, 343 (1991).

Journal 1991 Discusses why families of persistent vegetative state patients should not make decisions regarding whether to withdraw life support. Observes that leaving decisions to families creates the possibility they will decide in opposition of the patient. References Opinion 2.20. Baron, *Why Withdrawal of Life-Support for PVS Patients Is Not A Family Decision*, 19 Law, Med. & Health Care 73 (1991).

Journal 1991 Considers the issue of how courts should decide right-to-die cases in Massachusetts. Concludes that there are no clear standards for physicians to follow and recommends that physicians obtain court approval before withdrawing artificial nutrition and hydration from a patient in a persistent vegetative state. Quotes Opinion 2.20. Comment, *A Right to Die: Can a Massachusetts Physician Withdraw Artificial Nutrition and Hydration From a Persistently Vegetative Patient Following Cruzan v. Director, Missouri Department of Health?* 26 New Eng. L. Rev. 199, 216, 220 (1991).

Journal 1991 Discusses major neurologic syndromes in life-sustaining medical treatment decisions. Concludes with a survey of the major legal developments in the area since *Cruzan*. References Opinion 2.20. Cranford, *Neurologic Syndromes and Prolonged Survival: When Can Artificial Nutrition and Hydration Be Foregone?* 19 Law, Med. & Health Care 13, 14, 16, 17 (1991).

Journal 1991 Reports that most individuals surveyed favor use of advance directives and would not desire life-sustaining treatment if faced with a poor prognosis. Recommends that physicians routinely discuss advance directives with patients. Cites Opinion 2.20. Emanuel, Barry, Stoeckle, Ettelson, & Emanuel, *Advance Directives for Medical Care—A Case for Greater Use*, 324 New Eng. J. Med. 889 (1991).

Journal 1991 Discusses the "slippery slope" argument against expanding the right to die. Concludes that society seems to be sliding down the slippery slope toward euthanasia. Cites Opinion 2.18 (1986) [now Opinion 2.20]. Kamisar, *When is There A Constitutional "Right to Die"? When is There No Constitutional "Right to Live"?* 25 Georgia L. Rev. 1203, 1207, 1208, 1222 (1991).

Journal 1991 Discusses common misperceptions about legal implications of terminating life support. Emphasizes importance of educating physicians about these medical legal considerations. References Opinion 2.20. Meisel, *Legal Myths About Terminating Life Support*, 151 Arch. Intern. Med. 1497, 1499 (1991).

Journal 1991 Discusses health care decisionmaking for terminally ill incompetent patients in Ohio. Argues that Ohio is one of the few remaining states that does not adequately protect the rights of incompetent terminally ill patients. Cites Opinion 2.18 (1986) [now Opinion 2.20]. Mullins, *The Need for Guidance in Decisionmaking for Terminally Ill Incompetents: Is the Ohio Legislature in a "Persistent Vegetative State?,"* 17 Ohio No. Univ. L. Rev. 827, 844 (1991).

Journal 1991 Discusses the major issues contained in the *Cruzan* decision. Analyzes the legal predicates for an incompetent patient's right to refuse life-sustaining treatment. References Opinion 2.20. Note, *Cruzan v. Director, Missouri Department of Health: To Die or Not to Die: That is the Question—But Who Decides?*, 51 Louisiana L. Rev. 1307, 1327, 1333 (1991).

Journal 1991 Explores the growth of "right to die" jurisprudence with particular emphasis on post-*Cruzan* developments. Notes that the New York "Health Care Proxy Law" does not apply to situations in which a patient is incompetent, but did not appoint an agent. References Opinion 2.20. Note, *Health Care Proxies: New York's Attempt to Resolve the Right to Die Dilemma*, 57 Brooklyn L. Rev. 145, 168 (1991).

Journal 1991 Analyzes the Illinois Supreme Court case of *In re Estate of Longeway*, where the court decided that, absent an advance directive, the guardian of an incompetent patient could authorize the withdrawal of artificial nutrition and hydration. Concludes that written directives other than living wills may best secure patients' rights. Cites Opinion 2.18 (1986) [now Opinion 2.20]. Note, *Redefining the Right to Die in Illinois*, 15 So. Ill. Univ. L. J. 1261, 1273 (1991).

Journal 1991 Discusses applicable law regarding patients in a persistent vegetative state. Compares *Cruzan* with other right-to-die cases, arguing that the *Cruzan* decision makes it more difficult for individuals to secure this right. Quotes Opinion 2.20. Note, *Something Worth Writing Home About: Clear and Convincing Evidence, Living Wills, and Cruzan v. Director, Missouri Department of Health*, 22 Univ. Toledo L. Rev. 871, 879 (1991).

Journal 1991 Examines the living will and durable power of attorney as health care planning devices in South Carolina. Considers both statutory and nonstatutory forms of the living will. References Opinion 2.20. Patterson, *Planning for Health Care Using Living Wills and Durable Powers of Attorney: A Guide for the South Carolina Attorney*, 42 So. Carolina L. Rev. 525, 535, 541, 547, 548 (1991).

Journal 1991 Explains the contractual nature of the physician-patient relationship and how it has been ignored by many courts in right-to-die cases. Concludes there is a constitutional right to privacy in health care decisionmaking. Cites Opinion 2.18 (1986) [now Opinion 2.20]. Rich, *The Assault on Privacy on Healthcare Decisionmaking*, 68 Denver L. Rev. 1, 10 (1991).

Journal 1991 Considers the limits of patient autonomy in demanding treatment that the physician feels provides no medical benefit. Discusses these issues in light of the Helga Wanglie case. References Opinion 2.20. Rie, *The Limits of a Wish*, 21 Hastings Center Rep. 24 (July/August 1991).

Journal 1991 Analyzes three important right-to-die cases: *Cruzan*; *Wanglie*; and *Busalacchi*. Concludes that there should be a nationwide system to address right-to-die cases. References Opinion 2.20. Roach, *Paradox and Pandora's Box: The Tragedy of Current Right-to-Die Jurisprudence*, 25 Univ. Mich. J. Law Reform 133, 137, 158 (1991).

Journal 1990 Argues that *Roe v. Wade* not only protects a woman's right to choose, but also preserves a physician's right to treat. Observes that this protected relationship extends into the arena of right-to-die cases. Cites Opinion 2.20. Annas, Glantz, & Mariner, *The Right of Privacy Protects the Doctor-Patient Relationship*, 263 JAMA 858, 861 (1990).

Journal 1990 Discusses the connection between law and medicine in the context of health care decisionmaking. Presents several illustrations, noting the involvement of courts and judges. Quotes Opinion 2.18 [now Opinion 2.20]. Bellacosa, *The Fusion of Medicine and Law for In*

Extremis Health and Medical Decisions: Does It Produce Energy and Light or Just Cosmic Debris?, 18 *Bull. Am. Acad. Psychiatry Law* 5, 9 (1990).

Journal 1990 Finds that a vast majority of North Carolina nursing homes have written cardiopulmonary resuscitation policies, but that there is substantial variation among them. Concludes that such variations risk limiting or ignoring the personal rights of residents. References Opinions 2.20 and 2.22. Brunetti, Weiss, Studenski, & Clipp, *Cardiopulmonary Resuscitation Policies and Practices: A Statewide Nursing Home Study*, 150 Arch. Intern. Med. 121, 122 (1990).

Journal 1990 Discusses the importance of living wills and society's acceptance of terminating medical care in appropriate situations. Proposes a living will that addresses the shortcomings of current living will statutes. Cites Opinion 2.18 (1986) [now Opinion 2.20]. Cantor, *My Annotated Living Will*, 18 Law, Med. & Health Care 114 (1990).

Journal 1990 Discusses the "living will" and its role in American society. Concludes that legislators need to be more aware of the goals of living wills when drafting statutes. Quotes Opinion 2.20. Comment, *The Living Will: Preservation of the Right-To-Die Demands Clarity and Consistency*, 95 Dickinson L. Rev. 209, 217 (1990).

Journal 1990 Explores current law governing the right of a person to withdraw artificial hydration and nutrition, with emphasis on Oklahoma law, which omits artificial nutrition and hydration from the list of treatments that may be withdrawn. Concludes that individuals have a right to withdraw such treatment and that Oklahoma law may be unconstitutional. Quotes Opinion 2.18 (1986) [now Opinion 2.20]. Comment, *Right to Die: Oklahoma's Position on Nutrition and Hydration: Confusing or Unconstitutional?* 43 Okla. L. Rev. 143, 151 (1990).

Journal 1990 Examines the right of competent patients to refuse treatment on the basis of a common law right of bodily integrity, the right to privacy, and statutory provisions such as natural death acts. Concludes that the law is unsettled with respect to the right of incompetent, nonterminal patients to refuse medical care. Quotes Opinion 2.18 (1986) [now Opinion 2.20]. Comment, *The Right to Refuse Life Sustaining Medical Treatment and the Nonterminally Ill Patient: An Analysis of Abridgment and Anarchy*, 17 Pepperdine L. Rev. 461, 462 (1990).

Journal 1990 Discusses how the imprecise language of euthanasia muddles public discussion of the issue. Concludes that medical ethics must distinguish between acts and omissions undertaken to cause death and those considered reasonable treatment under the circumstances. Quotes Opinion 2.20 (1989). Devettere, *The Imprecise Language of Euthanasia and Causing Death*, 1 J. Clinical Ethics 268, 268 (1990).

Journal 1990 Discusses the proposition that an objective standard should govern end-of-life decisionmaking instead of living wills or similar instruments. Concludes that an objective standard is preferable and recommends that courts adopt such a standard. References Opinion 2.20. Dresser, *Relitigating Life and Death*, 51 Ohio St. L. J. 425, 436 (1990).

Journal 1990 Discusses the development of the law regarding the withdrawal of life-sustaining medical treatment from incompetent patients since the *Quinlan* case. Concludes that *Cruzan* did not resolve a number of important questions concerning the right to die. Quotes Opinion 2.18 (1986) [now Opinion 2.20]. McNoble, *The* Cruzan *Decision—A Surgeon's Perspective*, 20 Memphis State Univ. L. Rev. 569, 581, 600, 601 (1990).

Journal 1990 Considers how the case may be misperceived. Proposes that health care professionals should routinely advise patients of the necessity of making their wishes about life-sustaining treatment known. Quotes Opinion 2.18 (1986) [now Opinion 2.20]. Meisel, *Lessons from* Cruzan, 1 J. Clinical Ethics 245, 248 (1990).

Journal 1990 Discusses the right of physicians to refrain from participating in the withdrawal or removal of life-sustaining treatment. Concludes that federal and state legislation is needed to protect the right of conscience of medical personnel in this context. Quotes Opinion 2.20. Note, *I Have A Conscience, Too: The Plight of Medical Personnel Confronting the Right to Die*, 65 Notre Dame L. Rev. 699, 706 (1990).

Journal 1990 Discusses advance medical directives including living wills and durable powers of attorney. Concludes by examining the physician's role in implementing patient preferences. Cites Opinion 2.20. Orentlicher, *Advance Medical Directives*, 263 JAMA 2365 (1990).

Journal 1990 Discusses the moral dilemma in deciding whether to withdraw artificial nutrition and hydration from a patient and the appropriate role of the judiciary. Concludes that judicial decisions do not represent the moral viewpoint of society and that moral pronouncements should not be made in the courtroom. Quotes Preamble, Principles I, II, III, IV, V, VI, and VII, and Opinion 2.20. Peccarelli, *A Moral Dilemma: The Role of Judicial Intervention in Withholding or Withdrawing Nutrition and Hydration*, 23 John Marshall L. Rev. 537, 539, 540, 541 (1990).

Journal 1990 Explores how recent advances in medical science and technology have resulted in changing views concerning withdrawing and withholding of life support. Concludes that morality plays a key role in dealing with this issue and that physicians should rely upon fundamental principles of medicine for guidance. Quotes Opinion 2.20. Sprung, *Changing Attitudes and Practices in Forgoing Life-Sustaining Treatments*, 263 JAMA 2211, 2213 (1990).

Journal 1990 Looks into the appropriateness of terminating life-prolonging treatment for patients lacking decisionmaking abilities. Concludes that physicians do not risk serious liability for withdrawing life support. References Opinion 2.20. Weir & Gostin, *Decisions to Abate Life-Sustaining Treatment for Nonautonomous Patients: Ethical Standards and Legal Liability for Physicians After Cruzan*, 264 JAMA 1846, 1849, 1850 (1990).

Journal 1989 Challenges the notion that removal of artificial nutrition from permanently unconscious patients constitutes active euthanasia. Concludes by observing that the traditional judicial approach, which permits withdrawal of artificial nutrition, is entirely consistent with accepted medical legal and ethical doctrines. Cites Opinion 2.18 (1986) [now Opinion 2.20]. Cantor, *The Permanently Unconscious Patient, Non-Feeding and Euthanasia*, XV Am. J. Law & Med. 381, 385 (1989).

Journal 1989 Examines and criticizes the legal advice that was rendered by hospital counsel in the context of the Samuel Linares case which occurred at Rush-Presbyterian-St. Luke's Medical Center in Chicago, Illinois. Focusing on such issues as whether foregoing ventilator assistance constitutes murder or child abuse and neglect, concludes that ultraconservative legal advice led to moral paralysis, thereby precipitating the tragic and unnecessary action of the child's father. References Opinion 2.20. Nelson & Cranford, Legal Advice, *Moral Paralysis and the Death of Samuel Linares*, 17 Law, Med. & Health Care 316, 319 (1989).

Journal 1989 Observes that, while new policies regarding physician care of hopelessly ill patients have developed, there is a significant gap between development and implementation of those policies. Urges that this gap be closed and that an overall doctrine of flexible care be developed. References Opinion 2.20. Wanzer, Federman, Adelstein, Cassel, Cassem, Cranford, Hook, Lo, Moertel, Safar, Stone, & Van Eys, *The Physician's Responsibility Toward Hopelessly Ill Patients: A Second Look*, 320 New Eng. J. Med. 844, 844 (1989).

Journal 1988 Considers and challenges certain presumed implications of the definition of *death* as brain death. Points to the importance of the distinction between death of the person as contrasted with death of the body. References Opinion 2.18 (1986) [now Opinion 2.20]. Brody, *Ethical Questions Raised by the Persistent Vegetative Patient*, 18 Hastings Center Rep. 33, 34 (Feb./March 1988).

Journal 1988 Explores the revitalization of the hospice concept and the various structural models available for providing care to the terminally ill. Examines the cost effectiveness of hospice care and discusses various ethical and legal problems that arise in the context of providing hospice care, including withholding or withdrawing life-prolonging medical treatment. References Opinion 2.18 (1986) [now Opinion 2.20]. Comment, *The Hospice Movement: A Renewed View of the Death Process*, 4 J. Contemp. Health L. & Pol'y 295, 312 (1988).

Journal 1988 Focuses on the issue of removal of life-sustaining medical treatment from incompetent patients whose wishes are unknown. The importance of quality of life considerations as an aspect of surrogate decisionmaking in this context is emphasized. References Opinion 2.18 (1986) [now Opinion 2.20]. Quinn, *The Best Interests of Incompetent Patients: The Capacity for Interpersonal Relationships as a Standard for Decisionmaking*, 76 Cal. L. Rev. 897, 906 (1988).

Journal 1988 Examines the meaning and scope of the phrase *artificial* feeding, the distinction between ordinary and extraordinary care, and the impact of medical condition and competency on the patient's right to refuse treatment. Concludes that the value of patient autonomy is not the controlling factor in such cases, but only one factor that must be balanced against the nature and probable results of the proposed treatment. Quotes Opinion 2.18 (1986) [now Opinion 2.20]. Snyder, *Artificial Feeding and the Right to Die: The Legal Issues*, 9 J. Legal Med. 349, 351, 352, 357 (1988).

Journal 1988 Discusses numerous judicial decisions in which the courts have focused, among other things, on the withdrawal of artificial feeding from incompetent adult patients. Practical suggestions are offered to care givers and relevant policy implications and other unresolved issues are addressed. Quotes from Opinion 2.18 (1986) [now Opinion 2.20]. Steinbrook & Lo, *Artificial Feeding Solid Ground, Not a Slippery Slope*, 318 New Eng. J. Med. 286, 288 (1988).

Journal 1988 Discusses moral justification for limited respirator use in prolonging anencephalic infants as organ donors for neonates, problems in determining brain death, and the need for additional research relative to anencephalic newborns. Ethical justifications for withdrawal of artificial life support from adult patients who are permanently comatose are offered, by way of analogy, for the purpose of demonstrating the ethical and medical propriety of attaching volunteered, select anencephalic infants to respirators in an effort to obtain scarce organs. Cites Opinion 2.18 (1986) [now Opinion 2.20]. Walters & Ashwal, *Organ Prolongation in Anencephalic Infants: Ethical and Medical Issues*, 18 Hastings Center Rep. 19, 21 (Oct./Nov. 1988).

Journal 1987 Focuses on the issue of withholding nutrition and hydration from comatose patients with emphasis on the questions of what constitutes medical treeatment and when it may properly be withheld. Briefly discusses the often cited cases that have addressed these issues, noting the importance of the position of the AMA regarding withholding or withdrawing life-prolonging medical treatment. References Opinion 2.18 (1986) [now Opinion 2.20]. Comment, *Hold On Courts: May a Comatose Patient Be Denied Food and Water*, 31 St. Louis Univ. L. J. 749, 750 (1987).

Journal 1987 Following comprehensive analysis of existing common law, notes a trend toward granting families greater autonomy in making decisions for incompetent adult patients. Supports this trend and advocates recognition of a more prominent role for the family in these situations. References Opinion 2.18 (1986) [now Opinion 2.20]. Comment, *The Role of the Family in Medical Decisionmaking for Incompetent Adult Patients: A Historical Perspective and Case Analysis*, 48 U. Pittsburgh L. Rev. 539, 571, 607, 610-11 (1987).

Journal 1986 Discusses the distinction between the persistent vegetative state and coma, pointing out the confusion of these concepts in various leading right to die cases. Addresses philosophical and ethical predicates for withholding treatment noting that, in the final analysis, a balancing of the benefits and burdens of treatment should involve the patient, the family, and the physician. Cites Opinion 2.11 (1981) [now Opinion 2.20]. Berrol, *Considerations for Management of the Persistent Vegetative State*, 67 Arch. Phys. Med. Rehabil. 283, 285 (1986).

Journal 1986 Observes that life-sustaining medical treatment includes artificial nutrition and hydration and that patients have a right to forego such treatment under the Washington State Constitution, applicable common law, and the Washington Natural Death Act. Notes that available judicial standards for surrogate decisionmaking in this context are inadequate, and proposes substantive guidelines for the making of such decisions. References Opinion 2.18 (1986) [now Opinion 2.20]. Comment, *Artificial Nutrition and the Terminally Ill: How Should Washington Decide?*, 61 Wash. L. Rev. 419, 421, 447 (1986).

Journal 1986 Analyzes the law's approach to death by evaluating various legal issues that arise in the context of efforts to define death. Asserts that neocortical death should be viewed as death of the person for all legal purposes. References Opinion 2.18 (1986) [now Opinion 2.20]. Smith, *Legal Recognition of Neocortical Death*, 71 Cornell L. Rev. 850, 860, 876-77 (1986).

Journal 1985 Focuses on the issue of withholding medical care and treatment from infants for whom there is little reasonable expectation of normal development. Urges that parents should assume principal decisionmaking responsibility and offers framework for limited state intervention. References Opinion 2.18 (1986) [now Opinion 2.20]. Haddon, *Baby Doe Cases: Compromise and Moral Dilemma*, 34 Emory L. J. 545, 556 (1985).

Journal 1984 Evaluates two divergent approaches to the legal treatment of withdrawing nourishment. Favors the patient's rights to privacy and to treatment as the primary factors in resolving the issue of withdrawing nourishment. Quotes Opinion 2.11 (1982) [now Opinion 2.20]. Horan & Grant, *The Legal Aspects of Withdrawing Nourishment*, 5 J. Legal Med. 595, 626 (1984).

2.21   The previous Opinion 2.21, "Withholding or Withdrawing Life-Prolonging Medical Treatment—Patients' Preferences," was deleted in 1994 and combined with the current Opinion 2.20, "Withholding or Withdrawing Life-Sustaining Medical Treatment."

Euthanasia is the administration of a lethal agent by another person to a patient for the purpose of relieving the patient's intolerable and incurable suffering.

It is understandable, though tragic, that some patients in extreme duress—such as those suffering from a terminal, painful, debilitating illness—may come to decide that death is preferable to life. However, permitting physicians to engage in euthanasia would ultimately cause more harm than good. Euthanasia is fundamentally incompatible with the physician's role as healer, would be difficult or impossible to control, and would pose serious societal risks.

The involvement of physicians in euthanasia heightens the significance of its ethical prohibition. The physician who performs euthanasia assumes unique responsibility for the act of ending the patient's life. Euthanasia could also readily be extended to incompetent patients and other vulnerable populations.

Instead of engaging in euthanasia, physicians must aggressively respond to the needs of patients at the end of life. Patients should not be abandoned once it is determined that cure is impossible. Patients near the end of life must continue to receive emotional support, comfort care, adequate pain control, respect for patient autonomy, and good communication. (I, IV)

Issued June 1994 based on the report "Decisions Near the End of Life," adopted June 1991 (JAMA. 1992; 267: 2229-33).

Updated June 1996.

9th Cir. 1996 Suit was brought by several physicians and not-for-profit corporation which provides information, assistance, and counseling to competent terminally ill adult patients contemplating suicide, asserting that a state statute making it a crime to aid anyone in attempting to commit suicide unconstitutionally prevents terminally ill patients from exercising their protected liberty interests. Appeals court, en banc, held that the choice of how and when to die is a liberty interest and that the statute violates the due process rights of competent, terminally ill adults who wish to hasten their deaths by obtaining medication prescribed by their physicians. Stating that physician-assisted suicide runs counter to medical ethics, the dissent cited Opinions 2.20, 2.21, and 2.211 and quoted Opinion 2.211. *Compassion in Dying v. Washington,* 79 F.3d 790, 840, 855 *replacing,* 49 F.3d 586 (9th Cir. 1995).

Mich. App. 2001 State brought criminal action against physician for the murder of a patient by lethal injection. The trial court convicted the physician of second-degree murder and delivering a controlled substance. On appeal, the trial court decision was affirmed. The physician asked the appellate court to conclude that euthanasia is legal and to reverse his conviction on constitutional grounds. The appellate court relied on *Washington v. Glucksberg,* 521 U.S. 702 (1997) in determining there is no constitutional right to commit euthanasia, so that an individual can be free from intolerable and irremediable suffering. In discussing Glucksberg, the court observed that a state has a legitimate interest in protecting the integrity and ethics of the medical profession. The court noted *Glucksberg's* reference to Opinions 2.20, 2.21, and 2.211 in this regard. *People v. Kevorkian,* 248 Mich. App. 373, 639 N.W.2d 291, 305 n. 42.

Journal 2002 Examines key factors that led to the current palliative care crisis. Analyzes state legislative and judicial efforts to improve palliative care. Concludes with model legislation that holds physicians accountable for inadequate palliative care. Quotes Opinions 2.21 and 2.211. References Opinion 2.20. Oken, *Curing Healthcare Providers' Failure to Administer Opioids in the Treatment of Severe Pain,* 23 Cardozo L. Rev. 1917, 1925-26, 1952, 1954 (2002).

Journal 2002 Reviews the ethical and legal issues arising in connection with the development of standards for pain management. Concludes that appropriate guidelines for pain management should be established by the medical profession. Cites Opinions 2.21 and 2.211. Stark, *Bio-Ethics and Physician Liability: The Liability Effects of Developing Pain Management Standards,* 14 St. Thomas L. Rev. 601, 631 (2002).

Journal 2001 Explores the similarities and differences between active voluntary euthanasia, terminal sedation, and assisted suicide. Examines the problems with making moral distinctions based on physicians' intentions. Concludes that, with proper safeguards, active voluntary euthanasia and assisted suicide are more protective of patient self determination. Quotes Opinions 2.20 and 2.21. Gauthier, *Active Voluntary Euthanasia, Terminal Sedation, and Assisted Suicide, 12 J. Clinical Ethics 43, 43-44, 49 (2001)*.

Journal 2000 Examines questions regarding the legality of such practices as voluntary stopping of eating and drinking (VSED), use of risky analgesics, and terminal sedation. Explores the distinctions between physician-assisted suicide and other palliative interventions. Concludes VSED, risky analgesics, and certain types of terminal sedation are lawful and should be made available to dying patients who make informed decisions to accept the risks involved. Quotes Opinions 2.21 and 2.211. Cites Opinions 2.18 and 2.20. Cantor & Thomas, *The Legal Bounds of Physician Conduct Hastening Death, 48 Buff. L. Rev. 83, 110, 131, 158 (2000)*.

Journal 2000 Considers the question of whether physician-assisted suicide and euthanasia should be legalized. Concludes that, under basic moral and common law principles, the intentional taking of human life by a private person is wrong. References Opinions 2.20, 2.21, and 2.211. Gorsuch, *The Right to Assisted Suicide and Euthanasia, 23 Harv. J. L. & Pub. Pol'y 599, 653, 707 (2000)*.

Journal 2000 Explores the ongoing debate surrounding the legalization of assisted suicide. Defines and distinguishes assisted suicide and euthanasia from other ethical acts. Concludes most of the critical research questions that bear on current policy debates regarding legalization of assisted suicide remain unanswered. References Opinions 2.21 and 2.211. Rosenfeld, *Assisted Suicide, Depression, and the Right to Die, 6 Psychol. Pub. Pol'y & L. 467, 469 (2000)*.

Journal 1999 Examines legal and policy issues regarding physician-assisted suicide. Distinguishes between refusing treatment and assisted suicide. Concludes that there are too many dangers posed by physician-assisted suicide to warrant legalization. Quotes Opinion 2.211. Cites Opinions 2.20 and 2.21. Pratt, *Too Many Physicians: Physician-Assisted Suicide After Glucksberg/Quill, 9 Alb. L. J. Sci. & Tech. 161, 208 (1999)*.

Journal 1997 Considers the legal and ethical issues involved with physician-assisted suicide and euthanasia. Explores recent legal developments in the courts. Opines that Texas should allow physician-assisted suicide, at least for the terminally ill. Asserts that banning such a practice is unconstitutional. Quotes Opinion 2.211. References Opinion 2.21. Comment, *Physician-Assisted Suicide: Should Texas Be Different?, 33 Hous. L. Rev. 1475, 1480, 1488 (1997)*.

Journal 1997 Discusses goals of care included in advance directives and whether they can be used to predict specific interventions and results. Offers insights provided by survey of physicians at Massachusetts General Hospital. Cites Opinions 2.20 and 2.21. Fischer, Alpert, Stoeckle, & Emanuel, *Can Goals of Care Be Used to Predict Intervention Preferences in an Advance Directive?, 157 Arch. Intern. Med. 801, 807 (1997)*.

Journal 1996 Examines the issue of physician-assisted suicide. Observes that it is important not only to consider whether some form of physician-assisted suicide should enjoy legal and ethical support in our society, but whether physicians should be involved. Concludes that physicians, as a profession, probably are not the proper individuals to perform this function. Cites Opinions 2.21 and 2.211. Clark, *Autonomy and Death, 71 Tul. L. Rev. 45, 89 (1996)*.

Journal 1996 Explores the issue of legalizing physician-assisted suicide. Opines that the current state of technology increases life expectancy but with a concomitant decrease in dignity and autonomy surrounding one's death. Notes that the elderly are committing suicide at an increasing rate. Cites Opinions 2.20, 2.21, and 2.211. Morgan & Sutherland, *Last Rights? Confronting Physician-Assisted Suicide in Law and Society: Legal Liturgies on Physician-Assisted Suicide, 26 Stetson L. Rev. 481, 484 (1996)*.

Journal 1995 Analyzes the case of *Compassion in Dying v. Washington* in which a federal district court judge held that certain people have a constitutional right to physician-assisted suicide. Criticizes the decision for being too broad in that it would protect active euthanasia by physicians on patients who are physically unable to perform the act themselves. Quotes Opinion 2.21. References Opinion 2.211. Larson, *Prescription For Death: A Second Opinion, 44 DePaul L. Rev. 461, 472 (1995)*.

Journal 1995 Offers relevant historical perspectives and provides comprehensive ethical and legal discussion of physician-assisted suicide and euthanasia. Highlights important legislative developments, including the Oregon Death with Dignity Act, and analyzes significant judicial opinions. Quotes Principles III, IV, and VI and Opinions 2.21 and 9.12. Cites Opinions 2.20 and 8.11. Stone & Winslade, *Physician-Assisted Suicide and Euthanasia in the United States: Legal and Ethical Observations*, 16 J. Legal Med. 481, 483, 490, 497, 498, 499 (1995).

Journal 1993 Considers how life-sustaining treatments have led to prolonged life under unacceptable circumstances. Recommends quality assurance programs that promote discussion between physicians and patients regarding life-sustaining treatment problems. Cites Opinions 2.20 and 2.21. Pearlman, Cain, Patrick, Appelbaum-Maizel, Starks, Jecker, & Uhlmann, *Insights Pertaining to Patient Assessments of States Worse than Death*, 4 J. Clinical Ethics 33, 40 (1993).

Journal 1992 Analyzes the arguments for and against active euthanasia, including ethical concerns, the slippery slope argument, and the proper role of the physician. Suggests that active euthanasia may be acceptable when its administration is restricted to physicians. References Opinions 2.20 and 2.21. Brock, *Voluntary Active Euthanasia*, 22 Hastings Center Rep. 10 (March/April 1992).

Journal 1992 Considers the debate surrounding medical futility. Observes that this debate is encouraging reexamination of the nature of patient entitlement to medical care as well as the "ends of medicine." References Opinions 2.20, 2.21, and 2.22. Miles, *Medical Futility*, 20 Law, Med. & Health Care 310, 311, 313 (1992).

Journal 1992 Examines the history of the right an individual has over his or her own body, and how the right to commit suicide has evolved from that concept. Concludes that the right of an incurably ill person to commit suicide is a personal issue to be decided outside of the judicial system. References Opinions 2.21 and 2.211. Morgan, Marks, & Harty-Golder, *The Issue of Personal Choice: The Competent Incurable Patient and the Right to Commit Suicide?*, 57 Mo. L. Rev. 1, 44, 45 (1992).

2.211 Physician-Assisted Suicide

Physician-assisted suicide occurs when a physician facilitates a patient's death by providing the necessary means and/or information to enable the patient to perform the life-ending act (eg, the physician provides sleeping pills and information about the lethal dose, while aware that the patient may commit suicide).

It is understandable, though tragic, that some patients in extreme duress—such as those suffering from a terminal, painful, debilitating illness—may come to decide that death is preferable to life. However, allowing physicians to participate in assisted suicide would cause more harm than good. Physician-assisted suicide is fundamentally incompatible with the physician's role as healer, would be difficult or impossible to control, and would pose serious societal risks.

Instead of participating in assisted suicide, physicians must aggressively respond to the needs of patients at the end of life. Patients should not be abandoned once it is determined that cure is impossible. Multidisciplinary interventions should be sought including specialty consultation, hospice care, pastoral support, family counseling, and other modalities. Patients near the end of life must continue to receive emotional support, comfort care, adequate pain control, respect for patient autonomy, and good communication. (I, IV)

Issued 1994 based on the reports "Decisions Near the End of Life," adopted June 1991 (JAMA. 1992; 267: 2229-33) and "Physician-Assisted Suicide," adopted December 1993.

Updated June 1996.

U.S. 1997 Several physicians and terminally ill patients sued the state seeking a declaration that its prohibition against physician-assisted suicide violates the Fourteenth Amendment's Equal Protection Clause. The trial court disagreed, but the Second Circuit reversed, holding that the state accords different treatment to those terminally ill patients who wish to hasten their death by self-administering prescribed drugs and to those patients who wish to do so by directing the removal of life support systems. The Supreme Court reversed holding that the prohibition against assisting suicide does not violate the Equal Protection Clause. The Court concluded that there is a distinction between assisting suicide and withdrawing treatment quoting reports of the AMA Council on Ethical and Judicial Affairs [now Opinions 2.20 and 2.211]. *Vacco v. Quill, 117 S. Ct. 2293, 2298, 138 L. Ed. 2d 834.*

U.S. 1997 Several Washington physicians, terminally ill patients, and a not for profit organization that counsels people considering physician-assisted suicide sued the state seeking to have statutory ban on physician-assisted suicide declared unconstitutional. The trial court agreed and the Ninth Circuit affirmed. The Supreme Court, in reversing the decision, held that prohibition against causing or aiding a suicide does not violate the Due Process Clause. The Court also noted that the prohibition was rationally related to legitimate state interests in protecting the integrity and ethics of the medical profession quoting from Opinion 2.211. *Washington v. Glucksberg, 117 S. Ct. 2258, 2273, 138 L. Ed. 2d 772.*

9th Cir. 1996 Suit was brought by several physicians and not-for-profit corporation which provides information, assistance, and counseling to competent terminally ill adult patients contemplating suicide, asserting that a state statute making it a crime to aid anyone in attempting to commit suicide unconstitutionally prevents terminally ill patients from exercising their protected liberty interests. Appeals court, en banc, held that the choice of how and when to die is a liberty interest and that the statute violates the due process rights of competent, terminally ill adults who wish to hasten their deaths by obtaining medication prescribed by their physicians. Stating that physician-assisted suicide runs counter to medical ethics, the dissent cited Opinions 2.20, 2.21, and 2.211 and quoted Opinion 2.211. *Compassion in Dying v. Washington, 79 F.3d 790, 840, 855 replacing, 49 F.3d 586 (9th Cir. 1995).*

9th Cir. 1995 A not-for-profit corporation organized to assist terminally ill persons in committing suicide and several physicians alleged that a state statute making aiding a suicide attempt a crime violated 42 U.S.C. § 1983 and the Constitution. In upholding the statute, the court quoted Opinion 2.211 as articulating the ethical position of the medical profession against assisted suicide. In turn, the court found upholding the ethical integrity of the medical profession to be one of the many state interests outweighing the alleged liberty interest in medically-assisted suicide. *Compassion in Dying v. Washington, 49 F.3d 586, 592, replaced, 79 F.3d 790 (9th Cir. 1996).*

Alaska 2001 Two mentally competent, terminally ill adults filed suit, asking the superior court to declare Alaska's manslaughter statute invalid so that their physicians could assist them in committing suicide. The superior court entered summary judgment against the patients and the Alaska Supreme Court affirmed. In concluding that Alaska's constitutional rights of privacy and liberty do not afford terminally ill patients the right to a physician's assistance in committing suicide, the court quoted Opinion 2.211 in support of the state's interest in protecting the integrity of the medical profession. *Sampson v. State, 31 P.3d 88, 96, 97.*

Fla. 1997 A patient, suffering from acquired immune deficiency syndrome (AIDS), and his physician filed suit for a declaratory judgment that state law prohibiting assisted suicide, violated the privacy clause of the state constitution, as well as the due process and equal protection clauses of the Fourteenth Amendment to the United States Constitution. The trial court concluded that the law was unconstitutional. On appeal the state supreme court, relying on the United States Supreme Court's rulings in *Washington v. Glucksberg, 117 S.Ct. 2258 (1997)* and *Vacco v. Quill, 117 S.Ct. 2293 (1997),* held that the state's ban was not unconstitutional. In determining that the right to assisted suicide is not included in the state's guarantee of privacy, the court quoted from Opinion 2.211. *Krischer v. McIver, 697 So. 2d 97, 103.*

Mich. App. 2001 State brought criminal action against physician for the murder of a patient by lethal injection. The trial court convicted the physician of second-degree murder and delivering a controlled substance. On appeal, the trial court decision was affirmed. The physician asked the appellate court to conclude that euthanasia is legal and to reverse his conviction on constitutional grounds. The appellate court relied on *Washington v. Glucksberg, 521 U.S. 702 (1997)* in determining there is no constitutional right to commit euthanasia, so that an individual can be free from intolerable and irremediable suffering. In discussing *Glucksberg,* the court observed that a state has a legitimate interest in protecting the integrity and ethics of the medical profession. The court noted *Glucksberg's* reference to Opinions 2.20, 2.21, and 2.211 in this regard. *People v. Kevorkian, 248 Mich. App. 373, 639 N.W.2d 291, 305 n. 42.*

Journal 2003 Considers societal harm as a justification for statutes prohibiting otherwise harmless conduct. Concludes that moral reaction patterns, which typically prevent humans from injuring one another, are important fibers in the fabric of society. Quotes Opinion 2.211. Johnson, *Harm to the "Fabric of Society" as a Basis for Regulating Otherwise Harmless Conduct: Notes on a Theme from Ravin v. State*, 27 Seattle U. L. Rev. 41, 55 (2003).

Journal 2002 Considers the use of nonlegal materials in United States Supreme Court decisions. Concludes that law alone cannot answer complex legal questions. Cites Opinions 2.20 and 2.211. Hasko, *Persuasion in the Court: Nonlegal Materials in U.S. Supreme Court Opinions*, 94 Law Libr. J. 427, 444, 453 (2002).

Journal 2002 Examines key factors that led to the current palliative care crisis. Analyzes state legislative and judicial efforts to improve palliative care. Concludes with model legislation that holds physicians accountable for inadequate palliative care. Quotes Opinions 2.21 and 2.211. References Opinion 2.20. Oken, *Curing Healthcare Providers' Failure to Administer Opioids in the Treatment of Severe Pain*, 23 Cardozo L. Rev. 1917, 1925-26, 1952, 1954 (2002).

Journal 2002 Proposes an ethical argument for suppressing agonal respiration in dying patients under rare circumstances. Concludes that using neuromuscular block agents in terminally ill, well-sedated, gasping patients can allow for a good death. References Opinion 2.211. Perkin & Resnik, *The Agony of Agonal Respiration: Is the Last Gasp Necessary?* 28 J. Med. Ethics 164, 169 (2002).

Journal 2002 Reviews the ethical and legal issues arising in connection with the development of standards for pain management. Concludes that appropriate guidelines for pain management should be established by the medical profession. Cites Opinions 2.21 and 2.211. Stark, *Bio-Ethics and Physician Liability: The Liability Effects of Developing Pain Management Standards*, 14 St. Thomas L. Rev. 601, 631 (2002).

Journal 2000 Examines questions regarding the legality of such practices as voluntary stopping of eating and drinking (VSED), use of risky analgesics, and terminal sedation. Explores the distinctions between physician-assisted suicide and other palliative interventions. Concludes VSED, risky analgesics, and certain types of terminal sedation are lawful and should be made available to dying patients who make informed decisions to accept the risks involved. Quotes Opinions 2.21 and 2.211. Cites Opinions 2.18 and 2.20. Cantor & Thomas, *The Legal Bounds of Physician Conduct Hastening Death*, 48 Buff. L. Rev. 83, 110, 131, 158 (2000).

Journal 2000 Considers the question of whether physician-assisted suicide and euthanasia should be legalized. Concludes that, under basic moral and common law principles, the intentional taking of human life by a private person is wrong. References Opinions 2.20, 2.21, and 2.211. Gorsuch, *The Right to Assisted Suicide and Euthanasia*, 23 Harv. J. L. & Pub. Pol'y 599, 653, 707 (2000).

Journal 2000 Examines British pharmacists' views on physician-assisted suicide (PAS), including such topics as professional responsibility, personal beliefs, and relevant legal and ethical guidelines. Concludes that most pharmacists view their professional responsibilities regarding PAS differently from physicians. Cites Opinion 2.211. Hanlon, Weiss, & Rees, *British Community Pharmacists' Views of Physician-Assisted Suicide (PAS)*, 26 J. Med. Ethics 363, 367, 369 (2000).

Journal 2000 Discusses ways in which courts and society can take steps to ensure ethical integrity in the medical profession (EIMP). Reviews the case of *Washington v. Glucksberg*, discussing its role in advocating EIMP as a state interest in assisted suicide law. Quotes Opinion 2.211. Kalt, *Death, Ethics, and the State*, 23 Harv. J. L. & Pub. Pol'y 487, 537, 539 (2000).

Journal 2000 Discusses the debate regarding whether physicians should legally participate in hastening or causing death. Explores laws against assisted suicide. Evaluates ethical and social concerns associated with assisted suicide. Quotes Opinion 2.211. Larson, *Tales of Death: Storytelling in the Physician-Assisted Suicide Litigation*, 39 Washburn L. J. 159, 177 (2000).

Journal 2000 Explores the ongoing debate surrounding the legalization of assisted suicide. Defines and distinguishes assisted suicide and euthanasia from other ethical acts. Concludes most of the critical research questions that bear on current policy debates regarding legalization of assisted suicide remain unanswered. References Opinions 2.21 and 2.211. Rosenfeld, *Assisted Suicide, Depression, and the Right to Die*, 6 Psychol. Pub. Pol'y & L. 467, 469 (2000).

Journal 2000 Examines the background of assisted suicide and Michigan's attempt to ban it. Discusses *Cooley v. Granholm*, which is Michigan's most recent constitutional challenge. Concludes that the issue of physician-assisted suicide likely would not arise if society did a better job of providing end-of-life care. Quotes Opinion 2.211. Santayana, *The Michigan Legislature Persists in Prohibiting Assisted Suicide*, 77 U. Det. Mercy L. Rev. 875, 886 (2000).

Journal 2000 Explores the debate regarding physician-assisted suicide. Concludes that autonomy should be respected and that an individual's wishes for assisted suicide should be honored, unless the individual is misinformed or legally incompetent. Quotes Opinion 2.211. References Opinion 2.06. Urofsky, *Justifying Assisted Suicide: Comments on the Ongoing Debate*, 14 Notre Dame J. L. Ethics & Pub. Pol'y 893, 918, 923 (2000).

Journal 1999 Points out that a majority of people favor legalizing physician-assisted suicide. Discusses the right to die under the Ninth Amendment. Explains that a Ninth Amendment claim to the right to die has not been addressed by the United States Supreme Court. Quotes Opinion 2.211. Hardaway, Peterson, & Mann, *The Right to Die and the Ninth Amendment: Compassion and Dying after Glucksberg and Vacco*, 7 Geo. Mason L. Rev. 313, 342 (1999).

Journal 1999 Examines legal and policy issues regarding physician-assisted suicide. Distinguishes between refusing treatment and assisted suicide. Concludes that there are too many dangers posed by physician-assisted suicide to warrant legalization. Quotes Opinion 2.211. Cites Opinions 2.20 and 2.21. Pratt, *Too Many Physicians: Physician-Assisted Suicide After Glucksberg/Quill*, 9 Alb. L. J. Sci. & Tech. 161, 208 (1999).

Journal 1998 Evaluates recent Supreme Court decisions denying a constitutional right to physician-assisted suicide. Explains that, if society adopts Oregon's view on physician-assisted suicide, then the focus will shift to when it is acceptable to end someone's life. Suggests that the debate over physician-assisted suicide does not concern death, but rather how society will care for people at the end of their lives. Quotes Opinion 2.211. Chopko, *Responsible Public Policy at the End of Life*, 75 U. Det. Mercy L. Rev. 557, 573 (1998).

Journal 1998 Explains that the United States Supreme Court's decisions in *Washington* and *Vacco* left the door open for future constitutional challenges regarding the right to physician-assisted suicide. States that the Court did not explicitly deny the existence of a right to physician-assisted suicide. Quotes Opinion 2.20. Cites Opinion 2.211. Cohen, *The Open Door: Will the Right to Die Survive Washington v. Glucksberg and Vacco v. Quill?*, 16 In Pub. Interest 79, 94 (1998).

Journal 1998 Examines ethical issues surrounding physician-assisted suicide. Explores physician-assisted suicide in the context of the influence of psychodynamic psychiatry on the physician-patient relationship. Concludes that if physicians approved of physician-assisted suicide, then it would undermine the physician-patient relationship. Quotes Opinion 2.211. Hamilton, Edwards, Boehnlein, & Hamilton, *The Doctor-Patient Relationship and Assisted Suicide: A Contribution from Dynamic Psychiatry*, 19 Am. J. Forensic Psychiatry 59, 60 (1998).

Journal 1998 Analyzes recent United States Supreme Court decisions on physician-assisted suicide. Discusses amicus briefs that may have affected the Supreme Court's decisions. Theorizes that the Supreme Court will confront the subject of physician-assisted suicide in the future. References Opinion 2.211. Kamisar, *On the Meaning and Impact of the Physician-Assisted Suicide Cases*, 82 Minn. L. Rev. 895, 909, 918 (1998).

Journal 1998 Explains that a determination of mental capacity to consent must be made when a person requests physician-assisted suicide in a jurisdiction where such practice is legal. Explores the potential for liability in the context of making such a determination. Argues that standards regarding determination of mental capacity must be established by case law or legislation. Cites Opinion 2.211. References Opinion 2.06. Lipschitz, *Psychiatry and Consent for Physician-Assisted Suicide*, 19 Am. J. Forensic Psychiatry 91, 103, 104 (1998).

Journal 1998 Discusses legal aspects of physician-assisted suicide. Identifies acceptable end-of-life choices and compares them to physician-assisted suicide. Points out that physician-assisted suicide has the potential for abuse and that safeguards have not been implemented to protect people from that risk. Quotes Opinion 2.211. Cites Opinions 2.20 and 8.08. Mitchell, *Physician-Assisted Suicide: A Survey of the Issues Surrounding Legalization*, 74 N. D. L. Rev. 341, 349 (1998).

Journal 1998 Points out that the court in *Vacco v. Quill* did not reject the practice of physician-assisted suicide and left the subject open for state experimentation. Discusses routes some states have taken regarding assisted suicide. Concludes that access to assisted suicide is outweighed by the risk it will be utilized by depressed and mentally ill people. Quotes Opinions 2.20 and 2.211. Moore, *Physician-Assisted Suicide: Does "The End" Justify the Means?*, 40 Ariz. L. Rev. 1471, 1472, 1481-82, 1491 (1998).

Journal 1998 Points out that psychiatrists have a limited ability to make assessments regarding the requests of terminally ill patients for physician-assisted suicide. Argues that psychiatrists must oppose physician-assisted suicide because its practice would be detrimental to the profession of medicine and would adversely affect the practice of psychiatry. Quotes Opinion 2.211. Orr & Bishop, *Why Psychiatrists Should Not Participate in Euthanasia and Physician-Assisted Suicide*, 19 Am. J. Forensic Psychiatry 35, 36 (1998).

Journal 1998 Analyzes arguments for and against physician-assisted suicide. Distinguishes between killing and allowing a person to die. Concludes that the issue of assisted suicide should be addressed in the political arena rather than in the federal court system. Cites Opinion 2.211. Park, *Physician-Assisted Suicide: State Legislation Teetering at the Pinnacle of a Slippery Slope*, 7 Wm. & Mary Bill Rts. J. 277, 292, 293 (1998).

Journal 1998 Argues that physician-assisted suicide should be available for terminally ill patients whose pain is not alleviated through medications. Analyzes the effects of state regulation of physician-assisted suicide. Explores the possibility of using Thirteenth Amendment claims to abolish possible racially discriminatory use of physician-assisted suicide. Quotes Opinion 2.211. Pittman, *Physician-Assisted Suicide in the Dark Ward: The Intersection of the Thirteenth Amendment and Health Care Treatments Having Disproportionate Impacts on Disfavored Groups*, 28 Seton Hall L. Rev. 774, 784 (1998).

Journal 1998 Explains that physician-assisted suicide diametrically opposes the ideals of the medical profession. States that referendums are not good ways to make public policy. Suggests that patients should discuss their wishes regarding withholding or withdrawing life-sustaining medical treatment with their physicians and families. References Opinion 2.211. Reardon, *American Medical Association Perspective on Physician Assisted Suicide*, 75 U. Det. Mercy L. Rev. 515 (1998).

Journal 1998 Analyzes the Supreme Court's decision in *Washington v. Glucksberg*. Explains how the state's interest in preserving life can be viewed as an interest in preserving the sanctity of personal autonomy. Argues that physician-assisted suicide would preserve individual freedom and the sanctity of life. Quotes Opinion 2.211. Staihar, *The State's Unqualified Interest in Preserving Life: A Critique of the Formulations of Life's Sanctity in Washington v. Glucksberg*, 34 Idaho L. Rev. 401, 415 (1998).

Journal 1998 Discusses the United States Supreme Court's decision in *Washington v. Glucksberg*. Points out that the Supreme Court left many unresolved issues concerning physician-assisted suicide. Provides criteria that could be used by state legislatures in drafting pertinent statutes. Cites Opinion 2.211. Testa, *Sentenced to Life? An Analysis of the United States Supreme Court's Decision in Washington v. Glucksberg*, 22 Nova L. Rev. 821, 839 (1998).

Journal 1998 Examines society's increasing acceptance of the belief in an individual's right to die. Discusses issues surrounding physician-assisted suicide. Evaluates the impact of United States Supreme Court decisions on physician-assisted suicide. Quotes Opinion 2.211. Urofsky, *Leaving the Door Ajar: The Supreme Court and Assisted Suicide*, 32 U. Rich. L. Rev. 313, 336 (1998).

Journal 1997 Reviews the arguments made in *amicus curiae* briefs submitted to the Supreme Court on the topic of assisted suicide. Focuses on key insights into the debate offered by the various *amici curiae*. Quotes Opinion 2.211. Coleson, *The Glucksberg & Quill Amicus Curiae Briefs: Verbatim Arguments Opposing Assisted Suicide*, 13 Issues in Law & Med. 3, 67 (1997).

Journal 1997 Considers the legal and ethical issues involved with physician-assisted suicide and euthanasia. Explores recent legal developments in the courts. Opines that Texas should allow physician-assisted suicide, at least for the terminally ill. Asserts that banning such a practice is unconstitutional. Quotes Opinion 2.211. References Opinion 2.21. Comment, *Physician-Assisted Suicide: Should Texas Be Different?*, 33 Hous. L. Rev. 1475, 1480, 1488 (1997).

Journal 1997 Discusses the consequences of physician-assisted suicide. Argues that assisted suicide would divide the medical community. Concludes that physician-assisted suicide does not enhance freedom. Quotes Opinion 2.211. FitzGibbon, *The Failure of the Freedom-Based and Utilitarian Arguments for Assisted Suicide*, 42 Am. J. Juris. 211, 252 (1997).

Journal 1997 Explores a model physician-assisted suicide statute. Explains its history, provisions, and effects. Posits that the Act reaches further than one may suspect. Notes the AMA's position on assisted death and concludes that the Act fails to account for moral tradition. Quotes Opinion 2.211. FitzGibbon & Lai, *The Model Physician-Assisted Suicide Act and the Jurisprudence of Death*, 13 Issues in Law & Med. 173, 203-04 (1997).

Journal 1997 Considers United States Supreme Court decisions regarding physician-assisted suicide. Argues that state legislatures should enact statutes to legalize physician-assisted suicide. Proposes a model act on physician-assisted suicide. Cites Opinion 2.211. Glynn, *Turning to State*

Legislatures to Legalize Physician-Assisted Suicide for Seriously Ill, Non-Terminal Patients After Vacco v. Quill and Washington v. Glucksberg, 6 J. L. & Pol'y. 329, 345 (1997).

Journal 1997 Considers the right to die. Discusses the extension of the right to refuse treatment to decisions affecting life and death. Explains that courts distinguish between withdrawing life-sustaining treatment and euthanasia or assisted suicide. Emphasizes the importance of quality end-of-life care. Cites Opinion 2.211. Gostin, *Deciding Life and Death in the Courtroom: From Quinlan to Cruzan, Glucksberg, and Vacco—A Brief History and Analysis of Constitutional Protection of the Right to Die,'* 278 JAMA 1523, 1525, 1528 (1997).

Journal 1997 States that the United States Supreme Court has ended the *Roe v. Wade* era in which the Court made decisions on social policy based on normative judgments. Discusses the dangers posed by physician-assisted suicide. Argues that the decision in *Washington v. Glucksberg* averted the danger of abuse posed by physician-assisted suicide. Quotes Opinion 2.211. McConnell, *The Right to Die and the Jurisprudence of Tradition,* 1997 Utah L. Rev. 665, 703-04 (1997).

Journal 1997 Examines possible legalization of euthanasia, observing that any form of euthanasia will be a step toward horrible death. Posits that legalizing euthanasia will create unsolvable mortal dangers that conflict with universal values of life. Concludes that physician-assisted suicide would create many victims. Cites Opinion 2.211. McGonnigal, *This is Who Will Die When Doctors Are Allowed To Kill Their Patients,* 31 J. Marshall L. Rev. 95, 103 (1997).

Journal 1997 Explores the ethical and legal debate over assisted suicide. Examines cases dealing with prohibitions against physician-assisted suicide. Considers the Oregon Death with Dignity Act in light of the ruling in *Lee v. Oregon.* Quotes Opinion 2.211. Note, *Constitutional Aspects of Physician-Assisted Suicide After Lee v. Oregon,* XXIII Am. J. Law & Med. 69 (1997).

Journal 1997 Discusses the difference between physician-assisted suicide and the withdrawal of life-sustaining medical treatment. Posits that traditional moral arguments cannot justify the distinction. Examines how a right to assisted suicide for terminal patients brings right-to-die laws into alignment with underlying ethical precepts. References Opinion 2.211. Orentlicher, *The Legalization of Physician Assisted Suicide: A Very Modest Revolution,* 38 B.C.L. Rev. 443, 459-60 (1997).

Journal 1997 Considers the perspectives of medical residents about end-of-life issues. Investigates the differences of opinion held by residents in psychiatry, internal medicine, and emergency medicine. References Opinion 2.211. Roberts, Roberts, Warner, Solomon, Hardee, & McCarty, *Internal Medicine, Psychiatry, and Emergency Medicine Residents' Views of Assisted Death Practices,* 157 Arch. Intern. Med. 1603, 1609 (1997).

Journal 1996 Proposes a model state statute allowing and controlling physician-assisted suicide. Analyzes the constitutionality of the act and offers public policy justifications for the act's provisions. Concludes that proponents of physician-assisted suicide should provide precise, carefully tailored examples of regulations. Quotes Opinion 2.211. Cites Opinion 2.20. Baron, Bergstresser, Brock, Cole, Dorfman, Johnson, Schnipper, Vorenberg, & Wanzer, *A Model State Act to Authorize and Regulate Physician-Assisted Suicide,* 33 Harv. J. Legis. 1, 2, 7 (1996).

Journal 1996 Examines the issue of physician-assisted suicide. Observes that it is important not only to consider whether some form of physician-assisted suicide should enjoy legal and ethical support in our society, but whether physicians should be involved. Concludes that physicians, as a profession, probably are not the proper individuals to perform this function. Cites Opinions 2.21 and 2.211. Clark, *Autonomy and Death,* 71 Tul. L. Rev. 45, 89 (1996).

Journal 1996 Criticizes the circuit court's opinion in *Compassion in Dying.* Suggests that the opinion fails to fully consider the ethical prohibitions against physician-assisted suicide. Concludes that the court's opinion is not based on a complete and accurate presentation of historical views and attitudes about suicide. Quotes Opinion 2.211. Duncan & Lubin, *The Use and Abuse of History in Compassion in Dying,* 20 Harv. J.L. & Pub. Pol'y 175, 183 (1996).

Journal 1996 Examines ethical and legal issues involved in physician-assisted suicide. Asserts that the judiciary is not the proper forum for establishing guidelines regarding these issues. Concludes that individual state legislative enactments are the proper vehicles for delineating appropriate guidelines. Quotes Opinion 2.211. Kass & Lund, *Physician-Assisted Suicide, Medical Ethics and the Future of the Medical Profession,* 35 Duq. L. Rev. 395, 404 (1996).

Journal 1996 Discusses the historical development of the right to die. Considers patient autonomy and paternalism and the role physicians play in end-of-life decisions. Explains the issue in the context of federal cases. Examines the true extent of a protected right to die. Cites Opinion

2.211. Kelly, *The "Right to Die" in America: The Ninth Circuit's Decision in Compassion in Dying v. The State of Washington*, 29 J. Health & Hosp. L. 246, 255 (1996).

Journal 1996 Explores the issue of legalizing physician-assisted suicide. Opines that the current state of technology increases life expectancy but with a concomitant decrease in dignity and autonomy surrounding one's death. Notes that the elderly are committing suicide at an increasing rate. Cites Opinions 2.20, 2.21, and 2.211. Morgan & Sutherland, *Last Rights? Confronting Physician-Assisted Suicide in Law and Society: Legal Liturgies on Physician-Assisted Suicide*, 26 Stetson L. Rev. 481, 484 (1996).

Journal 1996 Considers the right to death with dignity. Suggests that the AMA's position undermines mitigation of suffering and the individuals' right to self-determination. Concludes that restrictions on the right to death with dignity may be constitutionally impermissible. Quotes Opinion 2.211. Cites Opinion 2.20. Note, *Who Decides if There is Triumph in the Ultimate Agony? Constitutional Theory and the Emerging Right to Die With Dignity*, 37 Wm. & Mary L. Rev. 827, 829 (1996).

Journal 1996 Explores ethical problems accompanying the power to prolong and preserve life past points previously achievable. Questions whether physician-assisted suicide is a proper and ethically desirable course of treatment. Discusses recent developments and arguments surrounding physician-assisted suicide. References Opinion 2.211. Thomasma, *When Physicians Choose to Participate in the Death of Their Patients: Ethics and Physician-Assisted Suicide*, 24 J. Law, Med. & Ethics 183, 184, 195 (1996).

Journal 1995 Suggests that people seeking suicide need life-affirming treatment, not aid in dying. Concludes that the US Constitution does not require society to stand by while a person seeks suicide. Cites Opinion 2.211. Bopp & Coleson, *The Constitutional Case Against Permitting Physician-Assisted Suicide for Competent Adults With Terminal Conditions*, 11 Issues in Law & Med. 239, 250 (1995).

Journal 1995 Examines four essential principles of bioethics–patient autonomy, nonmaleficence, beneficence. and justice–and describes the application of these in clinical settings according to bioethical norms and AMA opinions. Concludes that such an approach promotes compassionate medical caregiving and that laws should reflect these values. Quotes Opinions 2.01 and 8.18. References Opinion 2.211. Cohen, *Toward a Bioethics of Compassion*, 28 Ind. L. Rev. 667, 673, 681-82, 683 (1995).

Journal 1995 Analyzes the case of *Compassion in Dying v. Washington* in which a federal district court judge held that certain people have a constitutional right to physician-assisted suicide. Criticizes the decision for being too broad in that it would protect active euthanasia by physicians on patients who are physically unable to perform the act themselves. Quotes Opinion 2.21. References Opinion 2.211. Larson, *Prescription For Death: A Second Opinion*, 44 DePaul L. Rev. 461, 472 (1995).

Journal 1994 Argues that assisted suicide is not an implicit right under the fourteenth amendment's liberty guarantee. Suggests that giving physicians the authority to determine the appropriateness of assisted suicide furthers no legitimate state interest. Cites Opinion 2.06. References Opinion 2.211. Marzen, *Out, Out Brief Candle: Constitutionally Prescribed Suicide for the Terminally Ill*, 21 Hastings Const. L.Q. 799, 821 (1994).

Journal 1992 Examines the history of the right an individual has over his or her own body, and how the right to commit suicide has evolved from that concept. Concludes that the right of an incurably ill person to commit suicide is a personal issue to be decided outside of the judicial system. References Opinions 2.21 and 2.211. Morgan, Marks, & Harty-Golder, *The Issue of Personal Choice: The Competent Incurable Patient and the Right to Commit Suicide?*, 57 Mo. L. Rev. 1, 44, 45 (1992).

Journal 1992 Discusses the historical, legal, and social arguments both for and against assisted suicide and voluntary active euthanasia. Concludes that only physician-assisted suicide should be legalized. References Opinion 2.211. Note, *Aid-in-Dying: Should We Decriminalize Physician-Assisted Suicide and Physician-Committed Euthanasia?*, XVIII Am. J. Law & Med. 369, 370 (1992).

2.215 Treatment Decisions for Seriously Ill Newborns

The primary consideration for decisions regarding life-sustaining treatment for seriously ill newborns should be what is best for the newborn. Factors that should be weighed are (1) the chance that therapy will succeed, (2) the risks involved with treatment and nontreatment, (3) the degree to which the therapy, if successful, will extend life, (4) the pain and discomfort associated with the therapy, and (5) the anticipated quality of life for the newborn with and without treatment.

Care must be taken to evaluate the newborn's expected quality of life from the child's perspective. Life-sustaining treatment may be withheld or withdrawn from a newborn when the pain and suffering expected to be endured by the child will overwhelm any potential for joy during his or her life. When an infant suffers extreme neurological damage, and is consequently not capable of experiencing either suffering or joy, a decision may be made to withhold or withdraw life-sustaining treatment. When life sustaining treatment is withheld or withdrawn, comfort care must not be discontinued.

When an infant's prognosis is largely uncertain, as is often the case with extremely premature newborns, all life-sustaining and life-enhancing treatment should be initiated. Decisions about life-sustaining treatment should be made once the prognosis becomes more certain. It is not necessary to attain absolute or near absolute prognostic certainty before life-sustaining treatment is withdrawn, since this goal is often unattainable and risks unnecessarily prolonging the infant's suffering.

Physicians must provide full information to parents of seriously ill newborns regarding the nature of treatments, therapeutic options, and expected prognosis with and without therapy, so that parents can make informed decisions for their children about life-sustaining treatment. Counseling services and an opportunity to talk with persons who have had to make similar decisions should be available to parents. Ethics committees or infant review committees should also be utilized to facilitate parental decision making. These committees should help mediate resolutions of conflicts that may arise among parents, physicians, and others involved in the care of the infant. These committees should also be responsible for referring cases to the appropriate public agencies when it is concluded that the parents' decision is not a decision that could reasonably be judged to be in the best interests of the infant. (I, III, IV, V)

Issued June 1994 based on the report "Treatment Decisions for Seriously Ill Newborns," adopted June 1992.

N.Y. Sup. 2003 Mother petitioned court to remove her daughter from a respirator. Hospital policy denied mother the authorization to withdraw care. Court granted petition and held parents have a right to refuse medical treatment for their children. Applying the best interest test, the court held that the burdens of prolonging life exceeded the benefits and that, absent extraordinary circumstances or disagreement between parents, judicial intervention is not required to withhold medical treatment from a minor in a vegetative state. Quotes Opinion 2.215. References Opinion 2.20. *In re AB*, 196 *Misc.* 2d 940, 768 *N.Y.S.* 2d 256, 268-69.

Journal 2002 Explores the implications of withholding medical treatment when abortion results in a live birth. Concludes that, in these situations, abortive parents and physicians should not solely decide the child's best interest. Quotes Preamble, Principles I and III, and Opinions 2.035, 2.20, and 2.215. Casagrande, *Children Not Meant to Be: Protecting the Interests of the Child When Abortion Results in Live Birth*, 6 Quinnipiac Health L.J. 19, 44, 45, 47-48 (2002).

Journal 2001 Examines end-of-life care given to infants under the age of one. Concludes that palliative care consultations may improve the end-of-life care that terminally ill infants and their families currently receive. References Opinion 2.215. Pierucci, Kirby, & Leuthner, *End-of-Life Care for Neonates and Infants: The Experience and Effects of a Palliative Care Consultation Service*, 108 Pediatrics 653, 659 (2001).

Journal 2001 Discusses neonatal euthanasia and the related moral dilemmas. Explores the background and current legal status of neonatal euthanasia in the United States. Concludes that the moral and legal status of passive neonatal euthanasia is unclear and should be reviewed and clarified. Quotes Opinion 2.215. Sklansky, *Neonatal Euthanasia: Moral Considerations and Criminal Liability,* 27 J. Med. Ethics 5, 8, 9 (2001).

2.22   Do-Not-Resuscitate Orders

Efforts should be made to resuscitate patients who suffer cardiac or respiratory arrest except when circumstances indicate that cardiopulmonary resuscitation (CPR) would be inappropriate or not in accord with the desires or best interests of the patient.

Patients at risk of cardiac or respiratory failure should be encouraged to express in advance their preferences regarding the use of CPR, and this should be documented in the patient's medical record. These discussions should include a description of the procedures encompassed by CPR and, when possible, should occur in an outpatient setting when general treatment preferences are discussed or as early as possible during hospitalization. The physician has an ethical obligation to honor the resuscitation preferences expressed by the patient. Physicians should not permit their personal value judgments about quality of life to obstruct the implementation of a patient's preferences regarding the use of CPR.

If a patient is incapable of rendering a decision regarding the use of CPR, a decision may be made by a surrogate decision maker, based upon the previously expressed preferences of the patient or, if such preferences are unknown, in accordance with the patient's best interests.

If, in the judgment of the attending physician, it would be inappropriate to pursue CPR, the attending physician may enter a do-not-resuscitate (DNR) order into the patient's record. Resuscitative efforts should be considered inappropriate by the attending physician only if they cannot be expected either to restore cardiac or respiratory function to the patient or to meet established ethical criteria, as defined in the Principles of Medical Ethics and Opinions 2.03, "Allocation of Limited Medical Resources," and 2.095, "The Provision of Adequate Health Care." When there is adequate time to do so, the physician must first inform the patient, or the incompetent patient's surrogate, of the content of the DNR order, as well as the basis for its implementation. The physician also should be prepared to discuss appropriate alternatives, such as obtaining a second opinion (eg, consulting a bioethics committee) or arranging for transfer of care to another physician.

DNR orders, as well as the basis for their implementation, should be entered by the attending physician in the patient's medical record.

DNR orders only preclude resuscitative efforts in the event of cardiopulmonary arrest and should not influence other therapeutic interventions that may be appropriate for the patient. (I, IV)

Issued March 1992 based on the report "Guidelines for the Appropriate Use of Do-Not-Resuscitate Orders," adopted December 1990 (JAMA. 1991; 265: 1868-71).

Updated June 1994.

Kan. App. 1998 Physician was convicted of attempted murder of a terminally ill patient, and intentional and malicious second-degree murder of another terminally ill patient. The court quoted Opinion 2.22, to exemplify a physician's duty to provide cardiopulmonary resuscitation unless the physician believes that such action would be futile. Additionally, the court referenced Opinion 2.20, in support of a physician's duty to provide a terminally ill patient adequate pain relief. The court reversed the physician's convictions, stating that the jury could not disregard the testimony of several physicians who concurred with the defendant-physician's treatment of the deceased patients. *State v. Naramore*, 25 Kan. App. 2d 302, 965 P.2d 211, 214, 216.

Journal 2001 Observes that many aspects of managed care have increased the tensions between patients and their health care providers. Notes that patient dissatisfaction is on the rise for other reasons as well. Concludes that Congress should take a comprehensive legislative approach in addressing these issues. Quotes Opinion 2.17. Cites Opinion 2.035. References Opinions 2.037 and 2.22. Sanematsu, *Taking a Broader View of Treatment Disputes Beyond Managed Care: Are Recent Legislative Efforts the Cure?* 48 UCLA L. Rev. 1245, 1258, 1284 (2001).

Journal 2000 Discusses a medical-ethical strategy for managing iatrogenic cardiac arrests in DNR patients. Suggests that many factors must be taken into account before withholding resuscitation in certain unanticipated situations, such as an iatrogenic catastrophe. References Opinion 2.22. Christensen & Orlowski, *Iatrogenic Cardiopulmonary Arrests in DNR Patients*, 11 J. Clinical Ethics 14, 15, 20 (2000).

Journal 2000 Discusses euphemisms used through medical codes in hospitals regarding end-of-life patient care. Examines how the fear of medical failure and the fear of litigation mold decision-making in critical care units. Concludes that health care providers often lack the courage to let a patient die. References Opinion 2.22. Smith, *Euphemistic Codes and Tell-Tale Hearts: Humane Assistance in End-of-Life Cases*, 10 Health Matrix 175, 177 (2000).

Journal 2000 Discusses current law governing consent to sperm retrieval and insemination after death or persistent vegetative state. Identifies gaps in the law. Concludes that sperm retrieval and insemination in these situations should be permitted, provided there is express prior consent or sufficient evidence from which consent may be implied. Cites Opinion 2.22. Strong, *Consent to Sperm Retrieval and Insemination After Death or Persistent Vegetative State*, 14 J.L. & Health 243, 248 (2000).

Journal 1998 Explains when a surrogate is required to make health care decisions. Discusses limitations of a surrogate's authority. Emphasizes that the health care provider must recognize that ultimate decision-making regarding care first belongs to the patient, and then to the surrogate. Quotes Opinion 2.035. Cites Opinion 8.11. References Opinion 2.22. O'Neill, *Surrogate Health Care Decisions for Adults in Illinois—Answers to the Legal Questions That Health Care Providers Face on a Daily Basis*, 29 Loy. Univ. Chi. L. J. 411, 445, 448 (1998).

Journal 1998 Discusses various ways theorists define medical futility. Evaluates the impact of *In re Baby K* on the correct notion of medical futility. Examines how futility affects patient autonomy. Quotes Opinion 2.22. Strasser, *The Futility of Futility?: On Life, Death, and Reasoned Public Policy*, 57 Md. L. Rev. 505, 523, 552, 553 (1998).

Journal 1997 Examines case law pertaining to medical futility disputes. Reviews hospital policies regarding futility and notes a variety of definitions and guidelines. Concludes that, absent a clear consensus, physicians should not act solely to decide questions of futility. References Opinions 2.035 and 2.22. Johnson, Gibbons, Goldner, Wiener, & Eton, *Legal and Institutional Policy Responses to Medical Futility*, 30 J. Health & Hosp. L. 21, 26, 31, 35, 36 (1997).

Journal 1997 Explores the meaning of cardiopulmonary resuscitation and legal issues involving DNR orders. Considers problems created by DNR orders in operating rooms in light of patients' rights. Concludes that hospitals must adopt clear policies for their surgical teams to follow. Quotes Opinion 8.08. References Opinion 2.22. Lonchyna, *To Resuscitate or Not . . . In the Operating Room: The Need for Hospital Policies for Surgeons Regarding DNR Orders*, 6 Annals Health L. 209, 215, 217 (1997).

Journal 1997 Considers individuals' right to die and the value of a wrongful living tort. Proposes that courts should reject any cause of action for wrongful living in situations where patient advance directives are not honored by physicians. References Opinion 2.22. Milani, *Better Off Dead Than Disabled? Should Courts Recognize A Wrongful Living Cause of Action When Doctors Fail to Honor Patients' Advance Directives?*, 54 Wash. & Lee L. Rev. 149, 151-52 (1997).

Journal 1994 Considers how greater patient autonomy has led to situations in which medical care may be viewed as futile. Suggests that the law has intruded too far into this area of medicine.

Quotes Opinion 2.035. Cites Opinions 2.03, 2.095, 2.17, 2.19, 2.20, and 2.22. Cultice, *Medical Futility: When Is Enough, Enough?*, 27 J. Health & Hosp. Law 225, 230, 256 (1994).

Journal 1993 Discusses physician, patient, and societal concerns about futility. Concludes that futility decisions should be left to physicians. Cites Opinion 2.22. Bennett, *When Is Medical Treatment Futile?*, 9 Issues in Law & Med. 35, 39 (1993).

Journal 1993 Considers how patient self-determination may be affected by cardiopulmonary resuscitation and Do-Not-Resuscitate policies. Opposes a "futility" exception to informed consent as being violative of a physician's fiduciary duties to patients. Cites Opinion 8.07 (1986) [now Opinion 8.08]. References Opinion 2.22. Boozang, *Death Wish: Resuscitating Self-Determination for the Critically Ill*, 35 Ariz. L. Rev. 23, 24, 28, 52 (1993).

Journal 1993 Discusses the problem of physicians withholding needed medical treatment from HIV-infected infants. Concludes that current law should be expanded to eliminate this discrimination. Quotes Opinions 2.09, 2.17, 2.20, 2.22, 4.04, and 8.03. Crossley, *Of Diagnoses and Discrimination: Discriminatory Nontreatment of Infants With HIV Infection*, 93 Columbia L. Rev. 1581, 1620, 1621 (1993).

Journal 1993 Discusses the relationship between a physician's professional conscience and end of life decisionmaking. Considers the issue of futile medical treatment. Examines case law concerning a patient's right to demand treatment and a physician's obligation to provide it. References Opinions 2.20 and 2.22. Daar, *A Clash at the Bedside: Patient Autonomy v. A Physician's Professional Conscience*, 44 Hastings L. J. 1241, 1257, 1268, 1286 (1993).

Journal 1993 Discusses the American Heart Association's acknowledgment of medical futility, but questions whether its views adequately reflect current ethical perceptions. Proposes ways in which the guidelines should be reformed. References Opinion 2.22. Jecker & Schneiderman, *An Ethical Analysis of the Use of "Futility" in the 1992 American Heart Association Guidelines for Cardiopulmonary Resuscitation and Emergency Cardiac Care*, 153 Arch. Intern. Med. 2195, 2197 (1993).

Journal 1993 Examines the American Heart Association's guidelines for withholding cardiopulmonary resuscitation in emergency medical service systems and criticizes them for being too strict. Argues that a mechanism should be created to facilitate prehospital DNR orders and ensure that they are followed. References Opinion 2.22. McIntyre, *Loosening Criteria for Withholding Prehospital Cardiopulmonary Resuscitation*, 153 Arch. Intern. Med. 2189, 2190 (1993).

Journal 1992 Examines several issues regarding persistent vegetative state (PVS) patients, including whether PVS patients are really dead, whether nutrition and hydration should be withheld, whether life-sustaining treatments are futile or medically inappropriate, and whether ordinary standards for decisionmaking should be applied to PVS patients. Concludes that life-sustaining therapy may be withheld or continued, but that withdrawal of nutrition and hydration, as well as active euthanasia, present more difficult questions. References Opinions 2.20 and 2.22. Brody, *Special Ethical Issues in the Management of PVS Patients*, 20 Law, Med. & Health Care 104, 109 (1992).

Journal 1992 Discusses "Do-Not-Resuscitate" (DNR) orders in light of the Patient Self-Determination Act. Proposes a policy of required reconsideration of DNR orders in hospitals when a patient enters a treatment setting in which discreet, time-limited therapies are offered that may precipitate cardiac arrest. References Opinion 2.22. Cohen & Cohen, *Required Reconsideration of "Do-Not-Resuscitate" Orders in the Operating Room and Certain Other Treatment Settings*, 20 Law, Med. & Health Care 354, 356 (1992).

Journal 1992 Examines ethical and legal issues surrounding cardiopulmonary resuscitation and emergency cardiac care. Discusses advance directives and proxy decisionmaking, medical futility, resource allocation, and Do-Not-Resuscitate orders. References Opinions 2.20 and 2.22. Comment, *Ethical Considerations in Resuscitation*, 268 JAMA 2282, 2283, 2287 (1992).

Journal 1992 Considers the debate surrounding medical futility. Observes that this debate is encouraging reexamination of the nature of patient entitlement to medical care as well as the "ends of medicine." References Opinions 2.20, 2.21, and 2.22. Miles, *Medical Futility*, 20 Law, Med. & Health Care 310, 311, 313 (1992).

Journal 1992 Explains how the "terminal condition" requirement in natural death acts may reduce the number of people who fall within the scope of coverage. Also indicates that omission of nutrition and hydration from the list of treatments that may be withdrawn limits patient choices. Quotes Opinion 2.20. References Opinion 2.22. Note, *State Natural Death Acts: Illusory Protection of Individuals' Life-Sustaining Treatment Decisions*, 29 Harvard J. Legis. 175, 186, 194,

195, 201 (1992).

Journal 1992 Discusses the impact of physicians' values on end-of-life decision making for patients. Examines how and why physician values may become dominant. References Opinions 2.20, 2.22, and 9.121. Orentlicher, *The Illusion of Patient Choice in End-Of-Life Decisions*, 267 JAMA 2101, 2102 (1992).

Journal 1992 Discusses results of a study that evaluated the impact of ethics education on Do-Not-Resuscitate (DNR) practices by house officers. Concludes that educational programs improve care for DNR patients. References Opinion 2.22. Sulmasy, Geller, Faden, & Levine, *The Quality of Mercy: Caring for Patients With "Do Not Resuscitate" Orders*, 267 JAMA 682 (1992).

Journal 1991 Examines the involvement of the legal system in end-of-life medical decisionmaking. Questions whether the law should intrude into the domain. Concludes that judges should become involved primarily to address the "terms of reconciliation" between physicians and patients. References Opinion 2.22. Flick, *The Due Process of Dying*, 79 Cal. L. Rev. 1121, 1132 (1991).

Journal 1990 Finds that a vast majority of North Carolina nursing homes have written cardiopulmonary resuscitation policies, but that there is substantial variation among them. Concludes that such variations risk limiting or ignoring the personal rights of residents. References Opinions 2.20 and 2.22. Brunetti, Weiss, Studenski, & Clipp, *Cardiopulmonary Resuscitation Policies and Practices: A Statewide Nursing Home Study*, 150 Arch. Intern. Med. 121, 122 (1990).

2.225 Optimal Use of Orders-Not-to-Intervene and Advance Directives

More rigorous efforts in advance care planning are required in order to tailor end-of-life care to the preferences of patients so that they can experience a satisfactory last chapter in their lives. There is need for better availability and tracking of advance directives, and more uniform adoption of form documents that can be honored in all states of the United States. The discouraging evidence of inadequate end-of-life decision-making indicates the necessity of several improvement strategies:

(1) Patients and physicians should make use of advisory as well as statutory documents. Advisory documents aim to accurately represent a patient's wishes and are legally binding under law. Statutory documents give physicians immunity from malpractice for following a patient's wishes. If a form is not available that combines the two, an advisory document should be appended to the state statutory form.

(2) Advisory documents should be based on validated worksheets, thus ensuring reasonable confidence that preferences for end-of-life treatment can be fairly and effectively elicited and recorded, and that they are applicable to medical decisions.

(3) Physicians should directly discuss the patient's preferences with the patient and the patient's proxy. These discussions should be held ahead of time wherever possible. The key steps of structuring a core discussion and of signing and recording the document in the medical record should not be delegated to a junior member of the health care team.

(4) Central repositories should be established so that completed advisory documents, state statutory documents, identification of a proxy, and identification of the primary physician can be obtained efficiently in emergency and urgent circumstances as well as routinely.

(5) Health care facilities should honor, and physicians use, a range of orders on the Doctor's Order Sheet to indicate patient wishes regarding avoidable treatments that might otherwise be given on an emergency basis or by a

covering physician with less knowledge of the patient's wishes. Treatment avoidance orders might include, along with a Do Not Resuscitate (DNR) order, some of the following: Full Comfort Care Only (FCCO); Do Not Intubate (DNI); Do Not Defibrillate (DND); Do Not Leave Home (DNLH); Do Not Transfer (DNTransfer); No Intravenous Lines (NIL); No Blood Draws (NBD); No Feeding Tube (NFT); No Vital Signs (NVS); and so forth. One common new order, Do Not Treat (DNT), is specifically not included in this list, since it may unintentionally convey the message that no care should be given and the patient may lose the intense attention due to a dying person; FCCO serves the same purpose without the likely misinterpretation. As with DNR orders, these treatment avoidance orders should be revisited periodically to ensure their continued applicability. Active comfort care orders might include Allow Visitors Extended Hours (AVEH) and Inquire About Comfort (IAC) b.i.d. (twice daily). (I, IV)

Issued June 1998 based on the report "Optimal Use of Orders-Not-to-Intervene and Advance Directives," adopted June 1997 (*Psych, Pub Pol'y, and Law.* 1998; 4: 668-75).

Journal 2000 Discusses the process of advance care planning. Identifies five steps for success: appropriate introduction of the topic; structured discussions covering specific situations; documentation of patient preferences; updating of directives; and application of directives when indicated. References Opinion 2.225. Emanuel, von Gunten, & Ferris, *Advance Care Planning,* 9 Arch. Fam. Med. 1181, 1181 (2000).

Journal 1999 States that a distrust of the medical profession arose from changes in the health care system and federal law. Explains how legislation may help alleviate some of the distrust. Suggests that people need more access to information about their health plans. References Opinions 2.20 and 2.225. Cerminara, *Protecting Participants in and Beneficiaries of ERISA-Governed Managed Health Care Plans,* 29 U. Mem. L. Rev. 317, 324 (1999).

2.23   HIV Testing

Human immunodeficiency virus (HIV) testing is appropriate and should be encouraged for diagnosis and treatment of HIV infection or for medical conditions that may be affected by HIV. Treatment may prolong the lives of those with acquired immunodeficiency syndrome (AIDS) and prolong the symptom-free period in those with an asymptomatic HIV infection. Wider testing is imperative to ensure that individuals in need of treatment are identified and treated.

Physicians should ensure that HIV testing is conducted in a way that respects patient autonomy and assures patient confidentiality as much as possible.

The physician should secure the patient's informed consent specific for HIV testing before testing is performed. Because of the need for pretest counseling and the potential consequences of an HIV test on an individual's job, housing, insurability, and social relationships, the consent should be specific for HIV testing. Consent for HIV testing cannot be inferred from a general consent to treatment.

When a health care provider is at risk for HIV infection because of the occurrence of puncture injury or mucosal contact with potentially infected bodily fluids, it is acceptable to test the patient for HIV infection even if the patient refuses consent. When testing without consent is performed in accordance with the law, the patient should be given the customary pretest counseling.

The confidentiality of the results of HIV testing must be maintained as much as possible and the limits of a patient's confidentiality should be known to the patient before consent is given.

Exceptions to confidentiality are appropriate when necessary to protect the public health or when necessary to protect individuals, including health care workers, who are endangered by persons infected with HIV. If a physician knows that a seropositive individual is endangering a third party, the physician should, within the constraints of the law (1) attempt to persuade the infected patient to cease endangering the third party; (2) if persuasion fails, notify authorities; and (3) if the authorities take no action, notify the endangered third party.

In order to limit the public spread of HIV infection, physicians should encourage voluntary testing of patients at risk for infection.

It is unethical to deny treatment to HIV-infected individuals because they are HIV seropositive or because they are unwilling to undergo HIV testing, except in the instance where knowledge of the patient's HIV status is vital to the appropriate treatment of the patient. When a patient refuses to be tested after being informed of the physician's medical opinion, the physician may transfer the patient to a second physician who is willing to manage the patient's care in accordance with the patient's preferences about testing. (I, IV)

Issued March 1992 based on the report "Ethical Issues Involved in the Growing AIDS Crisis," adopted December 1987 (*JAMA*. 1988; 259: 1360-61).

Updated June 1994.

Journal 2001 Compares the American system of patient confidentiality to the Austrian system. Discusses the debate between patients' rights and public safety. Concludes that the duty to warn third parties of dangerous patients should be discretionary instead of mandatory, except in cases of HIV seropositivity, which should involve mandatory disclosure to public health officials. Quotes Opinions 2.23, 5.05 and 5.06. Kenworthy, *The Austrian Psychotherapy Act: No Legal Duty to Warn*, 11 Ind. Int'l & Comp. L. Rev. 469, 480-81, 485, 490, 496 (2001).

Journal 2000 Examines the effect of HIV/AIDS on the relationship between the general public and health care professionals (HCPs). Discusses the importance of creating an environment in which HIV-positive patients do not fear disclosing their HIV status. Discusses policies and guidelines that address methods to prevent transmission of HIV from HCPs to patients. Quotes Opinion 2.23. References Opinions 9.13 and 9.131. Rediger, *Living in a World with HIV: Balancing Privacy, Privilege and the Right to Know Between Patients and Health Care Professionals*, 21 Hamline J. Pub. L. & Pol'y 443, 456-57, 461, 472 (2000).

Journal 1999 Explores the possibility of genetic testing in the managed care setting. Points out that genetic testing is not likely to reduce health care costs, but may improve health. Recommends ways in which genetic medicine can be practiced in the managed care context. Quotes Opinion 2.23. Rothstein & Hoffman, *Genetic Testing, Genetic Medicine, and Managed Care*, 34 Wake Forest L. Rev. 849, 883 (1999).

Journal 1999 Discusses whether health care professionals have the right to refuse to treat patients under common law and federal statutes and regulations. Explores the impact of the Americans with Disabilities Act and the United States Supreme Court decision in *Bragdon v. Abbott* on the duties of health care professionals in the context of providing treatment to HIV-positive patients. Quotes Principle VI and Opinions 2.23 and 9.131. White, *Health Care Professionals and Treatment of HIV-Positive Patients*, 20 J. Legal Med. 67, 86 (1999).

Journal 1998 Compares the New York AIDS confidentiality statute with statutes that mandate testing for other communicable diseases. Discusses whether the legal response to AIDS will serve as a model for responses to undiscovered diseases. Suggests that the prohibition on involuntary HIV testing should be reconsidered. Cites Opinion 2.23. Fernandez, *Is AIDS Different?*, 61 Alb. L. Rev. 1053 (1998).

Journal 1996 Discusses conflict between physicians' duty of confidentiality to patients and physicians' obligation to warn third parties of foreseeable injuries. Examines physicians' current legal responsibility to breach confidentiality to prevent the spread of infectious diseases, including AIDS. Identifies guidelines for physicians. Cites Opinions 2.23 and 5.057. Comment, *Taking Tarasoff Where No One Has Gone Before: Looking at Duty to Warn Under the AIDS Crisis*, 15 St. Louis U. Pub. L. Rev. 471, 499 (1996).

Journal 1995 Observes that statutes criminalizing HIV transmission would pose a disincentive for testing and also infringe upon the patient's right to confidentiality because criminal prosecutions are a matter of public record. Concludes that legislatures must carefully consider such issues when drafting legislation to prevent the spread of HIV. Quotes Opinion 2.23. O'Toole, *HIV-Specific Crime Legislation: Targeting an Epidemic for Criminal Prosecution*, 10 J.L. & Health 183, 195, 199 (1995).

Journal 1990 Explores potential physician tort liability for failure to warn at-risk individuals of the danger of being infected by the physician's HIV-positive patient. Concludes that there is a legal duty requiring health care professionals to warn those persons foreseeably at risk of being infected by an HIV-positive patient. References Opinion 2.23. Labowitz, *Beyond Tarasoff: AIDS and the Obligation to Breach Confidentiality*, 9 St. Louis Univ. Pub. L. Rev. 495, 514 (1990).

Journal 1990 Considers the tension between confidentiality and the duty to warn in the context of AIDS and HIV. Considers the appropriateness of mandatory reporting and partner notification and proposes legal reforms in this area. References Opinion 2.23. Price, *Between Scylla and Charybdis: Charting a Course to Reconcile the Duty of Confidentiality and the Duty to Warn in the AIDS Context*, 94 Dickinson L. Rev. 435, 477 (1990).

2.24 Impaired Drivers and Their Physicians

The purpose of this report is to articulate physicians' responsibility to recognize impairments in patients' driving ability that pose a strong threat to public safety and which ultimately may need to be reported to the Department of Motor Vehicles. It does not address the reporting of medical information for the purpose of punishment or criminal prosecution.

(1) Physicians should assess patients' physical or mental impairments that might adversely affect driving abilities. Each case must be evaluated individually since not all impairments may give rise to an obligation on the part of the physician. Nor may all physicians be in a position to evaluate the extent or the effect of an impairment (eg, physicians who treat patients on a short-term basis). In making evaluations, physicians should consider the following factors:

(a) The physician must be able to identify and document physical or mental impairments that clearly relate to the ability to drive.

(b) The driver must pose a clear risk to public safety.

(2) Before reporting, there are a number of initial steps physicians should take. A tactful but candid discussion with the patient and family about the risks of driving is of primary importance. Depending on the patient's medical condition, the physician may suggest to the patient that he or she seek further treatment, such as substance abuse treatment or occupational therapy. Physicians also may encourage the patient and the family to decide on a restricted driving schedule. Efforts made by physicians to inform patients and their families, advise them of their options, and negotiate a workable plan may render reporting unnecessary.

(3) Physicians should use their best judgement when determining when to report impairments that could limit a patient's ability to drive safely. In situations where clear evidence of substantial driving impairment implies a

strong threat to patient and public safety, and where the physician's advice to discontinue driving privileges is ignored, it is desirable and ethical to notify the Department of Motor Vehicles.

(4) The physician's role is to report medical conditions that would impair safe driving as dictated by his or her state's mandatory reporting laws and standards of medical practice. The determination of the inability to drive safely should be made by the state's Department of Motor Vehicles.

(5) Physicians should disclose and explain to their patients this responsibility to report.

(6) Physicians should protect patient confidentiality by ensuring that only the minimal amount of information is reported and that reasonable security measures are used in handling that information.

(7) Physicians should work with their state medical societies to create statutes that uphold the best interests of patients and community and that safeguard physicians from liability when reporting in good faith. (I, III, IV, VII)

Issued June 2000 based on the report "Impaired Drivers and Their Physicians," adopted December 1999.

Journal 2002 Discusses issues regarding regulation of elderly drivers. Concludes that mandating physicians to report unfit elderly patients will protect the public and help resolve ethical and legal dilemmas. Quotes Opinions 1.02, 2.24, 5.05, and 10.01. Kane, *Driving into the Sunset: A Proposal for Mandatory Reporting to the DMV by Physicians Treating Unsafe Elderly Drivers*, 25 U. Haw. L. Rev. 59, 59, 61, 62, 67, 69, 82, 83 (2002).

Journal 2002 Discusses malpractice liability in connection with treatment and diagnosis of dementia. Concludes that physicians must stay aware of new diagnostic and treatment developments in order to reduce risk. Cites Opinion 2.24. Kapp, *Legal Standards for the Medical Diagnosis and Treatment of Dementia*, 23 J. Legal Med. 359, 382 (2002).

Journal 2000 Explores physician involvement in the care of cognitively impaired elderly people who operate motor vehicles. Discusses conflicts that arise in fulfilling obligations to the patient, while upholding obligations to the welfare of the community. Cites Opinion 2.24. Berger & Rosner, *Ethical Challenges Posed by Dementia and Driving*, 11 J. Clinical Ethics 304, 307, 308 (2000).

2.30   Information from Unethical Experiments

All proposed experiments using human subjects should undergo proper ethical evaluation by a human studies review board before being undertaken.

Responsibility for revealing that the data are from unethical experiments lies in the hands of authors, peer reviewers, and editors of medical texts that publish results of experimental studies. Each publication should adopt a standard regarding publication of data from unethical experiments.

If data from unethical experiments can be replaced by existing ethically sound data and achieve the same ends, then such must be done. If ethically tainted data that have been validated by rigorous scientific analysis are the only data of that nature available, and such data are necessary in order to save lives, then the utilization of such data by physicians and editors may be appropriate.

Should editors and/or authors decide to publish an experiment or data from an experiment that does not reach standards of contemporary ethical conduct, a disclaimer should be included. Such disclosure would by no means rectify unethical conduct or legitimize the methods of collection of data gathered from unethical experimentation. This disclaimer should: (1) clearly describe the unethical nature of the origin of any material being published; (2) clearly state that publication of the data is needed in order to save human lives; (3) pay respect to the victims; (4) avoid trivializing trauma suffered by the participants; (5) acknowledge the unacceptable nature of the experiments; and (6) endorse higher ethical standards.

Based on both scientific and moral grounds, data obtained from cruel and inhumane experiments, such as data collected from the Nazi experiments and data collected from the Tuskegee Study, should virtually never be published or cited. In the extremely rare case when no other data exist and human lives would certainly be lost without the knowledge obtained from use of such data, publication or citation is permissible. In such a case, the disclosure should cite the specific reasons and clearly justify the necessity for citation.

Certain generally accepted historical data may be cited without a disclaimer, though a disclosure of the ethical issues would be valuable and desirable. (II, V, VII)

Issued December 1998 based on the report "Information from Unethical Experiments," adopted June 1998.

Journal 2001 Focuses on the moral dilemmas raised by stem cell research. Concludes that problems arising as a result of use of embryonic stem cells may be avoided if adult stem cells are used instead. Quotes Opinions 2.30. Orr & Hook, *Stem Cell Research: Magical Promise v. Moral Peril,* 2 *Yale J. Health Pol'y, Law & Ethics* 189, 197 (2001).

3.00 Opinions on Interprofessional Relations

3.01 Nonscientific Practitioners

It is unethical to engage in or to aid and abet in treatment which has no scientific basis and is dangerous, is calculated to deceive the patient by giving false hope, or which may cause the patient to delay in seeking proper care.

Physicians should also be mindful of state laws which prohibit a physician from aiding and abetting an unlicensed person in the practice of medicine, aiding or abetting a person with a limited license in providing services beyond the scope of his or her license, or undertaking the joint medical treatment of patients under the foregoing circumstances.

Physicians are otherwise free to accept or decline to serve anyone who seeks their services, regardless of who has recommended that the individual see the physician. (III, VI)

Issued prior to April 1977.

Updated June 1994 and June 1996.

3d Cir. 1984 Osteopathic physician brought class action against hospital and medical staff alleging violation of antitrust statute after hospital refused to grant staff privileges. In determining that the per se rule should be used to determine whether the medical staff had violated restraint of trade section of antitrust statute, the court distinguished in a footnote an earlier case which had employed the rule of reason analysis in a boycott case involving physicians and chiropractors. The earlier case had concluded that since there was no per se illegal purpose for Principle 3 (1957) [now Opinion 3.01], rule of reason analysis was appropriate because defendants were asserting a public service/ethical norm justification for their actions; no such rationale for their discriminatory treatment was raised by defendants in the instant case. *Weiss v. York Hosp.*, 745 *F.2d* 786, 821 n.61, cert. denied, 470 US 1060 (1985).

6th Cir. 1989 Plaintiff, a chiropractic association, alleged that the American Medical Association and several other professional associations violated antitrust law by conspiring to contain and ultimately eliminate the practice of chiropractic. The court provided an historical overview of the Association's gradual, but incomplete, recognition of chiropractors and limited licensed practitioners referring specifically to Principle 3 (1957) as well as to the Opinions and Reports of the Judicial Council Sec. 3, Para. 8 (1969) and to the Opinions and Reports 3.60 and 3.70 (1977) [now Principles VI and Opinions 3.01 and 3.04]. Based on its reading of these Principles and Opinions, the court reversed the trial court's grant of summary judgment to the Association because there remained a material issue of fact of whether it had continued to illegally boycott chiropractic. *Chiropractic Coop. Ass'n v. AMA*, 867 *F.2d* 270, 272-75.

7th Cir. 1990 Appellate court affirmed district court ruling that American Medical Association and other national professional associations violated federal antitrust laws by illegal conspiracy against chiropractors. Plaintiff alleged in lower court that Association sought by means of boycott to eliminate chiropractic through application of Principle 3 (1957) [now Opinion 3.01] labeling chiropractors as unscientific practitioners. The appellate court traced the history of the

Association's position regarding chiropractic including references to Principle 3 and Opinion 3.50 (1977) as revised by Opinion 3.01 (1981). The court found the evidence supported finding of an illegal boycott and that injunctive relief was appropriate. *Wilk v. American Medical Ass'n*, 895 F.2d 352, 355 n.1, 356-58, 361-63, 364 n.2, 365-66, 368-69, 369 n.4.

7th Cir. 1983 Defendants in antitrust suit appealed the denial of their directed verdict, claiming that the evidence presented by plaintiff failed to show the existence of a conspiracy to eliminate the practice of chiropractic. The Seventh Circuit affirmed the lower court's decision, noting that the adoption of Principle 3 (1957) [now Opinion 3.01], which condemned professional association with any one practicing a method of healing that was not scientifically based, in concert with other actions, might have allowed a jury to reasonably conclude that the defendant orthopaedic association conspired to discourage medical doctors from associating with chiropractors. *Wilk v. American Medical Ass'n*, 735 F.2d 217, 219, cert. denied, 467 US 1210 (1984).

7th Cir. 1983 Plaintiff-chiropractors alleged that American Medical Association and others conspired to induce physicians to forego any professional association with chiropractors, to induce hospitals to deny access to chiropractors, and to induce patients to avoid chiropractors, all in violation of the Sherman Act. Plaintiffs argued that Principle 3 (1957) and a 1966 House of Delegates resolution later included in Opinions and Reports of the Judicial Council Sec. 3, Para. 8 (1969) [now Opinion 3.01] reflected defendants' behavior. In response, defendants asserted that their actions were non-commercial and had been taken in the interest of public health, safety, and welfare in the good faith belief that chiropractic was dangerous to patients. The appellate court found the case inappropriate for application of the per se rule applying instead the rule of reason focusing on whether the challenged activities were anticompetitive. Further, as to the rule of reason, the court found the defendants could possibly avoid antitrust liability by showing that the dominant motive in their actions was a genuine concern for patient care. However, the court held that only such patient care concerns, and not a generalized public interest motive could be used as an antitrust defense. *Wilk v. American Medical Ass'n*, 719 F.2d 207, 213-15, 225-27, 233, cert. denied, 467 US 1210 (1984).

N.D. Ill. 1987 Plaintiffs, licensed chiropractors, sued defendant medical associations for violation of antitrust laws. With regard to defendant American Medical Association, plaintiffs alleged that through Principle 3 (1957) [now Opinion 3.01], the Association had successfully precluded physicians from associating professionally with chiropractors. The Association asserted that with the 1980 revision of its Principles, which eliminated the offending portions of Principle 3, any alleged boycott activity directed toward chiropractors had ceased. The court found, however, that plaintiffs did in fact suffer professional rejections and lost opportunities due to lingering effects of the boycott, traceable to the Association's actions. The court also noted that the revised stance of the Association on the legitimacy of chiropractic as reflected in Opinion 3.01 fell short of being an affirmative statement that physicians could professionally associate with chiropractors without fear of reprisal. *Wilk v. American Medical Ass'n.*, 671 F. Supp 1465, 1470, 1473, 1474, 1475, aff'd, 895 F.2d 352 (7th Cir. 1990).

N.D. Ill. 1986 In case involving antitrust challenge to rule promulgated by American College of Surgeons, the court concluded that the rule was a facially legitimate ethical canon and therefore it would apply the rule of reason in deciding the case. The court also rejected defendant's argument that the modified rule of reason test in *Wilk v. AMA*, 719 F.2d 207 (7th Cir. 1983), cert. denied, 467 US 1210 (1984), allowing a defense based upon a patient care motive exception to otherwise illegal restraint, should be applicable in this case. The court found that the *Wilk* exception was limited to Principle 3 (1957) [now Opinion 3.01] pertaining to the importance of scientific method in patient care. *Koefoot v. American College of Surgeons*, 652 F. Supp. 882, 889, 890, 891.

E.D. Mich. 1986 Plaintiff-chiropractors claimed violation of the Sherman Antitrust Act alleging that the American Medical Association conspired with others to injure them professionally and financially. In support of their claim, plaintiffs cited Principle 3 (1957) and the Opinions and Reports of the Judicial Council Sec. 3, Para. 8 (1969) [now Principles VI and Opinions 3.01 and 3.04]. The court, noting the 1977 change in the Association's position regarding chiropractic, reflected in the Opinions and Reports of the Judicial Council 3.60 and 3.70 (1977) [now Opinion 3.04] held that plaintiffs failed to demonstrate evidence of an overt act by the Association within the statutory limitations period. Summary judgment entered for Association. *Chiropractic Coop. Ass'n v. AMA*, 1986-2 Trade Cas. (CCH) & 67,294, aff'd in part and rev'd in part, 867 F.2d 270 (6th Cir. 1989).

E.D. Mich. 1985 In an antitrust case brought by plaintiff-chiropractic association against the American Medical Association, plaintiffs presented the court with a motion in limine asking that the court strike defendant's affirmative defense of a good faith concern with public health and patient care. Plaintiffs argued that the defense was unprecedented, in conflict with existing law and dramatically wrong. Plaintiffs referred to Principle 3 (1957) [now Principle VI and Opinions 3.01 and 3.04] as the source of the AMA's antitrust violations. The court denied plaintiffs' motion to strike, stating that under the rule of reason test, the Association had the right to present evidence that its actions furthered the public interest and patient care. *Chiropractic Coop. Ass'n v. AMA*, 617 F. Supp. 264, 266, *aff'd in part and rev'd in part*, 867 F.2d 270 (6th Cir. 1989).

D.N.M. 1987 In an antitrust action against major health insurance provider and state medical society, group of chiropractors alleged that a conspiracy existed in which the insurer refused to provide health cost reimbursement coverage for chiropractic services. Plaintiffs urged court to apply a per se analysis, rather than the rule of reason analysis to determine the legality of defendants' restrictive practices. The court declined to apply the per se test. In part, court's conclusion was based on view that concerns of defendant-physicians about relationship with chiropractors because of ethical restrictions imposed by Principle 3 (1957) [now Principle VI and Opinions 3.01 and 3.04] deserved more consideration than the per se test would afford. *Johnson v. Blue Cross/Blue Shield*, 677 F. Supp. 1112, 1118.

Ariz. 1965 Physician appealed denial of medical license which was based on alleged violations of local medical society rules and Principles 3, 5, and 10 (1957) [now Principles III and VII, and Opinions 3.01, 8.11, and 9.06]. Alleged violations included treating a patient without first obtaining a prior treating physician's permission, inadequate patient care, performing operations without hospital privileges, and signing the medical record of a deceased patient who had been treated by interns. The court held that the evidence failed to show any clear violation of the Principles and that a local medical society had no right to prescribe a code of ethics for state licensing purposes. *Arizona State Bd. of Medical Examiners v. Clark*, 97 Ariz. 205, 398 P.2d 908, 914-915, 915 n.3.

N.J. 1963 Plaintiff, an osteopath fully licensed to practice medicine and surgery by the state, sought to apply for staff privileges at defendant-hospital, a private, not for profit, general hospital. Defendant refused application based on a bylaw requiring staff members to be graduates of medical schools approved by the American Medical Association and members of the county medical society. In plaintiff's action challenging refusal of the application, the court held that the hospital's power to pass upon staff applications was a fiduciary power, and that plaintiff's application was to be considered on its own merit without regard to the bylaw provision. In its opinion, the court noted the historic opposition of the American Medical Association to osteopathy. The court also referred to a position adopted by the Association in 1961, later reflected in Opinions and Reports of the Judicial Council Sec. 3, Para. 7 (1965) [now Opinion 3.01], allowing for association with osteopaths who follow scientific principles. *Greisman v. Newcomb Hosp.*, 40 N.J. 389, 192 A.2d 817, 819.

N.J. Super. 1960 Plaintiff, a graduate of a school of osteopathy and licensed to practice medicine and surgery in New Jersey, sought to compel the defendant medical society to admit him to full membership. Defendant claimed as an affirmative defense that to admit plaintiff would violate Principle 3 (1957) [now Principle VI and Opinion 3.01] because plaintiff possessed a degree in osteopathy rather than an MD. The court noted that the defendant society had virtually monopolistic control of medical practice in the state and that exclusion from membership caused substantial injury. In view of this, the court ordered the defendant society to admit plaintiff to its membership. To bar membership of a licensed graduate of an approved school of osteopathy would, the court held, violate public policy. *Falcone v. Middlesex County Medical Soc'y*, 62 N.J. Super. 184, 162 A.2d 324, 328-329, *aff'd*, 34 N.J. 582, 170 A.2d 791 (1961).

Journal 1999 Explores the use of alternative therapies in the Caribbean due to the high cost of medical care. Compares the American Medical Association and the Commonwealth Medical Association views on nonscientific practitioners. Observes that Caribbean societies should implement standards for conducting research on alternative forms of treatment and should establish practice guidelines for utilization of these types of therapy. Quotes Opinion 3.01. Aarons, *Medicine and Its Alternatives: Health Care Priorities in the Caribbean*, 29 Hastings Center Rep. 23, 25 (July-Aug. 1999).

Journal 1996 Explores the incorporation of holistic health care into modern medical practice. Observes that the AMA previously condemned association with chiropractors as unethical. Concludes that alternative health care methods need to be further integrated into patient treatment plans where warranted. Quotes Principle 3 (1956) [amended and now Opinion 3.01]. Cohen, *Holistic Health Care: Including Alternative and Complementary Medicine in Insurance and Regulatory Schemes*, 38 Ariz. L. Rev. 83, 92 (1996).

3.02   Nurses

The primary bond between the practices of medicine and nursing is mutual ethical concern for patients. One of the duties in providing reasonable care is fulfilled by a nurse who carries out the orders of the attending physician. Where orders appear to the nurse to be in error or contrary to customary medical and nursing practice, the physician has an ethical obligation to hear the nurse's concern and explain those orders to the nurse involved. The ethical physician should neither expect nor insist that nurses follow orders contrary to standards of good medical and nursing practice. In emergencies, when prompt action is necessary and the physician is not immediately available, a nurse may be justified in acting contrary to the physician's standing orders for the safety of the patient. Such occurrences should not be considered to be a breakdown in professional relations. (IV, V)

Issued June 1983.

Updated June 1994.

3.03   The previous Opinion 3.03, "Optometry," was deleted in June 1994.

3.03   Allied Health Professionals

Physicians often practice in concert with allied health professionals such as, but not limited to, optometrists, nurse anesthetists, nurse midwives, and physician assistants in the course of delivering appropriate medical care to their patients. In doing so, physicians should be guided by the following principles:
(1) It is ethical for a physician to work in consultation with or employ allied health professionals, as long as they are appropriately trained and duly licensed to perform the activities being requested.
(2) Physicians have an ethical obligation to the patients for whom they are responsible to ensure that medical and surgical conditions are appropriately evaluated and treated.
(3) Physicians may teach in recognized schools for the allied health professionals for the purpose of improving the quality of their education. The scope of teaching may embrace subjects which are within the legitimate scope of the allied health profession and which are designed to prepare students to engage in the practice of the profession within the limits prescribed by law.
(4) It is inappropriate to substitute the services of an allied health professional for those of a physician when the allied health professional is not appropriately trained and duly licensed to provide the medical services being requested. (I, V, VII)

Issued December 1997.

3.04   Referral of Patients

A physician may refer a patient for diagnostic or therapeutic services to another physician, limited practitioner, or any other provider of health care services permitted by law to furnish such services, whenever he or she believes that this may benefit the patient. As in the case of referrals to physician-specialists, referrals to limited practitioners should be based on their individual competence and ability to perform the services needed by the patient. A physician should not so refer a patient unless the physician is confident that the services provided on referral will be performed competently and in accordance with accepted scientific standards and legal requirements. (V, VI)

Issued prior to April 1977.

6th Cir. 1989 Plaintiff, a chiropractic association, alleged that the American Medical Association and several other professional associations violated antitrust law by conspiring to contain and ultimately eliminate the practice of chiropractic. The court provided an historical overview of the Association's gradual, but incomplete, recognition of chiropractors and limited licensed practitioners referring specifically to Principle 3 (1957) as well as to the Opinions and Reports of the Judicial Council Sec. 3, Para. 8 (1969) and to the Opinions and Reports 3.60 and 3.70 (1977) [now Principles VI and Opinions 3.01 and 3.04]. Based on its reading of these Principles and Opinions, the court reversed the trial court's grant of summary judgment to the Association because there remained a material issue of fact of whether it had continued to illegally boycott chiropractic. *Chiropractic Coop. Ass'n v. AMA, 867 F.2d 270, 272-75.*

E.D. Mich. 1986 Plaintiff-chiropractors claimed violation of the Sherman Antitrust Act alleging that the American Medical Association conspired with others to injure them professionally and financially. In support of their claim, plaintiffs cited Principle 3 (1957) and the Opinions and Reports of the Judicial Council Sec. 3, Para. 8 (1969) [now Principles VI and Opinions 3.01 and 3.04]. The court, noting the 1977 change in the Association's position regarding chiropractic reflected in the Opinions and Reports of the Judicial Council 3.60 and 3.70 (1977) [now Opinion 3.04] held that plaintiffs failed to demonstrate evidence of an overt act by the Association within the statutory limitations period. Summary judgment entered for Association. *Chiropractic Coop. Ass'n v. AMA, 1986-2 Trade Cas. (CCH) & 67,294, aff'd in part and rev'd in part, 867 F.2d 270 (6th Cir. 1989).*

E.D. Mich. 1985 In an antitrust case brought by plaintiff-chiropractic association against the American Medical Association, plaintiffs presented the court with a motion in limine asking that the court strike defendant's affirmative defense of a good faith concern with public health and patient care. Plaintiffs argued that the defense was unprecedented, in conflict with existing law and dramatically wrong. Plaintiffs referred to Principle 3 (1957) [now Principle VI and Opinions 3.01 and 3.04] as the source of the AMA's antitrust violations. The court denied plaintiffs' motion to strike, stating that under the rule of reason test, the Association had the right to present evidence that its actions furthered the public interest and patient care. *Chiropractic Coop. Ass'n v. AMA, 617 F. Supp. 264, 266, aff'd in part and rev'd in part, 867 F.2d 270 (6th Cir. 1989).*

D.N.M. 1987 In an antitrust action against major health insurance provider and state medical society, group of chiropractors alleged that a conspiracy existed in which the insurer refused to provide health cost reimbursement coverage for chiropractic services. Plaintiffs urged court to apply a per se analysis, rather than the rule of reason analysis to determine the legality of defendants' restrictive practices. The court declined to apply the per se test. In part, court's conclusion was based on view that concerns of defendant-physicians about relationship with chiropractors because of ethical restrictions imposed by Principle 3 (1957) [now Principle VI and Opinions 3.01 and 3.04] deserved more consideration than the per se test would afford. *Johnson v. Blue Cross/Blue Shield, 677 F. Supp. 1112, 1118.*

S.D. Ohio 1995 Physician accused of soliciting bribes in return for referring patients to Medicaid provider moved to dismiss the indictment which alleged mail fraud and violations of Medicaid antikickback statute. In denying physician's motion to dismiss indictment, the court noted that physician's fiduciary duty under Opinion 3.04 supported an intangible rights mail fraud charge. *United States v. Neufeld, 908 F. Supp. 491, 500.*

Journal 1994 Focuses on physicians' legal and ethical duties to pregnant women to provide medical information relevant to patient choice regarding abortion and to make referrals for services that physicians are unable or unwilling to perform. Concludes that medical educators, professional associations, women's groups, and state legislatures should address these issues. Cites

Opinions 3.04 and 8.04. Law, *Silent No More: Physicians' Legal and Ethical Obligations to Patients Seeking Abortions,* 21 N.Y.U. Rev. L. & Soc. Change 279, 289, 290, 300 (1994).

Journal 1993 Focuses on how antitrust laws might be used to prevent exclusion of chiropractors by health maintenance organizations (HMOs) by discussing two theories under which it might be illegal. Concludes that chiropractors challenging their exclusion from HMOs may establish an antitrust claim under the theories of "structural conspiracy" and "tacit collusion" if certain criteria are met. Quotes Opinion 3.04. Note, *HMO Exclusion of Chiropractors,* 66 So. Cal. L. Rev. 807, 823 (1993).

3.041 Chiropractic

It is ethical for a physician to associate professionally with chiropractors provided that the physician believes that such association is in the best interests of his or her patient. A physician may refer a patient for diagnostic or therapeutic services to a chiropractor permitted by law to furnish such services whenever the physician believes that this may benefit his or her patient. Physicians may also ethically teach in recognized schools of chiropractic. (V, VI)

Issued March 1992.

3.05   The previous Opinion 3.05, "Specialists," was deleted in June 1994.

3.06 Sports Medicine

Physicians should assist athletes to make informed decisions about their participation in amateur and professional contact sports which entail risks of bodily injury.

The professional responsibility of the physician who serves in a medical capacity at an athletic contest or sporting event is to protect the health and safety of the contestants. The desire of spectators, promoters of the event, or even the injured athlete that he or she not be removed from the contest should not be controlling. The physician's judgment should be governed only by medical considerations. (I, VII)

Issued June 1983.

Updated June 1994.

Journal 1999 Describes conflicts of interest faced by professional sports team physicians. Examines cases where athletes have sued team physicians for failing to follow the proper standard of care. Provides a clear standard of care and suggests ways team physicians can reduce conflicts of interest. Quotes Opinion 3.06. Keim, *Physicians for Professional Sports Teams: Health Care Under the Pressure of Economic and Commercial Interests,* 9 Seton Hall. J. Sport L. 196, 218-19 (1999).

Journal 1999 Discusses the need for physicians to advocate on behalf of patients' rights in the context of health care delivery. Evaluates the nature and scope of the physician's role as advocate, noting that physicians cannot be expected to engage in attorney-like advocacy. Quotes Principles IV and VI, Fundamental Elements (2), (4), and (6) [now Opinion 10.01], Patient Responsibilities 5 [now Opinion 10.02], and Opinions 2.03, 2.07, 2.09, 2.16, 2.19, 3.06, 4.01, 4.04, 6.01, 7.02, 8.02, 8.03, 8.13, 8.132, 9.06, 9.07, and 9.131. Cites Opinions 5.05, 5.09, 7.01, 8.135, and 9.02. Sage, *Physicians as Advocates,* 35 Hous. L. Rev. 1529, 1537, 1541, 1542, 1552-53, 1554, 1556, 1557, 1559, 1561-62, 1564, 1571, 1574, 1576, 1580 (1999).

Journal 1993 Discusses an athlete's rights to assume serious health risks by playing a sport, despite a physical abnormality or medical condition. Considers the team physician's conflicting duties toward the patient/player and the team. Concludes that physicians or athletes should bear legal responsibility if either violates their obligations in this context. Cites Opinion 3.06. Mitten, *Team Physicians and Competitive Athletes: Allocating Legal Responsibility for Athletic Injuries*, 55 U. Pitt. L. Rev. 129, 140 (1993).

3.07   The previous Opinion 3.07, "Teaching," was deleted in June 1994.

3.08   Sexual Harassment and Exploitation between Medical Supervisors and Trainees

Sexual harassment may be defined as sexual advances, requests for sexual favors, and other verbal or physical conduct of a sexual nature when (1) such conduct interferes with an individual's work or academic performance or creates an intimidating, hostile, or offensive work or academic environment or (2) accepting or rejecting such conduct affects or may be perceived to affect employment decisions or academic evaluations concerning the individual. Sexual harassment is unethical.

Sexual relationships between medical supervisors and their medical trainees raise concerns because of inherent inequalities in the status and power that medical supervisors wield in relation to medical trainees and may adversely affect patient care. Sexual relationships between a medical trainee and a supervisor even when consensual are not acceptable regardless of the degree of supervision in any given situation. The supervisory role should be eliminated if the parties involved wish to pursue their relationship. (II, IV, VII)

Issued March 1992 based on the report "Sexual Harassment and Exploitation Between Medical Supervisors and Trainees," adopted June 1989.

Updated June 1994.

Va. App. 2003 Physician appealed Board of Medicine's license probation order for unprofessional conduct. Board found the physician's pattern of inappropriate advances towards medical students violated medical ethical standards. Appellate court reversed, holding that the evidence was insufficient to support Board's finding, since the ethical standards by which the physician should be adjudicated were not established by competent evidence. Quotes Opinions 3.08 and 9.05. *Goad v. Virginia Board of Medicine*, 40 Va. App. 621, 580 S.E.2d 494, 498, n.7, 499, n.9.

3.09   Medical Students Performing Procedures on Fellow Students

(1) In the context of learning basic clinical skills, medical students must be asked specifically to consent to procedures being performed by fellow students. The stringency of standards for ensuring the explicit and non-coerced informed consent increases as the invasiveness and intimacy of the procedure increase.

(2) Instructors should explain to students how the procedures will be performed, making certain that students are not placed in situations that violate their privacy or sense of propriety. The confidentiality, consequences, and appropriate management of a diagnostic finding should also be discussed.

(3) Students should be given the choice of whether to participate prior to entering the classroom and there should be no requirement that the students provide a reason for their unwillingness to participate.

(4) Students should not be penalized for refusal to participate. Thus instructors must refrain from evaluating students' overall performance in terms of their willingness to volunteer as "patients." (IV, V)

Issued June 2000 based on the report "Medical Students Performing Procedures on Fellow Students," adopted December 1999.

4.00 **Opinions on Hospital Relations**

4.01 Admission Fee

Charging a separate and distinct fee for the incidental, administrative, non-medical service the physician performs in securing the admission of a patient to a hospital is unethical. Physicians should derive their income from medical services rendered, in keeping with the traditions of the American Medical Association. (IV)

Issued prior to April 1977.

Updated June 1994.

Journal 1999 Discusses the need for physicians to advocate on behalf of patients' rights in the context of health care delivery. Evaluates the nature and scope of the physician's role as advocate, noting that physicians cannot be expected to engage in attorney-like advocacy. Quotes Principles IV and VI, Fundamental Elements (2), (4), and (6) [now Opinion 10.01], Patient Responsibilities 5 [now Opinion 10.02], and Opinions 2.03, 2.07, 2.09, 2.16, 2.19, 3.06, 4.01, 4.04, 6.01, 7.02, 8.02, 8.03, 8.13, 8.132, 9.06, 9.07, and 9.131. Cites Opinions 5.05, 5.09, 7.01, 8.135, and 9.02. Sage, *Physicians as Advocates, 35 Hous. L. Rev. 1529, 1537, 1541, 1542, 1552-53, 1554, 1556, 1557, 1559, 1561-62, 1564, 1571, 1574, 1576, 1580 (1999).*

4.02 Assessments, Compulsory

It is improper to condition medical staff membership or privileges on compulsory assessments for any purpose. However, self-imposed assessments by vote of the medical staff are acceptable. (IV)

Issued prior to April 1977.

Updated June 1994.

4.03 Billing for Housestaff and Student Services

When a physician assumes responsibility for the services rendered to a patient by a resident or student, the physician may ethically bill the patient for services which were performed under the physician's direct personal observation, direction, and supervision. (II)

Issued prior to April 1977.

Updated June 1994.

The primary obligation of the hospital medical staff is to safeguard the quality of care provided within the institution. The medical staff has the responsibility to perform essential functions on behalf of the hospital in accordance with licensing laws and accreditation requirements. Treatment or hospitalization that is willfully excessive or inadequate constitutes unethical practice. The organized medical staff has an obligation to avoid wasteful practices and unnecessary treatment that may cause the hospital needless expense. In a situation where the economic interests of the hospital are in conflict with patient welfare, patient welfare takes priority. (I, II, IV, V, VI)

Issued June 1986.

Journal 1999 Discusses the need for physicians to advocate on behalf of patients' rights in the context of health care delivery. Evaluates the nature and scope of the physician's role as advocate, noting that physicians cannot be expected to engage in attorney-like advocacy. Quotes Principles IV and VI, Fundamental Elements (2), (4), and (6) [now Opinion 10.01], Patient Responsibilities 5 [now Opinion 10.02], and Opinions 2.03, 2.07, 2.09, 2.16, 2.19, 3.06, 4.01, 4.04, 6.01, 7.02, 8.02, 8.03, 8.13, 8.132, 9.06, 9.07, and 9.131. Cites Opinions 5.05, 5.09, 7.01, 8.135, and 9.02. Sage, *Physicians as Advocates, 35 Hous. L. Rev. 1529, 1537, 1541, 1542, 1552-53, 1554, 1556, 1557, 1559, 1561-62, 1564, 1571, 1574, 1576, 1580 (1999).*

Journal 1998 Discusses conflicts of interest in the physician-patient relationship arising out of use of financial incentives by managed care organizations. Considers how such conflicts are dealt with in the attorney-client relationship. Suggests that a financial incentive should be legally denounced if it unreasonably interferes with a physician's duty to properly care for and treat patients. Quotes Preamble, Fundamental Elements (1) [now Opinion 10.01] and Opinions 4.04, 5.01, 8.03, 8.13, and 9.06. Cites Fundamental Elements (4) [now Opinion 10.01] and Opinions 2.07, 2.08, and 2.132. Hall, *Third-Party Payor Conflicts of Interest in Managed Care: A Proposal for Regulation Based on the Model Rules of Professional Conduct, 29 Seton Hall L. Rev. 95, 96, 107, 108, 109, 110, 111, 112, 134, 135, 136 (1998).*

Journal 1996 Considers the change from traditional medical care systems to managed care, noting the conflicts of interest this creates between physicians' ethical obligations and financial concerns. Discusses these issues in the context of managed behavioral health care. Suggests community-based care and social supports as a solution. Quotes Opinion 2.03 and 4.04. Petrila, *Ethics, Money, and the Problem of Coercion in Managed Behavioral Health Care, 40 St. Louis U. L. J. 359, 377 (1996).*

Journal 1994 Observes that health care reform proposals present significant challenges to the role and ethics of attending physicians. Emphasizes that reform proposals must set forth the role envisioned for physicians and must articulate an acceptable ethical framework within which physicians may fulfill that role. Quotes Opinions 4.04, 9.121, and 9.122. Cites Opinions 2.03, 2.09, 5.01, and 8.03. Wolf, *Health Care Reform and the Future of Physician Ethics, 24 Hastings Center Rep. 28, 32, 40 (March/April 1994).*

Journal 1993 Discusses the problem of physicians withholding needed medical treatment from HIV-infected infants. Concludes that current law should be expanded to eliminate this discrimination. Quotes Opinions 2.09, 2.17, 2.20, 2.22, 4.04, and 8.03. Crossley, *Of Diagnoses and Discrimination: Discriminatory Nontreatment of Infants With HIV Infection, 93 Columbia L. Rev. 1581, 1620, 1621 (1993).*

Journal 1992 Examines the major health care rationing issues facing the United States including increasing costs and decreasing access. Concludes that the standard of care should not be changed and that rationing should be a separate enterprise undertaken pursuant to explicit criteria. Quotes Opinions 2.03, 2.09, and 4.04. Hirshfeld, *Should Ethical and Legal Standards for Physicians Be Changed to Accommodate New Models for Rationing Health Care?, 140 Univ. Pa. L. Rev. 1809, 1816 (1992).*

Journal 1990 Discusses efforts of third-party payors to control health care expenditures for beneficiaries. Concludes that financial incentives to limit care and other cost control techniques should be disclosed and that the rationale for such disclosure is compelling. Quotes Opinions 2.03, 2.09, and 8.03. Cites Opinions 2.19, 4.04, and 4.06. Hirshfeld, *Should Third Party Payors of Health Care Services Disclose Cost Control Mechanisms to Potential Beneficiaries?*, 14 Seton Hall Legis. J. 115, 130, 131, 144, 145, 146 (1990).

4.05 Organized Medical Staff

The organized medical staff performs essential hospital functions even though it may often consist primarily of independent practicing physicians who are not hospital employees. As a practical matter, however, the organized medical staff may enjoy a dual status. In addition to functioning as a division of the hospital, members of the organized medical staff may choose to act as a group for the purpose of communicating and dealing with the governing board and others with respect to matters that concern the interests of the organized medical staff and its members. This is ethical so long as there is no adverse interference with patient care or violation of applicable laws. (IV, VI)

Issued July 1983.

Updated June 1994.

4.06 Physician-Hospital Contractual Relations

There are various financial or contractual arrangements that physicians and hospitals may enter into and find mutually satisfactory. A physician may, for example, be a hospital employee, a hospital-associated medical specialist, or an independent practitioner with staff privileges. The form of the contractual or financial arrangement between physicians and hospitals depends on the facts and circumstances of each situation. A physician may be employed by a hospital for a fixed annual amount, for a certain amount per hour, or pursuant to other similar arrangements that are related to the professional services, skill, education, expertise, or time involved. (VI)

Issued March 1981.

Updated June 1994.

Journal 1990 Discusses efforts of third-party payors to control health care expenditures for beneficiaries. Concludes that financial incentives to limit care and other cost control techniques should be disclosed and that the rationale for such disclosure is compelling. Quotes Opinions 2.03, 2.09, and 8.03. Cites Opinions 2.19, 4.04, and 4.06. Hirshfeld, *Should Third Party Payors of Health Care Services Disclose Cost Control Mechanisms to Potential Beneficiaries?*, 14 Seton Hall Legis. J. 115, 130, 131, 144, 145, 146 (1990).

4.07 Staff Privileges

The mutual objective of both the governing board and the medical staff is to improve the quality and efficiency of patient care in the hospital. Decisions regarding hospital privileges should be based upon the training, experience, and demonstrated competence of candidates, taking into consideration the availability of facilities and the overall medical needs of the community, the hospital, and especially patients. Privileges should not be based on numbers of patients admitted to the facility or the economic or insurance status of the patient. Personal friendships, antagonisms, jurisdictional disputes, or fear of competition should not play a role in making these decisions. Physicians who are involved in the granting, denying, or termination of hospital privileges have an ethical responsibility to be guided primarily by concern for the welfare and best interests of patients in discharging this responsibility. (IV, VI, VII)

Issued July 1983.

Updated June 1994.

Journal 1990 Presents current issues, policies, legislation, and judicial decisions regarding impaired physicians. Concludes by proposing enhanced confidentiality requirements in disciplinary proceedings and nationwide adoption of a uniform law in this area. Quotes Opinion 4.07. References Principle IV. Walzer, *Impaired Physicians: An Overview and Update of the Legal Issues, 11 J. Legal Med. 131, 174, 192 (1990).*

5.00 Opinions on Confidentiality, Advertising, and Communications Media Relations

5.01 Advertising and Managed Care Organizations

A physician may provide medical services to members of a prepaid medical care plan or to members of a health maintenance organization which seeks members or subscribers through advertising. Physicians practicing in prepaid plans or managed care organizations are subject to the same ethical principles as other physicians. Advertising which would lead prospective members or subscribers to believe that the services of a named physician who has a reputation for outstanding skill would be routinely available to all members or subscribers, if in fact this is not so, is deceptive. However, the publication by name of the roster of physicians who provide services to members, the type of practice in which each is engaged, and biographical and other relevant information is not a deceptive practice. (II, VI)

Issued prior to April 1977.

Updated June 1996.

Journal 1998 Discusses conflicts of interest in the physician-patient relationship arising out of use of financial incentives by managed care organizations. Considers how such conflicts are dealt with in the attorney-client relationship. Suggests that a financial incentive should be legally denounced if it unreasonably interferes with a physician's duty to properly care for and treat patients. Quotes Preamble, Fundamental Elements (1) [now Opinion 10.01] and Opinions 4.04, 5.01, 8.03, 8.13, and 9.06. Cites Fundamental Elements (4) [now Opinion 10.01] and Opinions 2.07, 2.08, and 2.132. Hall, *Third-Party Payor Conflicts of Interest in Managed Care: A Proposal for Regulation Based on the Model Rules of Professional Conduct*, 29 Seton Hall L. Rev. 95, 96, 107, 108, 109, 110, 111, 112, 134, 135, 136 (1998).

Journal 1994 Observes that health care reform proposals present significant challenges to the role and ethics of attending physicians. Emphasizes that reform proposals must set forth the role envisioned for physicians and must articulate an acceptable ethical framework within which physicians may fulfill that role. Quotes Opinions 4.04, 9.121, and 9.122. Cites Opinions 2.03, 2.09, 5.01, and 8.03. Wolf, *Health Care Reform and the Future of Physician Ethics*, 24 Hastings Center Rep. 28, 32, 40 (March/April 1994).

5.015 Direct-to-Consumer Advertisements of Prescription Drugs

The medical profession needs to take an active role in ensuring that proper advertising guidelines are enforced and that the care patients receive is not compromised as a result of direct-to-consumer advertising. Since the Food and Drug Administration (FDA) has a critical role in determining future directions of direct-to-consumer advertising of prescription drugs, physicians should work to ensure that the FDA remains committed to advertising standards that protect patients' health and safety. Moreover, physicians should encourage and engage in studies regarding the effect of direct-to-consumer advertising on patient health and medical care. Such studies should examine whether direct-to-consumer advertising improves the communication of health information; enhances the patient-physician relationship; and contains accurate and reasonable information on risks, precautions, adverse reactions, and costs.

Physicians must maintain professional standards of informed consent when prescribing. When a patient comes to a physician with a request for a drug he or she has seen advertised, the physician and the patient should engage in a dialogue that would assess and enhance the patient's understanding of the treatment. Although physicians should not be biased against drugs that are advertised, physicians should resist commercially induced pressure to prescribe drugs that may not be indicated. Physicians should deny requests for inappropriate prescriptions and educate patients as to why certain advertised drugs may not be suitable treatment options, providing, when available, information on the cost effectiveness of different options.

Physicians must remain vigilant to assure that direct-to-consumer advertising does not promote false expectations. Physicians should be concerned about advertisements that do not enhance consumer education; do not convey a clear, accurate, and responsible health education message; do not refer patients to their physicians for more information; do not identify the target population at risk; and fail to discourage consumer self-diagnosis and self-treatment. Physicians may choose to report these concerns directly to the pharmaceutical company that sponsored the advertisement.

To assist the FDA in enforcing existing law and tracking the effects of direct-to-consumer advertising, physicians should, whenever reasonably possible, report to them advertisements that (1) do not provide a fair and balanced discussion of the use of the drug product for the disease, disorder, or condition; (2) do not clearly explain warnings, precautions, and potential adverse reactions associated with the drug product; (3) do not present summary information in language that can be understood by the consumer; (4) do not comply with applicable FDA rules, regulations, policies, and guidelines as provided by the FDA; or (5) do not provide collateral materials to educate both physicians and consumers. (II, III)

Issued June 1999 based on the report "Direct-to-Consumer Advertisements of Prescription Drugs," adopted December 1998 (*Food & Drug L. J.* 2000; 55: 119-24).

Journal 2002 Examines the legal, ethical, and social implications of internet direct-to-consumer advertising of health products. Concludes that such advertising may be worthwhile, but privacy, product liability, and corporate responsibility issues must be addressed. References Opinion 5.015. Kao & Linden, *Direct-to-Consumer Advertising and the Internet: Informational Privacy, Product Liability and Organizational Responsibility*, 46 St. Louis U. L.J. 157, 170 (2002).

5.02   Advertising and Publicity

There are no restrictions on advertising by physicians except those that can be specifically justified to protect the public from deceptive practices. A physician may publicize him or herself as a physician through any commercial publicity or other form of public communication (including any newspaper, magazine, telephone directory, radio, television, direct mail, or other advertising) provided that the communication shall not be misleading because of the omission of necessary material information, shall not contain any false or misleading statement, or shall not otherwise operate to deceive.

Because the public can sometimes be deceived by the use of medical terms or illustrations that are difficult to understand, physicians should design the form of communication to communicate the information contained therein to the public in a readily comprehensible manner. Aggressive, high-pressure advertising and publicity should be avoided if they create unjustified medical expectations or are accompanied by deceptive claims. The key issue, however, is whether advertising or publicity, regardless of format or content, is true and not materially misleading.

The communication may include (1) the educational background of the physician, (2) the basis on which fees are determined (including charges for specific services), (3) available credit or other methods of payment, and (4) any other nondeceptive information.

Nothing in this opinion is intended to discourage or to limit advertising and representations which are not false or deceptive within the meaning of Section 5 of the Federal Trade Commission Act. At the same time, however, physicians are advised that certain types of communications have a significant potential for deception and should therefore receive special attention. For example, testimonials of patients as to the physician's skill or the quality of the physician's professional services tend to be deceptive when they do not reflect the results that patients with conditions comparable to the testimoniant's condition generally receive.

Objective claims regarding experience, competence, and the quality of physicians and the services they provide may be made only if they are factually supportable. Similarly, generalized statements of satisfaction with a physician's services may be made if they are representative of the experiences of that physician's patients.

Because physicians have an ethical obligation to share medical advances, it is unlikely that a physician will have a truly exclusive or unique skill or remedy. Claims that imply such a skill or remedy therefore can be deceptive. Statements that a physician has an exclusive or unique skill or remedy in a particular geographic area, if true, however, are permissible. Similarly, a statement that a physician has cured or successfully treated a large number of cases involving a particular serious ailment is deceptive if it implies a certainty of result and creates unjustified and misleading expectations in prospective patients.

Consistent with federal regulatory standards which apply to commercial advertising, a physician who is considering the placement of an advertisement or publicity release, whether in print, radio, or television, should determine in advance that the communication or message is explicitly and implicitly truthful and not misleading. These standards require the advertiser to have a reasonable basis for claims before they are used in advertising. The reasonable basis must be established by those facts known to the advertiser, and those which a reasonable, prudent advertiser should have discovered. Inclusion of the physician's name in advertising may help to assure that these guidelines are being met. (II)

Issued prior to April 1977.

Updated June 1996.

US 1977 Disciplinary sanctions were imposed by state bar against attorneys who violated state rule prohibiting advertising. After state court upheld sanctions, attorneys appealed to Supreme Court arguing that state rule violated federal antitrust laws and was unconstitutional. State bar argued that rule prohibiting advertising was justified to prevent adverse impact on the legal profession. In questioning this assertion, the Court referred to the position of the American Medical Association announced in 235 JAMA 2328 (1976) and included in Opinions and Reports of the Judicial Council 6.00 (1977) [now Opinion 5.02], that the medical profession permits advertising by physicians. The Court held that the state may regulate some aspects of advertising, but that a blanket prohibition against advertising by attorneys was unconstitutional as a violation of the first amendment. *Bates v. State Bar of Ariz., 433 US 350, 369-70 n.20.*

1st Cir. 1966 Physician sued electric shaver manufacturer for libel on basis of its use of reprints of an article quoting a study favorably mentioning manufacturer which allegedly falsely indicated that physician was one of the co-authors of the research study. Plaintiff asserted that he had agreed to participate in the research only if his name was not used in advertising claims since this would be a violation of established rules of ethics of the American Medical Association, Opinions and Reports of the Judicial Council Sec. 5, Para. 29 (1965) [now Opinion 5.02]. These facts were considered sufficient to submit to the jury. *Sperry Rand Corp. v. Hill, 356 F.2d 181, 184, cert. denied, 384 US 973 (1966).*

2d Cir. 1980 Federal Trade Commission ordered American Medical Association and others to cease, with some exceptions, imposing restraints on advertising and contract practice by physicians, as well as on business relations between physicians and laypersons. Commission found restraints violated 15 U.S.C. Sec. 45 (a) (1). See 94 F.T.C. 701 (1979). Association petitioned for judicial review of Commission's order. Court reviewed order, noting specific ethical pronouncements of Association which Commission found improper, including the following: restrictions upon advertising and solicitation, Principle 5 (1957) and Opinions and Reports of the Judicial Council Sec. 5, Para. 11 (1971) [now Opinion 5.02]; restrictions on contract practice, Principle 6 (1957) and Opinions and Reports of the Judicial Council Sec. 6, Paras. 3, 4, and 5 (1971) [now Opinion 8.05]; and restrictions on business organizations and relations with laypersons, Opinions and Reports of the Judicial Council, Sec.6, Paras. 14 and 15 (1971). The court rejected the Association's argument that its ethical rules did not provide impetus for local and state medical societies to act against physicians violating its rules. Further, the court rejected the Association's position that liability should be precluded because of revisions in the Opinions in 1977 and the Principles in 1980. Specifically, the court found that removal of the ban on patient solicitation and changes reflected in Principles II and IV (1980) did not render Commission's order moot. The order was therefore enforced with modifications. Dissenting judge, referring to 1980 revisions in Principles and to Opinions and Reports of the Judicial Council 4.05 and 6.00 (1977) [now Opinions 5.02 and 8.05], concluded order should not be enforced on grounds of mootness. *American Medical Ass'n v. FTC, 638 F.2d 443, 446, 446 n.1, 448, 449, 449 n.5, 450, 451, 455-57, aff'd, 455 US 676 (1982).*

D.C. Cir. 1980 Professional associations, including American Medical Association, filed for judicial review of a Federal Trade Commission rule limiting the ability of states and professional associations to restrict advertising of eye exams as well as ophthalmic goods and services. Since the United States Supreme Court had found certain restrictions on lawyer advertising unconstitutional while the case was pending, the court remanded the case for further consideration by the Commission. In its analysis of advertising in the eye care profession, the court quoted Principle 5 (1957) and the Opinions and Reports of the Judicial Council Sec. 10, Para. 4 (1971) which prohibited solicitation and advertising. However, the court also noted the intervening changes in the American Medical Association's position regarding advertising, quoting the Opinions and

Reports of the Judicial Council 6.00 (1977) [now Opinion 5.02] which permitted nondeceptive advertising. *American Optometric Ass'n v. F.T.C.*, 626 F.2d 896, 900-01, 913, 914, 914 n.11.

E.D. Va. 1976 Health planning agency, which sought to compile directory of services and fees of community physicians, and consumer group interested in obtaining such information, challenged state statute which prohibited direct or indirect advertisement by physicians. In holding that the statute violated first amendment rights, court noted that to protect the public from being misled as to medical quality, directory was designed in conformity with American Medical Association advertising guidelines. Court quoted Judicial Council position published in 235 JAMA 2328 (1976), later included in Opinions and Reports of the Judicial Council 6.00 (1977) [now Opinion 5.02] to support analysis. *Health Sys. Agency v. Virginia State Bd. of Medicine*, 424 F. Supp. 267, 274, 275 n.11, 276 Appendix B.

Cal. App. 1968 Plaintiff-physician sought dissolution of a medical partnership with defendant's decedent, and also sought a larger percentage of the partnership receipts based upon an alleged oral agreement. Defendant crossclaimed to enjoin plaintiff from taking physical control of the partnership offices and patient records. The trial court enjoined plaintiff from treating previous patients, requiring that he return all medical records and pay defendant all fees received from patients he had treated during the time of dispute. The appellate court reversed insofar as the injunction prohibited plaintiff from treating the patient who desired to continue to receive his services or prevented access to medical records essential for this purpose, citing Opinions and Reports of the Judicial Council Sec. 7, Para. 16, Sec. 5, Para. 21, and Sec. 9 (1966) [now Opinions 6.08, 5.02, and 5.05] to support view that patients may not be regarded as the subject of ownership. *Jones v. Fakehany*, 261 Cal. App. 2d 298, 67 Cal. Rptr. 810, 815, 816 n.1.

Fla. App. 1968 Physician sued to enjoin county medical association and telephone company from eliminating medical specialty headings in classified section of directory pursuant to guidelines issued by American Medical Association's Judicial Council in June, 1966 [now Opinion 5.02]. The court held that where medical association had no statutory authority to dictate directory listings, association's restrictions interfered with individual physicians' right to contract and deprived them of due process. *Dade County Medical Ass'n v. Samartino*, 213 So. 2d 627, 629, n.2, 631.

Mich. Att'y Gen. 1978 Opinion was requested from state attorney general as to constitutionality of blanket statutory prohibition of advertising by physicians and as to legality of expulsion of a member of a professional society for advertising that is otherwise proper. In finding the statutory restrictions unconstitutional, the opinion refers to the Judicial Council's advertising statement at 235 JAMA 2328 (1976) included as Opinion 6.00 (1977) [now Opinion 5.02]. *Michigan Att'y. Gen. Opinion N. 5024*, 1977-78 Att'y Gen. Op. 299, 303.

N.Y. Sup. 1965 Physician sued publishing company to bar insertion of advertisement for baby and child care products in physician's book, seeking declaration that book contract was void to the extent that it allowed inclusion of such an advertisement. Physician asserted that the advertisement was contrary to public policy, citing Opinions and Reports of the Judicial Council Sec. 5, Para. 29 (1965) [now Opinion 5.02] which stated that a doctor should not lend his name to any product. In rejecting the physician's claim, the court was willing to give careful consideration to the American Medical Association's view but concluded that it did not, in itself, constitute an expression of public policy. *Spock v. Pocket Books, Inc.*, 48 Misc. 2d 812, 266 N.Y.S.2d 77, 79.

Journal 2001 Compares and contrasts certain ethical positions articulated by the legal and medical professions. Concludes that both professions generally agree on ethical principles, but sometimes differ in the manner of implementation. Quotes Principle II. Cites Opinion 5.02. Needell, *Legal Ethics in Medicine: Are Medical Ethics Different from Legal Ethics?* 14 St. Thomas L. Rev. 31, 35, 50 (2001).

Journal 1999 Explains modern jurisdictional analysis and how it applies in medical malpractice cases. Examines the impact of physician advertising, referrals, consultations, prescribing practices, and involvement in state programs on personal jurisdiction in medical malpractice cases. Cites Opinion 5.02. Booker, *Physicians, Malpractice, and State Lines: A Guide to Personal Jurisdiction in Medical Malpractice Lawsuits*, 20 J. Legal Med. 385, 394 (1999).

Journal 1990 Provides an overview of the recent developments in the area of physician advertising. Proposes alternative solutions to the practical and ethical problems raised. Quotes Opinion 5.02. Olson, *Physician Specialty Advertising: The Tendency to Deceive?*, 11 J. Legal Med. 351, 354 (1990).

Journal 1984 Discusses the AMA policy on physician advertising and identifies several factors that may affect the decision to advertise. Among the important factors are variations in prominence of physician advertising from region to region and state to state, local attitudes of patients and physicians toward physician advertising, and acceptable forms of physician advertising. Quotes Opinion 5.01 (1984) [now Opinion 5.02]. Porter, *Physician Advertising—What is Legal? What is Ethical? What is Acceptable?*, 80 *Ohio State Med. J.* 437, 437, 439 (1984).

5.025 Physician Advisory or Referral Services by Telecommunication

Telecommunication advisory services, by way of phone, fax, or computer, distinct from an existing patient-physician relationship can be a helpful source of medical information for the public. Often, people are not sure where to turn for information of a general medical nature or do not have easy access to other sources of information. Individuals also may be embarrassed about directly bringing up certain questions with their physicians. Although telecommunication advisory services can provide only limited medical services, they can be a useful complement to more comprehensive services, if used properly.

Any telecommunication advisory service should employ certain safeguards to prevent misuse. For example, the physician responding to the call should not make a clinical diagnosis. Diagnosis by telecommunication is done without the benefit of a physician examination or even a face-to-face meeting with the caller. Critical medical data may be unavailable to the physician. Physicians who respond to callers should therefore act within the limitations of telecommunication services and ensure that callers understand the limitations of the services. Under no circumstances should medications be prescribed.

Physicians who respond to the calls should elicit all necessary information from the callers. When callers are charged by the minute, they may try to hurry their calls to limit their costs. As a result, important information may not be disclosed to the physician. Physicians should also ensure that callers do not incur large bills inadvertently or without understanding the billing system.

Physician referral services can also offer important information to the public. Referral services are often provided by medical societies, hospitals, and for-profit entities. To ensure that the service bases its recommendation on medically legitimate considerations rather than the likelihood of being paid by the physician, when the service charges physicians a fee to participate, physicians should not pay the service per referral. Also, callers should be told how the list is created. For example, callers should be informed whether the list includes physicians who pay a flat fee to be listed, members of a particular hospital staff or medical society, or physicians who meet some general quality-based criteria.

While these safeguards are described as applying primarily to telephone services, they should be considered equally applicable to any other communication media, such as radio or television, in which the physician and patient do not meet face-to-face. (I, IV, VI)

Issued June 1994.

Updated June 1996.

5.026 The Use of Electronic Mail

Electronic mail (e-mail) can be a useful tool in the practice of medicine and can facilitate communication within a patient-physician relationship. When communicating with patients via e-mail, physicians should take the same precautions used when sending faxes to patients. These precautions are presented in the following considerations:

(1) E-mail correspondence should not be used to establish a patient-physician relationship. Rather, e-mail should supplement other, more personal, encounters.

(2) When using e-mail communication, physicians hold the same ethical responsibilities to their patients as they do during other encounters. Whenever communicating medical information, physicians must present the information in a manner that meets professional standards. To this end, specialty societies can provide specific guidance as to the appropriateness of offering specialty care or advice through e-mail communication.

(3) Physicians should engage in e-mail communication with proper notification of e-mail's inherent limitations. Such notice should include information regarding potential breaches of privacy and confidentiality, difficulties in validating the identity of the parties, and delays in responses. Patients should have the opportunity to accept these limitations prior to the communication of privileged information. Disclaimers alone cannot absolve physicians of the ethical responsibility to protect patients' interests.

(4) Proper notification of e-mail's inherent limitations can be communicated during a prior patient encounter or in the initial e-mail communication with a patient. This is similar to checking with a patient about the privacy or security of a particular fax machine prior to faxing sensitive medical information. If a patient initiates e-mail communication, the physician's initial response should include information regarding the limitations of e-mail and ask for the patient's consent to continue the e-mail conversation. Medical advice or information specific to the patient's condition should not be transmitted prior to obtaining the patient's authorization. (I, IV, VI, VIII)

Issued June 2003 based on the report "Ethical Guidelines for the Use of Electronic Mail between Patients and Physicians," adopted December 2002, (AJOB 2003; 3(3)).

5.027 Use of Health-Related Online Sites

As Internet prevalence and access rapidly increases, individuals turn to the Internet to find health-related information quickly and efficiently. Online users can access innumerable informational or interactive online sites, many of which are maintained by physicians or rely on their services. Physician involvement should be guided by the following considerations:

(1) Physicians responsible for the health-related content of an online site should ensure that the information is accurate, timely, reliable, and scientifically sound, and includes appropriate scientific references.

(2) The provision of diagnostic or therapeutic services through interactive online sites, including advice to online users with whom the physician does

not have a pre-existing relationship or the use of decision-support programs that generate personalized information directly transmitted to users, should be consistent with general and specialty-specific standards. General standards include truthfulness, protection of privacy, principles of informed consent, and disclosures such as limitations inherent in the technology.

(3) When participating in interactive online sites that offer email communication, physicians should follow guidelines established in Opinion 5.026, "The Use of Electronic Mail."

(4) Physicians who establish or are involved in health-related online sites must minimize conflicts of interest and commercial biases. This can be achieved through safeguards for disclosure and honesty in funding and advertising. It also requires that physicians not place commercial interests ahead of patient health; therefore, physicians must not use health-related online sites to promote unnecessary services, refer patients to entities in which they have ownership interests, or sell products outside of established ethical guidelines. (See Opinions 2.19, "Unnecessary Services;" 8.032, "Conflicts of Interest: Health Facility Ownership by a Physician;" 8.062, "Sale of Non-Health-Related Goods from Physicians' Offices;" and 8.063, "Sale of Health-Related Products from Physicians' Offices"). Promotional claims on online sites must conform to Opinion 5.02, "Advertising and Publicity."

(5) Physicians who establish or are involved in health-related online sites that use patient-specific information must provide high-level security protections, as well as privacy and confidentiality safeguards. (I, II, IV, V, VI)

Issued December 2003 based on the report "Use of Health-Related Online Sites," adopted June 2003, (AJOB 2003; 3(3)).

5.03   The previous Opinion 5.03, "Communications Media: Press Relations," issued prior to April 1977, was deleted in June 1996 and combined with Opinion 5.04, "Communications Media: Standard of Professional Responsibility."

5.04 Communications Media: Standards of Professional Responsibility

Physicians are ethically and legally required to protect the personal privacy and other legal rights of patients. When information concerning a specific patient is requested by the media, the physician must obtain the consent of the patient or an authorized representative before releasing such information. The physician may release only the authorized information or that which is public knowledge. The patient-physician relationship and its confidential nature must be maintained.

With these considerations in mind, the physician may assist the representatives of the media in every way possible. When the patient or authorized representative consents to the release of information, physicians should cooperate with the press to ensure that medical news is available more promptly and more accurately than would be possible without their assistance. Inasmuch as a diagnosis may be made only by a physician and may depend upon X-ray and laboratory studies, no statement regarding diagnosis should be made except by or on behalf of the attending physician. For the same reason, prognosis will be given only by the attending physician or at the attending physician's direction.

Statements regarding the circumstances surrounding shootings, knifings, and poisonings are properly police matters, and questions whether they were accidental should be referred to the appropriate authorities.

Certain news that is part of the public record, such as deaths, may be made available without the consent of the patient or authorized representative. (IV)

Issued prior to 1977.

Updated June 1994 and June 1996.

Journal 1999 Explores the increased use of physician-patient communication through e-mail. Analyzes current laws regarding medical privacy. Suggests that patients' communications to their physicians are part of their medical record and should be given the same protections. Quotes Opinions 5.05 and 5.07. Cites Opinions 5.04 and 5.06. Spielberg, *Online Without a Net: Physician-Patient Communication by Electronic Mail*, 25 Am. J. Law & Med. 267, 284-85 (1999).

Journal 1998 Examines the use of e-mail in the physician-patient relationship. Focuses on privacy concerns stemming from the use of e-mail in the medical context. Suggests that physicians should discuss the implications of communicating through e-mail with their patients and should obtain informed consent prior to communicating in this manner. Cites Opinions 5.04, 5.05, 5.057, 5.07, 5.075, and 5.08. Spielberg, *On Call and Online: Sociohistorical, Legal, and Ethical Implications of E-mail for the Patient-Physician Relationship*, 280 JAMA 1353, 1356 (1998).

Journal 1995 Addresses presidential disability, its past impact on American government, and possible solutions to potential problems. Proposes enhancement of the role of the President's physician. Quotes Opinion 8.03. Cites Opinions 5.04 and 5.05. Abrams, *The Vulnerable President and the Twenty-Fifth Amendment, with Observations on Guidelines, a Health Commission, and the Role of the President's Physician*, 30 Wake Forest L. Rev. 453, 466, 471 (1995).

Journal 1984 Observes that available ethical and legal guidelines are insufficient to aid physicians in addressing issues of patient privacy and confidentiality. Concludes that there is need for legislation in order to provide suitable guidance to physicians who fulfill an important role in protecting patient privacy. Cites 1982 Opinions 5.03 [now Opinion 5.04], 5.04, 5.05 [now Opinion 5.06], 5.06 [now Opinion 5.07], 5.07 [now Opinion 5.08], and 5.08 [now Opinion 5.09]. Gellman, *Prescribing Privacy: The Uncertain Role of the Physician in the Protection of Patient Privacy*, 62 No. Carolina L. Rev. 255, 271 (1984).

5.045 Filming Patients in Health Care Settings

The use of any medium to film, videotape, or otherwise record (hereafter film) patient interactions with their health care providers requires the utmost respect for the privacy and confidentiality of the patient. The following guidelines are offered to assure that the rights of the patient are protected. These guidelines specifically address filming with the intent of broadcast for public viewing, and do not address other uses such as in medical education, forensic or diagnostic filming, or the use of security cameras.

(1) Educating the public about the health care system should be encouraged, and filming of patients may be one way to accomplish this. This educational objective is not severely compromised by filming only patients who can consent; when patients cannot consent, dramatic reenactments utilizing actors should be considered instead of violating patient privacy.

(2) Filming patients without consent is a violation of the patient's privacy. Consent is therefore an ethical requirement for both initial filming and subsequent broadcast for public viewing. Because filming cannot benefit a

patient medically, and moreover has the potential of causing harm to the patient, it is appropriate to limit filming to instances where the party being filmed can explicitly consent. Consent by a surrogate decision-maker is not an ethically appropriate substitute for consent by the patient because the role of surrogates is to make medically necessary decisions in the best interest of the patient. A possible exception exists when the person in question is permanently or indefinitely incompetent (eg, persistent vegetative state or minor child). In such circumstances, if a parent or legal guardian provides consent, filming may occur.

(a) Patients should have the right to have filming stopped upon request at any time and the film crew removed from the area. Also, persons involved in the direct medical care of the patient who feel that the filming may jeopardize patient care should request that the film crew be removed from the patient care area.

(b) The initial granting of consent does not preclude the patient from withdrawing consent at a later time. After filming has occurred, patients who have been filmed should have the opportunity to rescind their consent up until a reasonable time period before broadcast for public viewing. The consent process should include a full disclosure of whether the tape will be destroyed if consent is rescinded, and the degree to which the patient is allowed to view and edit the final footage before broadcast for public viewing.

(c) Due to the potential conflict of interest, informed consent should be obtained by a disinterested third party, and not a member of the film crew or production team.

(3) Information obtained in the course of filming medical encounters between patients and physicians is confidential. Persons who are not members of the health care team, but who may be present for filming purposes, must demonstrate that they understand the confidential nature of the information and are committed to respecting it. Where possible, it is desirable for stationary cameras or health care professionals to perform the filming.

Physicians, as advocates for their patients, should not allow financial or promotional benefit to the health care institution to influence their advice to patients regarding participation in filming. Because physician compensation for participation in filming may cause an undue influence to recruit patients, physicians should not be compensated directly. To protect the best interests of patients, physicians should participate in institutional review of requests to film. (I, IV, VII, VIII)

Issued December 2001 based on the report "Filming Patients in Health Care Settings," adopted June 2001.

5.046 Filming Patients for the Education of Health Professionals

It is important to recognize that filming patients for educational purposes has direct implications in relation to privacy, which itself has become the object of recent detailed federal regulations. Therefore, filming for educational purposes in the health care setting should comply with relevant laws and regulations. In addition, filming for educational purposes should be analyzed from the perspective of the ethics of the patient-physician relationship. In this regard, an important distinction can be drawn between filming for commercial purposes (see Opinion 5.045, "Filming Patients in Health Care Settings") and filming for educational purposes, since the latter is performed and viewed by members of the health care team, who are bound by ethical responsibilities regarding patient autonomy, privacy, and confidentiality. Specifically:

(1) Informed consent should be obtained before filming whenever possible. If it is not possible to obtain consent from the patient before filming, then consent must be obtained before the film is used for educational purposes. A surrogate decision-maker may give consent for filming only if the patient temporarily lacks capacity to give consent before the filming. When the patient regains decision-making capacity, his or her consent should be obtained before the film is used. In the case of minor children or permanently incompetent adults, consent may be obtained from the patient's parent or guardian (see Opinion 5.045, "Filming Patients in Health Care Settings").

(2) When obtaining consent, physicians should disclose information similar to that provided for other medical interventions, including an explanation of the educational purpose of film, potential benefits and harms (such as breaches of privacy and confidentiality), as well as a clear statement that participation in filming is voluntary and that the decision will not affect the medical care the patient receives. Moreover, physicians should be aware that filming may affect patient behavior during a clinical encounter. The patient should be given ample opportunity to discuss concerns about the film, before and after filming, and a decision to withdraw consent must be respected.

(3) Information contained in educational films must be held to the same standards of confidentiality as other patient information. If filming requires the presence of non-clinical persons, these persons must agree to protect the patient's privacy and confidentiality. Viewing must be limited to health professionals, professionals-in-training, and students in the health professions, unless it has been disclosed to the patient that non-health professionals would view the film and the patient has consented to such viewing. If the film is to be distributed outside the institution in which it was produced, disclosure of the distribution must be made and explicit consent obtained.

(4) Films contain a record of personal patient information. Depending on its content, a film may or may not be considered part of the patient's medical record, and may be protected under privacy law. Irrespective of these legal standards, films should be securely stored and final disposal should ensure that they are properly destroyed. (I, IV, V, VIII)

Issued December 2003 based on the report "Filming Patients for Educational Purposes," adopted June 2003.

5.05 Confidentiality

The information disclosed to a physician during the course of the relationship between physician and patient is confidential to the greatest possible degree.

The patient should feel free to make a full disclosure of information to the physician in order that the physician may most effectively provide needed services. The patient should be able to make this disclosure with the knowledge that the physician will respect the confidential nature of the communication. The physician should not reveal confidential communications or information without the express consent of the patient, unless required to do so by law.

The obligation to safeguard patient confidences is subject to certain exceptions which are ethically and legally justified because of overriding social considerations. Where a patient threatens to inflict serious bodily harm to another person or to him or herself and there is a reasonable probability that the patient may carry out the threat, the physician should take reasonable precautions for the protection of the intended victim, including notification of law enforcement authorities. Also, communicable diseases and gun shot and knife wounds should be reported as required by applicable statutes or ordinances. (IV)

Issued December 1983.

Updated June 1994.

US 2001 Obstetrical patients at a state university hospital who were arrested after testing positive for cocaine, filed suit challenging the nonconsensual drug tests given to them by the hospital and later used for law enforcement purposes. The lower courts found for the respondents. The Supreme Court reversed, finding the searches unconstitutional and not within the "special needs" category of constitutional, nonconsensual searches. The Court quoted Opinion 5.05, noting that this was not a case where the physicians were required to report to law enforcement the threat of harm by a patient. *Ferguson v. City of Charleston, 532 US 67, 121 S. Ct. 1281, 1290.*

E.D. Ark. 1992 Plaintiff sought an injunction to prevent defendant's attorneys from contacting patient's non-party treating physicians and interviewing them privately without the patient's consent. Quoting Opinion 5.05, the court stated that patients have a right not to have privileged information disclosed by their physician without express authorization. While the privilege may be partially waived where the patient's medical condition is put in issue by the filing of a lawsuit, patients still retain the right to insist that disclosure be made pursuant to formal discovery methods, absent express consent to ex parte contact. *Harlan v. Lewis, 141 F.R.D. 107, 109 n.5.*

D. Kan. 1991 With apparent reliance on Principle IV and Opinion 5.05, plaintiff claimed that other than in discovery or judicial proceedings, the physician-patient privilege is absolute and precludes ex parte communications with defense counsel. While recognizing the confidential nature of the physician-patient relationship, the court held that the ethical standards promulgated by the AMA are not binding law and that, where a litigant-patient has placed his or her medical status in issue, the physician is released from the constraints imposed by the physician-patient relationship for the purposes of the litigation. *Bryant v. Hilst, 136 F.R.D. 487, 490.*

E.D. Pa. 1992 Patient sued state mental institution and psychiatrist for violation of her right to privacy under the Fourteenth Amendment. Defendants had disclosed to law enforcement personnel and to plaintiff's supervisor threats made by plaintiff during the course of her treatment. While recognizing a strong public policy against breaches of confidentiality, the court held that the state's interest in protecting its citizens from serious bodily harm was overriding. The court noted that the limits placed on patient-therapist confidentiality by Opinion 5.05 (1989) are in accordance with the judicially recognized duty that a mental health professional take reasonable steps to prevent harm to others threatened by his or her patient. *Ms. B. v. Montgomery County Emergency Service, Inc., 799 F. Supp. 534, 539 cert denied, 114 S.Ct. 174 (1993).*

M.D. Pa. 1987 Plaintiff in a medical malpractice action sought to preclude his treating physicians from serving as defendant's expert witnesses at trial. The court held that defense counsel's failure to provide prior notice of ex parte communication with plaintiff's treating physicians barred their use as defense experts. Referring to *Petrillo v. Syntex Laboratories, Inc.*, 148 Ill. App. 3d 581, 499 N.E.2d 952 (1986), the court noted that the court there favorably cited Principle IV and Opinions 5.05, 5.06, and 5.07 (1984) in support of a public policy protecting confidentiality between physician and patient and against ex parte discussion. *Manion v. N.P.W. Medical Center of N.E. Pa., Inc.*, 676 F. Supp. 585, 591.

Ala. 1973 Physician revealed patient information to the patient's employer, contrary to instructions of patient. Patient sued for breach of fiduciary duty. Citing Principle 9 (1957) [now Principle IV and Opinion 5.05] as well as cases from other states, the court held that even in the absence of a testimonial privilege statute, as a matter of public policy, a physician has a fiduciary duty not to make extrajudicial disclosures of patient information acquired in the course of treatment unless the public interest or the private interest of the patient demands otherwise. In holding that the physician had breached his contract with patient, the court found the Principles together with state licensing requirements sufficient to establish the public policy of confidentiality. *Horne v. Patton*, 291 Ala. 701, 287 So. 2d 824, 829, 832.

Alaska 1977 Physician-school board member failed to fully comply with state's conflict of interest law by refusing to reveal the names of patients from whom he had received over $100 in income. The physician claimed a legal privilege or ethical duty not to disclose the information under Principle 9 (1957) [now Principle IV and Opinion 5.05] and, alternatively, that the conflict of interest law unconstitutionally invaded a patient's right to privacy. The court held that disclosure was not barred by a legal privilege or ethical mandate, but that the conflict of interest law unconstitutionally invaded patient privacy due to the absence of protective regulations. In ruling on the ethical duty issue, the court noted that under Alaska law, a physician's license may be revoked for violating the Principles. However, the court found this licensing provision irrelevant to the privileged relationship exception in the conflict of interest law. The court found that otherwise the privilege exception in the statute could be changed by the American Medical Association, a private organization, simply by amending the Principles. *Falcon v. Alaska Pub. Offices Comm'n*, 570 P.2d 469, 474 n.13.

Ariz. App. 1989 In a medical malpractice action, defense counsel interviewed several of plaintiff's treating physicians ex parte and notified plaintiff of this in preparation for a medical liability review panel hearing. Plaintiff moved to bar all testimony by those physicians and to disqualify defense counsel from representing defendants. The appellate court noted a physician's obligation of confidentiality pursuant to Principle IV and Opinion 5.05 and held that defense counsel in a medical malpractice action may not engage in non-consensual ex parte communications with plaintiff's treating physicians. *Duquette v. Superior Court*, 161 Ariz. 269, 778 P.2d 634, 641.

Cal. 1994 Plaintiff alleged that treating physician and medical group violated her statutory and constitutional right to privacy by engaging in ex parte communications with original physician's insurance company during discovery in a medical malpractice action against her original physician. The court concluded that state law clearly exempts the defendants from liability and that plaintiff failed to allege a sufficiently serious invasion of privacy to warrant relief. The dissent quoted Opinion 5.05 to emphasize the fiduciary nature of the physician-patient relationship. *Heller v. Norcal Mutual Ins. Co.*, 8 Cal. 4th 30, 876 P.2d 999, 32 Cal. Rptr. 2d 200, 220, cert. denied, 115 S. Ct. 669, 130 L. Ed. 2d 602 (1994).

Cal. 1976 Parents sued psychotherapists to recover for murder of daughter by psychiatric patient, alleging that failure to warn victim of patient's violent threat was a proximate cause of her death. In considering whether such a revelation would have been a violation of professional ethics, the Court noted that Principle 9 (1957) [now Principle IV and Opinion 5.05] recognized that the confidential nature of a physician-patient communication must yield when disclosure is necessary to protect an individual or community as a whole. The court concluded that, in the circumstances of this case, disclosure would not have violated medical ethics and held that psychotherapists are under a duty to warn when they determine or should determine that a patient poses a serious danger of violence to someone else. *Tarasoff v. Regents of Univ. of Cal.*, 17 Cal. 3d 425, 551 P.2d 334, 347, 131 Cal. Rptr. 14, 27.

Cal. 1970 Psychiatrist-witness in civil assault case applied for writ of habeas corpus after being held in contempt of court for refusing to produce patient's psychiatric records. Patient, plaintiff in the assault action, neither expressly claimed nor waived the statutory psychotherapist-patient privilege. The court held that the litigant-patient exception to the statutory psychotherapist-patient privilege does not unconstitutionally infringe rights of privacy of either psychotherapists or their patients. The court noted that in such a context a psychiatrist does not violate Principle 9 (1957) [now Principle IV and Opinion 5.05] since the Principle allows for legally compelled disclosure. *In re Lifschutz*, 2 Cal. 3d 415, 467 P.2d 557, 565-66 n.9, 85 Cal. Rptr. 829, 837-38 n.9.

Cal. App. 1982 Defendant was convicted of lewd act with a child and child molestation or annoyance, after licensed clinical psychologist reported defendant's admission of sexual conduct to authorities. The court held that the psychologist's testimony was properly admitted since a statute requiring the reporting of actual or suspected child abuse expressly made the psychotherapist-patient privilege inapplicable. The court quoted Principle 9 (1957) [now Principle IV and Opinions 2.02 and 5.05] in concluding the disclosure was not a breach of professional ethics. *People v. Stritzinger, 126 Cal. App. 3d 135, 186 Cal. Rptr. 750, 752 rev'd, 34 Cal. 3d 505, 668 P.2d 738, 194 Cal. Rptr. 431 (1983)*.

Cal. App. 1968 Plaintiff-physician sought dissolution of a medical partnership with defendant's decedent, and also sought a larger percentage of the partnership receipts based upon an alleged oral agreement. Defendant crossclaimed to enjoin plaintiff from taking physical control of the partnership offices and patient records. The trial court enjoined plaintiff from treating previous patients, requiring that he return all medical records and pay defendant all fees received from patients he had treated during the time of dispute. The appellate court reversed insofar as the injunction prohibited the plaintiff from treating patient who desired to continue to receive his services or prevented access to medical records essential for this purpose, citing Opinions and Reports of the Judicial Council Sec. 7, Para. 16, Sec. 5, Para. 21, and Sec. 9 (1966) [now Opinions 6.08, 5.02, and 5.05] to support view that patients may not be regarded as the subject of ownership. *Jones v. Fakehany, 261 Cal. App. 2d 298, 67 Cal. Rptr. 810, 815, 816 n.1*.

Colo. 1989 Spouse of police officer killed by released psychiatric patient sued state mental hospital and psychiatrist for negligence. Patient had blamed police for his misfortunes during repeated involuntary commitments for paranoid schizophrenia, and psychiatrist knew that patient would have access to a gun after release. The court held that a psychiatrist owed a duty of care in determining whether patient had propensity for violence and posed unreasonable risk of serious bodily harm to others. In so holding, the court cited Principle 9 (1957) [now Principle IV and Opinion 5.05], in support of the view that there are situations in which the need to protect an individual or the community from the threat of harm from a patient may outweigh the strong policy in favor of non-disclosure of patient confidences. *Perreira v. State, 768 P.2d 1198, 1210 n.7*.

D.C. App. 1985 Patient sued plastic surgeon for breach of confidential physician-patient relationship following surgeon's use of before and after photographs of her plastic surgery in a department store presentation. In considering whether such a breach was an actionable tort, the court made reference to an earlier case quoting Principles Ch. II, Sec. 2 (1947) [erroneously cited in the earlier case as Ch. II, Sec. 1 (1943); [now Principle IV and Opinion 5.05], as evidence of the strong public policy which exists in favor of maintaining a patient's confidences. *Vassiliades v. Garfinckel's, Brooks Bros., 492 A.2d 580, 590, 591*.

Fla. App. 1995 The court considered the issue of the effect of § 455.241(2) of the Florida Statutes on right of defense in a medical malpractice action to engage in ex parte communications with plaintiff's non-party treating physician. The court held that a 1988 amendment to § 455.241(2) negated the applicability of the statute to medical malpractice cases. The dissent, citing *Petrillo v. Syntex Laboratories, Inc.*, 148 Ill. App. 3d 581, 499 N.E.2d 952 (1986), quoted Principles II and IV and Opinions 5.05, 5.06, and 5.08 as strong public policy support for its position that ex parte communications should be barred altogether. *Castillo-Plaza v. Green, 655 So. 2d 197, 206 n.4*.

Ill. 1997 Trial court held various statutory sections, including those permitting unlimited disclosure of a patient's medical records, unconstitutional. On appeal, state supreme court affirmed. Regarding provisions mandating consent to the disclosure of medical records, the court noted, with reference to Principle IV and Opinion 5.05, the crucial importance of confidentiality in the physician-patient relationship. *Best v. Taylor Machine Works, 179 Ill. 2d 367, 689 N.E. 2d 1057, 1099*.

Ill. App. 1987 In appeal of malpractice action, an issue was whether expert testimony of plaintiff's treating physician, based upon discussions with the defense counsel without patient's consent, was admissible. The court held that ex parte communications between a plaintiff's treating physician and legal adversary violated public policy. In determining the existence of such a policy favoring the sanctity of the doctor-patient relationship, the court noted *Petrillo v. Syntex Laboratories, Inc.*, 148 Ill. App. 3d 581, 499 N.E.2d 952 (1st Dist. 1986) and its reference to the Principles and Opinions, namely Principle IV and Opinion 5.05 (1984), which establish an ethical obligation to keep physician-patient communications confidential, generally requiring a patient's consent before information is released. *Yates v. El-Deiry, 160 Ill. App. 3d 198, 513 N.E.2d 519, 522*.

Ill. App. 1986 Defense attorney in product liability suit was held in contempt of court for conducting ex parte discussions with plaintiff-patient's treating physician without patient's consent and contrary to authorized methods of discovery. The court held that the strong public policy favoring physician-patient confidentiality articulated in Principles II and IV and Opinions 5.05, 5.06, 5.07, and 5.08 (1984) justified a rule against such ex parte discussions. Further, the court held that the public has the right to rely on physicians to faithfully execute their ethical obligations. *Petrillo v. Syntex Laboratories, Inc.*, 148 Ill. App. 3d 581, 499 N.E.2d 952, 957, 958, 959, cert. denied, 483 US 1007 (1987).

Ill. App. 1979 Patient filed suit against physician for breach of contract and breach of confidential relationship after physician's employee disclosed patient's name to police. Patient alleged that implied contract arose out of a statutory physician-patient privilege, and provisions of the Canons of Medical Ethics, with apparent reference to Principle 9 (1957) [now Principle IV and Opinion 5.05]. The court held that disclosure of patient's name alone by a physician or the physician's agents is insufficient to state a cause of action in contract and does not violate the physician-patient privilege. *Geisberger v. Willuhn*, 72 Ill. App. 3d 435, 390 N.E.2d 945, 946, 948.

Ind. App. 1996 A patient filed suit against a mental health counseling center for disclosing to a third party death threats made by the patient during therapy. The patient claimed this was a breach of the standard of care owed to her. The trial court found that the counseling center was not statutorily prohibited from disclosing death threats the patient made. On appeal, the court affirmed the decision. It noted, with apparent reference to Principle IV and Opinion 5.05, that physicians may disclose confidential information to ensure the safety of the public or of individuals. In clarifying its holding, the court observed that while free and frank communication should be promoted to aid proper diagnosis and treatment, public policy supports disclosure of confidential information when appropriate. *Rocca v. Southern Hills Counseling Center, Inc.*, 671 N.E. 2d 913, 916.

Ky. 2002 Patient appealed denial of writ to prevent release to grand jury of psychiatric treatment records. Records were requested to demonstrate that patient had visited multiple physicians to obtain the same prescription drugs. Trial judge reviewed the records *in camera* and denied writ. The Supreme Court of Kentucky reversed, holding that the evidence reviewed *in camera* was inadmissible. The court found that a sufficient evidentiary basis must be shown to permit *in camera* review of privileged records. Concurring judge quotes Opinion 5.05. *Stidham v. Clark*, 74 S.W.3d 719, 729, 730.

Md. Att'y Gen. 1977 Opinion addresses the obligation of a psychiatrist to report child abuse information obtained from a parent-patient. Referring to state statutes and to Principle 9 (1957) [now Principle IV and Opinions 2.02 and 5.05] the opinion concludes that the question of whether to disclose suspected child abuse is a matter left to the individual psychiatrist's professional and moral judgment. *Maryland Att'y. Gen. Opinion*, 62 Op. Att'y Gen. Md. 157, 160.

Mass. 1984 Employee sued employer for libel and invasion of privacy following disclosure of medical facts about employee to other employees. In part, claim involved disclosure of opinion about employee's mental state to his supervisor by physician retained by employer. Citing Principle 9 (1957) [now Principle IV and Opinions 5.05 and 5.09], the court held that a physician retained by an employer may disclose to the employer information concerning an employee if receipt of the information is reasonably necessary to serve a substantial and valid business interest of the employer. *Bratt v. Int'l Business Mach. Corp.*, 392 Mass. 508, 467 N.E.2d 126, 137 n.23.

Minn. 1976 Plaintiff-patient in malpractice action appealed trial court's order to provide authorization for private, informal interview between defense counsel and patient's treating physician. In holding that formal pretrial discovery provided the exclusive procedure by which defendant could obtain medical testimony, the court noted, without deciding the issue, that a physician who discloses confidential patient information in a private interview may be subject to tort liability for breach of patient's right to privacy or professional discipline for unprofessional conduct, citing Principle 9 (1957) [now Principle IV and Opinion 5.05]. *Wenninger v. Muesing*, 240 N.W.2d 333, 337 n.3.

Mo. 1993 Patient sued physicians alleging a breach of fiduciary duty of confidentiality for participating in an unauthorized ex parte discussion with defendant's attorney. While recognizing this duty, the court held that, where the plaintiff's medical condition is in issue, this constitutes a waiver of both the testimonial privilege and the physician's fiduciary duty in so far as the information is related to the medical issues. Quoting Opinion 5.05 and citing Principle IV, the court stated that courts may apply ethical principles to frame the specific limits of the legal duty of confidentiality. *Brandt v. Medical Defense Assoc.*, 856 S.W.2d 667, 671 n.1.

Mo. 1989 In a personal injury suit, plaintiff challenged trial court's authority to compel plaintiff to authorize ex parte meetings between defendant insurance company and plaintiff's treating physician. Applying a balancing test between preserving the physician-patient confidential and fiduciary relationship, the physician-patient testimonal privilege, and the quest for truth in civil litigation, the court held that such information could be obtained through the methods of formal discovery. The court quoted Principle IV and Opinion 5.05 (1984) as statements of the policy underlying medical confidentiality and a basis for a patient's affirmative right to rely on the confidential nature of disclosures to a treating physician. *State ex. rel. Woytus v. Ryan, 776 S.W.2d 389, 392-93.*

Mo. App. 1985 In a prohibition proceeding arising from a medical malpractice action, defense attorneys sought order compelling plaintiff to authorize a private interview between defense attorneys and physician who treated plaintiff for injuries allegedly caused by defendant-physician. The appellate court, after discussing Principle IV and Opinion 5.05 (1984), held that the defense attorneys had the right to seek an ex parte interview with the treating physician, subject to the willingness of the physician to grant the interview. Furthermore, the court noted that Opinion 5.05 prevents a physician from revealing a patient's confidences only where there is a lack of consent from the patient and found that consent did exist here in the form of a medical authorization executed by plaintiff during pendency of the malpractice action. *State ex rel. Stufflebam v. Appelquist, 694 S.W.2d 882, 886, 888 n.7, overruled by State ex. rel. Woytus v. Ryan, 776 S.W.2d 389 (Mo. 1989).*

N.J. 1985 Plaintiff provided authorization for release of decedent's medical records from former treating physicians but refused to consent to depositions or interviews between defense counsel and physicians. The court noted physicians' ethical duty to avoid unauthorized disclosure, as stated in Principle 9 (1957) [now Principle IV and Opinion 5.05], but recognized that a patient's right to confidentiality was not absolute. After balancing the competing interests involved, the court held that defense counsel had a right to seek ex parte interviews of decedent's other treating physicians regarding litigation matters, provided procedural safeguards were met including clear statements that participation in such an interview is voluntary on the part of a physician. *Stempler v. Speidell, 100 N.J. 368, 495 A.2d 857, 860, cert. denied, 483 US 1007 (1987).*

N.J. 1979 In wrongful death action against a psychiatrist whose patient murdered plaintiff's decedent, the court concluded, in accord with Principle 9 (1957) [now Principle IV], that a psychiatrist may owe a duty to warn potential victims of possible danger from psychiatrist's patient despite the general emphasis on confidentiality. The court also noted the Preamble and Principles 1 and 3 (1957) [now revised Preamble, Principle I and Opinion 5.05] in discussing the psychiatrist-patient relationship. *McIntosh v. Milano, 168 N.J. Super. 466, 403 A.2d 500, 510, 512-13.*

N.J. 1962 Parents sued pediatrician for unauthorized disclosure to life insurer of deceased infant's congenital heart defect. The court quoted Principle 9 (1957) [now Principle IV and Opinion 5.05] as an articulation of a physician's legal duty to his or her patient subject to exceptions of compelling social or patient interests. The court held that the parents had lost their limited right to nondisclosure by filing an insurance claim. *Hague v. Williams, 37 N.J. 328, 181 A.2d 345, 347.*

N.J. Super. 1991 Physician's estate sued hospital alleging that it violated state law against discrimination by restricting the physician's surgery privileges and requiring him to inform patients of his HIV-infected status before performing invasive procedures. The defendant hospital was also alleged to have breached its duty to maintain confidentiality of his seropositive diagnosis. The court held that the hospital had not discriminated against the physician since the hospital had relied on ethical and professional standards, including a report of the Council on Ethical and Judicial Affairs of the AMA dealing with the issue of AIDS [now Opinions 9.13 and 9.131]. However, the hospital was held to have breached its fiduciary duty to maintain the confidentiality of the physician's medical records. Referring to *McIntosh v. Milano,* 168 N.J. Super. 466, 403 A.2d 500 (1979) which had quoted AMA Principles of Medical Ethics sec. 9 (1957) [now Principle IV and Opinion 5.05] in applying the "duty to warn" exception, the court noted that the disclosure in this case went far beyond the medical personnel directly involved in the treatment of the physician and those patients entitled to informed consent. *Estate of Behringer v. Medical Ctr., 249 N.J. Super. 597, 614, 633, 592 A.2d 1251, 1259, 1268.*

N.J. Super. 1988 Several portions of state Department of Corrections regulations concerning exceptions to privileged communications between psychologist and inmates were invalidated by appellate court because they permitted disclosure of confidences that did not present clear and imminent danger to the inmate or others, or failed to identify any intended victim. Court made general reference (with erroneous quotation) to Principle 9 (1957) [now Principle IV and Opinion 5.05]. *In re Rules Adoption, 224 N.J. Super. 252, 540 A.2d 212, 215.*

N.J. Super. 1987 Defendant in a personal injury suit sought to offer testimony from plaintiff's treating physician regarding plaintiff's prognosis. The court denied plaintiff's motion to exclude that evidence, despite the ethical obligation of physicians to uphold patients' communications as confidential under Principle 9 (1957) [now Principle IV and Opinion 5.05]. The court's decision was based on New Jersey case law permitting disclosure of a patient's medical condition to someone having a legitimate interest where the physical condition of the patient is made an element of a claim. *Kurdek v. West Orange Bd. of Educ.*, 222 N.J. Super. 218, 536 A.2d 332, 335.

N.J. Super. 1967 In a suit for separate maintenance, communications between plaintiff-wife and her psychiatrist were not protected from disclosure during depositions, despite Principle 9 (1957) [now Principle IV and Opinion 5.05] which prohibited physicians from disclosing patient confidences except where necessary to protect the welfare of the individual or of the community. The court concluded that the patient had only a limited right of nondisclosure, subject to exceptions created by supervening interest of society and that the institution of litigation by the patient constituted a vitiation of that right. *Ritt v. Ritt*, 98 N.J. Super. 590, 238 A.2d 196, 199, rev'd, 52 N.J. 177, 244 A.2d 497 (1968).

N.Y. Sup. 2000 Physician brought wrongful discharge claim against corporate employer. The physician alleged she was discharged because she refused to reveal confidential medical information regarding employees. With apparent reference to Principle IV and Opinions 5.05 and 5.09, the affidavit filed by the physician claimed she had an ethical and legal duty to protect patient confidentiality. The court found termination of an employee at will based upon such grounds is sufficient to state a cause of action for breach of contract. The court ruled that obligations of good faith and fair dealing may be implied in a contract for the employment of a physician and that no physician should be placed in the position of choosing between retaining employment or violating ethical standards. *Horn v. New York Times*, 186 Misc. 2d 469, 719 N.Y.S. 2d 471, 474.

N.Y. Sup. 1977 Plaintiff, a psychiatric patient, sued her psychiatrist and the psychiatrist's spouse for violating several state statutes and her privacy rights by publishing a book about the intimate details of plaintiff's psychotherapy. The court found for plaintiff, basing its decision in part upon Principle 9 (1957) [now Principle IV and Opinion 5.05] which requires a physician to uphold the confidences of a patient. *Doe v. Roe*, 93 Misc. 2d 201, 400 N.Y.S.2d 668, 674.

N.Y. Surr. 1977 In a discovery proceeding, respondent-psychiatrist, who had treated some patients of deceased psychiatrist subsequent to his death, allegedly misappropriated decedent's patient records. Estate petitioned court for return of records and damages for injury to value of decedent's practice. Respondent sought dismissal of claim arguing that estate could not sell patient records. The court rejected respondent's request. In so ruling, the court noted that under Principle 9 (1957) [now Principle IV and Opinion 5.05] prohibiting physicians from revealing patient confidences, various guidelines had been issued regarding sale of a medical practice [now Opinion 7.04]. Whether respondent's actions had interfered with the estate's efforts to dispose of decedent's practice in keeping with these guidelines presented the court with factual issues for later resolution. *Estate of Finkle*, 90 Misc. 2d 550, 395 N.Y.S.2d 343, 346.

N.C. 1990 Plaintiff in a malpractice case was granted an order prohibiting ex parte conferences between defendant's attorney and non-party treating physicians. The court noted that both the Principles of Medical Ethics and Current Opinions affirm the physician's duty to protect patient confidentiality, in apparent reference to Principle IV and Opinion 5.05. In consideration of (1) the patient's right to privacy, (2) physician-patient confidentiality, (3) the adequacy of formal discovery procedures, and (4) the dilemma in which non-party treating physicians are placed by ex parte conferences, the court held that an attorney may not interview a patient's non-party treating physicians privately without express authorization. *Crist v. Moffatt*, 326 N.C. 326, 333, 389 S.E.2d 41, 46.

N. C. App. 1999 Plaintiff appealed Industrial Commission's finding for the plaintiff's employer on the grounds that there was insufficient medical evidence to find that the plaintiff's absence from work was attributed to injury. The plaintiff in part alleged that his employer engaged in ex parte communications with the plaintiff's treating physician. The court held that the Commission erroneously placed on the plaintiff the burden of proving that the medical treatment he sought related to his injury. The court quoted Opinion 5.05, noting that it is improper for a physician to engage in ex parte communications with a defendant. The court stated however, that the plaintiff failed to present evidence of such ex parte communications. *Reinninger v. Prestige Fabricators, Inc.*, 523 S.E.2d 720, 724.

Ohio 1999 Patients brought a class action suit against hospital on grounds that the hospital disclosed patients' confidential medical information to the hospital's law firm, in order to determine whether the patients were eligible for government benefits to pay for unpaid hospital bills. The trial court granted defendants' motion for summary judgment. On appeal, the court held that a physician or a hospital can be held liable for unauthorized out-of-court disclosure of patients' confidential information. Additionally, the court found that an independent tort exists for unauthorized, unprivileged disclosure of patients' private medical information to a third party. The court cited Principle 9 (1957) [now Principle IV and Opinion 5.05], noting that courts have looked to such sources in providing a cause of action for breach of patient confidentiality. *Biddle v. Warren General Hospital*, 86 Ohio St. 3d 395, 715 N.E.2d 518, 523.

Ohio 1997 Estates of victims who were killed by their mentally ill son brought suit against son's psychotherapist for failing to disclose potential for violence. Son had been institutionalized and treated for schizophrenia. After release, he continued to take medication and see a psychotherapist. Despite parents' objections and attempts to have him involuntarily recommitted, psychotherapist reduced his medication and continued to recommend outpatient treatment. The court held that the psychotherapist had a duty to exercise reasonable care to control the son so as to prevent him from causing harm to his family. The court expressed concern for safeguarding the confidentiality of psychotherapeutic communications but noted that Principle 9 (1957) [now Principle IV and Opinion 5.05] has long allowed breaches of confidence when it becomes necessary to protect the welfare of the individual or the community. *Estates of Morgan v. Fairfield Family Counseling Center*, 77 Ohio St. 3d 284, 303, 673 N.E.2d 1311, 1326.

Ohio 1988 Administrator sued psychiatrist for wrongful death after recently discharged patient killed her infant daughter. In determining whether a professional judgment rule should be adopted in the malpractice standard of care where the prediction of violent behavior is involved, the court referred favorably to Principle 9 (1957) [now Principle IV and Opinion 5.05] which allows breaches of patient confidences when necessary to protect potential victims. *Littleton v. Good Samaritan Hospital*, 39 Ohio St. 3d 86, 529 N.E.2d 449, 459 n.19.

Okla. 1988 In response to a police request, physician reported patient treated for a penile bite. Patient sued physician for negligence after information furnished by physician led to patient's arrest and conviction for rape. Patient alleged a tortious breach of the physician-patient confidential relationship, breach of contract, violation of licensing statute, and breach of Principle 9 (1957) [now Principle IV and Opinion 5.05]. The court reasoned that the benefit of the divulgence inured to the public at large and thus fell within the public policy exception to the testimonial privilege, created no liability in tort or contract, and was not a breach of medical ethics under the licensing statute or the Principles. *Bryson v. Tillinghast*, 749 P.2d 110, 113, 114.

Pa. 1999 Administratrix of estate of victim murdered by a mental patient filed suit against the mental health center and member of professional staff. The trial court found in favor of the defendants. The Pennsylvania Supreme Court held that mental health professionals have a duty to warn a third party who is the subject of patient's threats when there is a immediate risk of serious bodily harm. The court quoted Opinion 5.05, noting that the AMA allows an exception to the duty of confidentiality when safety is a reasonable concern. The court found that the defendants had the duty to warn the victim and had fulfilled that duty when the victim was warned not to go to the patient's apartment. *Emerich v. Philadelphia Center for Human Development, Inc.*, 554 Pa. 209, 720 A.2d 1032, 1043.

Pa. 1973 Plaintiff in personal injury suit resulting from auto accident claimed that trial court should have allowed showing on cross-examination that defendant's expert medical witness, who had treated plaintiff, violated Principle 9 (1957) [now Principle IV and Opinion 5.05] by ex parte communications with defense counsel, in order to impeach his medical testimony. The court held that any connection between an alleged breach of medical ethics and the credibility of a physician on the witness stand was tenuous. Therefore, the trial court's decision barring further inquiry in this regard was proper. *Downey v. Weston*, 451 Pa. 259, 301 A.2d 635, 638.

Pa. Super. 1998 The court denied a social worker's motion to quash a subpoena compelling her to testify before a grand jury regarding a client's murder. The court explained that the duty of confidentiality should be waived because the deceased client was not a crime suspect and because the information was necessary to solve a crime. The court further reasoned that disclosure of the confidential information was in the client's best interest because it would aid in solving the client's murder. The court, citing an earlier case, referenced Opinion 5.05, in support of the notion that confidentiality may be waived under special circumstances such as overriding public safety concerns. *In re Subpoena No. 22., Appeal of A.B.*, 709 A.2d 385, 391.

Pa. Super. 1988 Plaintiff-patient sued her physician for breach of confidentiality when physician conferred with defense counsel in plaintiff's malpractice suit against the hospital (physician's employer). In its majority opinion, the court cited Principle IV, commenting that it gave very little guidance to physicians but nonetheless was not violated by the physician. The court also noted Opinion 5.07 (1986) finding that the plaintiff's suit minimized her expectations of confidentiality. The dissent, however, interpreted these same provisions, along with Opinion 5.05 (1986), as protecting plaintiff's expectations of confidentiality. *Moses v. McWilliams*, 379 Pa. Super. 150, 549 A.2d 950, 956, 962 (dissent), appeal denied, 521 Pa. 630, 558 A.2d 532 (1989).

Tenn. App. 1994 Plaintiff sought damages for wrongful death from defendant-surgeon. Defendant requested that the court require plaintiff to sign a form authorizing release of medical records and information to defense counsel. Trial court denied defendant's motion noting, with apparent reference to Principle IV and Opinion 5.05, that confidential relationship exists between physician and patient. Appellate court affirmed although it did not reach the ethical issue of the propriety of disclosures by a physician. *Wright v. Wasudev*, 1994 Tenn. App. LEXIS 657.

Utah Att'y Gen. 1978 A physician who, acting in good faith, discloses confidential information to proper authorities concerning a patient's unfitness to drive is not liable for doing so. Reference is made to Principle 9 (1957) [now Principle IV and Opinion 5.05] to support propriety of such disclosure where the public interest is involved. *Utah Att'y Gen. Op. No. 77-294.*

Wash. 1988 Personal representative brought wrongful death action against decedent's physicians. At issue was whether defense counsel in a personal injury action may communicate ex parte with plaintiff's treating physician where plaintiff has waived the physician-patient relationship. In holding that defense counsel may not engage in ex parte communication, and is limited to formal discovery methods, the court cited Principle IV and Opinion 5.05 (1986) with approval, reasoning that the mere threat of disclosure of private conversations between a physician and defense counsel would chill the physician-patient relationship and hinder further treatment. *Loudon v. Mhyre*, 110 Wash. 2d 675, 756 P.2d 138, 141, 141 n.3.

W. Va. 1993 Plaintiff, in a malpractice action, sought a writ of prohibition to prevent the enforcement of a trial court order allowing ex parte interviews. The court, in granting the writ, held that any benefit from ex parte interviews that occurs is minimal compared to the danger that they will undermine the confidential nature of the physician-patient relationship. Quoting Principles of Medical Ethics Ch. II, sec. 1 (1943) [now Principle IV and Opinion 5.05], the court noted that the medical profession is well aware of the importance of patient confidentiality. *State ex. rel. Kitzmiller v. Henning*, 437 S.E.2d 452, 454.

Wis. 1995 In medical malpractice suit, the court held that (1) subject to restrictions, defense counsel may engage in ex parte communications with plaintiff's treating physician if the communications do not involve disclosure of confidential information; (2) outside a judicial proceeding, defendant-physician may communicate ex parte with plaintiff's treating physician subject to a physician's duty of confidentiality; and (3) if defense counsel elicits confidential information from a treating physician during ex parte communications, the appropriate sanction is within the discretion of the court. The court expressly overruled *State ex rel. Klieger v. Alby*, 125 Wis. 2d 468, 373 N.W.2d 57 (Ct. App. 1985) and the cases applying it. The majority and concurring opinions referred to Principle IV and Opinion 5.05. *Steinberg v. Jensen*, 194 Wis. 2d 440, 534 N.W.2d 361, 370, 377.

Wis. App. 1999 Defendant who pled guilty to carrying a concealed weapon appealed on grounds that the police officer's search of the defendant was based on information obtained from the defendant's psychotherapist. The appellate court held that the defendant's statements made to his psychotherapist could be considered in evaluating the reasonableness of the search because the defendant posed a threat of danger. The court quoted Opinion 5.05, regarding confidentiality and noted the exception where safety is a concern. *State v. Agacki*, 226 Wis. 2d 349, 595 N.W.2d 31, 37.

Wis. App. 1994 In medical malpractice suit, defense counsel engaged in ex parte communications with plaintiff's consulting physicians. Plaintiff amended her complaint seeking punitive damages for breach of confidentiality. The court concluded that the rule of *State ex rel. Klieger v. Alby*, 125 Wis. 2d 468, 373 N.W.2d 57 (Ct. App. 1985), which prohibits ex parte communications that have the potential to breach physician-patient confidentiality, was violated and sanctions were required. The court referred to *Petrillo v. Syntax Labs., Inc.*, 148 Ill. App. 3d 581, 499 N.E.2d 952 (1986) and its use of Principle IV and Opinion 5.05. *Steinberg v. Jensen*, 186 Wis. 2d 237, 519 N.W.2d 753, 761 n.9, rev'd, 194 Wis. 2d 440, 534 N.W.2d 361 (1995).

Wis. Att'y Gen. 1987 Physicians may report cases of suspected child abuse or neglect when a patient discloses that he or she has abused a child in some manner. Where report is made in good faith, physicians are immune from any civil or criminal liability. Passing reference is made to Principle 9 (1957) [now Principle IV and Opinions 2.02 and 5.05] in support of this position. *Wisconsin Att'y Gen. Op. 10-87 (March 16, 1987) (LEXIS, States library, Wis. file).*

Journal 2003 Argues the legal profession must become meaningfully involved in efforts to address the causes and effects of domestic violence. Concludes that lawyers must do more in an effort to protect the interests of clients. Quotes Opinion 5.05. Burman, *Lawyers and Domestic Violence: Raising the Standard of Practice,* 9 Mich. J. Gender & L. 207, 254 (2003).

Journal 2003 Highlights HIPAA privacy issues that need to be monitored and have yet to be resolved. Concludes that HIPAA poses many challenges and it remains unclear whether HIPAA will increase privacy protection. Cites Opinions 5.05, 5.055, 5.057, 5.06, 5.07, 5.075, 5.08, and 5.09. Kutzko, Boyer, Thoman, & Scott, *HIPAA in Real Time: Practical Implications of the Federal Privacy Rule,* 51 Drake L. Rev. 403, 408 (2003).

Journal 2003 Considers the legal, medical, and ethical issues of physician-patient confidentiality in disclosure of paternity. Concludes that a balancing test should be applied to making determinations regarding disclosure of paternity. Quotes Principles I, IV, and V, and Opinions 1.02, 5.055, and 10.01. Cites Principle II and Opinion 5.05. Richards & Wolf, *Medical Confidentiality and Disclosure of Paternity,* 48 S.D. L. Rev. 409, 411, 412, 413 (2003).

Journal 2003 Discusses legal principles governing electronic personal information and other digital media. Concludes that biometric security methods will become the standard for protecting private information. Quotes Opinion 5.05. Yang & Gorman, *What's Yours is Mine: Protection and Security in a Digital World,* 36 Md. B.J. 24, 28-29 (Nov./Dec. 2003).

Journal 2002 Discusses issues regarding regulation of elderly drivers. Concludes that mandating physicians to report unfit elderly patients will protect the public and help resolve ethical and legal dilemmas. Quotes Opinions 1.02, 2.24, 5.05, and 10.01. Kane, *Driving into the Sunset: A Proposal for Mandatory Reporting to the DMV by Physicians Treating Unsafe Elderly Drivers,* 25 U. Haw. L. Rev. 59, 59, 61, 62, 67, 69, 82, 83 (2002).

Journal 2002 Discusses legal and medical policies that protect confidentiality in the physician-patient relationship. Concludes that reducing the current level of privacy protection would jeopardize health care. Quotes Preamble and Opinions 2.136, 5.05, and 10.01. References Principles VIII and IX. Sciarrino, *Ferguson v. City of Charleston: "The Doctor Will See You Now, Be Sure to Bring Your Privacy Rights in With You!"* 12 Temp. Pol. & Civ. Rts. L. Rev. 197, 213, 215, 220, 221, 222 (2002).

Journal 2002 Discusses the lapse of Fourth Amendment protection in the collection of third-party records by the government. Concludes that a new paradigm is needed for regulating government collection of third-party information. Quotes Opinion 5.05. Solove, *Digital Dossiers and the Dissipation of Fourth Amendment Privacy,* 75 S. Cal. L. Rev. 1083, 1155 (2002).

Journal 2002 Considers issues of health information privacy in the electronic age. Concludes that protections afforded by the HIPAA privacy rules and common law will be increasingly important. Quotes Opinion 5.05. Winn, *Confidentiality in Cyberspace: The HIPAA Privacy Rules and the Common Law,* 33 Rutgers L.J. 617, 622 (2002).

Journal 2001 Examines ethical issues surrounding physician disclosure of information to attorneys. Observes that attorneys do not have an absolute right to interfere with the physician-patient relationship. Concludes that attorneys' efforts to obtain information may give rise to lawsuits for aiding and abetting the physician's breach of a fiduciary duty to preserve confidentiality. Quotes Opinion 5.05. Freeman, *Dealing with Doctors,* 13 S. C. Law 11, 11 (July/Aug. 2001).

Journal 2001 Explores the Uniform Mediation Act (UMA). Describes how certain exceptions to confidentiality in mediation arise from an inability to balance the means of confidentiality and the ends of self-determination. Concludes that, under the UMA, confidentiality does not promote self-determination. Quotes Opinion 5.05. Hughes, *The Uniform Mediation Act: To the Spoiled Go the Privileges,* 85 Marq. L. Rev. 9, 26 (2001).

Journal 2001 Compares the American system of patient confidentiality to the Austrian system. Discusses the debate between patients' rights and public safety. Concludes that the duty to warn third parties of dangerous patients should be discretionary instead of mandatory, except in cases of HIV seropositivity, which should involve mandatory disclosure to public health officials. Quotes Opinions 2.23, 5.05 and 5.06. Kenworthy, *The Austrian Psychotherapy Act: No Legal Duty to Warn,* 11 Ind. Int'l & Comp. L. Rev. 469, 480-81, 485, 490, 496 (2001).

Journal 2001 Considers whether or not it is ethical for physicians to prescribe, and pharmacists to dispense, syringes for use by injection drug users. Concludes that ethical considerations suggest such actions are permissible but not obligatory. Quotes Principle III and Opinion 1.02. References Opinion 5.05. Lazzarini, *An Analysis of Ethical Issues in Prescribing and Dispensing Syringes to*

Injection Drug Users, 11 Health Matrix 85, 107, 119 (2001).

Journal 2001 Focuses on the case of *Weld v. CVS Pharmacy, Inc.* Examines whether an individual's privacy is invaded when pharmacies disclose prescription information about customers to aid other private organizations with implementation of marketing activities. Quotes Opinion 5.05. Schawbel, *Are You Taking Any Prescription Medication?: A Case Comment on Weld v. CVS Pharmacy, Inc., 35 New Eng. L. Rev. 909, 957 (2001).*

Journal 2001 Evaluates current forms of cybermedicine and Internet resources that support it. Explores patient and regulatory concerns, including privacy issues, insurance reimbursement problems, licensure, and liability, which may thwart the growth of cybermedicine. Concludes that cybermedicine may facilitate delivery of cost-effective, quality medical care. Quotes Opinions 5.05, 6.02, and 6.03. Scott, *Cybermedicine and Virtual Pharmacies, 103 W. Va. L. Rev. 407, 441, 451 (2001).*

Journal 2001 Discusses the history of fetal abuse prosecution and the Medical University of South Carolina's Interagency Policy of Management of Substance Abuse During Pregnancy. Concludes that, although the *Ferguson v. City of Charleston* decision will continue to allow pregnant drug users to access prenatal care, it leaves open questions regarding the future of fetal abuse prosecutions. Quotes Opinion 5.05. Toll, *For My Doctor's Eyes Only: Ferguson v. City of Charleston, 33 Loy. U. Chi. L.J. 267, 305 (2001).*

Journal 2000 Explores confidentiality and discusses the legal standards pertaining to attorneys, physicians, and social workers. Concludes that the concept of confidentiality is the backbone of each profession and without privileged communications such professions would fail the American public. Quotes Opinion 5.05. Clark, *Confidential Communications in a Professional Context: Attorney, Physician, and Social Worker, 24 J. Legal Prof. 79, 92 (2000).*

Journal 2000 Describes possible solutions designed to improve post-approval regulation of prescription drugs so that fewer patients will suffer from adverse drug reactions. Concludes that the FDA along with physicians and clinical researchers should rethink the existing approach to monitoring of unexpected side effects. Quotes Principle V and Opinion 9.032. Cites Opinion 5.05. Noah, *Adverse Drug Reactions: Harnessing Experimental Data to Promote Patient Welfare, 49 Cath. U. L. Rev. 449, 477, 497-98 (2000).*

Journal 2000 Addresses the philosophical conflict between free speech and privacy. Examines the commercial speech doctrine and discusses the constitutional and human rights implications of use of private sector data. Cites Opinion 5.05. Singleton, *Privacy Versus the First Amendment: A Skeptical Approach, 11 Fordham Intell. Prop. Media & Ent. L. J. 97, 122 (2000).*

Journal 2000 Defines and explores current and future applications of telemedicine. Considers issues of cost, quality, access, and regulation. Concludes that telemedicine holds tremendous promise for improving the United States health care system. Quotes Opinions 5.05 and 5.07. Volkert, *Telemedicine: RX for the Future of Health Care, 6 Mich. Telecomm. & Tech. L. Rev. 147, 214, 225 (2000).*

Journal 1999 Explores changes in technology and the resulting impact on privacy of medical information. Observes that current federal and state laws inadequately protect medical information privacy and suggests that Congress needs to enact legislation addressing this issue. Quotes Opinion 5.05. References Opinions 7.02 and 7.05. Carter, *Health Information Privacy: Can Congress Protect Confidential Medical Information in the "Information Age"?, 25 Wm. Mitchell L. Rev. 223, 236, 273 (1999).*

Journal 1999 Discusses the "ever-expanding" disclosure of confidential medical record information regarding patients. Emphasizes organizational problems relating to access and security in medical record systems. Argues in favor of stronger regulations limiting access to and use of information. Quotes Opinion 5.05. Hall, *Confidentiality as an Organizational Ethics Issue, 10 J. Clinical Ethics 230, 232 (1999).*

Journal 1999 Discusses the need for physicians to advocate on behalf of patients' rights in the context of health care delivery. Evaluates the nature and scope of the physician's role as advocate, noting that physicians cannot be expected to engage in attorney-like advocacy. Quotes Principles IV and VI, Fundamental Elements (2), (4), and (6) [now Opinion 10.01], Patient Responsibilities 5 [now Opinion 10.02], and Opinions 2.03, 2.07, 2.09, 2.16, 2.19, 3.06, 4.01, 4.04, 6.01, 7.02, 8.02, 8.03, 8.13, 8.132, 9.06, 9.07, and 9.131. Cites Opinions 5.05, 5.09, 7.01, 8.135, and 9.02. Sage, *Physicians as Advocates, 35 Hous. L. Rev. 1529, 1537, 1541, 1542, 1552-53, 1554, 1556, 1557, 1559, 1561-62, 1564, 1571, 1574, 1576, 1580 (1999).*

Journal 1999 Explores the increased use of physician-patient communication through e-mail. Analyzes current laws regarding medical privacy. Suggests that patients' communications to their physicians are part of their medical record and should be given the same protections. Quotes Opinions 5.05 and 5.07. Cites Opinions 5.04 and 5.06. Spielberg, *Online Without a Net: Physician-Patient Communication by Electronic Mail*, 25 Am. J. Law & Med. 267, 284-85 (1999).

Journal 1999 Explores Model Rules of Professional Conduct focusing on the attorney-client relationship. Compares confidentiality provisions in the Model Rules with the rules of confidentiality governing the medical profession. Observes that existing confidentiality rules are incomplete and ambiguous. Concludes that one remedy is to embrace a discretionary confidentiality rule. Quotes Opinion 5.05. Cites Principle IV and Opinion 5.07. Zer-Gutman, *Revising the Ethical Rules of Attorney-Client Confidentiality: Towards a New Discretionary Rule*, 45 Loy. L. Rev. 669, 683-84, 699, 709, 718 (1999).

Journal 1998 Describes the special nature of confidentiality in the relationship between the psychotherapist and patient. States that not many breach of confidentiality cases involve psychotherapists. Concludes that patients and psychotherapists must better understand their rights and responsibilities in this context. Quotes Opinion 5.05. Cites Opinions 5.06, 5.07, 5.08, and 5.09. Grabois, *The Liability of Psychotherapists for Breach of Confidentiality*, 12 J. Law & Health 39, 53-54 (1998).

Journal 1998 Explains risks involved with the use of electronic medical records. States that patients need to be aware of who has access to their medical records. Concludes that health care providers should equalize the risks and benefits related to the use of electronic medical records. Cites Opinion 5.05. References Opinion 5.07. Jurevic, *When Technology and Health Care Collide: Issues with Electronic Medical Records and Electronic Mail*, 66 UMKC L. Rev. 809, 819-20 (1998).

Journal 1998 Discusses issues of patient consent regarding disclosure of medical information. Points out that recent changes in the health care system have presented medical record privacy concerns. Discloses findings of a study regarding hospital consent forms and calls for more research to be conducted. Cites Principle IV and Opinion 5.05. Merz, Sankar, & Yoo, *Hospital Consent for Disclosure of Medical Records*, 26 J. Law, Med. & Ethics 241, 248 (1998).

Journal 1998 Points out that most victims of elder abuse are socially isolated and thus few incidents of elder abuse are reported to authorities. Argues that current protections against elder abuse are inadequate. Suggests that the legal system and health professionals can make a difference in reducing elder abuse. Quotes Opinion 5.05. References Opinion 2.02. Moskowitz, *Saving Granny from the Wolf: Elder Abuse and Neglect—The Legal Framework*, 31 Conn. L. Rev. 77, 116, 120, 121, 122 (1998).

Journal 1998 Discusses issues of privacy concerning the collection and use of computerized pharmacy records by pharmaceutical companies. Concludes that federal legislation is needed to protect the privacy of prescription information. Quotes Opinion 5.05. Mowery, *A Patient's Right of Privacy in Computerized Pharmacy Records*, 66 U. Cin. L. Rev. 697, 717 (1998).

Journal 1998 Discusses the ramifications of physician license revocation for failing to pay child support. Points out that patients stand to lose access to trusted physicians and confidence in the health care system. Concludes that children need the most protection and that patients will have an easier time finding another physician than children will have finding another means for support. Quotes Opinion 5.05. Cites Opinions 9.02 and 9.06. Noyes, *Higher Penalties for Failing to Pay Child Support: A Look at Medical License Revocation*, 19 J. Legal Med. 127, 138 (1998).

Journal 1998 Explores the role of pharmacy benefits managers. Discusses the impact of pharmacy benefits managers on patients, consumers, and the medical field. Analyzes potential privacy problems stemming from pharmacy benefits managers. Cites Opinion 5.05. Rosoff, *The Changing Face of Pharmacy Benefits Management: Information Technology Pursues a Grand Mission*, 42 St. Louis U. L. J. 1, 25-26 (1998).

Journal 1998 Examines the use of e-mail in the physician-patient relationship. Focuses on privacy concerns stemming from the use of e-mail in the medical context. Suggests that physicians should discuss the implications of communicating through e-mail with their patients and should obtain informed consent prior to communicating in this manner. Cites Opinions 5.04, 5.05, 5.057, 5.07, 5.075, and 5.08. Spielberg, *On Call and Online: Sociohistorical, Legal, and Ethical Implications of E-mail for the Patient-Physician Relationship*, 280 JAMA 1353, 1356 (1998).

Journal 1998 Explores the increased use and benefits of telemedicine. Points out that there is inadequate protection of privacy rights regarding electronic medical information. Concludes that federal law does not uniformly address medical record privacy and that Missouri law lacks adequate specificity. Quotes Principle IV. References Opinion 5.05. Young, *Telemedicine: Patient Privacy Rights of Electronic Medical Records*, 66 UMKC L. Rev. 921, 926 (1998).

Journal 1997 Compares past ethical opinions to current opinions and notes the differences. Comments on the forces that have changed medical ethics through the years. Notes differing theories on the future course of medical ethics. Quotes Fundamental Elements (Preamble) and Opinions 5.05, 5.057, 7.01, 8.12, 9.12, and 9.131. Cites Fundamental Elements (5) and Opinions 8.115 and 8.13. Buchanan, *Medical Ethics at the Millennium: A Brief Retrospective*, 26 Colo. Law. 141, 142, 143, 144, 145 (1997).

Journal 1997 Describes the DNA profile and its use in the scientific community. Examines common misconceptions about the DNA profile. Considers implication of the DNA profile as a unique identifier in the context of Community Health Information Networks. Quotes Principle 9 (1957) [now Opinion 5.05]. Dahm, *Using DNA Profile as the Unique Patient Identifier in the Community Health Information Network: Legal Implications*, 15 J. Marshall J. Computer & Info. L. 227, 266, 275 (1997).

Journal 1997 Considers how breast cancer has given rise to numerous medical malpractice lawsuits. Discusses trial techniques and strategies for litigating these types of claims. Quotes Opinions 5.05 and 5.06. Hillerich, Ellerin, & Frieder, *Selecting and Presenting a Failure to Diagnose Breast Cancer Case*, 20 Am. J. Trial Advoc. 253, 271 (1996-97).

Journal 1997 Considers principles of confidentiality in the physician-patient relationship. Notes the current trend emphasizing public reporting obligations of physicians to protect members of society. Emphasizes need for balance between patient rights and societal interests. Quotes Principle IV and Opinion 5.05. References Preamble. Jozefowicz, *The Case Against Having Professional Privilege in the Physician-Patient Relationship*, 16 Med. & L. 385, 386-87, 391 (1997).

Journal 1997 Suggests that ex parte conferences between treating physicians and opposing counsel undermine the physician-patient relationship. Notes that there are no significant benefits within the fact-finding process that justify the conflicts of interest created. Concludes that ex parte conferences are unnecessary. Quotes Principle IV and Opinion 5.05. Kassel, *Counterpoint . . . Defense Counsel's Ex Parte Communication with Plaintiff's Doctors: A Bad One-Sided Deal*, 9 S.C. Law. 42, 43 (Sept./Oct. 1997).

Journal 1997 Discusses the practice of ex parte communications between treating physicians and their patients' legal adversaries without informing the patient or obtaining consent. Examines harms that may occur in these situations. Argues that Oklahoma needs to prohibit treating physicians from communicating ex parte with their patients' legal adversaries. Quotes Opinions 5.05, 5.07, 5.08, 8.02, 8.03, and 9.07. Cites Opinion 7.02. McNaughton & McNaughton, *Divided Loyalty: The Dilemma of the Treating Physician Advocate*, 22 Okla. City U. L. Rev. 1051, 1052, 1054, 1056, 1058, 1059, 1062 (1997).

Journal 1997 Considers Connecticut AIDS statute, which relates to testing and confidentiality of patient medical information. Discusses statutory construction of provisions of this law by the Connecticut Supreme Court in *Doe v. Marselle*. Quotes Opinion 5.05. Note, *A Case Study of New Textualism in State Courts: Doe v. Marselle and the Confidentiality of HIV-Related Information*, 30 Conn. L. Rev. 295, 297 (1997).

Journal 1997 Considers whether the physician-patient privilege should be extended to protect communications to alternative health practitioners. Suggests that these practitioners treat and diagnose patients within the meaning of the privilege. Advocates an extension of the privilege to recognize the importance of confidentiality. Quotes Opinion 5.05. Note, *Healer-Patient Privilege: Extending the Physician-Patient Privilege to Alternative Health Practitioners in California*, 48 Hastings L. J. 633, 657 (1997).

Journal 1996 Explains the benefits of high-tech access to patient information by pharmacists. Considers related issues of patient confidentiality. Advocates a pharmacist-patient privilege. Quotes Opinion 5.05. Berger, *Patient Confidentiality in a High Tech World*, 5 J. Pharmacy & L., 139, 141 (1996).

Journal 1996 Suggests that attorneys representing HIV-infected and sexually active adolescents face an ethical conflict between their duty of client confidentiality and the duty to protect third parties. Notes that attorneys failing to warn third parties may face liability. Concludes that clients should be informed of potential limitations on the right to confidentiality. Quotes Opinion 5.05. Katner, *The Ethical Dilemma Awaiting Counsel Who Represent Adolescents with HIV/AIDS: Criminal*

Law and Tort Suits Pressure Counsel to Breach the Confidentiality of the Clients' Medical Status, 70 *Tul. L. Rev.* 2311, 2341 (1996).

Journal 1996 Discusses sexual abuse litigation in which accusers have recovered memories of molestation in psychotherapy sessions. Observes that, to successfully defend against such claims, it is necessary for the accused to have access to the clinical record. Posits that confidentiality problems can be eliminated with *in camera* record inspections. References Principle IV and Opinion 5.05. Loftus, Paddock, & Guernsey, *Patient-Psychotherapist Privilege: Access to Clinical Records in the Tangled Web of Repressed Memory Litigation*, 30 *U. Rich L. Rev.* 109, 127 (1996).

Journal 1996 Reviews two Washington state supreme court decisions in which subsequent treating physicians testified against their patients and on behalf of defendant physicians in malpractice litigation. Observes that these decisions erode the physician-patient privilege. Posits that the decisions are inconsistent with current medical ethics and proposes a statutory enactment as a solution. Quotes Opinion 5.05. Cites Principle 9 (1957) [now Principle IV]. Oppenheim, *Physicians as Experts Against Their Own Patients? What Happened to the Privilege?*, 63 *Def. Couns. J.* 254, 257, 261 (1996).

Journal 1996 Considers prearraignment forensic evaluations. Notes the prohibition against use of such evaluations. Examines underlying ethical precepts. Observes that principles of beneficence are misapplied to forensic psychiatry in this context. Advocates a new ethical framework. Quotes Preamble. References Principle IV and Opinion 5.05. Ornish, Mills, & Ornish, *Prearraignment Forensic Evaluations: Toward a New Policy*, 24 *Bull. Am. Acad. Psychiatry Law* 453, 454, 469 (1996).

Journal 1996 Examines the psychiatrist-patient duty of confidentiality. Notes that Principles of Medical Ethics prohibit the disclosure of patient confidences and medical records. Observes that exceptions to this prohibition exist when required by law or to protect the community. Quotes Principle 9 (1957) [now Principle IV and Opinion 5.05]. Sadoff, *Ethical Obligations for the Psychiatrist: Confidentiality, Privilege, and Privacy in Psychiatric Treatment*, 29 *Loy. L.A. L. Rev.* 1709, 1710, 1711 (1996).

Journal 1995 Addresses presidential disability, its past impact on American government, and possible solutions to potential problems. Proposes enhancement of the role of the President's physician. Quotes Opinion 8.03. Cites Opinions 5.04 and 5.05. Abrams, *The Vulnerable President and the Twenty-Fifth Amendment, with Observations on Guidelines, a Health Commission, and the Role of the President's Physician*, 30 *Wake Forest L. Rev.* 453, 466, 471 (1995).

Journal 1995 Discusses the belief of health care providers that they have an ethical obligation to warn the partners of HIV-positive patients. Examines both the scope of a Massachusetts statute that prevents providers from releasing HIV test results of patients and possible defenses that providers may assert. Quotes Principle IV and Opinion 5.05. Friedland, *HIV Confidentiality and the Right to Warn The Health Care Provider's Dilemma*, 80 *Mass. L. Rev.* 3, 4 (March 1995).

Journal 1995 Considers how the use of health care identification cards and medical record databases would threaten privacy rights. Concludes that federal legislation should be enacted to protect health care record privacy and prevent misuse of health care identification cards. Quotes Opinion 5.05. Minor, *Identity Cards and Databases in Health Care: The Need for Federal Privacy Protections*, 28 *Colum. J.L. & Soc. Probs.* 253, 279 (1995).

Journal 1995 Examines the impact of health care reform on physician-patient relationships. Discusses how reform may threaten the physician's fiduciary duty of loyalty by forcing physicians to make rationing decisions and giving physicians financial incentives to limit use of health care resources. Quotes Fundamental Elements (5) [now Opinion 10.0]. Cites Opinion 5.05. Orentlicher, *Health Care Reform and the Patient-Physician Relationship*, 5 *Health Matrix* 141, 143, 148 (1995).

Journal 1995 Analyzes the secular approach to the duty to treat HIV-infected individuals and the duty to warn those who are sexual partners of, or who share needles with, people infected with HIV. Observes that the secular approach leaves these issues unresolved; but indicates that Jewish law compels physicians both to treat and to warn. Quotes Opinions 5.05 and 9.131. Shorr, *AIDS, Judaism, and the Limits of the Secular Society*, 20 *Second Opinion* 23, 24, 27 (1995).

Journal 1994 Considers whether an exception should be made to physician-patient confidentiality that would allow a physician to reveal parental medical history to a child. Concludes that such an exception would not completely erode physician-patient confidentiality. Quotes Principles IV, Fundamental Elements (4), and Opinion 5.05. Cites Principle I and Fundamental Elements (1).

Friedland, *Physician-Patient Confidentiality: Time to Re-Examine a Venerable Concept in Light of Contemporary Society and Advances in Medicine*, 15 J. Legal Med. 249, 257, 264, 276 (1994).

Journal 1994 Explores the ethical issues involved in a multidisciplinary team working with children in legal proceedings. Focuses on the relationships between professionals and the conflicts that arise regarding disclosure of confidential information and forced disclosure of non-privileged information. Quotes Principles III, IV, Fundamental Elements (4) and Opinions 1.02 (1992) and 5.07 (1992) [now Opinion 5.05]. Cites Opinions 2.02. Glynn, *Multidisciplinary Representation of Children: Conflicts Over Disclosures of Client Communications*, 27 J. Marshall L. Rev. 617, 625, 626, 630-32, 637, 639, 643 (1994).

Journal 1994 Compares Texas law with Illinois law on the issue of ex parte communications between defense counsel and the patient/plaintiff's physician in civil litigation. Argues that preservation of the physician-patient relationship requires prohibition of such contact. Quotes Principles II and IV and Opinion 5.05. Comment, *From the Land of Lincoln a Healing Rule: Proposed Texas Rule of Civil Procedure Prohibiting Ex Parte Contact Between Defense Counsel and a Plaintiff's Treating Physician*, 25 Tex. Tech L. Rev. 1081, 1081, 1082 (1994).

Journal 1994 Considers how computerized medical records might threaten patient confidentiality. Explores proposed legislation for computerized records and the potential need for new legal standards in this area. Cites Opinion 5.05. Field, *Overview: Computerized Medical Records Create New Legal and Business Confidentiality Problems*, 11 HealthSpan 3, 4 (1994).

Journal 1993 Discusses family privacy rights and considers the meaning of justice, self respect, and the fundamental principles of physician ethics. Concludes that physicians have an ethical duty to intervene in domestic violence so long as such intervention does not breach confidentiality or violate patient autonomy. Quotes Principle IV and Opinion 5.05. References Opinions 8.14 and 9.131. Jecker, *Privacy Beliefs and the Violent Family: Extending the Ethical Argument for Physician Intervention*, 269 JAMA 776, 778, 779 (1993).

Journal 1993 Evaluates the legal issues surrounding AIDS and HIV. Examines various aspects of the law that would be relevant to a medical or health care lawyer. Quotes Opinion 5.05. Skiver & Hickey, *AIDS: Legal Issues 1992*, 19 Ohio No. Univ. L. Rev. 839, 860 (1993).

Journal 1991 Discusses current law protecting confidential genetic information obtained in the workplace and presents several safeguard mechanisms. Analyzes the legal grounds upon which various parties may access this information. References Opinion 5.05. Andrews & Jaeger, *Confidentiality of Genetic Information in the Workplace*, XVII Am. J. Law & Med. 75, 78 (1991).

Journal 1991 Examines the problem of AIDS in this country and the risk of HIV transmission via sexual assault. Concludes that state laws requiring HIV testing for sex offenders are necessary to preserve the rights of victims of sexual assault. Quotes Opinion 5.05. McGuire, *AIDS and the Sexual Offender: The Epidemic Now Poses New Threats to the Victim and the Criminal Justice System*, 96 Dickinson L. Rev. 95, 109, 110 (1991).

Journal 1991 Focuses on the case *Crist v. Moffatt*, where a court permitted ex parte interview of a plaintiff's physician only after the plaintiff signed a written authorization. Concludes that *Crist* was correctly decided, but warns against expanding the decision to the point of unduly restricting discovery. Quotes Opinion 5.05. Note, *Restricting Ex Parte Interviews With Nonparty Treating Physicians: Crist v. Moffatt*, 69 No. Carolina L. Rev. 1381, 1391, 1392 (1991).

Journal 1991 Discusses confidentiality with respect to a patient's HIV status. Notes how confidentiality may be lost in the hospital setting and emphasizes importance of heightened attention to this issue by institutional health care providers. Quotes Opinion 5.05. Obade, *Whisper Down the Lane: AIDS, Privacy, and the Hospital Grapevine*, 2 J. Clinical Ethics 133, 133 (1991).

Journal 1990 Discusses the legal and ethical considerations associated with genetic research, including recombinant DNA technology. Offers case examples illustrating issues raised by the application of this technology in the clinical setting. Quotes Opinion 5.05. Elsas, *A Clinical Approach to Legal and Ethical Problems in Human Genetics*, 39 Emory L.J. 811, 816, 820 (1990).

Journal 1990 Advocates physician liability for failure to warn third parties of the potential risk of being infected with HIV from the physician's patient. Concludes that there should be no liability for disclosure because public health concerns outweigh an individual patient's right to confidentiality. References Opinion 5.05. Note, *AIDS: Establishing a Physician's Duty to Warn*, 21 Rutgers L.J. 645, 652 (1990).

Journal 1989 Discusses the history of the physician-patient privilege up through changes implemented under the Ohio Tort Reform Act of 1987. Aspects of the physician-patient privilege that are most significantly affected by this Tort Reform Act are highlighted, with recommendations for further refinement of the privilege in Ohio. Quotes Principles II and IV and Opinion 5.05. Note, *The Ohio Physician-Patient Privilege: Modified, Revised, and Defined*, 49 Ohio St. L. J. 1147, 1167 (1989).

5.051   Confidentiality of Medical Information Postmortem

All medically related confidences disclosed by a patient to a physician and information contained within a deceased patient's medical record, including information entered postmortem, should be kept confidential to the greatest possible degree. However, the obligation to safeguard patient confidences is subject to certain exceptions that are ethically and legally justifiable because of overriding societal considerations (Opinion 5.05, "Confidentiality"). At their strongest, confidentiality protections after death would be equal to those in force during a patient's life. Thus, if information about a patient may be ethically disclosed during life, it likewise may be disclosed after the patient has died.

Disclosure of medical information postmortem for research and educational purposes is appropriate as long as confidentiality is maintained to the greatest possible degree by removing any individual identifiers. Otherwise, in determining whether to disclose identified information after the death of a patient, physicians should consider the following factors:

(1) The imminence of harm to identifiable individuals or the public health

(2) The potential benefit to at-risk individuals or the public health (eg, if a communicable or inherited disease is preventable or treatable)

(3) Any statement or directive made by the patient regarding postmortem disclosure

(4) The impact disclosure may have on the reputation of the deceased patient

(5) Personal gain for the physician that may unduly influence professional obligations of confidentiality

When a family member or other decision maker has given consent to an autopsy, physicians may disclose the results of the autopsy to the individual(s) that granted consent to the procedure. (IV)

Issued December 2000 based on the report "Confidentiality of Medical Information Postmortem," adopted June 2000.

Updated December 2001 (*Arch Pathol Lab Med.* 2001; 125:1189-92).

Journal 2001 Analyzes postmortem patient confidentiality and proposes a framework for appropriate information disclosure. Concludes that, following death, decisions regarding disclosure of confidential information should be made on a case-by-case basis. Quotes Opinions 5.051 and 7.02. Berg, *Grave Secrets: Legal and Ethical Analysis of Postmortem Confidentiality*, 34 Conn. L. Rev. 81, 87, 117 (2001).

5.055   Confidential Care for Minors

Physicians who treat minors have an ethical duty to promote the autonomy of minor patients by involving them in the medical decision-making process to a degree commensurate with their abilities.

When minors request confidential services, physicians should encourage them to involve their parents. This includes making efforts to obtain the minor's reasons for not involving their parents and correcting misconceptions that may be motivating their objections.

Where the law does not require otherwise, physicians should permit a competent minor to consent to medical care and should not notify parents without the patient's consent. Depending on the seriousness of the decision, competence may be evaluated by physicians for most minors. When necessary, experts in adolescent medicine or child psychological development should be consulted. Use of the courts for competence determinations should be made only as a last resort.

When an immature minor requests contraceptive services, pregnancy-related care (including pregnancy testing, prenatal and postnatal care, and delivery services), or treatment for sexually transmitted disease, drug and alcohol abuse, or mental illness, physicians must recognize that requiring parental involvement may be counterproductive to the health of the patient. Physicians should encourage parental involvement in these situations. However, if the minor continues to object, his or her wishes ordinarily should be respected. If the physician is uncomfortable with providing services without parental involvement, and alternative confidential services are available, the minor may be referred to those services. In cases when the physician believes that without parental involvement and guidance, the minor will face a serious health threat, and there is reason to believe that the parents will be helpful and understanding, disclosing the problem to the parents is ethically justified. When the physician does breach confidentiality to the parents, he or she must discuss the reasons for the breach with the minor prior to the disclosure.

For minors who are mature enough to be unaccompanied by their parents for their examination, confidentiality of information disclosed during an exam, interview, or in counseling should be maintained. Such information may be disclosed to parents when the patient consents to disclosure. Confidentiality may be justifiably breached in situations for which confidentiality for adults may be breached, according to Opinion 5.05, "Confidentiality." In addition, confidentiality for immature minors may be ethically breached when necessary to enable the parent to make an informed decision about treatment for the minor or when such a breach is necessary to avert serious harm to the minor. (IV)

Issued June 1994 based on the report "Confidential Care for Minors," adopted June 1992.

Updated June 1996.

Journal 2003 Highlights HIPAA privacy issues that need to be monitored and have yet to be resolved. Concludes that HIPAA poses many challenges and it remains unclear whether HIPAA will increase privacy protection. Cites Opinions 5.05, 5.055, 5.057, 5.06, 5.07, 5.075, 5.08, and 5.09. Kutzko, Boyer, Thoman, & Scott, *HIPAA in Real Time: Practical Implications of the Federal Privacy Rule*, 51 Drake L. Rev. 403, 408 (2003).

Journal 2003 Considers the legal, medical, and ethical issues of physician-patient confidentiality in disclosure of paternity. Concludes that a balancing test should be applied to making determinations regarding disclosure of paternity. Quotes Principles I, IV, and V, and Opinions 1.02, 5.055, and 10.01. Cites Principle II and Opinion 5.05. Richards & Wolf, *Medical Confidentiality and Disclosure of Paternity*, 48 S.D. L. Rev. 409, 411, 412, 413 (2003).

5.057 Confidentiality of HIV Status on Autopsy Reports

Physicians should maintain the confidentiality of human immunodeficency virus (HIV) status on autopsy reports to the greatest extent possible.

Physicians who perform autopsies or who have access to autopsy information regarding a patient's HIV status should be familiar with state law governing (1) the reporting of HIV and acquired immunedeficiency syndrome (AIDS) to public health authorities; (2) obligations to inform third parties who may be at risk for HIV infection through contact with an HIV-infected decedent; (3) other parties to whom reporting may be required (ie, funeral directors, health care personnel involved in the care of the patient); and (4) the extent of confidentiality of autopsy records.

HIV status which appears on autopsy records performed under the authority of a hospital are part of the decedent's medical record and should be held confidential. The physician should comply with state laws regarding disclosure to public health authorities and at-risk third parties and, where such laws are absent, fulfill ethical obligations to notify endangered third parties (eg, identified sexual or needle-sharing partners). This includes reporting to organ or tissue procurement agencies if any parts of the decedent's body were taken for use in transplantation.

HIV status which appears on autopsy records performed by a medical examiner in the case of suspicious, accidental, or unexplained death should be kept confidential where autopsy records are not accessible to the public. The physician should comply with state laws regarding disclosure to public health authorities and at-risk third parties, and, where such laws are absent, fulfill ethical obligations to notify endangered third parties (eg, sexual and needle-sharing partners). This includes reporting to organ or tissue procurement agencies if any parts of the decedent's body were taken for use in transplantation.

In cases where autopsies are done under the auspices of the medical examiner's office and state law mandates that the autopsy information be accessible to the public, then physicians should comply with state law. However, in these instances, HIV status should only be recorded when the HIV status of the decedent would be relevant to determining the patient's cause of death. In addition, although a patient's HIV status may be learned from public records in some jurisdictions, it is still unethical for a physician to make a public disclosure of an individual patient's HIV status independent of the legal requirements governing the filing or processing of autopsy records. The physician should comply with state laws regarding disclosure to public health authorities and at-risk third parties, and, where such laws are absent, fulfill ethical obligations to notify endangered third parties (eg, sexual and needle-sharing partners). This includes reporting to organ or tissue procurement agencies if any parts of the decedent's body were taken for use in transplantation. (IV)

Issued June 1994 based on the report "Confidentiality of HIV Status on Autopsy Reports," adopted June 1992 (*Arch Pathol Lab Med.* 1992; 116: 1120-23).

Journal 2003 Highlights HIPAA privacy issues that need to be monitored and have yet to be resolved. Concludes that HIPAA poses many challenges and it remains unclear whether HIPAA will increase privacy protection. Cites Opinions 5.05, 5.055, 5.057, 5.06, 5.07, 5.075, 5.08, and

5.09. Kutzko, Boyer, Thoman, & Scott, *HIPAA in Real Time: Practical Implications of the Federal Privacy Rule*, 51 Drake L. Rev. 403, 408 (2003).

Journal 1998 Examines the use of e-mail in the physician-patient relationship. Focuses on privacy concerns stemming from the use of e-mail in the medical context. Suggests that physicians should discuss the implications of communicating through e-mail with their patients and should obtain informed consent prior to communicating in this manner. Cites Opinions 5.04, 5.05, 5.057, 5.07, 5.075, and 5.08. Spielberg, *On Call and Online: Sociohistorical, Legal, and Ethical Implications of E-mail for the Patient-Physician Relationship*, 280 JAMA 1353, 1356 (1998).

Journal 1997 Compares past ethical opinions to current opinions and notes the differences. Comments on the forces that have changed medical ethics through the years. Notes differing theories on the future course of medical ethics. Quotes Fundamental Elements (Preamble) and Opinions 5.05, 5.057, 7.01, 8.12, 9.12, and 9.131. Cites Fundamental Elements (5) and Opinions 8.115 and 8.13. Buchanan, *Medical Ethics at the Millennium: A Brief Retrospective*, 26 Colo. Law. 141, 142, 143, 144, 145 (1997).

Journal 1996 Discusses conflict between physicians' duty of confidentiality to patients and physicians' obligation to warn third parties of foreseeable injuries. Examines physicians' current legal responsibility to breach confidentiality to prevent the spread of infectious diseases, including AIDS. Identifies guidelines for physicians. Cites Opinions 2.23 and 5.057. Comment, *Taking Tarasoff Where No One Has Gone Before: Looking at Duty to Warn Under the AIDS Crisis*, 15 St. Louis U. Pub. L. Rev. 471, 499 (1996).

5.059 Privacy in the Context of Health Care

In the context of health care, emphasis has been given to confidentiality, which is defined as information told in confidence or imparted in secret. However, physicians also should be mindful of patient privacy, which encompasses information that is concealed from others outside of the patient-physician relationship.

Physicians must seek to protect patient privacy in all of its forms, including (1) physical, which focuses on individuals and their personal spaces, (2) informational, which involves specific personal data, (3) decisional, which focuses on personal choices, and (4) associational, which refers to family or other intimate relations. Such respect for patient privacy is a fundamental expression of patient autonomy and is a prerequisite to building the trust that is at the core of the patient-physician relationship.

Privacy is not absolute, and must be balanced with the need for the efficient provision of medical care and the availability of resources. Physicians should be aware of and respect the special concerns of their patients regarding privacy. Patients should be informed of any significant infringement on their privacy of which they may otherwise be unaware. (I, IV)

Issued June 2002 based on the report "Privacy in the Context of Health Care," adopted December 2001.

5.06 Confidentiality: Attorney-Physician Relation

The patient's history, diagnosis, treatment, and prognosis may be discussed with the patient's lawyer with the consent of the patient or the patient's lawful representative.

A physician may testify in court or before a worker's compensation board or the like in any personal injury or related case. (IV)

Issued prior to April 1977.

M.D. Pa. 1987 Plaintiff in a medical malpractice action sought to preclude his treating physicians from serving as defendant's expert witnesses at trial. The court held that defense counsel's failure to provide prior notice of ex parte communication with plaintiff's treating physicians barred their use as defense experts. Referring to *Petrillo v. Syntex Laboratories, Inc.*, 148 Ill. App. 3d 581, 499 N.E.2d 952 (1986), the court noted that the court there favorably cited Principle IV and Opinions 5.05, 5.06, and 5.07 (1984) in support of a public policy protecting confidentiality between physician and patient and against ex parte discussion. *Manion v. N.P.W. Medical Center of N.E. Pa., Inc.*, 676 F. Supp. 585, 591.

Fla. App. 1995 The court considered the issue of the effect of § 455.241(2) of the Florida Statutes on right of defense in a medical malpractice action to engage in ex parte communications with plaintiff's non-party treating physician. The court held that a 1988 amendment to § 455.241(2) negated the applicability of the statute to medical malpractice cases. The dissent, citing *Petrillo v. Syntex Laboratories, Inc.*, 148 Ill. App. 3d 581, 499 N.E.2d 952 (1986), quoted Principles II and IV and Opinions 5.05, 5.06, and 5.08 as strong public policy support for its position that ex parte communications should be barred altogether. *Castillo-Plaza v. Green*, 655 So. 2d 197, 206 n.4.

Ill. App. 1986 Defense attorney in product liability suit was held in contempt of court for conducting ex parte discussions with plaintiff-patient's treating physician without patient's consent and contrary to authorized methods of discovery. The court held that the strong public policy favoring physician-patient confidentiality articulated in Principles II and IV and Opinions 5.05, 5.06, 5.07, and 5.08 (1984) justified a rule against such ex parte discussions. Further, the court held that the public has the right to rely on physicians to faithfully execute their ethical obligations. *Petrillo v. Syntex Laboratories, Inc.*, 148 Ill. App. 3d 581, 499 N.E.2d 952, 957, 958, 959 cert. denied, 483 US 1007 (1987).

Journal 2003 Highlights HIPAA privacy issues that need to be monitored and have yet to be resolved. Concludes that HIPAA poses many challenges and it remains unclear whether HIPAA will increase privacy protection. Cites Opinions 5.05, 5.055, 5.057, 5.06, 5.07, 5.075, 5.08, and 5.09. Kutzko, Boyer, Thoman, & Scott, *HIPAA in Real Time: Practical Implications of the Federal Privacy Rule*, 51 Drake L. Rev. 403, 408 (2003).

Journal 1999 Explores the increased use of physician-patient communication through e-mail. Analyzes current laws regarding medical privacy. Suggests that patients' communications to their physicians are part of their medical record and should be given the same protections. Quotes Opinions 5.05 and 5.07. Cites Opinions 5.04 and 5.06. Spielberg, *Online Without a Net: Physician-Patient Communication by Electronic Mail*, 25 Am. J. Law & Med. 267, 284-85 (1999).

Journal 1998 Describes the special nature of confidentiality in the relationship between the psychotherapist and patient. States that not many breach of confidentiality cases involve psychotherapists. Concludes that patients and psychotherapists must better understand their rights and responsibilities in this context. Quotes Opinion 5.05. Cites Opinions 5.06, 5.07, 5.08, and 5.09. Grabois, *The Liability of Psychotherapists for Breach of Confidentiality*, 12 J. Law & Health 39, 53-54 (1998).

Journal 1997 Considers how breast cancer has given rise to numerous medical malpractice lawsuits. Discusses trial techniques and strategies for litigating these types of claims. Quotes Opinions 5.05 and 5.06. Hillerich, Ellerin, & Frieder, *Selecting and Presenting a Failure to Diagnose Breast Cancer Case*, 20 Am. J. Trial Advoc. 253, 271 (1996-97).

Journal 1991 Discusses the case of *Crist v. Moffat*, which prohibits ex parte communications with a plaintiff's treating physician in North Carolina. Examines the physician-patient privilege and looks at various jurisdictions that permit and forbid ex parte communications. Quotes Principle IV and Opinion 5.06. Comment, *Shielding the Plaintiff and Physician: The Prohibition of Ex Parte Contacts With a Plaintiff's Treating Physician*, 13 Campbell L. Rev. 233, 243, 248 (1991).

Journal 1984 Observes that available ethical and legal guidelines are insufficient to aid physicians in addressing issues of patient privacy and confidentiality. Concludes that there is need for legislation in order to provide suitable guidance to physicians who fulfill an important role in protecting patient privacy. Cites 1982 Opinions 5.03 [now Opinion 5.04], 5.04, 5.05 [now Opinion 5.06], 5.06 [now Opinion 5.07], 5.07 [now Opinion 5.08], and 5.08 [now Opinion 5.09]. Gellman, *Prescribing Privacy: The Uncertain Role of the Physician in the Protection of Patient Privacy*, 62 No. Carolina L. Rev. 255, 271 (1984).

5.07 Confidentiality: Computers

The utmost effort and care must be taken to protect the confidentiality of all medical records, including computerized medical records.

The guidelines below are offered to assist physicians and computer service organizations in maintaining the confidentiality of information in medical records when that information is stored in computerized data bases:

(1) Confidential medical information should be entered into the computer-based patient record only by authorized personnel. Additions to the record should be time and date stamped, and the person making the additions should be identified in the record.

(2) The patient and physician should be advised about the existence of computerized data bases in which medical information concerning the patient is stored. Such information should be communicated to the physician and patient prior to the physician's release of the medical information to the entity or entities maintaining the computer data bases. All individuals and organizations with some form of access to the computerized data bases, and the level of access permitted, should be specifically identified in advance. Full disclosure of this information to the patient is necessary in obtaining informed consent to treatment. Patient data should be assigned a security level appropriate for the data's degree of sensitivity, which should be used to control who has access to the information.

(3) The physician and patient should be notified of the distribution of all reports reflecting identifiable patient data prior to distribution of the reports by the computer facility. There should be approval by the patient and notification of the physician prior to the release of patient-identifiable clinical and administrative data to individuals or organizations external to the medical care environment. Such information should not be released without the express permission of the patient.

(4) The dissemination of confidential medical data should be limited to only those individuals or agencies with a bona fide use for the data. Only the data necessary for the bona fide use should be released. Patient identifiers should be omitted when appropriate. Release of confidential medical information from the data base should be confined to the specific purpose for which the information is requested and limited to the specific time frame requested. All such organizations or individuals should be advised that authorized release of data to them does not authorize their further release of the data to additional individuals or organizations, or subsequent use of the data for other purposes.

(5) Procedures for adding to or changing data on the computerized data base should indicate individuals authorized to make changes, time periods in which changes take place, and those individuals who will be informed about changes in the data from the medical records.

(6) Procedures for purging the computerized data base of archaic or inaccurate data should be established and the patient and physician should be notified before and after the data has been purged. There should be no mixing of a physician's computerized patient records with those of other computer service bureau clients. In addition, procedures should be developed to pro-

tect against inadvertent mixing of individual reports or segments thereof.

(7) The computerized medical data base should be online to the computer terminal only when authorized computer programs requiring the medical data are being used. Individuals and organizations external to the clinical facility should not be provided online access to a computerized data base containing identifiable data from medical records concerning patients. Access to the computerized data base should be controlled through security measures such as passwords, encryption (encoding) of information, and scannable badges or other user identification.

(8) Back-up systems and other mechanisms should be in place to prevent data loss and downtime as a result of hardware or software failure.

(9) Security:

(a) Stringent security procedures should be in place to prevent unauthorized access to computer-based patient records. Personnel audit procedures should be developed to establish a record in the event of unauthorized disclosure of medical data. Terminated or former employees in the data processing environment should have no access to data from the medical records concerning patients.

(b) Upon termination of computer services for a physician, those computer files maintained for the physician should be physically turned over to the physician. They may be destroyed (erased) only if it is established that the physician has another copy (in some form). In the event of file erasure, the computer service bureau should verify in writing to the physician that the erasure has taken place. (IV)

Issued prior to April 1977.

Updated June 1994 and June 1998.

M.D. Pa. 1987 Plaintiff in a medical malpractice action sought to preclude his treating physicians from serving as defendant's expert witnesses at trial. The court held that defense counsel's failure to provide prior notice of ex parte communication with plaintiff's treating physicians barred their use as defense experts. Referring to *Petrillo v. Syntex Laboratories, Inc.*, 148 Ill. App. 3d 581, 499 N.E.2d 952 (1986), the court noted that the court there favorably cited Principle IV and Opinions 5.05, 5.06, and 5.07 (1984) in support of a public policy protecting confidentiality between physician and patient and against ex parte discussion. *Manion v. N.P.W. Medical Center of N.E. Pa., Inc.*, 676 F.Supp. 585, 591.

Ill. App. 1986 Defense attorney in product liability suit was held in contempt of court for conducting ex parte discussions with plaintiff-patient's treating physician without patient's consent and contrary to authorized methods of discovery. The court held that the strong public policy favoring physician-patient confidentiality articulated in Principles II and IV and Opinions 5.05, 5.06, 5.07, and 5.08 (1984) justified a rule against such ex parte discussions. Further, the court held that the public has the right to rely on physicians to faithfully execute their ethical obligations. *Petrillo v. Syntex Laboratories, Inc.*, 148 Ill. App. 3d 581, 499 N.E.2d 952, 957, 958, 959, cert. denied 483 US 1007 (1987).

Pa. Super. 1988 Plaintiff-patient sued her physician for breach of confidentiality when physician conferred with defense counsel in plaintiff's malpractice suit against the hospital (physician's employer). In its majority opinion, the court cited Principle IV, commenting that it gave very little guidance to physicians but nonetheless was not violated by the physician. The court also noted Opinion 5.07 (1986) finding that the plaintiff's suit minimized her expectations of confidentiality. The dissent, however, interpreted these same provisions, along with Opinion 5.05 (1986), as protecting plaintiff's expectations of confidentiality. *Moses v. McWilliams, 379 Pa. Super. 150, 549 A.2d 950, 956, 962 (dissent) appeal denied 521 Pa. 630, 558 A.2d 532 (1989).*

Journal 2003 Highlights HIPAA privacy issues that need to be monitored and have yet to be resolved. Concludes that HIPAA poses many challenges and it remains unclear whether HIPAA will increase privacy protection. Cites Opinions 5.05, 5.055, 5.057, 5.06, 5.07, 5.075, 5.08, and 5.09. Kutzko, Boyer, Thoman, & Scott, *HIPAA in Real Time: Practical Implications of the Federal Privacy Rule*, 51 Drake L. Rev. 403, 408 (2003).

Journal 2000 Defines and explores current and future applications of telemedicine. Considers issues of cost, quality, access, and regulation. Concludes that telemedicine holds tremendous promise for improving the United States health care system. Quotes Opinions 5.05 and 5.07. Volkert, *Telemedicine: RX for the Future of Health Care*, 6 Mich. Telecomm. & Tech. L. Rev. 147, 214, 225 (2000).

Journal 1999 Explores the increased use of physician-patient communication through e-mail. Analyzes current laws regarding medical privacy. Suggests that patients' communications to their physicians are part of their medical record and should be given the same protections. Quotes Opinions 5.05 and 5.07. Cites Opinions 5.04 and 5.06. Spielberg, *Online Without a Net: Physician-Patient Communication by Electronic Mail*, 25 Am. J. Law & Med. 267, 284-85 (1999).

Journal 1999 Explores Model Rules of Professional Conduct focusing on the attorney-client relationship. Compares confidentiality provisions in the Model Rules with the rules of confidentiality governing the medical profession. Observes that existing confidentiality rules are incomplete and ambiguous. Concludes that one remedy is to embrace a discretionary confidentiality rule. Quotes Opinion 5.05. Cites Principle IV and Opinion 5.07. Zer-Gutman, *Revising the Ethical Rules of Attorney-Client Confidentiality: Towards a New Discretionary Rule*, 45 Loy. L. Rev. 669, 683-84, 699, 709, 718 (1999).

Journal 1998 Describes the special nature of confidentiality in the relationship between the psychotherapist and patient. States that not many breach of confidentiality cases involve psychotherapists. Concludes that patients and psychotherapists must better understand their rights and responsibilities in this context. Quotes Opinion 5.05. Cites Opinions 5.06, 5.07, 5.08, and 5.09. Grabois, *The Liability of Psychotherapists for Breach of Confidentiality*, 12 J. Law & Health 39, 53-54 (1998).

Journal 1998 Explains risks involved with the use of electronic medical records. States that patients need to be aware of who has access to their medical records. Concludes that health care providers should equalize the risks and benefits related to the use of electronic medical records. Cites Opinion 5.05. References Opinion 5.07. Jurevic, *When Technology and Health Care Collide: Issues with Electronic Medical Records and Electronic Mail*, 66 UMKC L. Rev. 809, 819-20 (1998).

Journal 1998 Examines the use of e-mail in the physician-patient relationship. Focuses on privacy concerns stemming from the use of e-mail in the medical context. Suggests that physicians should discuss the implications of communicating through e-mail with their patients and should obtain informed consent prior to communicating in this manner. Cites Opinions 5.04, 5.05, 5.057, 5.07, 5.075, and 5.08. Spielberg, *On Call and Online: Sociohistorical, Legal, and Ethical Implications of E-mail for the Patient-Physician Relationship*, 280 JAMA 1353, 1356 (1998).

Journal 1998 Examines the transition from paper medical records to electronic medical records. Identifies issues of confidentiality and privacy that arise as a result of the move to electronic medical records. Concludes that federal protection is needed to safeguard personal medical information. Quotes Principle IV and Opinions 5.07 and 5.075. Cites Opinion 8.061. Tsai, *Cheaper and Better: The Congressional Administrative Simplification Mandate Facilitates the Transition to Electronic Medical Records*, 19 J. Legal Med. 549, 570, 581 (1998).

Journal 1997 Discusses the practice of ex parte communications between treating physicians and their patients' legal adversaries without informing the patient or obtaining consent. Examines harms that may occur in these situations. Argues that Oklahoma needs to prohibit treating physicians from communicating ex parte with their patients' legal adversaries. Quotes Opinions 5.05, 5.07, 5.08, 8.02, 8.03, and 9.07. Cites Opinion 7.02. McNaughton & McNaughton, *Divided Loyalty: The Dilemma of the Treating Physician Advocate*, 22 Okla. City U. L. Rev. 1051, 1052, 1054, 1056, 1058, 1059, 1062 (1997).

Journal 1997 Examines the benefits of unconstrained access to personal medical information. Discusses drawbacks to full disclosure and absolute confidentiality of medical information. Advocates increased awareness of how medical data are used. Proposes guidelines for the best approach to regulation of health care data. Cites Opinion 5.07. Schwartz, *Privacy and the Economics of Personal Health Care Information*, 76 Tex. L. Rev. 1, 59 (1997).

Journal 1997 Considers new data-collection technology enabling collection, storage, and dissemination of data, including medical records information. Discusses the confidentiality problems triggered by increased utilization of computers in health care delivery. Quotes Opinion 5.07. Woodward, *Medical Record Confidentiality and Data Collection: Current Dilemmas, 25 J. Law, Med. & Ethics 88, 90, 95 (1997).*

Journal 1995 Examines federal legislative proposals intended to protect confidentiality of computerized medical records. Concludes that proposed legislation will significantly undermine confidentiality. Cites Opinion 5.07. References Principle IV. Hoge, *Proposed Federal Legislation Jeopardizes Patient Privacy, 23 Bull. Am. Acad. Psychiatry Law 495, 498, 500 (1995).*

Journal 1993 Discusses the issues surrounding the confidentiality of electronic and computerized medical records. Concludes that any legal standard addressing this problem should balance the need to protect patient confidentiality with the practical constraints limiting ideal security. References Principle IV and Opinion 5.07. Waller & Fulton, *The Electronic Chart; Keeping it Confidential and Secure, 26 J. Health & Hosp. L. 104, 105 (April 1993).*

Journal 1984 Observes that available ethical and legal guidelines are insufficient to aid physicians in addressing issues of patient privacy and confidentiality. Concludes that there is need for legislation in order to provide suitable guidance to physicians who fulfill an important role in protecting patient privacy. Cites 1982 Opinions 5.03 [now Opinion 5.04], 5.04, 5.05 [now Opinion 5.06], 5.06 [now Opinion 5.07], 5.07 [now Opinion 5.08], and 5.08 [now Opinion 5.09]. Gellman, *Prescribing Privacy: The Uncertain Role of the Physician in the Protection of Patient Privacy, 62 No. Carolina L. Rev. 255, 271 (1984).*

5.075   Confidentiality: Disclosure of Records to Data Collection Companies

Data collection from computerized or other patient records for marketing purposes raises serious ethical concerns. In some cases, firms have sought to amass information on physicians' prescribing practices on behalf of pharmaceutical houses for marketing purposes. Often, physicians are offered incentives such as computer hardware and software packages in return for agreeing to such an arrangement. They may be told that data-collecting software does not capture patients' names.

These arrangements may violate principles of informed consent and patient confidentiality. Patients divulge information to their physicians only for purposes of diagnosis and treatment. If other uses are to be made of the information, patients must give their permission after being fully informed about the purpose of such disclosures. If permission is not obtained, physicians violate patient confidentiality by sharing specific and intimate information from patients' records with commercial interests.

Arrangements of this kind may also violate Opinion 8.061, "Gifts to Physicians From Industry."

Finally, these arrangements may harm the integrity of the patient-physician relationship. The trust that is fundamental to this relationship is based on the principle that the physicians are the agents first and foremost of their patients. (I, II, IV)

Issued June 1994.

Updated June 1998.

Journal 2003 Highlights HIPAA privacy issues that need to be monitored and have yet to be resolved. Concludes that HIPAA poses many challenges and it remains unclear whether HIPAA will increase privacy protection. Cites Opinions 5.05, 5.055, 5.057, 5.06, 5.07, 5.075, 5.08, and 5.09. Kutzko, Boyer, Thoman, & Scott, *HIPAA in Real Time: Practical Implications of the Federal Privacy Rule, 51 Drake L. Rev. 403, 408 (2003).*

Journal 1998 Examines the use of e-mail in the physician-patient relationship. Focuses on privacy concerns stemming from the use of e-mail in the medical context. Suggests that physicians should discuss the implications of communicating through e-mail with their patients and should obtain informed consent prior to communicating in this manner. Cites Opinions 5.04, 5.05, 5.057, 5.07, 5.075, and 5.08. Spielberg, *On Call and Online: Sociohistorical, Legal, and Ethical Implications of E-mail for the Patient-Physician Relationship*, 280 JAMA 1353, 1356 (1998).

Journal 1998 Examines the transition from paper medical records to electronic medical records. Identifies issues of confidentiality and privacy that arise as a result of the move to electronic medical records. Concludes that federal protection is needed to safeguard personal medical information. Quotes Principle IV and Opinions 5.07 and 5.075. Cites Opinion 8.061. Tsai, *Cheaper and Better: The Congressional Administrative Simplification Mandate Facilitates the Transition to Electronic Medical Records*, 19 J. Legal Med. 549, 570, 581 (1998).

5.08 Confidentiality: Insurance Company Representative

History, diagnosis, prognosis, and the like acquired during the physician-patient relationship may be disclosed to an insurance company representative only if the patient or a lawful representative has consented to the disclosure. A physician's responsibilities to patients are not limited to the actual practice of medicine. They also include the performance of some services ancillary to the practice of medicine. These services might include certification that the patient was under the physician's care and comment on the diagnosis and therapy in the particular case. See also Opinion 2.135, "Insurance Companies and Genetic Information." (IV)

Issued prior to April 1977.

N.D. Ohio 1965 Plaintiff-patient alleged that the defendant-malpractice insurer induced physician to reveal confidential information about plaintiff on pretext that plaintiff filed a malpractice suit. In denying defendant's motion for reconsideration of the court's earlier opinion, the court confirmed its holding that actions of a third party inducing a physician to divulge confidential information may result in liability to the patient. In so holding, the court quoted (with incorrect citation to Ch. II, Sec.1) Principles Ch. I, Sec.2 (1912), [now Principle IV and Opinion 5.08], to emphasize the medical profession's established views regarding confidentiality. *Hammonds v. Aetna Casualty & Sur. Co.*, 243 F. Supp. 793, 803.

Fla. App. 1995 The court considered the issue of the effect of § 455.241(2) of the Florida Statutes on right of defense in a medical malpractice action to engage in ex parte communications with plaintiff's non-party treating physician. The court held that a 1988 amendment to § 455.241(2) negated the applicability of the statute to medical malpractice cases. The dissent, citing *Petrillo v. Syntex Laboratories, Inc.*, 148 Ill. App. 3d 581, 499 N.E.2d 952 (1986), quoted Principles II and IV and Opinions 5.05, 5.06, and 5.08 as strong public policy support for its position that ex parte communications should be barred altogether. *Castillo-Plaza v. Green*, 655 So. 2d 197, 206 n.4.

Ill. App. 1986 Defense attorney in product liability suit was held in contempt of court for conducting ex parte discussions with plaintiff-patient's treating physician without patient's consent and contrary to authorized methods of discovery. The court held that the strong public policy favoring physician-patient confidentiality articulated in Principles II and IV and Opinions 5.05, 5.06, 5.07, and 5.08 (1984) justified a rule against such ex parte discussions. Further, the court held that the public has the right to rely on physicians to faithfully execute their ethical obligations. *Petrillo v. Syntex Laboratories, Inc.*, 148 Ill. App. 3d 581, 499 N.E.2d 952, 957, 958, 959, cert. denied, 483 US 1007 (1987).

Journal 2003 Highlights HIPAA privacy issues that need to be monitored and have yet to be resolved. Concludes that HIPAA poses many challenges and it remains unclear whether HIPAA will increase privacy protection. Cites Opinions 5.05, 5.055, 5.057, 5.06, 5.07, 5.075, 5.08, and 5.09. Kutzko, Boyer, Thoman, & Scott, *HIPAA in Real Time: Practical Implications of the Federal Privacy Rule*, 51 Drake L. Rev. 403, 408 (2003).

Journal 2001 Discusses same-sex marriages in the transgender community. Explores Defense of Marriage Act statutes. Considers whether same-sex transgender marriages can prevail against attacks brought under such statutes. Cites Opinions 2.132, 2.135, 2.137, 5.08, and 5.09. Frye & Meiselman, *Same-Sex Marriages Have Existed Legally in the United States for a Long Time Now*, 64 *Alb. L. Rev.* 1031, 1053 (2001).

Journal 2000 Evaluates transgender legal and political activity in the United States. Discusses the International Bill of Gender Rights against the background of the Texas case, *Littleton v. Prange.* Cites Opinions 2.132, 2.135, 2.137, 5.08, and 5.09. Frye, *The International Bill of Gender Rights vs. the Cider House Rules: Transgenders Struggle with the Courts Over What Clothing They Are Allowed to Wear on the Job, Which Restroom They are Allowed to Use on the Job, Their Right to Marry, and the Very Definition of Their Sex*, 7 *Wm. & Mary J. Women & L.* 133, 149 (2000).

Journal 1998 Describes the special nature of confidentiality in the relationship between the psychotherapist and patient. States that not many breach of confidentiality cases involve psychotherapists. Concludes that patients and psychotherapists must better understand their rights and responsibilities in this context. Quotes Opinion 5.05. Cites Opinions 5.06, 5.07, 5.08, and 5.09. Grabois, *The Liability of Psychotherapists for Breach of Confidentiality*, 12 *J. Law & Health* 39, 53-54 (1998).

Journal 1998 Examines the use of e-mail in the physician-patient relationship. Focuses on privacy concerns stemming from the use of e-mail in the medical context. Suggests that physicians should discuss the implications of communicating through e-mail with their patients and should obtain informed consent prior to communicating in this manner. Cites Opinions 5.04, 5.05, 5.057, 5.07, 5.075, and 5.08. Spielberg, *On Call and Online: Sociohistorical, Legal, and Ethical Implications of E-mail for the Patient-Physician Relationship*, 280 *JAMA* 1353, 1356 (1998).

Journal 1997 Discusses the practice of ex parte communications between treating physicians and their patients' legal adversaries without informing the patient or obtaining consent. Examines harms that may occur in these situations. Argues that Oklahoma needs to prohibit treating physicians from communicating ex parte with their patients' legal adversaries. Quotes Opinions 5.05, 5.07, 5.08, 8.02, 8.03, and 9.07. Cites Opinion 7.02. McNaughton & McNaughton, *Divided Loyalty: The Dilemma of the Treating Physician Advocate*, 22 *Okla. City U. L. Rev.* 1051, 1052, 1054, 1056, 1058, 1059, 1062 (1997).

Journal 1984 Observes that available ethical and legal guidelines are insufficient to aid physicians in addressing issues of patient privacy and confidentiality. Concludes that there is need for legislation in order to provide suitable guidance to physicians who fulfill an important role in protecting patient privacy. Cites 1982 Opinions 5.03 [now Opinion 5.04], 5.04, 5.05 [now Opinion 5.06], 5.06 [now Opinion 5.07], 5.07 [now Opinion 5.08], and 5.08 [now Opinion 5.09]. Gellman, *Prescribing Privacy: The Uncertain Role of the Physician in the Protection of Patient Privacy*, 62 *No. Carolina L. Rev.* 255, 271 (1984).

5.09   The previous Opinion 5.09, "Confidentiality: Physicians in Industry," issued July 1983, was deleted in June 2000 and combined with Opinion 5.09, "Confidentiality: Industry-Employed Physicians and Dependent Medical Examiners."

5.09   Confidentiality: Industry-Employed Physicians and Independent Medical Examiners

Where a physician's services are limited to performing an isolated assessment of an individual's health or disability for an employer, business, or insurer, the information obtained by the physician as a result of such examinations is confidential and should not be communicated to a third party without the individual's prior written consent, unless required by law. If the individual authorized the release of medical information to an employer or a potential employer, the physician should release only that information which is reasonably relevant to the employer's decision regarding that individual's ability to perform the work required by the job.

When a physician renders treatment to an employee with a work-related illness or injury, the release of medical information to the employer as to the treatment provided may be subject to the provisions of worker's compensation laws. The physician must comply with the requirements of such laws, if applicable. However, the physician may not otherwise discuss the employee's health condition with the employer without the employee's consent or, in the event of the employee's incapacity, the appropriate proxy's consent.

Whenever statistical information about employees' health is released, all employee identities should be deleted. (IV)

Issued July 1983.

Updated June 1994; updated June 1996; updated December 1999 based on the report "Patient-Physician Relationship in the Context of Work-Related and Independent Medical Examinations," adopted June 1999.

Mass. 1984 Employee sued employer for libel and invasion of privacy following disclosure of medical facts about employee to other employees. In part, claim involved disclosure of opinion about employee's mental state to his supervisor by physician retained by employer. Citing Principle 9 (1957) [now Principle IV and Opinions 5.05 and 5.09], the court held that a physician retained by an employer may disclose to the employer information concerning an employee if receipt of the information is reasonably necessary to serve a substantial and valid business interest of the employer. *Bratt v. International Business Mach. Corp.*, 392 Mass. 508, 467 N.E.2d 126, 137 n.23.

N.Y. Sup. 2000 Physician brought wrongful discharge claim against corporate employer. The physician alleged she was discharged because she refused to reveal confidential medical information regarding employees. With apparent reference to Principle IV and Opinions 5.05 and 5.09, the affidavit filed by the physician claimed she had an ethical and legal duty to protect patient confidentiality. The court found termination of an employee at will based upon such grounds is sufficient to state a cause of action for breach of contract. The court ruled that obligations of good faith and fair dealing may be implied in a contract for the employment of a physician and that no physician should be placed in the position of choosing between retaining employment or violating ethical standards. *Horn v. New York Times*, 186 Misc. 2d 469, 719 N.Y.S. 2d 471, 474.

Journal 2003 Highlights HIPAA privacy issues that need to be monitored and have yet to be resolved. Concludes that HIPAA poses many challenges and it remains unclear whether HIPAA will increase privacy protection. Cites Opinions 5.05, 5.055, 5.057, 5.06, 5.07, 5.075, 5.08, and 5.09. Kutzko, Boyer, Thoman, & Scott, *HIPAA in Real Time: Practical Implications of the Federal Privacy Rule*, 51 Drake L. Rev. 403, 408 (2003).

Journal 2001 Discusses same-sex marriages in the transgender community. Explores Defense of Marriage Act statutes. Considers whether same-sex transgender marriages can prevail against attacks brought under such statutes. Cites Opinions 2.132, 2.135, 2.137, 5.08, and 5.09. Frye & Meiselman, *Same-Sex Marriages Have Existed Legally in the United States for a Long Time Now*, 64 Alb. L. Rev. 1031, 1053 (2001).

Journal 2000 Evaluates transgender legal and political activity in the United States. Discusses the International Bill of Gender Rights against the background of the Texas case, *Littleton v. Prange*. Cites Opinions 2.132, 2.135, 2.137, 5.08, and 5.09. Frye, *The International Bill of Gender Rights vs. the Cider House Rules: Transgenders Struggle with the Courts Over What Clothing They Are Allowed to Wear on the Job, Which Restroom They are Allowed to Use on the Job, Their Right to Marry, and the Very Definition of Their Sex*, 7 Wm. & Mary J. Women & L. 133, 149 (2000).

Journal 1999 Discusses the need for physicians to advocate on behalf of patients' rights in the context of health care delivery. Evaluates the nature and scope of the physician's role as advocate, noting that physicians cannot be expected to engage in attorney-like advocacy. Quotes Principles IV and VI, Fundamental Elements (2), (4), and (6) [now Opinion 10.01], Patient Responsibilities 5 [now Opinion 10.02], and Opinions 2.03, 2.07, 2.09, 2.16, 2.19, 3.06, 4.01, 4.04, 6.01, 7.02, 8.02, 8.03, 8.13, 8.132, 9.06, 9.07, and 9.131. Cites Opinions 5.05, 5.09, 7.01, 8.135, and 9.02. Sage, *Physicians as Advocates*, 35 Hous. L. Rev. 1529, 1537, 1541, 1542, 1552-53, 1554, 1556, 1557, 1559, 1561-62, 1564, 1571, 1574, 1576, 1580 (1999).

Journal 1998 Analyzes the decision in *Spaulding v. Zimmerman*. Discusses the issue of an attorney's obligation to disclose information to protect a third-party's health or safety. Includes in this discussion consideration of the duty of an "examining" physician to disclose such information to an examinee. Cites Opinion 5.09. Cramton & Knowles, *Professional Secrecy and its Exceptions: Spaulding v. Zimmerman Revisited*, 83 Minn. L. Rev. 63, 98 (1998).

Journal 1998 Describes the special nature of confidentiality in the relationship between the psychotherapist and patient. States that not many breach of confidentiality cases involve psychotherapists. Concludes that patients and psychotherapists must better understand their rights and responsibilities in this context. Quotes Opinion 5.05. Cites Opinions 5.06, 5.07, 5.08, and 5.09. Grabois, *The Liability of Psychotherapists for Breach of Confidentiality*, 12 J. Law & Health 39, 53-54 (1998).

Journal 1991 Explores ethical problems unique to the field of forensic psychiatry. Presents the results of a survey of members of the American Academy of Psychiatry and the Law (AAPL), asking their opinions regarding proposed ethical guidelines. Quotes Opinions 1.02 and 5.09. Weinstock, Leong, & Silva, *Opinions by AAPL Forensic Psychiatrists on Controversial Ethical Guidelines: A Survey*, 19 Bull. Am. Acad. Psychiatry Law 237, 238 (1991).

Journal 1984 Observes that available ethical and legal guidelines are insufficient to aid physicians in addressing issues of patient privacy and confidentiality. Concludes that there is need for legislation in order to provide suitable guidance to physicians who fulfill an important role in protecting patient privacy. Cites 1982 Opinions 5.03 [now Opinion 5.04], 5.04, 5.05 [now Opinion 5.06], 5.06 [now Opinion 5.07], 5.07 [now Opinion 5.08], and 5.08 [now Opinion 5.09]. Gellman, *Prescribing Privacy: The Uncertain Role of the Physician in the Protection of Patient Privacy*, 62 No. Carolina L. Rev. 255, 271 (1984).

6.00 Opinions on Fees and Charges

6.01 Contingent Physician Fees

If a physician's fee for medical service is contingent on the successful outcome of a claim, such as a malpractice or worker's compensation claim, there is the ever-present danger that the physician may become less of a healer and more of an advocate or partisan in the proceedings. Accordingly, a physician's fee for medical services should be based on the value of the service provided by the physician to the patient and not on the uncertain outcome of a contingency that does not in any way relate to the value of the medical service.

A physician's fee should not be made contingent on the successful outcome of medical treatment. Such arrangements are unethical because they imply that successful outcomes from treatment are guaranteed, thus creating unrealistic expectations of medicine and false promises to consumers. (VI)

Issued prior to April 1977.

Updated June 1994.

Cal. App. 1992 Lower court held that a contingent fee agreement between plaintiff and a medical-legal consulting service violated public policy and was void. In reversing, appellate court referred to *Polo v. Gotchel* 225 N.J. Super. 492, 542 A.2d 947 (1987) and *Dupree v. Malpractice Research, Inc.*, 179 Mich. App. 254, 445 N.W.2d 498 (1989) which had relied on Opinion 8.04 (1984) [now Opinion 6.01] to hold that contingent fee consulting contracts were per se invalid. The court was unpersuaded by the reasoning of these decisions, stating that (1) the contingent fee agreement was with a company, not with a physician, and (2) the term "medical services" in the Opinion refers to patient treatment and not to consulting services provided in conjunction with the services of an attorney. *Ojeda v. Sharp Cabrillo Hosp.*, 8 Cal. App. 4th 1, 12, 13 n.11, 14, 10 Cal. Rptr. 2d 230, 237 n.11, 238.

Mich. App. 1989 Plaintiffs, who settled an underlying medical malpractice suit, sought to invalidate contingent fee contract with expert witness service. Plaintiffs had paid witness and report fees, travel costs, and other expenses in advance according to a fee schedule but objected to a charge of 20 percent of their recovery. The court, citing Opinion 8.04 (1984) [now Opinion 6.01], held that the contingent fee contract for expert witnesses was repugnant to the public policy of preserving the plaintiff's recovery and preventing the exaggeration of favorable testimony and would not be enforced. Further, the court refused to consider defendant's quantum meruit claim, since some fees had been paid in advance, and any further attempt to collect fees would fail to deter such contracts. *Dupree v. Malpractice Research, Inc.*, 179 Mich. App. 254, 445 N.W.2d 498, 501.

N.J. Super. 1987 Contingent fee agreement between plaintiff's attorney in a medical malpractice action and a medical-legal consulting service which linked plaintiff with potential expert witnesses violated public policy and was void. The court cited with approval Opinion 8.04 (1984) [now Opinion 6.01], which states that a physician's fees should not be based upon the outcome of litigation because of the risk that the physician may become more of an advocate than a healer. *Polo v. Gotchel*, 225 N.J. Super. 429, 542 A.2d 947, 948.

Tenn. 1998 Physician sued patient and patient's attorney for breach of contract after the patient settled a personal injury claim. Physician claimed that under contract, he was entitled to receive a contingency fee for services as the medical expert in the patient's case and contingency fees for medical services rendered. Alternatively, the physician claimed that he could recover under the theory of quantum meruit. The court held that the contingency fee both for the physician acting as a medical expert and for medical services violated public policy. The court quoted Opinions 6.01 and 9.07, stating that the Tennessee Board of Medical Examiners, that governs state medical licenses, had adopted the AMA's stance on contingency fees. The court also rejected the physician's argument that he should be allowed to recover under the theory of quantum meruit because the underlying contracts were void as against public policy. *Swafford v. Harris*, 967 S.W.2d 319, 321-323.

Journal 2001 Considers result-based compensation arrangements for medical services. Focuses on a 1994 AMA amendment to Opinion 6.01 that prohibits payment of physicians contingent upon outcome. Concludes that such arrangements may be appropriate in some circumstances. Quotes Opinion 6.01. Hyman & Silver, *Just What the Patient Ordered: The Case for Result-Based Compensation Arrangements*, 29 J. L. Med. & Ethics 170, 170 (2001).

Journal 2001 Explains the design and potential benefits of result-based compensation arrangements for health care. Concludes that a more reliable and efficient health care delivery system is fostered by such arrangements. Quotes Opinion 6.01. References Opinions 9.121 and 9.122. Hyman & Silver, *You Get What You Pay For: Result-Based Compensation for Health Care*, 58 Wash. & Lee L. Rev. 1427, 1459, 1460, 1461, 1481-82 (2001).

Journal 2000 Considers the rules governing expert testimony. Explores professional ethical standards affecting expert witnesses and concludes that codes of ethics have not succeeded in eliminating biased expert testimony. Recommends creation of an organization to assist courts in obtaining reliable expert witness testimony. Quotes Principle III and Opinion 6.01. Cites Principles I, II, and V and Opinions 1.02 and 9.07. Murphy, *Expert Witnesses at Trial: Where are the Ethics?* 14 Geo. J. Legal Ethics 217, 231-32 (2000).

Journal 1999 Discusses the need for physicians to advocate on behalf of patients' rights in the context of health care delivery. Evaluates the nature and scope of the physician's role as advocate, noting that physicians cannot be expected to engage in attorney-like advocacy. Quotes Principles IV and VI, Fundamental Elements (2), (4), and (6) [now Opinion 10.01], Patient Responsibilities 5 [now Opinion 10.02], and Opinions 2.03, 2.07, 2.09, 2.16, 2.19, 3.06, 4.01, 4.04, 6.01, 7.02, 8.02, 8.03, 8.13, 8.132, 9.06, 9.07, and 9.131. Cites Opinions 5.05, 5.09, 7.01, 8.135, and 9.02. Sage, *Physicians as Advocates*, 35 Hous. L. Rev. 1529, 1537, 1541, 1542, 1552-53, 1554, 1556, 1557, 1559, 1561-62, 1564, 1571, 1574, 1576, 1580 (1999).

Journal 1998 Examines mechanisms of oversight for expert witness testimony by medical, legal, legislative, and regulatory agencies. Points out that the amount of malpractice litigation will increase the need for medical expert witnesses. Concludes that improvements in this context must uphold principles of due process and be acceptable to the medical and legal communities. Cites Opinions 6.01, 8.04, and 9.07. McAbee, *Improper Expert Medical Testimony: Existing and Proposed Mechanisms of Oversight*, 19 J. Legal Med. 257, 265 (1998).

Journal 1991 Looks at the problem of high expert witness fees and lack of access to expert testimony by those who may need it. Proposes revamping the current system to allow certain types of contingent fee arrangements. Quotes Opinion 8.04 (1984) [now Opinion 6.01]. Note, *Contingent Expert Witness Fees: Access and Legitimacy*, 64 So. Cal. L. Rev. 1363, 1374, 1382 (1991).

Journal 1990 Examines conflicting court decisions that have addressed the appropriateness of medical-legal consulting services and their use of contingent fee arrangements. Concludes by discussing the need for a less troublesome solution to the problems plaintiffs face in malpractice and personal injury cases. Quotes Opinion 6.01. Cites Opinions 6.12 (1989) [now Opinion 6.05] and 9.07. Dillon, *Contingent Fees and Medical-Legal Consulting Services: Economical or Unethical?*, 11 J. Legal Med. 93, 101, 111 (1990).

6.02   Fee Splitting

Payment by or to a physician solely for the referral of a patient is fee splitting and is unethical.

A physician may not accept payment of any kind, in any form, from any source, such as a pharmaceutical company or pharmacist, an optical company, or the manufacturer of medical appliances and devices, for prescribing or referring a patient to said source.

In each case, the payment violates the requirement to deal honestly with patients and colleagues. The patient relies upon the advice of the physician on matters of referral. All referrals and prescriptions must be based on the skill and quality of the physician to whom the patient has been referred or the quality and efficacy of the drug or product prescribed. (II)

Issued prior to April 1977.

Updated June 1994.

Kan. App. 1985 Members of a medical partnership sought an injunction to enforce a covenant not to compete against defendant-physician, a former partner. Defendant asserted that the covenant was void as against public policy relying on Opinion 9.02 (1984). The court however ruled that the covenant was reasonable as defined by precedent and that it was bound to follow this precedent as opposed to the American Medical Association's position regarding such covenants. Defendant further argued enforcement of the covenant was precluded because the partnership had violated ethical norms, apparently referring to Opinions 6.03 and 6.04 (1984) [now Opinions 6.02 and 6.03] which were part of partnership contract. The court held that defendant was estopped from complaining about the partnership's actions due to his own conduct. *Axtell Clinic v. Cranston, No. 56,745 (Kan. Ct. App. June 20, 1985) (LEXIS, States Library, Kan. file).*

Mass. 1955 Plaintiff-physician was charged under state licensing statute by defendant-board with conspiracy and fee-splitting. Both parties sought a declaratory judgment as to whether the defendant-board had jurisdiction to determine plaintiff's guilt or innocence. In holding that the board was qualified to determine if plaintiff's actions constituted gross misconduct under the statute, the court referred to Principles Ch. I, Secs. 1 and 6 (1947) [now Principle II and Opinion 6.02] delineating, in part, limitations on payment for medical services. These provisions, the court said, reflected the medical profession's understanding of its peculiar obligations. *Forziati v. Board of Registration in Medicine, 333 Mass. 125, 128 N.E.2d 789, 791.*

Mass. Super. 1998 Plaintiff surgeon filed suit against a medical group practice claiming that the defendants reduced referrals to him because he declined to join the group. Plaintiff claimed that the decline harmed his surgical practice. He alleged that the group's practice of taking 10 percent of members' income constituted unethical and illegal kickbacks. The court held that the decline in referrals was not connected to plaintiff not being a member of the group. The court also found that the plaintiff had not presented evidence that the decline in referrals harmed his practice. Finally, the court found that the fees paid by members of the group practice were gatekeeper fees rather than referral fees. The court quoted Opinion 6.02, in support of its decision that the defendants' fees did not constitute fee splitting. Further, the court referenced Opinion 8.032 concluding that a self-referral was not necessarily unethical if disclosed to the patient. *Boman v. Southeast Medical Services Group, 1998 WL 1182063, 11-12.*

Journal 2002 Suggests a reconceptualization for bioethics that integrates an analysis of the history of moral change. Concludes that bioethical textbooks should include discussion about the history of bioethics and medical ethics. Quotes Opinion 2.20. References Opinions 6.02, 6.03, 6.04 [now Opinion 8.06], and 8.032. Baker, *Bioethics and History, 27 J. Med. & Phil. 447, 455, 469 (2002).*

Journal 2001 Evaluates current forms of cybermedicine and Internet resources that support it. Explores patient and regulatory concerns, including privacy issues, insurance reimbursement problems, licensure, and liability, which may thwart the growth of cybermedicine. Concludes that cybermedicine may facilitate delivery of cost-effective, quality medical care. Quotes Opinions 5.05, 6.02, and 6.03. Scott, *Cybermedicine and Virtual Pharmacies, 103 W. Va. L. Rev. 407, 441, 451 (2001).*

Journal 1999 Provides a historical account of fee splitting and the corporate practice of medicine doctrine. Suggests that legislation on kickbacks should allow an exception for goods and services supplied at fair market value. Concludes that the legislature's approach to fee splitting should be revised to fit contemporary circumstances. References Opinion 6.02. Jacobs & Goodman, *Splitting Fees or Splitting Hairs? Fee Splitting and Health Care—The Florida Experience, 8 Annals Health L. 239, 244 (1999).*

Journal 1998 Explores aspects of trust in physician-patient relations. Discusses the transformation of the health care system and the need for regulation. Points out that too much involvement by politicians and legislators will put the health care system at risk. References Opinions 6.02 and 8.03. Mechanic, *The Functions and Limitations of Trust in the Provision of Medical Care*, 23 J. Health Pol'y & Law 661, 667 (1998).

Journal 1985 Initially describes how existing doctrines protect the value of autonomy in the context of the physician-patient relationship, then examines various problems in the current protective scheme. Concludes by recommending the creation of an independent articulable protected interest in patient autonomy. Quotes Principles II and IV. Cites Opinions 4.04 (1984) [now Opinion 8.03 and 8.032] and 6.03 (1984) [now Opinion 6.02]. Shultz, *From Informed Consent to Patient Choice: A New Protected Interest*, 95 Yale L. J. 219, 275 (1985).

6.03   Fee Splitting: Referrals to Health Care Facilities

Clinics, laboratories, hospitals, or other health care facilities that compensate physicians for referral of patients are engaged in fee splitting which is unethical.

Health care facilities should not compensate a physician who refers patients there for the physician's cognitive services in prescribing, monitoring, or revising the patient's course of treatment. Payment for these cognitive services is acceptable when it comes from patients, who are the beneficiaries of the physician's services, or from the patient's designated third-party payer.

Offering or accepting payment for referring patients to research studies (finder's fees) is also unethical. (II)

Issued prior to April 1977.

Updated June 1994 and updated June 1996 based on the report "Finder's Fees: Payment for the Referral of Patients to Clinical Research Studies," adopted December 1994.

Kan. App. 1985 Members of a medical partnership sought an injunction to enforce a covenant not to compete against defendant-physician, a former partner. Defendant asserted that the covenant was void as against public policy relying on Opinion 9.02 (1984). The court however ruled that the covenant was reasonable as defined by precedent and that it was bound to follow this precedent as opposed to the American Medical Association's position regarding such covenants. Defendant further argued enforcement of the covenant was precluded because the partnership had violated ethical norms, apparently referring to Opinions 6.03 and 6.04 (1984) [now Opinions 6.02 and 6.03] which were part of partnership contract. The court held that defendant was estopped from complaining about the partnership's actions due to his own conduct. *Axtell Clinic v. Cranston*, No. 56,745 (Kan. Ct. App. June 20, 1985) (LEXIS, States Library, Kan. file).

Journal 2002 Suggests a reconceptualization for bioethics that integrates an analysis of the history of moral change. Concludes that bioethical textbooks should include discussion about the history of bioethics and medical ethics. Quotes Opinion 2.20. References Opinions 6.02, 6.03, 6.04 [now Opinion 8.06], and 8.032. Baker, *Bioethics and History*, 27 J. Med. & Phil. 447, 455, 469 (2002).

Journal 2001 Evaluates current forms of cybermedicine and Internet resources that support it. Explores patient and regulatory concerns, including privacy issues, insurance reimbursement problems, licensure, and liability, which may thwart the growth of cybermedicine. Concludes that cybermedicine may facilitate delivery of cost-effective, quality medical care. Quotes Opinions 5.05, 6.02, and 6.03. Scott, *Cybermedicine and Virtual Pharmacies*, 103 W. Va. L. Rev. 407, 441, 451 (2001).

6.04   "Fee Splitting: Drug or Device Prescription Rebates," issued March 1980, was deleted in June 2002 and combined with Opinion 8.07, "Gifts to Physicians: Offers of Indemnity" and Opinion 8.06, "Drugs and Devices:

Prescribing," into the current Opinion 8.06, "Prescribing and Dispensing Drugs and Devices."

| 6.05 | **Fees for Medical Services** |

A physician should not charge or collect an illegal or excessive fee. For example, an illegal fee occurs when a physician accepts an assignment as full payment for services rendered to a Medicare patient and then bills the patient for an additional amount. A fee is excessive when after a review of the facts a person knowledgeable as to current charges made by physicians would be left with a definite and firm conviction that the fee is in excess of a reasonable fee. Factors to be considered as guides in determining the reasonableness of a fee include the following:

(1) The difficulty and/or uniqueness of the services performed and the time, skill, and experience required
(2) The fee customarily charged in the locality for similar physician services
(3) The amount of the charges involved
(4) The quality of performance
(5) The experience, reputation, and ability of the physician in performing the kind of services involved (II)

Issued prior to April 1977.

Updated June 1994.

Journal 1990 Examines conflicting court decisions that have addressed the appropriateness of medical-legal consulting services and their use of contingent fee arrangements. Concludes by discussing the need for a less troublesome solution to the problems plaintiffs face in malpractice and personal injury cases. Quotes Opinion 6.01. Cites Opinions 6.12 (1989) [now Opinion 6.05] and 9.07. Dillon, *Contingent Fees and Medical-Legal Consulting Services: Economical or Unethical?*, 11 J. Legal Med. 93, 101, 111 (1990).

| 6.06 | The previous Opinion 6.06, "Fees: Group Practice," issued in March 1981, was deleted in June 1994. |

| 6.07 | **Insurance Form Completion Charges** |

The attending physician should complete without charge the appropriate "simplified" insurance claim form as a part of service to the patient to enable the patient to receive his or her benefits. A charge for more complex or multiple forms may be made in conformity with local custom. (II)

Issued prior to April 1977.

Updated June 1994.

Journal 1992 Discusses the ethical and legal boundaries of medical treatment. Concludes that minor boundary violations occur frequently, but warns that if they become too frequent or serious, physicians risk substantial liability. Quotes Opinion 6.06 [sic] 6.07. Simon, *Treatment Boundary Violations: Clinical, Ethical, and Legal Considerations*, 20 Bull. Am. Acad. Psychiatry Law 269, 282 (1992).

6.08 Interest Charges and Finance Charges

Although harsh or commercial collection practices are discouraged in the practice of medicine, a physician who has experienced problems with delinquent accounts may properly choose to request that payment be made at the time of treatment or add interest or other reasonable charges to delinquent accounts. The patient must be notified in advance of the interest or other reasonable finance or service charges by such means as the posting of a notice in the physician's waiting room, the distribution of leaflets describing the office billing practices, and appropriate notations on the billing statement. The physician must comply with state and federal laws and regulations applicable to the imposition of such charges. Physicians are encouraged to review their accounting/collection policies to ensure that no patient's account is sent to collection without the physician's knowledge. Physicians who choose to add an interest or finance charge to accounts not paid within a reasonable time are encouraged to use compassion and discretion in hardship cases. (II)

Issued prior to April 1977.

Updated June 1994.

Cal. App. 1968 Plaintiff-physician sought dissolution of a medical partnership with defendant's decedent, and also sought a larger percentage of the partnership receipts based upon an alleged oral agreement. Defendant crossclaimed to enjoin plaintiff from taking physical control of the partnership offices and patient records. The trial court enjoined plaintiff from treating previous patients, requiring that he return all medical records and pay defendant all fees received from patients he had treated during the time of dispute. The appellate court reversed insofar as the injunction prohibited the plaintiff from treating patient who desired to continue to receive his services or prevented access to medical records essential for this purpose, citing Opinions and Reports of the Judicial Council Sec. 7, Para. 16, Sec. 5, Para. 21 and Sec. 9 (1966) [now Opinions 6.08, 5.02, and 5.05] to support view that patients may not be regarded as the subject of ownership. *Jones v. Fakehany, 261 Cal. App. 2d 298, 67 Cal. Rptr. 810, 815, 816 n.1.*

6.09 Laboratory Bill

When it is not possible for the laboratory bill to be sent directly to the patient, the referring physician's bill to the patient should indicate the actual charges for laboratory services, including the name of the laboratory, as well as any separate charges for the physician's own professional services. (II)

Issued prior to April 1977.

6.10 Services Provided by Multiple Physicians

Each physician engaged in the care of the patient is entitled to compensation commensurate with the value of the service he or she has personally rendered.

No physician should bill or be paid for a service which is not performed; mere referral does not constitute a professional service for which a professional charge should be made or for which a fee may be ethically paid or received.

When services are provided by more than one physician, each physician should submit his or her own bill to the patient and be compensated separately, if possible. A physician should not charge a markup, commission, or profit on the services rendered by others.

It is ethically permissible in certain circumstances, however, for a surgeon to engage other physicians to assist in the performance of a surgical procedure and to pay a reasonable amount for such assistance, provided the nature of the financial arrangement is made known to the patient. This principle applies whether regardless of the assisting physician is the referring physician. (II)

Issued prior to April 1977.

Updated June 1994.

6.11   Competition

Competition between and among physicians and other health care practitioners on the basis of competitive factors such as quality of services, skill, experience, miscellaneous conveniences offered to patients, credit terms, fees charged, etc, is not only ethical but is encouraged. Ethical medical practice thrives best under free market conditions when prospective patients have adequate information and opportunity to choose freely between and among competing physicians and alternate systems of medical care. (VII)

Issued July 1983.

Ohio App. 1991 Medical corporation sought an injunction to enforce a covenant not to compete against defendant-physician. The lower court granted summary judgment based on a referee's report which concluded that, under Principle VI and Opinions 6.11, 9.02, and 9.06 (1989) restrictive covenants were *per se* unenforceable as a matter of public policy. While recognizing a strong public interest in allowing open access to health care, the appellate court in reversing held that Opinion 9.02, which applied specifically to restrictive covenants, only "discouraged" such covenants. *Ohio Urology, Inc. v. Poll, 72 Ohio. App. 446, 450, 451, 594 N.E.2d 1027, 1030, 1031.*

Journal 1998 Explores changes in the health care reimbursement system and the impact on the recovery of damages for medical expenses. Discusses the historical development of the collateral source rule. Suggests that the collateral source rule should not be applied to allow recovery for sums that were not actually paid for medical services. Cites Opinion 6.11. Beard, *The Impact of Changes in Health Care Provider Reimbursement Systems on the Recovery of Damages for Medical Expenses in Personal Injury Suits, 21 Am. J. Trial Advoc. 453, 484 (1998).*

Journal 1997 Examines noncompetition clauses in the medical field. Reviews policy concerns and historical and common-law analyses of agreements not to compete. Posits that, the more commercialized the medical profession becomes, the more noncompetition clauses infringe upon the physician-patient relationship and patients' rights. Quotes Opinions 9.02 and 9.06. Cites Preamble and Opinion 6.11. Comment, *Noncompetition Clauses in Physician Employment Contracts in Oregon, 76 Or. L. Rev. 195, 204-06 (1997).*

Journal 1993 Discusses the controversies surrounding advertising in medicine and physician self-referral. Proposes adoption of the model of the physician as either professional or honest businessman. Quotes Opinion 6.11. Brody, *The Physician as Professional and the Physician as Honest Businessman, 119 Arch. Otolaryngol. Head Neck Surg. 495, 496 (1993).*

Journal 1991 Considers the question of whether physicians should provide medical treatment to those who come to them for second opinions. Concludes that each physician must individually decide whether to treat these patients. Quotes Opinions 6.11, 9.06, and 9.12. Cites Opinion 9.02. Ile, *Should Physicians Treat Patients Who Seek Second Opinions?, 266 JAMA 273, 274 (1991).*

Forgiveness or Waiver of Insurance Copayments

Under the terms of many health insurance policies or programs, patients are made more conscious of the cost of their medical care through co-payments. By imposing co-payments for office visits and other medical services, insurers hope to discourage unnecessary health care. In some cases, financial hardship may deter patients from seeking necessary care if they would be responsible for a co-payment for the care. Physicians commonly forgive or waive co-payments to facilitate patient access to needed medical care. When a co-payment is a barrier to needed care because of financial hardship, physicians should forgive or waive the copayment.

A number of clinics have advertised their willingness to provide detailed medical evaluations and accept the insurer's payment but waive the co-payment for all patients. Cases have been reported in which some of these clinics have conducted excessive and unnecessary medical testing while certifying to insurers that the testing is medically necessary. Such fraudulent activity exacerbates the high cost of health care, violates Opinion 2.19, "Unnecessary Services," and is unethical.

Physicians should be aware that forgiveness or waiver of co-payments may violate the policies of some insurers, both public and private; other insurers may permit forgiveness or waiver if they are aware of the reasons for the forgiveness or waiver. Routine forgiveness or waiver of co-payments may constitute fraud under state and federal law. Physicians should ensure that their policies on copayments are consistent with applicable law and with the requirements of their agreements with insurers. (II)

Issued June 1993.

Journal 2000 Examines civil and criminal liability in connection with the practice of professional courtesy fee waivers and discounts. Discusses conflicts between the long-standing traditional practice of professional courtesy and a prudent and ethical course under current law. Quotes Opinion 6.12. Cites Opinion 6.13. Schmidt, *Professional Courtesy Discounts Under Siege—Part II*, 29 Colo. Law. 59, 62 (Jan. 2000).

Professional Courtesy

Professional courtesy refers to the provision of medical care to physician colleagues or their families free of charge or at a reduced rate. While professional courtesy is a long-standing tradition in the medical profession, it is not an ethical requirement. Physicians should use their own judgment in deciding whether to waive or reduce their fees when treating fellow physicians or their families. Physicians should be aware that accepting insurance payments while waiving patient co-payments may violate Opinion 6.12, "Forgiveness or Waiver of Insurance Copayments." (II, IV)

Issued June 1994.

Journal 2000 Examines civil and criminal liability in connection with the practice of professional courtesy fee waivers and discounts. Discusses conflicts between the long-standing traditional practice of professional courtesy and a prudent and ethical course under current law. Quotes Opinion 6.12. Cites Opinion 6.13. Schmidt, *Professional Courtesy Discounts Under Siege—Part II*, 29 Colo. Law. 59, 62 (Jan. 2000).

Opinions on Physician Records

Records of Physicians: Availability of Information to Other Physicians

The interest of the patient is paramount in the practice of medicine, and everything that can reasonably and lawfully be done to serve that interest must be done by all physicians who have served or are serving the patient. A physician who formerly treated a patient should not refuse for any reason to make records of that patient promptly available on request to another physician presently treating the patient. Proper authorization for the use of records must be granted by the patient. Medical reports should not be withheld because of an unpaid bill for medical services. (IV)

Issued prior to April 1977.

Del. Super. 2002 Medical group sued physician for misappropriation of trade secrets and solicitation of patients while still employed with group. Group authorized physician to notify his patients of his departure. The physician used group's records and insurance data to send a mass-mail letter to about 900 patients. Appeals court held that the letter sent went beyond a notification and was instead a solicitation and that the group had not authorized him to use trade secrets to solicit patients. In so ruling the court quoted Opinions 7.01 and 7.03. *Total Care Physicians v. O'Hara, 2002 Del. Super. LEXIS 493, *19.*

Me. 1999 Physician appealed decision of the Board of Licensure in Medicine imposing a civil penalty for his failure to release medical records to patient's physicians. Physician argued that the Board did not specify the ethical standards that his conduct violated. The court vacated the Board's decision on the grounds that the physician was denied the opportunity to refute evidence of a violation of professional standards or to develop a defense predicated on those standards. The Board, in defense of its decision, presented Opinions 7.01 and 7.02 to the court. The court, in vacating the decision, pointed out that the hearing record did not demonstrate which Opinions the Board applied. Furthermore, the court, quoting Principle IV, stated that the physician had a responsibility to protect the patient's medical records. *Balian v. Board of Licensure in Medicine, 722 A.2d 364, 368.*

N.Y. Surr. 1968 Patients of a deceased physician filed an action seeking to obtain or copy records maintained by the decedent during his lifetime regarding them. The executor had refused to deliver the records by reason of a provision in the decedent's will directing that his "office records" be destroyed. Quoting Opinions and Reports of the Judicial Council, Sec. 9 Paras. 3, 4, 5, 6, and 7 (1966) [now Opinions 7.01, 7.02, 7.03, and 7.05], the court ruled that, while patient records are the property of the physician, it would be against public policy to permit their destruction. As a result, the court ordered the executor to make the records available to the patients' succeeding physicians at their request. *In re Culbertson's Will, 57 Misc. 2d 391, 292 N.Y.S.2d 806, 808-10.*

S.C. Att'y Gen. 1978 Citing Opinions 5.61, 5.62, and 5.63 (1977) [now Opinions 7.01, 7.02, and 7.03], state attorney general found that patient medical records are the property of the physician or hospital which compiled them and that patients have no ownership rights in them. Further, the opinion concludes that patients have a right to information contained in their records and the right to have records sent to another physician. Patients do not, however, have the right to unlimited direct access to their medical records. *South Carolina Att'y Gen. Op., 1978 S.C. AG LEXIS 806.*

Journal 1999 Discusses the need for physicians to advocate on behalf of patients' rights in the context of health care delivery. Evaluates the nature and scope of the physician's role as advocate, noting that physicians cannot be expected to engage in attorney-like advocacy. Quotes Principles IV and VI, Fundamental Elements (2), (4), and (6) [now Opinion 10.01], Patient Responsibilities 5 [now Opinion 10.02], and Opinions 2.03, 2.07, 2.09, 2.16, 2.19, 3.06, 4.01, 4.04, 6.01, 7.02, 8.02, 8.03, 8.13, 8.132, 9.06, 9.07, and 9.131. Cites Opinions 5.05, 5.09, 7.01, 8.135, and 9.02. Sage, *Physicians as Advocates*, 35 Hous. L. Rev. 1529, 1537, 1541, 1542, 1552-53, 1554, 1556, 1557, 1559, 1561-62, 1564, 1571, 1574, 1576, 1580 (1999).

Journal 1997 Compares past ethical opinions to current opinions and notes the differences. Comments on the forces that have changed medical ethics through the years. Notes differing theories on the future course of medical ethics. Quotes Fundamental Elements (Preamble) and Opinions 5.05, 5.057, 7.01, 8.12, 9.12, and 9.131. Cites Fundamental Elements (5) and Opinions 8.115 and 8.13. Buchanan, *Medical Ethics at the Millennium: A Brief Retrospective*, 26 Colo. Law. 141, 142, 143, 144, 145 (1997).

| 7.02 | **Records of Physicians: Information and Patients** |

Notes made in treating a patient are primarily for the physician's own use and constitute his or her personal property. However, on request of the patient, a physician should provide a copy or a summary of the record to the patient or to another physician, an attorney, or other person designated by the patient.

Most states have enacted statutes that authorize patient access to medical records. These statutes vary in scope and mechanism for permitting patients to review or copy medical records. Access to mental health records, particularly, may be limited by statute or regulation. A physician should become familiar with the applicable laws, rules, or regulations on patient access to medical records.

The record is a confidential document involving the patient-physician relationship and should not be communicated to a third party without the patient's prior written consent, unless required by law or to protect the welfare of the individual or the community. Medical reports should not be withheld because of an unpaid bill for medical services. Physicians may charge a reasonable fee for copying medical records. (IV)

Issued prior to April 1977.

Updated June 1994.

Me. 1999 Physician appealed decision of the Board of Licensure in Medicine imposing a civil penalty for his failure to release medical records to patient's physicians. Physician argued that the Board did not specify the ethical standards that his conduct violated. The court vacated the Board's decision on the grounds that the physician was denied the opportunity to refute evidence of a violation of professional standards or to develop a defense predicated on those standards. The Board, in defense of its decision, presented Opinions 7.01 and 7.02 to the court. The court, in vacating the decision, pointed out that the hearing record did not demonstrate which Opinions the Board applied. Furthermore, the court, quoting Principle IV, stated that the physician had a responsibility to protect the patient's medical records. *Balian v. Board of Licensure in Medicine*, 722 A.2d 364, 368.

N.Y. Surr. 1968 Patients of a deceased physician filed an action seeking to obtain or copy records maintained by the decedent during his lifetime regarding them. The executor had refused to deliver the records by reason of a provision in the decedent's will directing that his "office records" be destroyed. Quoting Opinions and Reports of the Judicial Council, Sec. 9 Paras. 3, 4, 5, 6, and 7 (1966) [now Opinions 7.01, 7.02, 7.03, and 7.05], the court ruled that, while patient records are the property of the physician, it would be against public policy to permit their destruction. As a result, the court ordered the executor to make the records available to the patients' succeeding physicians at their request. *In re Culbertson's Will*, 57 Misc. 2d 391, 292 N.Y.S.2d 806, 808-10.

S.C. Att'y Gen. 1978 Citing Opinions 5.61, 5.62, and 5.63 (1977) [now Opinions 7.01, 7.02, and 7.03], state attorney general found that patient medical records are the property of the physician or hospital which compiled them and that patients have no ownership rights in them. Further, the opinion concludes that patients have a right to information contained in their records and the right to have records sent to another physician. Patients do not, however, have the right to unlimited direct access to their medical records. *South Carolina Att'y Gen. Op., 1978 S.C. AG LEXIS 806.*

Journal 2001 Analyzes postmortem patient confidentiality and proposes a framework for appropriate information disclosure. Concludes that, following death, decisions regarding disclosure of confidential information should be made on a case-by-case basis. Quotes Opinions 5.051 and 7.02. Berg, *Grave Secrets: Legal and Ethical Analysis of Postmortem Confidentiality,* 34 Conn. L. Rev. 81, 87, 117 (2001).

Journal 1999 Explores changes in technology and the resulting impact on privacy of medical information. Observes that current federal and state laws inadequately protect medical information privacy and suggests that Congress needs to enact legislation addressing this issue. Quotes Opinion 5.05. References Opinions 7.02 and 7.05. Carter, *Health Information Privacy: Can Congress Protect Confidential Medical Information in the "Information Age"?,* 25 Wm. Mitchell L. Rev. 223, 236, 273 (1999).

Journal 1999 Discusses the need for physicians to advocate on behalf of patients' rights in the context of health care delivery. Evaluates the nature and scope of the physician's role as advocate, noting that physicians cannot be expected to engage in attorney-like advocacy. Quotes Principles IV and VI, Fundamental Elements (2), (4), and (6) [now Opinion 10.01], Patient Responsibilities 5 [now Opinion 10.02], and Opinions 2.03, 2.07, 2.09, 2.16, 2.19, 3.06, 4.01, 4.04, 6.01, 7.02, 8.02, 8.03, 8.13, 8.132, 9.06, 9.07, and 9.131. Cites Opinions 5.05, 5.09, 7.01, 8.135, and 9.02. Sage, *Physicians as Advocates,* 35 Hous. L. Rev. 1529, 1537, 1541, 1542, 1552-53, 1554, 1556, 1557, 1559, 1561-62, 1564, 1571, 1574, 1576, 1580 (1999).

Journal 1997 Discusses the practice of ex parte communications between treating physicians and their patients' legal adversaries without informing the patient or obtaining consent. Examines harms that may occur in these situations. Argues that Oklahoma needs to prohibit treating physicians from communicating ex parte with their patients' legal adversaries. Quotes Opinions 5.05, 5.07, 5.08, 8.02, 8.03, and 9.07. Cites Opinion 7.02. McNaughton & McNaughton, *Divided Loyalty: The Dilemma of the Treating Physician Advocate,* 22 Okla. City U. L. Rev. 1051, 1052, 1054, 1056, 1058, 1059, 1062 (1997).

7.025   Records of Physicians: Access by Non-Treating Medical Staff

Physicians who use or receive information from medical records share in the responsibility for preserving patient confidentiality and should play an integral role in the designing of confidentiality safeguards in health care institutions. Physicians have a responsibility to be aware of the appropriate guidelines in their health care institution, as well as the applicable federal and state laws.

Informal case consultations that involve the disclosure of detailed medical information are appropriate in the absence of consent only if the patient cannot be identified from the information.

Only physicians or other health care professionals who are involved in managing the patient, including providing consultative, therapeutic, or diagnostic services, may access the patient's confidential medical information. All others must obtain explicit consent to access the information.

Monitoring user access to electronic or written medical information is an appropriate and desirable means for detecting breaches of confidentiality. Physicians should encourage the development and use of such monitoring systems.

This opinion focuses on the issue of access to medical records by medical staff not involved in the treatment or diagnosis of patients. It does not address the need to access medical records for clinical research, epidemiological research, quality assurance, or administrative purposes. (IV)

Issued December 1999 based on the report "Records of Physicians: Access by Non-Treating Medical Staff," adopted June 1999.

7.03 Records of Physicians upon Retirement or Departure from a Group

A patient's records may be necessary to the patient in the future not only for medical care but also for employment, insurance, litigation, or other reasons. When a physician retires or dies, patients should be notified and urged to find a new physician and should be informed that upon authorization, records will be sent to the new physician. Records which may be of value to a patient and which are not forwarded to a new physician should be retained, either by the treating physician, another physician, or such other person lawfully permitted to act as a custodian of the records.

The patients of a physician who leaves a group practice should be notified that the physician is leaving the group. Patients of the physician should also be informed of the physician's new address and offered the opportunity to have their medical records forwarded to the departing physician at his or her new practice location. It is unethical to withhold such information upon request of a patient. If the responsibility for notifying patients falls to the departing physician rather than to the group, the group should not interfere with the discharge of these duties by withholding patient lists or other necessary information. (IV)

Issued prior to April 1977.

Updated June 1994, June 1996, and February 2002.

N.D. Ill. 1996 A corporation which provided hair transplants brought suit against a physician group under contract to provide medical services to the corporation. The complaint alleged that the defendants had breached the contract in bad faith by attempting to start their own company, by hiring staff members away, and by threatening to enforce noncompetition covenants in their contracts should any physicians attempt to remain with the corporation. The court referred to Opinion 9.02 as explicitly discouraging the use of restrictive covenants in contracts with physicians. Additionally, with apparent reference to Opinion 7.03, the court noted that defendants had not sent notices advising patients of the departure of physicians from the corporation, or of the departing physicians' new practice locations. *Cleveland Hair Clinic, Inc. v. Puig*, 968 F. Supp. 1227, 1246.

Ark. App. 2003 Clinic appealed summary judgment for a medical group that hired two physicians previously practicing in the clinic. Clinic did not pay the physicians and had no noncompetition agreement with them. Physicians notified their patients of their departure. Clinic alleged the medical group solicited its patients by employing the physicians and using patient lists. Appeals court found the clinic failed to establish an employment relationship or rights to the records. The court held the physicians had a right to terminate their association with the clinic and that their patients had a right to follow them. Cites Opinion 7.03. *Springdale Diagnostic Clinic v. Northwest Physicians*, 2003 Ark. App. LEXIS 697, *13, n.1.

Del. Super. 2002 Medical group sued physician for misappropriation of trade secrets and solicitation of patients while still employed with group. Group authorized physician to notify his patients of his departure. The physician used group's records and insurance data to send a mass-mail letter to about 900 patients. Appeals court held that the letter sent went beyond a notification and was instead a solicitation and that the group had not authorized him to use trade secrets to solicit patients. In so ruling the court quoted Opinions 7.01 and 7.03. *Total Care Physicians v. O'Hara*, 2002 Del. Super. LEXIS 493, *19.

N.Y. Surr. 1968 Patients of a deceased physician filed an action seeking to obtain or copy records maintained by the decedent during his lifetime regarding them. The executor had refused to deliver the records by reason of a provision in the decedent's will directing that his "office records" be destroyed. Quoting Opinions and Reports of the Judicial Council, Sec. 9 Paras. 3, 4, 5, 6, and 7 (1966) [now Opinions 7.01, 7.02, 7.03, and 7.05], the court ruled that, while patient records are the property of the physician, it would be against public policy to permit their destruction. As a result, the court ordered the executor to make the records available to the patients' succeeding physicians at their request. *In re Culbertson's Will, 57 Misc. 2d 391, 292 N.Y.S.2d 806, 808-10.*

S.C. Att'y Gen. 1978 Citing Opinions 5.61, 5.62, and 5.63 (1977) [now Opinions 7.01, 7.02, and 7.03], state attorney general found that patient medical records are the property of the physician or hospital which compiled them and that patients have no ownership rights in them. Further, the opinion concludes that patients have a right to information contained in their records and the right to have records sent to another physician. Patients do not, however, have the right to unlimited direct access to their medical records. *South Carolina Att'y Gen. Op., 1978 S.C. AG LEXIS 806.*

7.04 Sale of a Medical Practice

A physician or the estate of a deceased physician may sell the elements that comprise his or her practice, such as furniture, fixtures, equipment, office leasehold, and goodwill. In the sale of a medical practice, the purchaser is buying not only furniture and fixtures, but also goodwill, ie, the opportunity to take over the patients of the seller. A patient's records may be necessary to the patient in the future not only for medical care but also for employment, insurance, litigation, matriculation, or other reasons. Therefore, the transfer of records of patients is subject to the following:

(1) The physician (or the estate) must ensure that all medical records are transferred to another physician or entity who is held to the same standards of confidentiality and is lawfully permitted to act as custodian of the records.

(2) All active patients should be notified that the physician (or the estate) is transferring the practice to another physician or entity who will retain custody of their records and that at their written request, within a reasonable time as specified in the notice, the records (or copies) will be sent to another physician or entity of their choice.

(3) A reasonable charge may be made for the cost of locating, duplicating, and mailing records. (IV)

Issued July 1983.

Updated June 2000.

N.Y. Surr. 1977 In a discovery proceeding, respondent-psychiatrist, who had treated some patients of deceased psychiatrist subsequent to his death, allegedly misappropriated decedent's patient records. Estate petitioned court for return of records and damages for injury to value of decedent's practice. Respondent sought dismissal of claim arguing that estate could not sell patient records. The court rejected respondent's request. In so ruling, the court noted that under Principle 9 (1957) [now Principle IV and Opinion 5.05] prohibiting physicians from revealing patient confidences, various guidelines had been issued regarding sale of a medical practice [now Opinion 7.04]. Whether respondent's actions had interferred with the estate's efforts to dispose of decedent's practice in keeping with these guidelines presented the court with factual issues for later resolution. *Estate of Finkle, 90 Misc. 2d 550, 395 N.Y.S.2d 343, 346.*

Retention of Medical Records

Physicians have an obligation to retain patient records which may reasonably be of value to a patient. The following guidelines are offered to assist physicians in meeting their ethical and legal obligations:

(1) Medical considerations are the primary basis for deciding how long to retain medical records. For example, operative notes and chemotherapy records should always be part of the patient's chart. In deciding whether to keep certain parts of the record, an appropriate criterion is whether a physician would want the information if he or she were seeing the patient for the first time.

(2) If a particular record no longer needs to be kept for medical reasons, the physician should check state laws to see if there is a requirement that records be kept for a minimum length of time. Most states will not have such a provision. If they do, it will be part of the statutory code or state licensing board.

(3) In all cases, medical records should be kept for at least as long as the length of time of the statute of limitations for medical malpractice claims. The statute of limitations may be three or more years, depending on the state law. State medical associations and insurance carriers are the best resources for this information.

(4) Whatever the statute of limitations, a physician should measure time from the last professional contact with the patient.

(5) If a patient is a minor, the statute of limitations for medical malpractice claims may not apply until the patient reaches the age of majority.

(6) Immunization records always must be kept.

(7) The records of any patient covered by Medicare or Medicaid must be kept at least five years.

(8) In order to preserve confidentiality when discarding old records, all documents should be destroyed.

(9) Before discarding old records, patients should be given an opportunity to claim the records or have them sent to another physician, if it is feasible to give them the opportunity. (IV, V)

Issued June 1994.

N.Y. Surr. 1968 Patients of a deceased physician filed an action seeking to obtain or copy records maintained by the decedent during his lifetime regarding them. The executor had refused to deliver the records by reason of a provision in the decedent's will directing that his "office records" be destroyed. Quoting Opinions and Reports of the Judicial Council, Sec. 9 Paras. 3, 4, 5, 6, and 7 (1966) [now Opinions 7.01, 7.02, 7.03, and 7.05], the court ruled that, while patient records are the property of the physician, it would be against public policy to permit their destruction. As a result, the court ordered the executor to make the records available to the patients' succeeding physicians at their request. *In re Culbertson's Will*, 57 Misc. 2d 391, 292 N.Y.S.2d 806, 808-10.

Tex. 1998 Plaintiff, whose daughter was injured at birth, sued physician for intentional spoliation of medical records pertinent to lawsuit against hospital. The Texas Supreme Court refused to recognize a separate cause of action for intentional or negligent spoliation of evidence by parties to litigation. The court stated that creating a new cause of action for spoliation would result in duplicative litigation. Concurring judge explained other remedies available to the plaintiff. Quoting Opinion 7.05, judge stated that the ethical duty to retain medical records could be treated as a legal duty. *Trevino v. Ortega*, 41 Tex. Sup. Ct. J. 907, 969 S.W.2d 950, 955.

Journal 1999 Explores changes in technology and the resulting impact on privacy of medical information. Observes that current federal and state laws inadequately protect medical information privacy and suggests that Congress needs to enact legislation addressing this issue. Quotes Opinion 5.05. References Opinions 7.02 and 7.05. Carter, *Health Information Privacy: Can Congress Protect Confidential Medical Information in the "Information Age"?*, 25 Wm. Mitchell L. Rev. 223, 236, 273 (1999).

8.00 **Opinions on Practice Matters**

8.01 | **Appointment Charges**

A physician may charge a patient for a missed appointment or for one not cancelled 24 hours in advance if the patient is fully advised that the physician will make such a charge. (VI)

Issued prior to April 1977.

Updated June 1994.

8.02   The previous Opinion 8.02, "Clinics," was deleted in June 1994.

8.02 | **Ethical Guidelines for Physicians in Management Positions and Other Non-Clinical Roles**

Physicians in administrative and other non-clinical roles must put the needs of patients first. At least since the time of Hippocrates, physicians have cultivated the trust of their patients by placing patient welfare before all other concerns. The ethical obligations of physicians are not suspended when a physician assumes a position that does not directly involve patient care. (I, VII)

Issued June 1994 based on the report "Ethical Guidelines for Medical Consultants," adopted December 1992.

Updated June 1998.

Journal 2001 Examines issues relating to health care cost containment. Concludes that, if physicians are to meet the goals assigned to them in a cost-constrained health care system, then professional standards must be reevaluated and modified to afford meaningful guidance for clinical decision-making in the face of health care spending controls. Quotes Opinions 2.03, 2.09, 2.095, 8.032, and 9.04. Cites Opinions 8.02, 8.021, 8.051, and 8.13. Agrawal, *Resuscitating Professionalism: Self-Regulation in the Medical Marketplace*, 66 Mo. L. Rev. 341, 354, 355, 360, 361, 378, 388 (2001).

Journal 2001 Discusses the prohibition on non-lawyer ownership of legal service providers. Considers how ethical rules and standards governing physicians have been directed toward preserving independent judgment. Concludes that ethical conflicts created by abandoning the prohibition on non-lawyer ownership of legal service providers may be managed by following the medical ethics model. Quotes Principle VI and Opinions 2.03, 2.09, 8.02, 8.021, 8.03, 8.05, 8.051, 8.054, 8.13, and 8.132. Harris & Foran, *The Ethics of Middle-Class Access to Legal Services and What We Can Learn from the Medical Profession's Shift to a Corporate Paradigm*, 70 Fordham L. Rev. 775, 817, 821, 822, 823, 824 (2001).

Journal 1999 Discusses the need for physicians to advocate on behalf of patients' rights in the context of health care delivery. Evaluates the nature and scope of the physician's role as advocate, noting that physicians cannot be expected to engage in attorney-like advocacy. Quotes Principles IV and VI, Fundamental Elements (2), (4), and (6) [now Opinion 10.01], Patient Responsibilities

5 [now Opinion 10.02], and Opinions 2.03, 2.07, 2.09, 2.16, 2.19, 3.06, 4.01, 4.04, 6.01, 7.02, 8.02, 8.03, 8.13, 8.132, 9.06, 9.07, and 9.131. Cites Opinions 5.05, 5.09, 7.01, 8.135, and 9.02. Sage, *Physicians as Advocates*, 35 *Hous. L. Rev. 1529, 1537, 1541, 1542, 1552-53, 1554, 1556, 1557, 1559, 1561-62, 1564, 1571, 1574, 1576, 1580 (1999).*

Journal 1997 Discusses the practice of ex parte communications between treating physicians and their patients' legal adversaries without informing the patient or obtaining consent. Examines harms that may occur in these situations. Argues that Oklahoma needs to prohibit treating physicians from communicating ex parte with their patients' legal adversaries. Quotes Opinions 5.05, 5.07, 5.08, 8.02, 8.03, and 9.07. Cites Opinion 7.02. McNaughton & McNaughton, *Divided Loyalty: The Dilemma of the Treating Physician Advocate, 22 Okla. City U. L. Rev. 1051, 1052, 1054, 1056, 1058, 1059, 1062 (1997).*

8.021   Ethical Obligations of Medical Directors

Assuming a title or position that removes the physician from direct patient-physician relationships does not override professional ethical obligations. The term "medical directors," as used here, refers to physicians who are employed by third-party payers in the health care delivery system (ie, insurance companies, managed care organizations, self-insured employers) or by entities that perform medical appropriateness determinations on behalf of payers. These types of medical directors have specific functions, such as making coverage determinations, which go beyond mere administrative responsibility. The following stem from this understanding.

Whenever physicians employ professional knowledge and values gained through medical training and practice, and in so doing affect individual or group patient care, they are functioning within the professional sphere of physicians and must uphold ethical obligations, including those articulated by the AMA's *Code of Medical Ethics.*

Medical directors acting within the professional sphere, such as when making decisions regarding medical appropriateness, have an overriding ethical obligation to promote professional medical standards. Adherence to professional medical standards includes:

(1) Placing the interests of patients above other considerations, such as personal interests (eg, financial incentives) or employer business interests (eg, profit). This entails applying the plan parameters to each patient equally and engaging in neither discrimination nor favoritism.

(2) Using fair and just criteria when making care-related determinations. This entails contributing professional expertise to help craft plan guidelines that ensure fair and equal consideration of all plan enrollees. In addition, medical directors should review plan policies and guidelines to ensure that decision-making mechanisms are objective, flexible, and consistent, and apply only ethically appropriate criteria, such as those identified by the Council in Opinion 2.03, "Allocation of Limited Medical Resources."

(3) Working towards achieving access to adequate medical services. This entails encouraging employers to provide services that would be considered part of an adequate level of health care, as articulated in Opinion 2.095, "The Provision of Adequate Health Care." (I, III, VII)

Issued December 1999 based on the report "Ethical Obligations of Medical Directors," adopted June 1999.

173

Journal 2001 Examines issues relating to health care cost containment. Concludes that, if physicians are to meet the goals assigned to them in a cost-constrained health care system, then professional standards must be reevaluated and modified to afford meaningful guidance for clinical decision-making in the face of health care spending controls. Quotes Opinions 2.03, 2.09, 2.095, 8.032, and 9.04. Cites Opinions 8.02, 8.021, 8.051, and 8.13. Agrawal, *Resuscitating Professionalism: Self-Regulation in the Medical Marketplace*, 66 Mo. L. Rev. 341, 354, 355, 360, 361, 378, 388 (2001).

Journal 2001 Discusses the prohibition on non-lawyer ownership of legal service providers. Considers how ethical rules and standards governing physicians have been directed toward preserving independent judgment. Concludes that ethical conflicts created by abandoning the prohibition on non-lawyer ownership of legal service providers may be managed by following the medical ethics model. Quotes Principle VI and Opinions 2.03, 2.09, 8.02, 8.021, 8.03, 8.05, 8.051, 8.054, 8.13, and 8.132. Harris & Foran, *The Ethics of Middle-Class Access to Legal Services and What We Can Learn from the Medical Profession's Shift to a Corporate Paradigm*, 70 Fordham L. Rev. 775, 817, 821, 822, 823, 824 (2001).

8.03   Conflicts of Interest: Guidelines

Under no circumstances may physicians place their own financial interests above the welfare of their patients. The primary objective of the medical profession is to render service to humanity; reward or financial gain is a subordinate consideration. For a physician to unnecessarily hospitalize a patient, prescribe a drug, or conduct diagnostic tests for the physician's financial benefit is unethical. If a conflict develops between the physician's financial interest and the physician's responsibilities to the patient, the conflict must be resolved to the patient's benefit. (II)

Issued July 1986.

Updated June 1994.

7th Cir. 1984 Plaintiff brought medical malpractice suit against several physicians appointed to the Veterans Administration Department of Medicine and Surgery. The court held that strict control test for determining whether defendants ought to be considered employees or independent contractors under the Federal Tort Claims Act was not appropriate because the ethical obligation of a physician to a patient, evidenced by Principle 6 (1957) [now Opinions 8.03 and 8.05], required that independent judgment be exercised, preventing a physician from being strictly controlled by the Veterans Administration. *Quilico v. Kaplan*, 749 F.2d 480, 483-84.

10th Cir. 1983 Pursuant to the Federal Tort Claims Act, plaintiff sued the federal government for the negligence of a neurosurgeon, allegedly an employee of a Veteran's Administration hospital. Plaintiff argued that applying the traditional control test to determine a physician's employment status was inappropriate because physicians are bound by Principle 6 (1957) [now Opinions 8.03 and 8.05] requiring them to have free and complete exercise of [their] medical judgment and skill.... However, the court did not reach the merits of that argument because the contractual agreement between the neurosurgeon and the VA hospital was outside the parameters of an employer-employee relationship with the government, thus precluding plaintiff's claim. *Lurch v. United States*, 719 F.2d 333, 337, cert. denied, 466 US 927 (1984).

Cal. App. 1967 Physician-stockholders of publicly-owned pharmaceutical corporations and physicians whose medical partnerships owned and operated pharmacies challenged statutory prohibition of physician membership, proprietory interest, and co-ownership of pharmacies. The court quoted Principles Ch. I, Sec. 6 (1947) and a 1960 Judicial Council rule, later included in Opinions and Reports of the Judicial Council Sec. 7, Para. 38 (1965) [now Opinions 8.03, 8.032, and 8.06] in its discussion of the potential conflict of interest created by such ownership. The court held that the statute prohibited physician partnerships from directly owning pharmacies but did not apply to an individual physician or a partnership of physicians who own stock in a corporation which owns and operates a pharamacy. *Magan Medical Clinic v. California State Bd. of Medical Examiners*, 249 Cal. App. 2d 124, 57 Cal. Rptr. 256, 262.

Mich. Att'y Gen. 1977 State attorney general determined that, within limits, it was not illegal for physicians to refer patient specimens to clinical laboratories which they own or in which they have a financial interest. Opinion observes however that, under the Opinions and Reports of the Judicial Council Sec. 7, Paras. 21 and 22 (1972) [now Opinions 8.03 and 8.032] such referrals may be unethical. *Mich. Att'y Gen. Opinion No. 5229, 1977-78 Att'y. Gen. Op. 234.*

Miss. 2003 Patient's estate appealed summary judgment in favor of physician and hospital in wrongful death action. Supreme court affirmed, holding that physician was a state employee and that purchase of liability insurance did not waive immunity. In examining physician's status, the court found that the exercise of professional judgment and discretion are not determinative of employment status. Quotes Principle 6 (1957) [now Opinions 8.03 and 8.05]. *Corey v. Skelton, 834 So.2d 681, 685.*

Miss. 2002 Plaintiff in malpractice action appealed grant of summary judgment in favor of neurosurgeon who allegedly performed a thoracic diskectomy on the wrong disc. A resident performed the patient's physical and wrote the majority of the chart notes. The Mississippi Supreme Court affirmed the lower court. The court held that as a state employee the physician was immune from liability and that his exercise of professional judgment in treating patients did not change his status and insurance did not waive immunity. Quotes Principle 6 (1957) [now Opinions 8.03 and 8.05]. *Clayton v. Harkey, 826 So.2d 1283, 1287.*

Miss. 2001 Patient filed suit asserting that a physician was negligent in performing surgery. The trial court granted the physician's summary judgment motion and held that the physician, employed by a state university medical center, was immune under state law. Finding genuine issues of fact, the state supreme court reversed and remanded the case for further proceedings. In a separate opinion, one justice quoted Principle 6 (1957) [now Opinions 8.03 and 8.05], in evaluating the degree of control exercised by the state over the physician. This justice, stressing that the physician exercised discretion in treating the patient independent of the state's control, found no basis to hold the physician an employee for immunity purposes. *Conley v. Warren, 797 So. 2d 881, 886.*

Miss. 2000 Beneficiaries of patient's estate appealed summary judgment in malpractice action for a physician on sovereign immunity grounds. The court reversed and remanded the case finding issues of fact to be resolved at trial. The majority set out a five part test to determine the employment status of a physician working at a state healthcare facility, including the degree of control and direction exercised by the state over the physician. In a separate opinion one justice quoted Principle 6 (1957) [now Opinion 8.03 and 8.05], stating that, "A physician should not dispose of his services under terms or conditions which tend to interfere with or impair the free and complete exercise of his medical judgment and skill...." This justice reasoned that the physician could not claim the state controlled his medical discretion or treatment of patients and thus was clearly not an employee entitled to immunity. *Miller v. Meeks, 762 So. 2d 302, 314.*

Miss. 2000 Patient brought a medical malpractice action against physicians after receiving treatment at a state university medical center. The jury returned a verdict against the physicians. The Mississippi Supreme Court reversed, finding that the physicians were immune from liability as state employees. In determining the status of the physicians, the court noted that the physicians retained a considerable amount of professional discretion in treating the patient, quoting Principle 6 (1957) [now Opinions 8.03 and 8.05]. However, this alone was not determinative, and in the court's view the physicians were state employees. *Sullivan v. Washington, 768 So. 2d 881, 885.*

Miss. App. 2003 Patient brought malpractice action against physicians working at a state university teaching hospital. Patient argued that the physicians were independent contractors and sovereign immunity did not apply. Appellate court, citing the Mississippi Supreme Court's decision in *Miller v. Mecks*, 762 So.2d 302 (Miss. 2000), affirmed the trial court and held that sovereign immunity applied because the physicians were state employees. Quotes Principle 6 (1957) [now Opinions 8.03 and 8.05]. *Brown v. Warren, 858 So.2d 168, 175 (2003).*

Ohio Att'y Gen. 1999 State attorney general concluded that physicians who render opinions regarding the necessity of medical services for health insuring corporations are not engaged in the practice of medicine. Additionally, physicians who render opinions regarding medical necessity for appeals of adverse determinations do not fall under the regulatory, investigatory, or enforcement authority of the Ohio State Medical Board. Quoting Opinions 8.03, 8.11, and 8.13, the attorney general stated that physicians have an ethical duty to provide appropriate treatment for patients. *Ohio Att'y Gen. Op. No. 99-044, 1999 WL 692623.*

Journal 2003 Discusses conflicts of interest caused when managed care organizations provide financial incentives to physicians. Concludes that the focus of managed care is not well-suited for the doctor-patient relationship. Quotes Opinion 8.03. Cites Principle VII. References Opinion 8.051. Hall, *Bargaining with Hippocrates: Managed Care and the Doctor-Patient Relationship*, 54 S.C. L. Rev. 689, 696, 735 (2003).

Journal 2002 Examines how managed care has adversely affected information disclosure in the physician-patient relationship. Concludes that, unless courts expand applicability of principles of informed consent, patient self-determination and autonomy will continue to be undermined. Quotes Principle VIII and Opinions 8.03, 8.053, 8.054, and 8.08. Morris, *Dissing Disclosure: Just What the Doctor Ordered*, 44 Ariz. L. Rev. 313, 344, 349, 362, 363, 366 (2002).

Journal 2001 Considers conflicts of interest in clinical research and other types of medical practice. Compares the way in which doctors and lawyers address conflicts of interest in professional practice. Concludes that physicians are unaware of the need to create a meaningful conflict-of-interest doctrine for medical practice. Quotes Preamble, Principle IV, and Opinions 2.07, 8.03, 8.031, and 10.01. Moore, *What Doctors Can Learn from Lawyers about Conflicts of Interest*, 81 B.U.L. Rev. 445, 447, 449-50 (2001).

Journal 2001 Examines financial conflict of interest issues that arise in the context of clinical research. Concludes that open communication among stakeholders is necessary to resolve these issues. Quotes Opinions 8.03 and 8.031. Rose, *Financial Conflicts of Interest: How Are We Managing?* 8 Wid. L. Symp. J. 1, 24 (2001).

Journal 2000 Discusses patent law and policy. Examines whether or not those who practice medicine should be excused from patent laws because of the conflict that medical procedure patents create with respect to the practice of medicine. Concludes that Congress should repeal section 287(c) of the Patent Act. Quotes Principle V and Opinions 9.08 and 9.09. Cites Opinion 8.03. References Opinion 10.01. Ho, *Patents, Patients, and Public Policy: An Incomplete Intersection at 35 U.S.C. § 287(c)*, 33 U.C. Davis L. Rev. 601, 603, 623, 624, 625, 631 (2000).

Journal 2000 Examines issues relating to parental consent to circumcision. Identifies legal and ethical requirements for consent when medical professionals are treating adult patients. Analyzes the implications of those requirements for routine circumcision of infant males. Concludes that only when the male is an adult and capable of making decisions can circumcision be ethically and legally performed. Quotes Opinion 8.08. References Opinions 8.03 and 9.011. Svoboda, Van Howe, & Dwyer, *Informed Consent for Neonatal Circumcision: An Ethical and Legal Conundrum*, 17 J. Contemp. Health L. & Pol'y 61, 67, 73, 82 (2000).

Journal 1999 Asserts that patient autonomy is closely linked to patient-doctor discourse. Proposes a constitutional framework for evaluating how governmental regulations may interfere with such discourse. Concludes by emphasizing the importance of protecting the quality of doctor-patient discourse. Quotes Preamble and Opinion 8.03. Gatter, *Protecting Patient-Doctor Discourse: Informed Consent and Deliberative Autonomy*, 78 Or. L. Rev. 941, 956 (1999).

Journal 1999 Explores ethical and legal issues surrounding physician incentives in managed care. Concludes that successful ERISA claims for breach of fiduciary duty will hold managed care organizations accountable for controlling medical costs. Quotes Opinion 8.03. Marsh, *Sacrificing Patients for Profits: Physician Incentives to Limit Care and ERISA Fiduciary Duty*, 77 Wash. U. L. Q. 1323, 1332 (1999).

Journal 1999 Discusses the need for physicians to advocate on behalf of patients' rights in the context of health care delivery. Evaluates the nature and scope of the physician's role as advocate, noting that physicians cannot be expected to engage in attorney-like advocacy. Quotes Principles IV and VI, Fundamental Elements (2), (4), and (6) [now Opinion 10.01], Patient Responsibilities 5 [now Opinion 10.02], and Opinions 2.03, 2.07, 2.09, 2.16, 2.19, 3.06, 4.01, 4.04, 6.01, 7.02, 8.02, 8.03, 8.13, 8.132, 9.06, 9.07, and 9.131. Cites Opinions 5.05, 5.09, 7.01, 8.135, and 9.02. Sage, *Physicians as Advocates*, 35 Hous. L. Rev. 1529, 1537, 1541, 1542, 1552-53, 1554, 1556, 1557, 1559, 1561-62, 1564, 1571, 1574, 1576, 1580 (1999).

Journal 1999 Explores the impact managed care organizations have had on health care. Explains that patients may not understand restrictions and incentives imposed by their managed care organizations when entering the program. Argues that such information should be disclosed at various times during the period of plan coverage. Cites Opinions 2.03, 8.03, 8.032, 8.051, 8.13 and 8.132. Wolf, *Toward a Systemic Theory of Informed Consent in Managed Care*, 35 Hous. L. Rev. 1631, 1641, 1658, 1661, 1662, 1679 (1999).

Journal 1998 Discusses conflicts of interest in the physician-patient relationship arising out of use of financial incentives by managed care organizations. Considers how such conflicts are dealt with in the attorney-client relationship. Suggests that a financial incentive should be legally denounced if it unreasonably interferes with a physician's duty to properly care for and treat patients. Quotes Preamble, Fundamental Elements (1) [now Opinion 10.01] and Opinions 4.04, 5.01, 8.03, 8.13, and 9.06. Cites Fundamental Elements (4) [now Opinion 10.01] and Opinions 2.07, 2.08, and 2.132. Hall, *Third-Party Payor Conflicts of Interest in Managed Care: A Proposal for Regulation Based on the Model Rules of Professional Conduct*, 29 Seton Hall L. Rev. 95, 96, 107, 108, 109, 110, 111, 112, 134, 135, 136 (1998).

Journal 1998 Discusses the physician's fiduciary duty to the patient. Explores the expansion of the "honest services" mail fraud statute to prosecute undisclosed fiduciary breaches. Concludes that the mail fraud statute may be used to prosecute physicians who fail to disclose financial incentives to their patients. Quotes Opinion 8.03. Cites Opinions 2.03 and 8.07 [now Opinion 8.06]. Jones, *Primum Non Nocere: The Expanding "Honest Services" Mail Fraud Statute and the Physician-Patient Fiduciary Relationship*, 51 Vand. L. Rev. 139, 161, 164 (1998).

Journal 1998 Explores aspects of trust in physician-patient relations. Discusses the transformation of the health care system and the need for regulation. Points out that too much involvement by politicians and legislators will put the health care system at risk. References Opinions 6.02 and 8.03. Mechanic, *The Functions and Limitations of Trust in the Provision of Medical Care*, 23 J. Health Pol'y & Law 661, 667 (1998).

Journal 1997 Discusses physician-patient trust in the managed care environment. Explores options for enhancing trustworthiness in this context. Quotes Opinion 8.03. Gray, *Trust and Trustworthy Care in the Managed Care Era*, 16 Health Affairs 34, 38, 47-48 (1997).

Journal 1997 Discusses the practice of ex parte communications between treating physicians and their patients' legal adversaries without informing the patient or obtaining consent. Examines harms that may occur in these situations. Argues that Oklahoma needs to prohibit treating physicians from communicating ex parte with their patients' legal adversaries. Quotes Opinions 5.05, 5.07, 5.08, 8.02, 8.03, and 9.07. Cites Opinion 7.02. McNaughton & McNaughton, *Divided Loyalty: The Dilemma of the Treating Physician Advocate*, 22 Okla. City U. L. Rev. 1051, 1052, 1054, 1056, 1058, 1059, 1062 (1997).

Journal 1995 Addresses presidential disability, its past impact on American government, and possible solutions to potential problems. Proposes enhancement of the role of the President's physician. Quotes Opinion 8.03. Cites Opinions 5.04 and 5.05. Abrams, *The Vulnerable President and the Twenty-Fifth Amendment, with Observations on Guidelines, a Health Commission, and the Role of the President's Physician*, 30 Wake Forest L. Rev. 453, 466, 471 (1995).

Journal 1994 Discusses the issue of whom physicians must serve first: themselves, their patients, insurers, or society. Focuses on risks arising out of provider economic arrangements and risks arising out of other individual physician characteristics. Quotes Opinions 8.03 and 9.13. Cites Opinion 8.15. Dobinski, *Autonomy and Privacy: Protecting Patients from Their Physicians*, 55 U. Pitt. L. Rev. 291, 302, 313 (1994).

Journal 1994 Observes that health care reform proposals present significant challenges to the role and ethics of attending physicians. Emphasizes that reform proposals must set forth the role envisioned for physicians and must articulate an acceptable ethical framework within which physicians may fulfill that role. Quotes Opinions 4.04, 9.121, and 9.122. Cites Opinions 2.03, 2.09, 5.01, and 8.03. Wolf, *Health Care Reform and the Future of Physician Ethics*, 24 Hastings Center Rep. 28, 32, 40 (March/April 1994).

Journal 1993 Discusses the problem of physicians withholding needed medical treatment from HIV-infected infants. Concludes that current law should be expanded to eliminate this discrimination. Quotes Opinions 2.09, 2.17, 2.20, 2.22, 4.04, and 8.03. Crossley, *Of Diagnoses and Discrimination: Discriminatory Nontreatment of Infants With HIV Infection*, 93 Columbia L. Rev. 1581, 1620, 1621 (1993).

Journal 1992 Examines issues related to the responsibility of HIV-infected health care workers to protect patients from infection, including mandatory testing, disclosure to co-workers and supervisors, and the degree to which the practice of an HIV-infected health care worker should be modified. Concludes that courts likely will impose a requirement to disclose HIV-positive status to patients when there is a substantial risk of HIV transmission. Quotes Opinions 8.03 (1989) [now Opinion 8.032], and 8.07 (1989) [now Opinion 8.03]. References Opinion 9.131. Lieberman & Derse, *HIV-*

Positive Health Care Workers and the Obligation to Disclose: Do Patients Have a Right to Know?, 13 J. Legal Med. 333, 353, 354 (1992).

Journal 1990 Explains how the federal Medicare and Medicaid Anti-Fraud and Abuse statute limits the ability of physicians to adapt investment and referral strategies to an increasingly competitive health care marketplace. Proposes giving regulatory power over physician investments back to the states, which are more able to recognize and exempt beneficial arrangements from otherwise restrictive statutory schemes. Cites Opinion 8.03. Comment, *Regulating Physician Investment and Referral Behavior in the Competitive Health Care Marketplace of the '90s—An Argument for Decentralization*, 65 Wash. L. Rev. 657, 658 (1990).

Journal 1990 Examines various cost control mechanisms utilized by prepaid health plans and other managed care programs and considers the impact of such mechanisms on clinical decision making. Emphasis is placed on the possible existence of conflicts of interest on the part of health care providers in this context. Quotes Opinions 8.03 [now Opinions 8.03 and 8.032] and 8.13 [now Opinion 8.132]. Hirshfeld, *Defining Full and Fair Disclosure in Managed Care Contracts*, 60 The Citation 67, 70 (1990).

Journal 1990 Discusses efforts of third-party payors to control health care expenditures for beneficiaries. Concludes that financial incentives to limit care and other cost control techniques should be disclosed and that the rationale for such disclosure is compelling. Quotes Opinions 2.03, 2.09, and 8.03 [now Opinions 8.03 and 8.032]. Cites Opinions 2.19, 4.04, and 4.06. Hirshfeld, *Should Third Party Payors of Health Care Services Disclose Cost Control Mechanisms to Potential Beneficiaries?*, 14 Seton Hall Legis. J. 115, 130, 131, 144, 145, 146 (1990).

Journal 1989 Analyzes the Medicare and Medicaid Patient and Program Protection Act of 1987 and discusses the complexity of fraud and abuse issues that confront hospitals and health care providers who undertake financially attractive business arrangements. Concludes that the 1987 Act, along with its implementing regulations, can offer meaningful guidance in an area of uncertainty for the health care industry. Quotes Opinion 4.05 (1986) [now Opinion 8.03]. Comment, *Curing the Health Care Industry: Government Response to Medicare Fraud and Abuse*, 5 J. Contemp. Health L. & Pol'y 175, 189 (1989).

Journal 1985 Initially describes how existing doctrines protect the value of autonomy in the context of the physician-patient relationship, then examines various problems in the current protective scheme. Concludes by recommending the creation of an independent articulable protected interest in patient autonomy. Quotes Principles II and IV. Cites Opinions 4.04 (1984) [now Opinions 8.03 and 8.032] and 6.03 (1984) [now Opinion 6.02]. Shultz, *From Informed Consent to Patient Choice: A New Protected Interest*, 95 Yale L. J. 219, 275 (1985).

8.031 Conflicts of Interest: Biomedical Research

Avoidance of real or perceived conflicts of interest in clinical research is imperative if the medical community is to ensure objectivity and maintain individual and institutional integrity. All medical centers should develop specific guidelines for their clinical staff on conflicts of interest. These guidelines should include the following rules: (1) once a clinical investigator becomes involved in a research project for a company or knows that he or she might become involved, she or he, as an individual, cannot ethically buy or sell the company's stock until the involvement ends and the results of the research are published or otherwise disseminated to the public; (2) any remuneration received by the researcher from the company whose product is being studied must be commensurate with the efforts of the researcher on behalf of the company; and (3) clinical investigators should disclose any material ties to companies whose products they are investigating, including financial ties, participation in educational activities supported by the companies, participation in other research projects funded by the companies, consulting arrangements, and any other ties. The disclosures should be made in writing to the medical center where the research is conducted, organizations that are funding the research, and journals that publish the results of the research. An explanatory statement that discloses conflicts of interest should accompany all published research. Other types of publications, such as a letters to the editor, should also include an explanatory statement that discloses any potential conflict of interest.

In addition, medical centers should form review committees to examine disclosures by clinical staff about financial associations with commercial corporations. (II, IV)

Issued March 1992 based on the report "Conflicts of Interest in Biomedical Research," adopted December 1989 (JAMA. 1990; 263: 2790-93).

Updated June 1999 based on the report "Conflicts of Interest: Biomedical Research," adopted December 1998.

Journal 2002 Considers the implications of using pharmacogenomics in drug development and health care delivery. Emphasizes various legal, economic, and social issues. Concludes that these issues must be meaningfully addressed given the benefits of pharmacogenomics. Cites Opinion 8.031. Malinowski, *Law, Policy, and Market Implications of Genetic Profiling in Drug Development*, 2 *Hous. J. Health L. & Pol'y* 31, 51 (2002).

Journal 2002 Discusses ethical and legal issues involving acquisition of biological specimens by commercial biobanks. Sets forth areas of inquiry for institutional review boards in evaluating the propriety of research collaborations with commercial biobanks. Cites Opinion 8.031. Rothstein, *The Role of IRBs in Research Involving Commercial Biobanks*, 30 *J. Law, Med. & Ethics* 105, 106, 108 (2002).

Journal 2001 Explores institutional conflicts of interest arising from the impact of biotechnology and the genetics revolution on clinical research. Concludes that federal oversight changes should be implemented in order to maintain the public's trust in health science. Quotes Opinion 8.031. Malinowski, *Conflicts of Interest in Clinical Research: Legal and Ethical Issues: Institutional Conflicts and Responsibilities in an Age of Academic-Industry Alliances*, 8 *Wid. L. Symp. J.* 47, 70 (2001).

Journal 2001 Considers conflicts of interest in clinical research and other types of medical practice. Compares the way in which doctors and lawyers address conflicts of interest in professional practice. Concludes that physicians are unaware of the need to create a meaningful conflict-of-interest doctrine for medical practice. Quotes Preamble, Principle IV, and Opinions 2.07, 8.03, 8.031, and 10.01. Moore, *What Doctors Can Learn from Lawyers about Conflicts of Interest*, 81 *B.U.L. Rev.* 445, 447, 449-50 (2001).

Journal 2001 Examines financial conflict of interest issues that arise in the context of clinical research. Concludes that open communication among stakeholders is necessary to resolve these issues. Quotes Opinions 8.03 and 8.031. Rose, *Financial Conflicts of Interest: How Are We Managing?* 8 *Wid. L. Symp. J.* 1, 24 (2001).

Journal 1996 Explores biotechnology advances made possible through cooperation between universities and industries. Observes that clinical investigators involved in company research are ethically prohibited from buying or selling company stock, until results are published. Concludes that cooperation in the biotechnology field will benefit society. Cites Opinion 8.031. Comment, *Alliances for the Future: Cultivating a Cooperative Environment for Biotech Success*, 11 *Berkeley Tech. L. J.* 311, 344 (1996).

Journal 1991 Considers whether patients should be permitted or required to pay for research in which they participate. Concludes that patient-funded research may be useful, so long as the potential for individual harm and abuse can be minimized. References Opinion 8.031. Morreim, *Patient-Funded Research: Paying the Piper or Protecting the Patient?*, 13 *IRB* 1, 2 (May/June 1991).

Journal 1991 Discusses the ethical issues involved when physicians and scientists enroll patients in drug company-sponsored clinical trials in exchange for reimbursement. Concludes that financial arrangements between drug companies and scientists give the appearance and the opportunity for conflict of interest; thus physicians should be required to disclose funding sources to patients. References Opinion 8.031. Shimm & Spece, *Conflict of Interest and Informed Consent in Industry-Sponsored Clinical Trials*, 12 *J. Legal Med.* 477, 481, 507, 510 (1991).

8.0315 Managing Conflicts of Interest in the Conduct of Clinical Trials

As the biotechnology and pharmaceutical industries continue to expand research activities and funding of clinical trials, and as increasing numbers of physicians both within and outside academic health centers become involved in partnerships with industry to perform these activities, greater safeguards against conflicts of interest are needed to ensure the integrity of the research and to protect the welfare of human subjects. Physicians should be mindful of the conflicting roles of investigator and clinician and of the financial conflicts of interest that arise from incentives to conduct trials and to recruit subjects. In particular, physicians involved in clinical research should heed the following guidelines:

(1) Physicians should agree to participate as investigators in clinical trials only when it relates to their scope of practice and area of medical expertise. They should have adequate training in the conduct of research and should participate only in protocols which they are satisfied are scientifically sound.

(2) Physicians should be familiar with the ethics of research and should agree to participate in trials only if they are satisfied that an Institutional Review Board has reviewed the protocol, that the research does not impose undue risks upon research subjects, and that the research conforms to government regulations.

(3) When a physician has treated or continues to treat a patient who is eligible to enroll as a subject in a clinical trial that the physician is conducting, the informed consent process must differentiate between the physician's roles as clinician and investigator. This is best achieved when someone other than the treating physician obtains the participant's informed consent to participate in the trial. This individual should be protected from the pressures of financial incentives, as described in the following section.

(4) Any financial compensation received from trial sponsors must be commensurate with the efforts of the physician performing the research. Financial compensation should be at fair market value and the rate of compensation per patient should not vary according to the volume of subjects enrolled by the physician, and should meet other existing legal requirements. Furthermore, according to Opinion 6.03, "Fee Splitting: Referral to Health Care Facilities," it is unethical for physicians to accept payment solely for referring patients to research studies.

(5) Physicians should ensure that protocols include provisions for the funding of subjects' medical care in the event of complications associated with the research. Also, a physician should not bill a third-party payor when he or she has received funds from a sponsor to cover the additional expenses related to conducting the trial.

(6) The nature and source of funding and financial incentives offered to the investigators must be disclosed to a potential participant as part of the informed consent process. Disclosure to participants also should include information on uncertainties that may exist regarding funding of treatment for possible complications that may arise during the course of the trial. Physicians should ensure that such disclosure is included in any written informed consent.

(7) When entering into a contract to perform research, physicians should ensure themselves that the presentation or publication of results will not be unduly delayed or otherwise obstructed by the sponsoring company. (II, V)

Issued June 2001 based on the report "Managing Conflicts of Interest in the Conduct of Clinical Trials," adopted December 2000 (JAMA. 2002; 287: 78-84).

8.032 Conflicts of Interest: Health Facility Ownership by a Physician

Physician ownership interests in commercial ventures can provide important benefits in patient care. Physicians are free to enter lawful contractual relationships, including the acquisition of ownership interests in health facilities, products, or equipment. However, when physicians refer patients to facilities in which they have an ownership interest, a potential conflict of interest exists. In general, physicians should not refer patients to a health care facility which is outside their office practice and at which they do not directly provide care or services when they have an investment interest in that facility. The requirement that the physician *directly* provide the care or services should be interpreted as commonly understood. The physician needs to have personal involvement with the provision of care on site.

There may be situations in which a needed facility would not be built if referring physicians were prohibited from investing in the facility. Physicians may invest in and refer to an outside facility, whether or not they provide direct care or services at the facility, if there is a demonstrated need in the community for the facility and alternative financing is not available. Need might exist when there is no facility of reasonable quality in the community or when use of existing facilities is onerous for patients. Self-referral based on demonstrated need cannot be justified simply if the facility would offer some marginal improvement over the quality of services in the community. The potential benefits of the facility should be substantial. The use of existing facilities may be considered onerous when patients face undue delays in receiving services, delays that compromise the patient's care or affect the curability or reversibility of the patient's condition. The requirement that alternative financing not be available carries a burden of proof. The builder would have to undertake efforts to secure funding from banks, other financial institutions, and venture capitalists before turning to self-referring physicians.

Where there is a true demonstrated need in the community for the facility, the following requirements should also be met: (1) physicians should disclose their investment interest to their patients when making a referral, provide a list of effective alternative facilities if they are available, inform their patients that they have free choice to obtain the medical services elsewhere, and assure their patients that they will not be treated differently if they do not choose the physician-owned facility; (2) individuals not in a position to refer patients to the facility should be given a bona fide opportunity to invest in the facility on the same terms that are offered to referring physicians; (3) the opportunity to invest and the terms of investment should not be related to the past or expected volume of referrals or other business generated by the physician investor or owner; (4) there should be no requirement that a physician investor make referrals to the entity or otherwise generate business as a condition for remaining an investor; (5) the return on the physician's investment should be tied to the physician's equity in the facility rather than to the volume of referrals; (6) the entity should not loan funds or guarantee a loan for physicians in a position to refer to the entity; (7) investment contracts should not include "noncompetition clauses" that prevent physicians from investing in other facilities; (8) the physician's ownership interest should be disclosed to third party payers upon request; (9) an internal utilization review program should be established to ensure that investing physicians do not exploit their patients in any way, as by inappropriate or unnecessary utilization; (10) when a physician's commercial interest conflicts to the detriment of the patient, the physician should make alternative arrangements for the care of the patient. (II, III, IV)

Issued prior to April 1977.

Updated 1989; updated March 1992 based on the report "Conflicts of Interest: Physician Ownership of Medical Facilities," adopted December 1991 (JAMA. 1992; 267: 2366-69); and updated June 1994.

C.D. Ill. 1992 A contractual agreement between a clinic and hospital providing undisclosed financial incentives for referrals constituted a "business" aspect of the medical profession and was not exempt from state's Consumer Fraud Act. Reference is made to Council on Ethical Judicial Affairs, Conflicts of Interest Physician Ownership of Medical Facilities, 267 JAMA 2366 (1992) [now Opinion 8.032], which mandates that a physician disclose his financial interest to his patient when making a referral. *Gadson v. Newman, 807 F. Supp. 1412, 1416.*

E.D. N.Y. 1975 Medical laboratories sought injunction against city's award of exclusive contracts for Medicaid services. The court granted a preliminary injunction and held that the laboratories had a substantial probability of success on the merits of the claim that Medicaid recipients would be deprived of statutory right of free choice of providers. In balancing the equities, the court also noted that the contracts would create an ethical dilemma for physicians who are required to provide patients with free choice of ancillary services under Opinions and Reports of the Judicial Council Sec. 1, Paras. 6 and 14 (1971) [now Opinions 8.032, 8.06, and 9.06]. *Bay Ridge Diagnostic Laboratory, Inc. v. Dumpson, 400 F. Supp. 1104, 1109-10.*

E.D. Va. 1995 Claimants sustained personal injuries when ships collided. In an admiralty action, court had to determine the extent of probable injuries sustained by the claimants. The court observed that a treating physician had referred one of the claimants for tests to a facility in which the physician had a substantial ownership interest. In finding that these tests and procedures were unnecessary and unreasonable, the court quoted Opinion 8.032. *In re Capt. Wool, Inc., 1995 US Dist. LEXIS 20128.*

Cal. App. 1967 Physician-stockholders of publicly-owned pharmaceutical corporations and physicians whose medical partnerships owned and operated pharmacies challenged statutory prohibition of physician membership, proprietory interest, and co-ownership of pharmacies. The court quoted Principles Ch. I, Sec. 6 (1947) and a 1960 Judicial Council rule, later included in Opinions and Reports of the Judicial Council Sec. 7, Para. 38 (1965) [now Opinions 8.03, 8.032 and 8.06] in its discussion of the potential conflict of interest created by such ownership. The court held that the statute prohibited physician partnerships from directly owning pharmacies, but did not apply to an individual physician or a partnership of physicians who own stock in a corporation which owns and operates a pharmacy. *Magan Medical Clinic v. California State Bd. of Medical Examiners, 249 Cal. App. 2d 124, 57 Cal. Rptr. 256, 262.*

Mass. Super. 1998 Plaintiff surgeon filed suit against a medical group practice claiming that the defendants reduced referrals to him because he declined to join the group. Plaintiff claimed that the decline harmed his surgical practice. He alleged that the group's practice of taking 10 percent of members' income constituted unethical and illegal kick backs. The court held that the decline in referrals was not connected to plaintiff not being a member of the group. The court also found that the plaintiff had not presented evidence that the decline in referrals harmed his practice. Finally, the court found that the fees paid by members of the group practice were gatekeeper fees rather than referral fees. The court quoted Opinion 6.02, in support of its decision that the defendants' fees did not constitute fee splitting. Further, the court referenced Opinion 8.032 concluding that a self-referral was not necessarily unethical if disclosed to the patient. *Boman v. Southeast Medical Services Group, 1998 WL 1182063, 11-12.*

Mich. Att'y Gen. 1977 State attorney general determined that, within limits, it was not illegal for physicians to refer patient specimens to clinical laboratories which they own or in which they have a financial interest. Opinion observes however that, under the Opinions and Reports of the Judicial Council Sec. 7, Paras. 21 and 22 (1972) [now Opinions 8.03 and 8.032] such referrals may be unethical. *Mich. Att'y Gen. Opinion No. 5229, 1977-78 Att'y. Gen. Op. 234.*

Journal 2002 Suggests a reconceptualization for bioethics that integrates an analysis of the history of moral change. Concludes that bioethical textbooks should include discussion about the history of bioethics and medical ethics. Quotes Opinion 2.20. References Opinions 6.02, 6.03, 6.04 [now Opinion 8.06], and 8.032. Baker, *Bioethics and History,* 27 J. Med. & Phil. 447, 455, 469 (2002).

Journal 2001 Examines issues relating to health care cost containment. Concludes that, if physicians are to meet the goals assigned to them in a cost-constrained health care system, then professional standards must be reevaluated and modified to afford meaningful guidance for clinical decision-making in the face of health care spending controls. Quotes Opinions 2.03, 2.09, 2.095, 8.032, and 9.04. Cites Opinions 8.02, 8.021, 8.051, and 8.13. Agrawal, *Resuscitating Professionalism: Self-Regulation in the Medical Marketplace,* 66 Mo. L. Rev. 341, 354, 355, 360, 361, 378, 388 (2001).

Journal 2001 Considers ethical aspects of physician conflicts of interest in the context of human subjects research. Focuses on conflicts that are associated with clinical trials of new drugs and devices. Concludes by discussing the impact of these conflicts of interest on trust in the physician-patient relationship. References Principle IV and Opinion 8.032. Miller, *Trusting Doctors: Tricky Business When It Comes to Clinical Research,* 81 B.U.L. Rev. 423, 427-28 (2001).

Journal 2000 Examines physician value neutrality (PVN). Defines PVN as providing a foundation to suggest physicians must keep their values—religious, political, or otherwise—out of the patient-physician relationship. Concludes it is not clear how values can be removed from the patient-physician relationship without removing the very thing PVN supporters are trying to protect, the intrinsic value of persons. References Opinions 2.01, 2.02, 8.032, 8.05, 8.08, and 8.132. Beckwith & Peppin, *Physician Value Neutrality: A Critique,* 28 J. L. Med. & Ethics 67, 72-73 (2000).

Journal 2000 Examines justice in health care by focusing on concepts of access and allocation. Presents four principles for the just allocation of health care resources: improving health; informing patients about the manner in which resources are allocated in the context of managed care; affording patients an opportunity to consent to such allocation of resources; and minimization of conflicts of interest. References Opinion 8.032. Emanuel, *Justice and Managed Care: Four Principles for the Just Allocation of Health Care Resources,* 30 Hastings Center Rep. 8, 16 (May/June 2000).

Journal 2000 Explores the legal, ethical, social, and economic considerations associated with use of new genetic techniques in the prediction and diagnosis of Alzheimer Disease. Outlines the potential responsibilities and liabilities of physicians in connection with use of these techniques. References Opinions 2.132, 2.139, and 8.032. Kapp, *Physicians' Legal Duties Regarding the Use of Genetic Tests to Predict and Diagnose Alzheimer Disease,* 21 J. Legal Med. 445, 456-57, 465-66 (2000).

Journal 2000 Compares the changes in physician roles in Japan and the United States that exacerbate their conflicts of interest. Examines American physicians' dispensing practices and relations with pharmaceutical firms and hospital ownership. Concludes the United States is reducing one of the main strengths it had in addressing physician conflicts: institutions of countervailing power and countervailing incentives. References Opinions 8.032 and 8.061, Rodwin & Okamoto, *Physicians' Conflicts of Interest in Japan and the United States: Lessons for the United States,* 25 J. Health Pol. Pol'y & L. 343, 355, 358 (2000).

Journal 1999 Discusses issues surrounding ambulatory surgical centers. Focuses on self-referral laws, the federal antikickback statute, and tax issues. Outlines legal requirements pertaining to ambulatory surgical centers. Cites Opinion 8.032. DeMuro, *A Review of Key Legal Requirements Affecting Ambulatory Surgical Centers,* 11 Health Law. 1, 7 (1999).

Journal 1999 Explores the increased push toward mandatory disclosure laws regarding financial incentives imposed by managed care organizations. Discusses current laws and ethical guidelines.

Emphasizes that efforts to mandate disclosure force physicians to focus on the effects of imposed incentives and the essence of the physician-patient relationship. References Opinions 8.032, 8.13, and 8.132. Miller & Sage, *Disclosing Physician Financial Incentives*, 281 JAMA 1424, 1425 (1999).

Journal 1999 Discusses the practice of physicians using nonpublic information to invest in stocks. Provides guidelines on insider trading laws for physicians. Observes that insider trading damages the public perception of the medical profession. References Opinion 8.032. Prentice, *Clinical Trial Results, Physicians, and Insider Trading*, 20 J. Legal Med. 195, 221 (1999).

Journal 1999 Discusses the push to mandate disclosure in managed care programs. Explains the dangers of disclosing too much information. Provides objectives and goals for disclosure. Quotes Opinion 8.051. References Opinions 8.032 and 8.13. Sage, *Regulating Through Information: Disclosure Laws and American Health Care*, 99 Colum. L. Rev. 1701, 1753, 1758, 1760 (1999).

Journal 1999 Explores the impact managed care organizations have had on health care. Explains that patients may not understand restrictions and incentives imposed by their managed care organizations when entering the program. Argues that such information should be disclosed at various times during the period of plan coverage. Cites Opinions 2.03, 8.03, 8.032, 8.051, 8.13 and 8.132. Wolf, *Toward a Systemic Theory of Informed Consent in Managed Care*, 35 Hous. L. Rev. 1631, 1641, 1658, 1661, 1662, 1679 (1999).

Journal 1998 Discusses conflicts of interest in the physician-patient relationship arising out of use of financial incentives by managed care organizations. Considers how such conflicts are dealt with in the attorney-client relationship. Suggests that a financial incentive should be legally denounced if it unreasonably interferes with a physician's duty to properly care for and treat patients. Quotes Preamble, Fundamental Elements (1) [now Opinion 10.01] and Opinions 4.04, 5.01, 8.03, 8.13, and 9.06. Cites Fundamental Elements (4) [now Opinion 10.01] and Opinions 2.07, 2.08, and 2.132. Hall, *Third-Party Payor Conflicts of Interest in Managed Care: A Proposal for Regulation Based on the Model Rules of Professional Conduct*, 29 Seton Hall L. Rev. 95, 96, 107, 108, 109, 110, 111, 112, 134, 135, 136 (1998).

Journal 1997 Discusses the quality of neurological care and the ethical conflicts that are created by the drive to contain costs. Focuses on quality management and cost-containment programs and the conflicts created when neurologists attempt to reconcile the interests of patients and society. References Opinions 8.032 and 8.13. Bernat, *Quality of Neurological Care: Balancing Cost Control and Ethics*, 54 Arch. Neurol. 1341, 1343, 1345 (1997).

Journal 1995 Examines the metaphor of physicians as fiduciaries. Considers how the law holds physicians accountable in this regard. Quotes Preamble. Cites Opinion 8.03 (1986) [now Opinion 8.032]. Rodwin, *Strains in the Fiduciary Metaphor: Divided Physician Loyalties and Obligations in a Changing Health Care System*, XXI Am. J. Law & Med. 241, 246, 250 (1995).

Journal 1993 Argues that legislative efforts to curb or prohibit physician investment and self-referral are misdirected. Proposes a more effective solution to this problem: enforcement of existing laws. Quotes Opinion 8.032. Morreim, *Blessed Be the Tie That Binds? Antitrust Perils of Physician Investment and Self-Referral*, 14 J. Legal Med. 359, 367, 374, 377, 394, 409 (1993).

Journal 1993 Examines financial conflicts of interest involving physicians. Discusses ways to identify conflicts and possible remedies. References Opinion 8.032. Thompson, *Understanding Financial Conflicts of Interest*, 329 New Eng. J. Med. 573 (1993).

Journal 1992 Discusses the safe harbor regulations under the Medicare and Medicaid Antikickback Statute; examines the *Hanlester Network* case; and describes the problem of physician self-referral. Concludes that a societal consensus is evolving against self-referral. References Opinion 8.032. Crane, *The Problem of Physician Self-Referral Under the Medicare and Medicaid Antikickback Statute: The Hanlester Network Case and the Safe Harbor Regulation*, 268 JAMA 85, 89, 90 (1992).

Journal 1992 Analyzes the Medicare Antifraud Statute and the safe harbor regulations in light of recent criticisms. Concludes that the antifraud statute is an appropriate way to deal with fraud, but that other steps also should be taken. References Opinion 8.032. Farley, *The Medicare Antifraud Statute and Safe Harbor Regulations: Suggestions for Change*, 81 Georgetown L.J. 167, 184 (1992).

Journal 1992 Examines issues related to the responsibility of HIV-infected health care workers protect patients from infection, including mandatory testing, disclosure to co-workers and supervisors, and the degree to which the practice of an HIV-infected health care worker should be modified. Concludes that courts likely will impose a requirement to disclose HIV-positive status to patients when there is a substantial risk of HIV transmission. Quotes Opinions 8.03 (1989) [now Opinion 8.032], and 8.07 (1989) [now Opinion 8.03]. References Opinion 9.131. Lieberman & Derse, *HIV-Positive Health Care Workers and the Obligation to Disclose: Do Patients Have a Right to Know?, 13 J. Legal Med. 333, 353, 354 (1992).*

Journal 1992 Examines a memorandum issued by the Chief Counsel of the Internal Revenue Service, which clearly identified certain transactions that could jeopardize the tax exempt status of hospitals. Concludes that the memorandum provides valuable guidance for hospitals in spite of its shortcomings. References Opinion 8.032. Mancino, *New GCM Suggests Rules for Ventures Between Nonprofit Hospitals and Doctors, 76 J. Taxation 164, 167 (1992).*

Journal 1992 Analyzes the controversy over physician ownership of health care facilities. Considers a study of physician joint ventures in Florida and finds that current legislation prohibiting or restricting such arrangements is inadequate. Quotes Opinion 8.032. Mitchell & Scott, *Evidence on Complex Structures of Physician Joint Ventures, 9 Yale J. Regulation 489, 503 (1992).*

Journal 1992 Discusses the problem of physician joint ventures and examines their prevalence in Florida. Concludes that these arrangements may cause physicians to prioritize economic incentives over patients' medical needs. References Opinion 8.032. Mitchell & Scott, *New Evidence of the Prevalence and Scope of Physician Joint Ventures, 268 JAMA 80, 84 (1992).*

Journal 1992 Examines the issue of physician joint ventures in the context of physical therapy and rehabilitation services. Finds that facility utilization, patient cost, and physician profits were higher at joint venture facilities. References Opinion 8.032. Mitchell & Scott, *Physician Ownership of Physical Therapy Services: Effects on Charges, Utilization, Profits, and Service Characteristics, 268 JAMA 2055, 2058 (1992).*

Journal 1992 Presents results of a study indicating that joint ventures in radiation therapy increase the use and cost of these services and reduce access to care in inner city and rural areas. Concludes that physician joint ventures have negative consequences and proposes that carefully crafted legislation be enacted to ban such arrangements. Quotes Opinion 8.032. Mitchell & Sunshine, *Consequences of Physicians' Ownership of Health Care Facilities—Joint Ventures in Radiation Therapy, 327 New Eng. J. Med. 1497, 1500 (1992).*

Journal 1992 Examines the debate regarding physician self-referral. Argues in favor of the AMA's statement in general, but urges an even stronger and more comprehensive position in this context. References Opinion 8.032. Relman, *"Self-Referral"—What's at Stake?, 327 New Eng. J. Med. 1522, 1524 (1992).*

Journal 1992 Explores the problem of physician self-referral and overuse of physician-owned facilities. Concludes that in cases studied, physician ownership of a facility increased the use and cost of services. Quotes Opinion 8.032. Swedlow, Johnson, Smithline, & Milstein, *Increased Costs and Rates of Use in the California Workers' Compensation System as a Result of Self-Referral By Physicians, 327 New Eng. J. Med. 1502 (1992).*

Journal 1991 Looks at the physician as a fiduciary and the law governing fiduciary relationships. Concludes that fiduciary concepts are a valuable basis for establishing ethical and legal guidelines for physician behavior. Quotes Opinions 2.19, 8.03 (1989) [now Opinion 8.032], and 8.06. Healey & Dowling, *Controlling Conflicts of Interest in the Doctor-Patient Relationship: Lessons From Moore v. Regents of the University of California, 42 Mercer L. Rev. 989, 997, 998 (1991).*

Journal 1991 Discusses the issue of HIV-infected surgeons in light of the New Jersey case decision in *Behringer v. Medical Center.* Considers future developments. References Opinions 8.032 and 9.131. Orentlicher, *HIV-Infected Surgeons: Behringer v. Medical Center, 266 JAMA 1134, 1136 (1991).*

Journal 1990 Discusses efforts of third-party payors to control health care expenditures for beneficiaries. Concludes that financial incentives to limit care and other cost control techniques should be disclosed and that the rationale for such disclosure is compelling. Quotes Opinions 2.03, 2.09, and 8.03 [now Opinions 8.03 and 8.032]. Cites Opinions 2.19, 4.04, and 4.06. Hirshfeld, *Should Third Party Payors of Health Care Services Disclose Cost Control Mechanisms to Potential Beneficiaries?, 14 Seton Hall Legis. J. 115, 130, 131, 144, 145, 146 (1990).*

Journal 1990 Examines various cost control mechanisms utilized by prepaid health plans and other managed care programs and considers the impact of such mechanisms on clinical decision making. Emphasis is placed on the possible existence of conflicts of interest on the part of health care providers in this context. Quotes Opinions 8.03 [now Opinions 8.03 and 8.032] and 8.13 [now Opinion 8.132]. Hirshfeld, *Defining Full and Fair Disclosure in Managed Care Contracts*, 60 The Citation 67, 70 (1990).

Journal 1990 Balances the "laissez-faire" concerns of individual freedom and personal choice with the "Prohibitionists" desire to protect patients from poor quality care and unnecessary referrals. Concludes that civil remedies should be emphasized by extending the doctrines of "bad faith" and "breach of contract" into this arena. References Opinion 8.032. Morreim, *Physician Investment and Self-Referral: Philosophical Analysis of a Contentious Debate*, 15 J. Med. & Phil. 425, 428, 429, 430, 431 (1990).

Journal 1985 Initially describes how existing doctrines protect the value of autonomy in the context of the physician-patient relationship, then examines various problems in the current protective scheme. Concludes by recommending the creation of an independent articulable protected interest in patient autonomy. Quotes Principles II and IV. Cites Opinions 4.04 (1984) [now Opinions 8.03 and 8.032] and 6.03 (1984) [now Opinion 6.02]. Shultz, *From Informed Consent to Patient Choice: A New Protected Interest*, 95 Yale L. J. 219, 275 (1985).

Clarification of Opinion 8.032, "Conflicts of Interest: Health Facility Ownership by a Physician"

(1) **If physicians who share office space want to share a clinical lab, may they refer their patients there?**

The Council does not view self-referral to a shared clinical lab as inappropriate when the facility is a true extension of the physician's practice. Thus, the Council's guidelines permit two or more solo practicing physicians to share a clinical laboratory to avoid duplication and limit overhead costs, as long as several conditions are met: (a) the physicians have office space in the same building or complex where the laboratory is located, (b) the laboratory is not a separate corporate entity, (c) the physicians actively supervise the testing provided by the laboratory, (d) the physicians are equally responsible for the actions of the laboratory or are responsible for the services to their patients, (e) the laboratory provides services only for patients of the physicians, (f) all testing is performed on site, and (g) all services are billed by the ordering physician under that physician's provider number. While self-referral to shared clinical laboratories is permissible, there is still an obligation to comply with the Council's guidelines in Opinion 8.032, "Conflicts of Interest: Health Facility Ownership by a Physician."

(2) **May a physician refer patients to an outside pharmacy if the physician has a financial interest in the pharmacy?**

A pharmacy is a health care facility for the purposes of the Council's guidelines. Hence, when a physician has a financial interest in a pharmacy, it is inappropriate to refer patients to the pharmacy unless the demonstrated need or direct provision of care requirements of the Council's guidelines are met. (Opinion 8.06, "Prescribing and Dispensing Drugs and Devices.")

(3) **May physicians self-refer patients to outside physical therapy facilities, optical shops, or other health care facilities if they directly provide or supervise the care or services provided there?**

Physicians may self-refer to an outside facility if they directly provide care at that facility. For instance, a surgeon may operate at an ambulatory surgical facility in which the surgeon has an investment interest. In general, the provision of care is "direct" only if it entails the personal, hands-on involvement of the physician on site when care is being provided to the patient.

The physician need not be present the entire time on every visit of a patient's care. However, the physician must be participating in the patient's care on site for a significant percentage of visits and a significant portion of the time during which services are rendered. The appropriate degree of physician involvement is a medical decision that will vary according to patients' needs, making it difficult to give explicit guidelines in this area. Sometimes, physician participation will be required every third episode of patient care; for other cases, every sixth visit would be adequate. However, the Council feels that physicians who directly provide care to the patient on site at least every fourth patient visit may confidently be considered to have fulfilled the direct provision of care requirement, though there will be many patients for whom more or less on-site physician care will be medically indicated.

(4) May physicians self-refer patients to an outside home infusion company or dialysis center if they continue to be responsible for the management of the patient's case?

Continuing responsibility for the patient's overall course of treatment does not necessarily mean that the physician is actively involved in the care provided to the patient by the home infusion company or dialysis center. In home infusion, for instance, the physician directly provides care only if he or she regularly travels to the patients' homes and is personally involved in the patient's care. In a dialysis center, the physician directly provides care only if he or she is personally involved in the dialysis treatment. As discussed in question 3, the physician need not be on site during the entire time that care is being delivered or during every administration of care. However, there has to be significant on-site involvement.

(5) If physicians are part owners of a hospital, may they refer patients to a physical therapy facility, laboratory, or MRI located within that hospital?

A physician may refer an inpatient to needed hospital-based facilities, as long as the physician is providing care to the patient in the hospital. However, for outpatients seen in the physician's office practice, hospital-based facilities are no different from the other outside facilities the physician may own. Thus, referral of outpatients to a hospital-based facility in which the physician has an ownership interest is inappropriate self-referral, unless it meets the demonstrated need or direct provision of care requirements.

Furthermore, physicians with an ownership interest in a hospital may admit their own patients there, but only if they continue to directly provide care to those patients while the patients are in the hospital. Physicians may not admit patients to a hospital in which they have an ownership interest if the patients' care will be turned over to other members of the hospital's staff, unless the hospital meets a demonstrated need in the community.

(6) May physicians refer patients to physical therapists or opticians they employ if they are located next door to the physicians' offices, or within the same office building?

If physicians employ therapists, opticians, or other allied professionals as part of their practice, then they can have their patients see the allied professionals, regardless of the allied professions' physical location. However, if the allied professional is employed by a physical therapy facility, optical shop, or other health care facility in which the physician has an investment interest, but which is legally separate from the physician's practice, then self-referral is generally not appropriate unless the facility meets the demonstrated need or direct provision of care requirements.

(7) If a group of physicians owns some vacant office space next door to their own group practice, may they lease that space to an independent physical therapist or optician and refer their patients there?

This would be acceptable as long as the office space is leased at its fair market value, and the amount of rent paid is not tied to the profits of the facility.

(8) If a physician serves as the medical director of his or her own outside health care facility, does this constitute the direct provision of care at that facility?

The position of "Medical Director" of a facility does not in itself necessarily mean that the physician is directly involved in the care or services there. For instance, providing only administrative duties or serving as a figurehead or spokesperson for the facility would not constitute the direct provision of care or services. The relevant factor is the physician's activity, not his or her title.

(9) If the physician-owned facility can provide higher quality services to patients at a lower price than competitors, does this indicate that the facility meets a demonstrated need in the community, thereby allowing the physician-owners to refer their own patients there?

When existing facilities do not provide medically appropriate services, this demonstrates a need for the facility in the community that is strong enough to justify self-referral. For instance, if the quality of services provided by competing facilities is so poor that they cannot be considered adequate, or competitors charge substantially higher fees than the physician-owned facility, then a demonstrated need for the physician-owned facility may exist. However, the advantages of the physician-owned facility for patients must be truly substantial; a demonstrated need would not exist if the differences in quality and price were only marginal. Moreover, the builder of the facility would still have to show that alternative financing for the facility was unavailable.

(10) If physicians start their own outside facility in response to a demonstrated need in the community, and then some years later a few competitors enter the market, are the physicians obligated to divest from their own facility?

Yes. The risks inherent in self-referral require divestment when the need for self-referral no longer exists. However, physicians who invested in facilities to meet a demonstrated need in the community should not be damaged by the requirement to later divest. If the investor were able to recover his or her original investment, plus a reasonable rate of return, there would appear to be no loss or hardship. The Council expects that, generally, physicians can fully divest within three years after the entry of competitors into the market. In the meantime, there is still an obligation to comply with the Council's guidelines in Opinion 8.032, "Conflicts of Interest: Health Facility Ownership by a Physician."

Issued June 1993 as "Addendum I: Council on Ethical and Judicial Affairs Clarification of Self-Referral (E-8.032)."

Updated June 2004.

8.035 Conflicts of Interest in Home Health Care

Physicians who refer patients to home care providers or any other outside facility should avoid possible conflicts of interest by not accepting payment from those providers or facilities for referrals or as compensation for their cognitive services in prescribing, monitoring, or revising a patient's course of treatment. Payment for these cognitive services is acceptable when it comes from patients who are the beneficiaries of the physician's services, or from the patients' designated third-party payers.

In accordance with Opinion 8.032, "Conflicts of Interest: Health Facility Ownership by a Physician," physicians may refer patients to home care facilities in which they have an ownership interest if they actively participate on-site in the care provided to patients. Since the appropriate frequency and duration of home visits is a medical decision that should be made on a case-by-case basis, there is no specific minimum number of home visits that may be identified as a conclusive test of the physician's involvement in the patient's home care regimen. Although different patients will have different needs, physicians who directly provide care in the patient's home on at least every fourth visit may presumptively be considered to have made home care a true extension of practice. (II, III, IV)

Issued June 1994 based on the report "Conflicts of Interest: Update on Home Care," adopted December 1993.

Updated 1998.

189

8.04 Consultation

Physicians should obtain consultation whenever they believe that it would be medically indicated in the care of the patient or when requested by the patient or the patient's representative. When a patient is referred to a consultant, the referring physician should provide a history of the case and such other information as the consultant may need, calling to the attention of the consultant any specific questions about which guidance is sought, and the consultant should advise the referring physician of the results of the consultant's examination and recommendations. (V)

Issued prior to April 1977.

Updated June 1992 and June 1996.

D.S.C. 1968 Military dependent sued government physicians under Federal Tort Claims Act where child with acute abdominal pain was twice referred to naval hospital with diagnosis of possible appendicitis and twice sent home without treatment, eventually suffering ruptured appendix and serious complications. In finding for the plaintiff, the court quoted Principle 8 (1957) [now Principle V and Opinion 8.04] in considering whether the physicians had a duty to seek consultation in such a situation. *Steeves v. United States, 294 F. Supp. 446, 454.*

Wash. 1951 Plaintiff, a charitable, not for profit medical corporation, offered prepaid health care services to members and their families. Suit was filed against county medical society and others for damages and injunction for defendants' alleged efforts to monopolize prepaid medical care in area and unlawfully restrain competition by plaintiff and its physicians. Defendants alleged as affirmative defense that their efforts were designed to curb unethical prepaid contract practice by plaintiff. Court examined at length American Medical Association's position regarding contract practice including Principles Ch. III, Art. VI, Secs. 3 and 4 (1947) [now Principle VI and Opinions 8.05 and 9.06] concluding nothing in plaintiff's practice violated the Association's ethical guidelines. Further, quoting Principles Ch. III, Art. III, Sec.1 (1947) [now Opinion 8.04] dealing with consultations, court noted that defendants' efforts impeded plaintiff's physicians from obtaining consultations. Court concluded defendants' actions constituted unlawful, monopolistic behavior and issued an injunction, although it declined to award damages. *Group Health Coop. v. King County Medical Soc'y, 39 Wash. 2d 586, 237 P.2d 737, 744, 750-51, 759-60.*

Journal 1998 Examines mechanisms of oversight for expert witness testimony by medical, legal, legislative, and regulatory agencies. Points out that the amount of malpractice litigation will increase the need for medical expert witnesses. Concludes that improvements in this context must uphold principles of due process and be acceptable to the medical and legal communities. Cites Opinions 6.01, 8.04, and 9.07. McAbee, *Improper Expert Medical Testimony: Existing and Proposed Mechanisms of Oversight, 19 J. Legal Med. 257, 265 (1998).*

Journal 1994 Focuses on physicians' legal and ethical duties to pregnant women to provide medical information relevant to patient choice regarding abortion and to make referrals for services that physicians are unable or unwilling to perform. Concludes that medical educators, professional associations, women's groups, and state legislatures should address these issues. Cites Opinions 3.04 and 8.04. Law, *Silent No More: Physicians' Legal and Ethical Obligations to Patients Seeking Abortions, 21 N.Y.U. Rev. L. & Soc. Change 279, 289, 290, 300 (1994).*

8.041 Second Opinions

Physicians should recommend that a patient obtain a second opinion whenever they believe it would be helpful in the care of the patient. When recommending a second opinion, physicians should explain the reasons for the recommendation and inform their patients that patients are free to choose a second-opinion physician on their own or with the assistance of the first physician. Patients are also free to obtain second opinions on their own initiative, with or without their physician's knowledge.

With the patient's consent, the first physician should provide a history of the case and such other information as the second-opinion physician may need, including the recommendations about management. The second-opinion physician should maintain the confidentiality of the evaluation and should report to the first physician if the consent of the patient has been obtained.

After evaluating the patient, a second-opinion physician should provide the patient with a clear understanding of the opinion, whether or not it agrees with the recommendations of the first physician.

When a patient initiates a second opinion, it is inappropriate for the primary physician to terminate the patient-physician relationship solely because of the patient's decision to obtain a second opinion.

In some cases, patients may ask the second-opinion physician to provide the needed medical care. In general, second-opinion physicians are free to assume responsibility for the care of the patient. It is not unethical to enter into a patient-physician relationship with a patient who has been receiving care from another physician. By accepting second-opinion patients for treatment, physicians affirm the right of patients to have free choice in the selection of their physicians.

There are situations in which physicians may choose not to treat patients for whom they provide second opinions. Physicians may decide not to treat the patient in order to avoid any perceived conflict of interest or loss of objectivity in rendering the requested second opinion. However, the concern about conflicts of interest does not require physicians to decline to treat second-opinion patients. This inherent conflict in the practice of medicine is resolved by the responsible exercise of professional judgment.

Physicians may agree not to treat second-opinion patients as part of their arrangements with insurers or other third party payers. Physicians who enter into such contractual agreements must honor their commitments.

Physicians must decide independently of their colleagues whether to treat second-opinion patients. Physicians may not establish an agreement or understanding among themselves that they will refuse to treat each others' patients when asked to provide a second opinion. Such agreements compromise the ability of patients to receive care from the physicians of their choice and are therefore not only unethical but also unlawful. (IV, V)

Issued June 1992.

Updated June 1996.

8.043   Ethical Implications of Surgical Co-Management

For the purpose of this report, the term "surgical co-management" refers to the practice of allotting specific responsibilities of patient care to designated caregivers. The following guidelines stem from this understanding:

(1) Physicians should engage in co-management arrangements only to assure the highest quality of care.

(2) When surgical co-management arrangements are made between duly licensed physicians, their responsibilities should be delineated according

to the scope of the physicians' expertise. Likewise, when physicians enter into surgical co-management arrangements with allied health professionals, each caregiver's responsibility should correspond to his or her qualifications.

(3) Even though different caregivers will be responsible for rendering specific portions of the patient's care, a single physician should be ultimately responsible for ensuring that the care is delivered in a coordinated and appropriate manner. Other caregivers should support this obligation by communicating with this physician.

(4) The treating physicians are responsible for ensuring that the patient has consented not only to take part in the surgical co-management arrangement but also to the services that will be provided within the arrangement. In addition to disclosing medical facts to the patient, the patient should also be informed of other significant aspects of the surgical co-management arrangement such as the credentials of the other caregivers, the specific services each will provide, and the billing arrangement.

(5) Physicians should ensure that their surgical co-management arrangements do not violate the ethical or legal restrictions on self-referral.

(6) Referrals to another caregiver should be based only on that caregiver's skill and ability to meet the patient's needs and not on expected further referrals or other self-serving bases. Physicians who participate in surgical co-management arrangements must avoid such financial agreements as fee-splitting, which are both unethical and illegal.

Physicians who participate in surgical co-management arrangements should employ appropriate safeguards to ensure that confidential information is protected. (I, II, IV, V, VI)

Issued June 2000 based on the report "Ethical Implications of Surgical Co-Management," adopted December 1999.

8.05   Contractual Relationships

The contractual relationships that physicians assume when they join or affiliate with group practices or agree to provide services to the patients of an insurance plan are varied.

Income arrangements may include hourly wages for physicians working part time, annual salaries for those working full time, and share of group income for physicians who are partners in groups that are somewhat autonomous and contract with plans to provide the required medical care. Arrangements also usually include a range of fringe benefits, such as paid vacations, insurance, and pension plans.

Physicians may work directly for plans or may be employed by the medical group or the hospital that has contracted with the plan to provide services. In the operation of such plans, physicians should not be subjected to lay interference in professional medical matters and their primary responsibility should be to the patients they serve. (VI)

Issued prior to April 1977.

Updated June 1994 and June 1996.

1st Cir. 1984 Plaintiff-physicians sued defendant-insurer, alleging defendant's ban on balance billing practice violated antitrust law. That practice required defendant to pay the physicians treating defendant's insureds only if the physicians agreed not to make any additional charges to the insureds. In holding that defendant's billing practice did not violate antitrust law, the court noted in passing a 1954 law journal article that cited, with an incorrect reference, Principles Ch. III, Art. VI, Sec. 3 (1947) in arguing that selling services to third parties . . . might interfere with the absolute ethical obligation that a doctor owes to the patient. The specific concept treated by this Principle is no longer directly treated although Opinion 8.05 reflects similar concerns. *Kartell v. Blue Shield of Mass., Inc., 749 F.2d 922, 926, cert. denied, 471 US 1029 (1985).*

2d Cir. 1980 Federal Trade Commission ordered American Medical Association and others to cease, with some exceptions, imposing restraints on advertising and contract practice by physicians, as well as on business relations between physicians and laypersons. Commission found restraints violated 15 U.S.C. Sec. 45(a)(1). See 94 F.T.C. 701 (1979). Association petitioned for judicial review of Commission's order. Court reviewed order, noting specific ethical pronouncements of Association which Commission found improper, including the following: restrictions upon advertising and solicitation, Principle 5 (1957) and Opinions and Reports of the Judicial Council Sec. 5, Para. 11 (1971) [now Opinion 5.02]; restrictions on contract practice, Principle 6 (1957) and Opinions and Reports of the Judicial Council Sec. 6, Paras. 3, 4, and 5 (1971) [now Opinion 8.05]; and restrictions on business organizations and relations with laypersons, Opinions and Reports of the Judicial Council Sec. 6, Paras. 14 and 15 (1971). Court rejected Association's argument that its ethical rules did not provide impetus for local and state medical societies to act against physicians violating its rules. Further, court rejected Association's position that liability should be precluded because of revisions in the Opinions in 1977 and the Principles in 1980. Specifically, the court found that removal of the ban on patient solicitation and changes reflected in Principles II and IV (1980) did not render Commission's order moot. The order was therefore enforced with modifications. Dissenting judge, referring to 1980 revisions in Principles and to Opinions and Reports of the Judicial Council 4.05 and 6.00 (1977) [now Opinions 5.02 and 8.05], concluded order should not be enforced on grounds of mootness. *American Medical Ass'n v. FTC, 638 F.2d 443, 446, 446 n.1, 448, 449, 449 n.5, 450, 451, 455-57, aff'd, 455 US 676 (1982).*

7th Cir. 1984 Plaintiff brought medical malpractice suit against several physicians appointed to the Veterans Administration Department of Medicine and Surgery. The court held that strict control test for determining whether defendants ought to be considered employees or independent contractors under the Federal Tort Claims Act was not appropriate because the ethical obligation of a physician to a patient, evidenced by Principle 6 (1957) [now Opinions 8.03 and 8.05], required that independent judgment be exercised, preventing a physician from being strictly controlled by the Veterans Administration. *Quilico v. Kaplan, 749 F.2d 480, 483-84.*

10th Cir. 1983 Pursuant to the Federal Tort Claims Act, plaintiff sued the federal government for the negligence of a neurosurgeon, allegedly an employee of a Veteran's Administration hospital. Plaintiff argued that applying the traditional control test to determine a physician's employment status was inappropriate because physicians are bound by Principle 6 (1957) [now Opinions 8.03 and 8.05] requiring them to have free and complete exercise of [their] medical judgment and skill.... However, the court did not reach the merits of that argument because the contractual agreement between the neurosurgeon and the VA hospital was outside the parameters of an employer-employee relationship with the government, thus precluding plaintiff's claim. *Lurch v. United States, 719 F.2d 333, 337, cert. denied, 466 US 927. (1984).*

D.C. Cir. 1942 Medical associations appealed conviction on charges of conspiracy to restrain trade or commerce where associations attempted to prevent competition by elimination of prepaid, low cost medical and hospital care. Principles Ch. III, Art. VI, Secs. 2 and 3 [now Opinion 8.05] limiting contract practice had been used as a basis to discipline members of medical association employed by prepaid medical organization. The court held that the associations were subject to the Sherman Antitrust Act and that the evidence sustained the conviction. *American Medical Ass'n v. United States, 130 F.2d 233, 238-239 n.23, aff'd, 317 US 519 (1943).*

Miss. 2003 Patient's estate appealed summary judgment in favor of physician and hospital in wrongful death action. Supreme court affirmed, holding that physician was a state employee and that purchase of liability insurance did not waive immunity. In examining physician's status, the court found that the exercise of professional judgment and discretion are not determinative of employment status. Quotes Principle 6 (1957) [now Opinions 8.03 and 8.05]. *Corey v. Skelton, 834 So.2d 681, 685.*

Miss. 2002 Plaintiff in malpractice action appealed grant of summary judgment in favor of neurosurgeon who allegedly performed a thoracic diskectomy on the wrong disc. A resident performed the patient's physical and wrote the majority of the chart notes. The Mississippi Supreme Court affirmed the lower court. The court held that as a state employee the physician was immune from liability and that his exercise of professional judgment in treating patients did not change his status and insurance did not waive immunity. Quotes Principle 6 (1957) [now Opinions 8.03 and 8.05]. *Clayton v. Harkey, 826 So.2d 1283, 1287.*

Miss. 2001 Patient filed suit asserting that a physician was negligent in performing surgery. The trial court granted the physician's summary judgment motion and held that the physician, employed by a state university medical center, was immune under state law. Finding genuine issues of fact, the state supreme court reversed and remanded the case for further proceedings. In a separate opinion, one justice quoted Principle 6 (1957) [now Opinions 8.03 and 8.05], in evaluating the degree of control exercised by the state over the physician. This justice, stressing that the physician exercised discretion in treating the patient independent of the state's control, found no basis to hold the physician an employee for immunity purposes. *Conley v. Warren, 797 So. 2d 881, 886.*

Miss. 2000 Beneficiaries of patient's estate appealed summary judgment in malpractice action for a physician on sovereign immunity grounds. The court reversed and remanded the case finding issues of fact to be resolved at trial. The majority set out a five part test to determine the employment status of a physician working at a state healthcare facility, including the degree of control and direction exercised by the state over the physician. In a separate opinion one justice quoted Principle 6 (1957) [now Opinion 8.03 and 8.05], stating that, "A physician should not dispose of his services under terms or conditions which tend to interfere with or impair the free and complete exercise of his medical judgment and skill…." This justice reasoned that the physician could not claim the state controlled his medical discretion or treatment of patients and thus was clearly not an employee entitled to immunity. *Miller v. Meeks, 762 So. 2d 302, 314.*

Miss. 2000 Patient brought a medical malpractice action against physicians after receiving treatment at a state university medical center. The jury returned a verdict against the physicians. The Mississippi Supreme Court reversed, finding that the physicians were immune from liability as state employees. In determining the status of the physicians, the court noted that the physicians retained a considerable amount of professional discretion in treating the patient, quoting Principle 6 (1957) [now Opinions 8.03 and 8.05]. However, this alone was not determinative, and in the court's view the physicians were state employees. *Sullivan v. Washington, 768 So. 2d 881, 885.*

Miss. App. 2003 Patient brought malpractice action against physicians working at a state university teaching hospital. Patient argued that the physicians were independent contractors and sovereign immunity did not apply. Appellate court, citing the Mississippi Supreme Court's decision in *Miller v. Mecks, 762 So.2d 302 (Miss. 2000),* affirmed the trial court and held that sovereign immunity applied because the physicians were state employees. Quotes Principle 6 (1957) [now Opinions 8.03 and 8.05]. *Brown v. Warren, 858 So.2d 168, 175 (2003).*

Wash. 1951 Plaintiff, a charitable, not for profit medical corporation, offered prepaid health care services to members and their families. Suit was filed against county medical society and others for damages and injunction for defendants' alleged efforts to monopolize prepaid medical care in area and unlawfully restrain competition by plaintiff and its physicians. Defendants alleged as affirmative defense that their efforts were designed to curb unethical prepaid contract practice by plaintiff. Court examined at length American Medical Association's position regarding contract practice including Principles Ch. III, Art. VI, Secs. 3 and 4 (1947) [now Principle VI and Opinions 8.05 and 9.06] concluding nothing in plaintiff's practice violated the Association's ethical guidelines. Further, quoting Principles Ch. III, Art. III, Sec. 1 (1947) [now Opinion 8.04] dealing with consultations, court noted that defendants' efforts impeded plaintiff's physicians from obtaining consultations. Court concluded defendants' actions constituted unlawful, monopolistic behavior and issued an injunction, although it declined to award damages. *Group Health Coop. v. King County Medical Soc'y, 39 Wash. 2d 586, 237 P.2d 737, 744, 750-51, 759-60.*

Journal 2001 Discusses the prohibition on non-lawyer ownership of legal service providers. Considers how ethical rules and standards governing physicians have been directed toward preserving independent judgment. Concludes that ethical conflicts created by abandoning the prohibition on non-lawyer ownership of legal service providers may be managed by following the medical ethics model. Quotes Principle VI and Opinions 2.03, 2.09, 8.02, 8.021, 8.03, 8.05, 8.051, 8.054, 8.13, and 8.132. Harris & Foran, *The Ethics of Middle-Class Access to Legal Services* *and What We Can Learn from the Medical Profession's Shift to a Corporate Paradigm, 70 Fordham L. Rev. 775, 817, 821, 822, 823, 824 (2001).*

Journal 2000 Examines physician value neutrality (PVN). Defines PVN as providing a foundation to suggest physicians must keep their values—religious, political, or otherwise—out of the patient-physician relationship. Concludes it is not clear how values can be removed from the patient-physician relationship without removing the very thing PVN supporters are trying to protect, the intrinsic value of persons. References Opinions 2.01, 2.02, 8.032, 8.05, 8.08, and 8.132. Beckwith & Peppin, *Physician Value Neutrality: A Critique, 28 J. L. Med. & Ethics 67*, 72-73 (2000).

Journal 1997 Discusses the practice of physician deselection by managed care organizations. Suggests that deselection harms the physician-patient relationship and creates a conflict of interest. Argues that solutions to deselection should consider effects on the patient rather than on the physician. Quotes Principle III. Cites Principle I and Opinions 8.05 and 8.13. Liner, *Physician Deselection: The Dynamics of a New Threat to the Physician-Patient Relationship, 23 Am. J. Law & Med. 511, 513, 527 (1997).*

8.051   Conflicts of Interest under Capitation

The application of capitation to physicians' practices can result in the provision of cost-effective, quality medical care. It is important to note, however, that the potential for conflict exists under such systems. Physicians who contract with health care plans should attempt to minimize these conflicts and to ensure that capitation is applied in a manner consistent patients' interests.

(1) Physicians have an obligation to evaluate a health plan's capitation payments prior to contracting with that plan to ensure that the quality of patient care is not threatened by inadequate rates of capitation. Physicians should advocate that capitation payments be calculated primarily on the basis of relevant medical factors, available outcomes data, the costs associated with involved providers, and consensus-oriented standards of necessary care. Furthermore, the predictable costs resulting from existing conditions of enrolled patients should be considered when determining the rate of capitation. Different populations of patients have different medical needs and the costs associated with those needs should be reflected in the per member per month payment. Physicians should seek agreements with plans that provide sufficient financial resources for all care that is the physician's obligations to deliver and should refuse to sign agreements that fail in this regard.

(2) Physicians must not assume inordinate levels of financial risk and should therefore consider a number of factors when deciding whether or not to sign a provider agreement. The size of the plan and the time period over which the rate is figured should be considered by physicians evaluating a plan as well as in determinations of the per member per month payment. The capitation rate for large plans can be calculated more accurately than for smaller plans because of the mitigating influence of probability and the behavior of large systems. Similarly, length of time will influence the predictability of the cost of care. Therefore, physicians should advocate for capitation rates calculated for large plans over an extended period of time.

(3) Stop-loss plans can prevent the potential of catastrophic expenses from influencing physician behavior. Physicians should ensure that such arrangements are finalized prior to signing an agreement to provide services in a health plan.

(4) Physicians must be prepared to discuss with patients any financial arrangements which could impact patient care. Physicians should avoid reimbursement systems that, if disclosed to patients, could negatively affect the
patient-physician relationship. (II, III, VI)

Issued December 1997 based on the report "The Ethical Implications of Capitation," adopted
June 1997.

Updated June 2002.

Journal 2003 Discusses conflicts of interest caused when managed care organizations provide
financial incentives to physicians. Concludes that the focus of managed care is not well-suited for
the doctor-patient relationship. Quotes Opinion 8.03. Cites Principle VII. References Opinion
8.051. Hall, *Bargaining with Hippocrates: Managed Care and the Doctor-Patient Relationship*, 54 S.C.
L. Rev. 689, 696, 735 (2003).

Journal 2001 Discusses the prohibition on non-lawyer ownership of legal service providers.
Considers how ethical rules and standards governing physicians have been directed toward preserving independent judgment. Concludes that ethical conflicts created by abandoning the prohibition on non-lawyer ownership of legal service providers may be managed by following the
medical ethics model. Quotes Principle VI and Opinions 2.03, 2.09, 8.02, 8.021, 8.03, 8.05,
8.051, 8.054, 8.13, and 8.132. Harris & Foran, *The Ethics of Middle-Class Access to Legal Services
and What We Can Learn from the Medical Profession's Shift to a Corporate Paradigm*, 70 Fordham L.
Rev. 775, 817, 821, 822, 823, 824 (2001).

Journal 1999 Discusses the push to mandate disclosure in managed care programs. Explains the
dangers of disclosing too much information. Provides objectives and goals for disclosure. Quotes
Opinion 8.051. References Opinions 8.032 and 8.13. Sage, *Regulating Through Information:
Disclosure Laws and American Health Care*, 99 Colum. L. Rev. 1701, 1753, 1758, 1760 (1999).

Journal 1999 Explores the impact managed care organizations have had on health care. Explains
that patients may not understand restrictions and incentives imposed by their managed care organizations when entering the program. Argues that such information should be disclosed at various
times during the period of plan coverage. Cites Opinions 2.03, 8.03, 8.032, 8.051, 8.13 and 8.132.
Wolf, *Toward a Systemic Theory of Informed Consent in Managed Care*, 35 Hous. L. Rev. 1631,
1641, 1658, 1661, 1662, 1679 (1999).

8.052 Negotiating Discounts for Specialty Care

Patients are entitled to all the benefits outlined in their insurance plan.
Therefore, it is unethical for a referring physician to restrict the referral
options of patients who have chosen a plan that provides for access to an
unlimited or broad selection of specialist physicians. It is also unethical to base
the referral of these patients on a discount for the capitated patients in a primary care physician's practice. (II)

Issued December 1997 based on the report "Ethical Issues in Negotiating Discounts for Specialty
Care," adopted June 1996.

The previous Opinion 8.053, "Restrictions on Disclosure in Managed Care
Contracts," issued June 1998, was replaced by the current Opinion 8.053,
"Restrictions on Disclosure in Health Care Plan Contracts."

8.053 Restrictions on Disclosure in Health Care Plan Contracts

Despite ethical requirements demanding full disclosure of treatment options
regardless of limitations imposed by plan coverage, some health care plans

include clauses in their employment contracts that directly inhibit the ability of physicians to keep their patients fully informed. These types of contract clauses erect inappropriate barriers to necessary communications between physicians and patients, labeled "gag clauses" by some observers. Restrictive clauses of this type impact the ability of physicians to provide information to their patients and to act effectively as a patient advocate. They also threaten to undermine individual and public trust in the profession of medicine.

(1) Health care plans have the right to protect proprietary information. However, physicians should oppose any such protection that inhibits them from disclosing relevant information to patients. For this reason, physicians should advocate for the elimination of contract clauses that could prevent them from raising or discussing matters relevant to patients' medical care.

(2) The right of patients to be informed of all pertinent medical information must be reaffirmed by the medical profession, and individual physicians must continue to uphold their ethical obligation to disclose such information.

(3) Physicians, individually or through their representative, should review their contracts carefully to ensure that they are able to fulfill their ethical obligations to patients. (II, III, VI)

Issued June 1998 based on the report "Restrictions on Disclosure in Managed Care Contracts," adopted June 1996.

Updated June 2002.

S.D. Fla. 2001 Insured patients under health care plans sued managed care companies alleging improper nondisclosure of policies and procedures imposing restrictions on physicians' judgment as to appropriate medical treatment. The insureds sued under both the Racketeer Influenced and Corrupt Organizations Act (RICO) and the Employee Retirement Income Security Act (ERISA). The court, with one exception, dismissed without prejudice both the RICO and ERISA claims. Among the plaintiffs' arguments was that the defendants had included "gag clauses" in their physician contracts in violation of Opinion 8.053. *In Re Managed Care Litigation,* *150 F.Supp.2d 1330, 1335.*

Journal 2002 Examines how managed care has adversely affected information disclosure in the physician-patient relationship. Concludes that, unless courts expand applicability of principles of informed consent, patient self-determination and autonomy will continue to be undermined. Quotes Principle VIII and Opinions 8.03, 8.053, 8.054, and 8.08. Morris, *Dissing Disclosure: Just What the Doctor Ordered,* 44 Ariz. L. Rev. 313, 344, 349, 362, 363, 366 (2002).

8.054　Financial Incentives and the Practice of Medicine

In order to achieve the necessary goals of patient care and to protect the role of physicians as advocates for individual patients, the following statement is offered for the guidance of physicians:

(1) Although physicians have an obligation to consider the needs of broader patient populations within the context of the patient-physician relationship, their first duty must be to the individual patient. This obligation must override considerations of the reimbursement mechanism or specific financial incentives applied to a physician's clinical practice.

(2) Physicians, individually or through their representatives, should evaluate the financial incentives associated with participation in a health plan before contracting with that plan. The purpose of the evaluation is to ensure that the quality of patient care is not compromised by unrealistic

expectations for utilization or by placing that physician's payments for care at excessive risk. In the process of making judgments about the ethical propriety of such reimbursement systems, physicians should refer to the following general guidelines:

(a) Monetary incentives may be judged in part on the basis of their size. Large incentives may create conflicts of interest that can in turn compromise clinical objectivity. While an obligation has been established to resolve financial conflicts of interest to the benefit of patients, it is important to recognize that sufficiently large incentives can create an untenable position for physicians,

(b) The proximity of large financial incentives to individual treatment decisions should be limited in order to prevent physicians' personal financial concerns from creating a conflict with their role as individual patient advocates. When the proximity of incentives cannot be mitigated, as in the case of fee-for-service payments, physicians must behave in accordance with prior Council recommendations limiting the potential for abuse. This includes the Council's prohibitions on fee-splitting arrangements, the provision of unnecessary services, unreasonable fees, and self-referral. For incentives that can be distanced from clinical decisions, physicians should consider the following factors in order to evaluate the correlation between individual act and monetary reward or penalty:

(i) In general, physicians should favor incentives that are applied across broad physician groups. This dilutes the effect any one physician can have on his or her financial situation through clinical recommendations, thus allowing physicians to provide those services they feel are necessary in each case. Simultaneously, however, physicians are encouraged by the incentive to practice efficiently.

(ii) The size of the patient pool considered in calculations of incentive payments will affect the proximity of financial motivations to individual treatment decisions. The laws of probability dictate that in large populations of patients, the overall level of utilization remains relatively stable and predictable. Physicians practicing in plans with large numbers of patients in a risk pool therefore have greater freedom to provide the care they feel is necessary based on the likelihood that the needs of other plan patients will balance out decisions to provide extensive care.

(iii) Physicians should advocate for the time period over which incentives are determined to be long enough to accommodate fluctuations in utilization resulting from the random distribution of patients and illnesses. For example, basing incentive payments on an annual analysis of resource utilization is preferable to basing them on monthly review.

(iv) Financial rewards or penalties that are triggered by specific points of utilization may create enormous incentives as a physician's practice approaches the established level. Therefore, physicians should advocate that incentives be calculated on a continuum of utilization rather than a bracketed system with tiers of widely varied bonuses or penalties.

    (v) Physicians should ascertain that a stop-loss plan is in place to prevent the costs associated with unusual outliers from significantly impacting the reward or penalty offered to a physician.

(3) Physicians also should advocate for incentives that promote efficient practice, but are not be designed to realize cost savings beyond those attainable through efficiency. As a counterbalance to the focus on utilization reduction, physicians also should advocate for incentives based on quality of care and patient satisfaction.

(4) Patients must be informed of financial incentives that could impact the level or type of care they receive. Although this responsibility should be assumed by the health plan, physicians, individually or through their representatives, must be prepared to discuss with patients any financial arrangements that could impact patient care. Physicians should avoid reimbursement systems that, if disclosed to patients, could negatively affect the patient-physician relationship. (II, III)

Issued June 1998 based on the report "Financial Incentives and the Practice of Medicine," adopted December 1997.

Updated June 2002

Journal 2002 Examines how managed care has adversely affected information disclosure in the physician-patient relationship. Concludes that, unless courts expand applicability of principles of informed consent, patient self-determination and autonomy will continue to be undermined. Quotes Principle VIII and Opinions 8.03, 8.053, 8.054, and 8.08. Morris, *Dissing Disclosure: Just What the Doctor Ordered, 44 Ariz. L. Rev. 313, 344, 349, 362, 363, 366 (2002).*

Journal 2001 Discusses the prohibition on non-lawyer ownership of legal service providers. Considers how ethical rules and standards governing physicians have been directed toward preserving independent judgment. Concludes that ethical conflicts created by abandoning the prohibition on non-lawyer ownership of legal service providers may be managed by following the medical ethics model. Quotes Principle VI and Opinions 2.03, 2.09, 8.02, 8.021, 8.03, 8.05, 8.051, 8.054, 8.13, and 8.132. Harris & Foran, *The Ethics of Middle-Class Access to Legal Services and What We Can Learn from the Medical Profession's Shift to a Corporate Paradigm, 70 Fordham L. Rev. 775, 817, 821, 822, 823, 824 (2001).*

8.055 Retainer Practices

Individuals are free to select and supplement insurance for their health care on the basis of what appears to them to be an acceptable tradeoff between quality and cost. Retainer contracts, whereby physicians offer special services and amenities (such as longer visits, guaranteed availability by phone or pager, counseling for healthy lifestyles, and various other customized services) to patients who pay additional fees distinct from the cost of medical care, are consistent with pluralism in the delivery and financing of health care. However, they also raise ethical concerns that warrant careful attention, particularly if retainer practices become so widespread as to threaten access to care.

(1) When entering into a retainer contract, both parties must be clear about the terms of the relationship and must agree to them. Physicians must present the terms of the contract in an honest manner, and must not exert

undue pressure on patients to agree to the arrangement. If a physician has knowledge that the patient's health care insurance coverage will be compromised by the retainer contract, the information must be discussed with the patient before reaching an agreement on the terms of the retainer contract. Also, patients must be able to opt out of a retainer contract without undue inconveniences or financial penalties.

(2) Concern for quality of care the patient receives should be the physician's first consideration. However, it is important that a retainer contract not be promoted as a promise for more or better diagnostic and therapeutic services. Physicians must always ensure that medical care is provided only on the basis of scientific evidence, sound medical judgment, relevant professional guidelines, and concern for economic prudence. Physicians who engage in mixed practices, in which some patients have contracted for special services and amenities and others have not, must be particularly diligent to offer the same standard of diagnostic and therapeutic services to both categories of patients. All patients are entitled to courtesy, respect, dignity, responsiveness, and timely attention to their needs.

(3) In accord with medicine's ethical mandate to provide for continuity of care and the ethical imperative that physicians not abandon their patients, physicians converting their traditional practices into retainer practices must facilitate the transfer of their non-participating patients, particularly their sickest and most vulnerable ones, to other physicians. If no other physicians are available to care for non-retainer patients in the local community, the physician may be ethically obligated to continue caring for such patients.

(4) Physicians who enter into retainer contracts will usually receive reimbursement from their patients' health care plans for medical services. Physicians are ethically required to be honest in billing for reimbursement, and must observe relevant laws, rules, and contracts. It is desirable that retainer contracts separate clearly special services and amenities from reimbursable medical services. In the absence of such clarification, identification of reimbursable services should be determined on a case-by-case basis.

(5) Physicians have a professional obligation to provide care to those in need, regardless of ability to pay, particularly to those in need of urgent care. Physicians who engage in retainer practices should seek specific opportunities to fulfill this obligation. (I, II, VI, VIII, IX)

Issued December 2003 based on the report "Retainer Practices," adopted June 2003.

The previous Opinion 8.06, "Drugs and Devices: Prescribing," issued prior to April 1977, was combined with Opinion 6.04, "Fee Splitting: Drug or Device Prescription Rebates," and Opinion 8.07, "Gifts to Physicians: Offers of Indemnity," into the current Opinion 8.06 in June 2002.

8.06 Prescribing and Dispensing Drugs and Devices

(1) Physicians should prescribe drugs, devices, and other treatments based solely upon medical considerations and patient need and reasonable

expectations of the effectiveness of the drug, device or other treatment for the particular patient.

(2) Physicians may not accept any kind of payment or compensation from a drug company or device manufacturer for prescribing its products. Furthermore, physicians should not be influenced in the prescribing of drugs, devices, or appliances by a direct or indirect financial interest in a firm or other supplier, regardless of whether the firm is a manufacturer, distributor, wholesaler, or repackager of the products involved.

(3) Physicians may own or operate a pharmacy, but generally may not refer their patients to the pharmacy. Exceptionally, a physician may refer patients to his or her pharmacy in accord with guidelines established in Opinion 8.032, "Conflicts of Interest: Health Facility Ownership by a Physician." Physicians may dispense drugs within their office practices provided such dispensing primarily benefits the patient.

(4) In all instances, physicians should respect the patient's freedom of choice in selecting who will fill their prescriptions as they are in the choice of a physician and, therefore, have the right to have a prescription filled wherever they wish. (See Opinions 9.06, "Free Choice," and 8.03, "Conflicts of Interest: Guidelines.") Physicians should not urge patients to fill prescriptions from an establishment which has entered into a business or other preferential arrangement with the physician with respect to the filling of the physician's prescriptions.

(5) A third party's offer to indemnify a physician for lawsuits arising from the physician's prescription or use of the third party's drug, device, or other product, introduces inappropriate incentives into medical decision making. Such offers, regardless of their limitations, therefore constitute unacceptable gifts. This does not address contractual assignments of liability between employers or in research arrangements, nor does it address government indemnification plans.

(6) Patients have an ethically and legally recognized right to prompt access to the information contained in their individual medical records. Since a prescription is part of the patient's medical record, the patient is entitled to a copy of the physician's prescription for drugs or devices, including eyeglasses and contact lenses. Therefore, physicians should not discourage patients from requesting a written copy of a prescription. (II, III, IV, V)

Issued June 2002. This opinion is a consolidation of previous Opinions 6.04, "Fee Splitting: Drug or Device Prescription Rebates;" 8.06, "Drugs and Devices: Prescribing;" and 8.07, "Gifts to Physicians: Offers of Indemnity."

E.D. N.Y. 1975 Medical laboratories sought injunction against city's award of exclusive contracts for Medicaid services. The court granted a preliminary injunction and held that the laboratories had a substantial probability of success on the merits of the claim that Medicaid recipients would be deprived of statutory right of free choice of providers. In balancing the equities, the court also noted that the contracts would create an ethical dilemma for physicians who are required to provide patients with free choice of ancillary services under Opinions and Reports of the Judicial Council Sec. 1, Paras. 6 and 14 (1971) [now Opinions 8.03, 8.06, and 9.06]. *Bay Ridge Diagnostic Laboratory, Inc. v. Dumpson, 400 F. Supp. 1104, 1109-10.*

Cal. App. 1967 Physician-stockholders of publicly-owned pharmaceutical corporations and physicians whose medical partnerships owned and operated pharmacies challenged statutory prohibition of physician membership, proprietory interest, and co-ownership of pharmacies. The court quoted Principles Ch. I, Sec. 6 (1947) and a 1960 Judicial Council rule, later included in Opinions and Reports of the Judicial Council Sec. 7, Para. 38 (1965) [now Opinions 8.03, 8.032, and 8.06] in its discussion of the potential conflict of interest created by such ownership. The court held that the statute prohibited physician partnerships from directly owning pharmacies but did not apply to an individual physician or a partnership of physicians who own stock in a corporation which owns and operates a pharamacy. *Magan Medical Clinic v. California State Bd. of Medical Examiners*, 249 Cal. App. 2d 124, 57 Cal. Rptr. 256, 262.

Minn. App. 1997 Patients brought suit against physician for prescribing a growth hormone drug while receiving kickbacks, in violation of the physician-patient fiduciary duty and the Minnesota Consumer Fraud Act. The distributor of the drug induced physicians to refer patients for the drug. The court cited Opinion 8.06 for the proposition that patients are entitled to receive medical opinions and referrals which are not motivated by physician gain. The court found, however, that the complaint sounded in medical malpractice and declined to allow a new cause of action based on breach of a fiduciary duty. Because the malpractice limitations had expired and the patients had failed to allege sufficient injury under the Consumer Fraud Act, the court affirmed dismissal with prejudice. *D.A.B v. Brown*, 570 N.W. 2d 168, 170.

Ohio 1980 A physician, charged with violating the state medical licensing statute by distributing controlled substances without a proper license and writing prescriptions for narcotics in the name of one person when they were intended for another, challenged the state medical board's decision to suspend his license and place him on two years probation. Under the statute, a physician could be disciplined for various activities including violation of any provision of a code of ethics of a national professional organization such as the American Medical Association. The board found in part that the physician's actions violated Principles 4 and 7 (1957) [now Principles II and III and Opinions 8.06 and 9.04]. The trial court reversed, holding that the board had insufficient evidence for its decision, and the court of appeals affirmed. On appeal, the supreme court held that expert testimony was not required at a hearing before a medical licensing board because they were experts and could determine for themselves whether the Principles had been violated. *Arlen v. State*, 61 Ohio St. 2d 168, 399 N.E.2d 1251, 1252, 1253-54.

Mo. Att'y Gen. 1982 State attorney general, citing Opinion 8.06 (1982), concluded that a physician who requires a patient to accept drugs dispensed by the physician and refuses to provide the patient with a prescription for the patient's use elsewhere violates state antitrust law and has engaged in professional misconduct. A similar conclusion, again based in part on Opinion 8.06, was rendered regarding a physician who requires a patient to fill a prescription at a pharmacy in which the physician has a personal interest. *Missouri Att'y Gen. Op. No. 6 (July 8, 1982) (LEXIS, States library, Mo. file)*.

Journal 2002 Suggests a reconceptualization for bioethics that integrates an analysis of the history of moral change. Concludes that bioethical textbooks should include discussion about the history of bioethics and medical ethics. Quotes Opinion 2.20. References Opinions 6.02, 6.03, 6.04 [now Opinion 8.06], and 8.032. Baker, *Bioethics and History*, 27 J. Med. & Phil. 447, 455, 469 (2002).

Journal 2001 Explores how the Pegram case restricted the protection provided to HMOs by ERISA's state law preemption. Concludes that HMOs will be subject to increased litigation under two areas of state law–breach of statutory fiduciary duty and medical malpractice claims. Cites Opinion 8.06. McLean & Richards, *Managed Care Liability for Breach of Fiduciary Duty after Pegram v. Herdrich: The End of ERISA Preemption for State Law Liability for Medical Care Decision Making*, 53 Fla. L. Rev. 1, 38 (2001).

Journal 2001 Considers office dispensing of products within the dermatology practice. Examines related ethical issues. Concludes that the primary reasons patients buy products from their physicians are trust and knowledge, not convenience. Quotes Opinion 8.06. Ogbogu, Fleischer, Brodell, Bhalla, Draelos, & Feldman, *Physicians' and Patients' Perspectives on Office-Based Dispensing: The Central Role of the Physician-Patient Relationship*, 137 Arch. Dermatol. 151, 151 (2001).

Journal 2001 Explores the extent to which pediatricians should rely on their expertise when prescribing therapies and durable medical equipment for children with special health care needs. Emphasizes the importance of the pediatrician's role in this context and urges pediatricians to comply with pertinent AMA guidelines and relevant state and federal laws. Quotes Opinion 8.06. References Opinion 9.132. Sneed, May, & Stencel, *Physicians' Reliance on Specialists, Therapists, and Vendors When Prescribing Therapies and Durable Medical Equipment for Children with Special Health Care Needs*, 107 Pediatrics 1283, 1287, 1288, 1289 (2001).

Journal 1998 Discusses the physician's fiduciary duty to the patient. Explores the expansion of the "honest services" mail fraud statute to prosecute undisclosed fiduciary breaches. Concludes that the mail fraud statute may be used to prosecute physicians who fail to disclose financial incentives to their patients. Quotes Opinion 8.03. Cites Opinions 2.03 and 8.07 [now Opinion 8.06]. Jones, *Primum Non Nocere: The Expanding "Honest Services" Mail Fraud Statute and the Physician-Patient Fiduciary Relationship, 51 Vand. L. Rev. 139, 161, 164 (1998).*

Journal 1992 Surveys federal and state antikickback and antireferral statutes pertaining to drug and device marketing activities. Considers the effectiveness of regulatory safe harbors. Quotes Opinion 6.04 [now Opinion 8.06]. References Opinion 8.061. Kirschenbaum & Kuhlik, *Federal and State Laws Affecting Discounts, Rebates, and Other Marketing Practices for Drugs and Devices, 47 Food & Drug L. J. 533, 560 (1992).*

Journal 1991 Looks at the physician as a fiduciary and the law governing fiduciary relationships. Concludes that fiduciary concepts are a valuable basis for establishing ethical and legal guidelines for physician behavior. Quotes Opinions 2.19, 8.03 (1989) [now Opinion 8.032], and 8.06. Healey & Dowling, *Controlling Conflicts of Interest in the Doctor-Patient Relationship: Lessons From Moore v. Regents of the University of California, 42 Mercer L. Rev. 989, 997, 998 (1991).*

8.061   Gifts to Physicians from Industry

Many gifts given to physicians by companies in the pharmaceutical, device, and medical equipment industries serve an important and socially beneficial function. For example, companies have long provided funds for educational seminars and conferences. However, there has been growing concern about certain gifts from industry to physicians. Some gifts that reflect customary practices of industry may not be consistent with the Principles of Medical Ethics. To avoid the acceptance of inappropriate gifts, physicians should observe the following guidelines:

(1) Any gifts accepted by physicians individually should primarily entail a benefit to patients and should not be of substantial value. Accordingly, textbooks, modest meals, and other gifts are appropriate if they serve a genuine educational function. Cash payments should not be accepted. The use of drug samples for personal or family use is permissible as long as these practices do not interfere with patient access to drug samples. It would not be acceptable for non-retired physicians to request free pharmaceuticals for personal use or use by family members.

(2) Individual gifts of minimal value are permissible as long as the gifts are related to the physician's work (eg, pens and notepads).

(3) The Council on Ethical and Judicial Affairs defines a legitimate "conference" or "meeting" as any activity, held at an appropriate location, where (a) the gathering is primarily dedicated, in both time and effort, to promoting objective scientific and educational activities and discourse (one or more educational presentation(s) should be the highlight of the gathering), and (b) the main incentive for bringing attendees together is to further their knowledge on the topic(s) being presented. An appropriate disclosure of financial support or conflict of interest should be made.

(4) Subsidies to underwrite the costs of continuing medical education conferences or professional meetings can contribute to the improvement of patient care and therefore are permissible. Since the giving of a subsidy directly to a physician by a company's representative may create a relationship that could influence the use of the company's products, any subsidy

should be accepted by the conference's sponsor who in turn can use the money to reduce the conference's registration fee. Payments to defray the costs of a conference should not be accepted directly from the company by the physicians attending the conference.

(5) Subsidies from industry should not be accepted directly or indirectly to pay for the costs of travel, lodging, or other personal expenses of physicians attending conferences or meetings, nor should subsidies be accepted to compensate for the physicians' time. Subsidies for hospitality should not be accepted outside of modest meals or social events held as a part of a conference or meeting. It is appropriate for faculty at conferences or meetings to accept reasonable honoraria and to accept reimbursement for reasonable travel, lodging, and meal expenses. It is also appropriate for consultants who provide genuine services to receive reasonable compensation and to accept reimbursement for reasonable travel, lodging, and meal expenses. Token consulting or advisory arrangements cannot be used to justify the compensation of physicians for their time or their travel, lodging, and other out-of-pocket expenses.

(6) Scholarship or other special funds to permit medical students, residents, and fellows to attend carefully selected educational conferences may be permissible as long as the selection of students, residents, or fellows who will receive the funds is made by the academic or training institution. Carefully selected educational conferences are generally defined as the major educational, scientific or policy-making meetings of national, regional, or specialty medical associations.

(7) No gifts should be accepted if there are strings attached. For example, physicians should not accept gifts if they are given in relation to the physician's prescribing practices. In addition, when companies underwrite medical conferences or lectures other than their own, responsibility for and control over the selection of content, faculty, educational methods, and materials should belong to the organizers of the conferences or lectures. (II)

Issued June 1992 based on the report "Gifts to Physicians from Industry," adopted December 1990 (JAMA. 1991; 265: 501).

Updated June 1996 and June 1998.

Journal 2000 Compares the changes in physician roles in Japan and the United States that exacerbate their conflicts of interest. Examines American physicians' dispensing practices and relations with pharmaceutical firms and hospital ownership. Concludes the United States is reducing one of the main strengths it had in addressing physician conflicts: institutions of countervailing power and countervailing incentives. References Opinions 8.032 and 8.061, Rodwin & Okamoto, *Physicians' Conflicts of Interest in Japan and the United States: Lessons for the United States*, 25 J. Health Pol. Pol'y & L. 343, 355, 358 (2000).

Journal 2000 Examines the practice of gift-giving by the health care technology industry as incentives in the context of continuing medical education activities. Concludes that industry-wide standards must be developed governing interactions between physicians and representatives of health care technology industry companies. Cites Opinions 8.061 and 9.011. Tenery, *Interactions Between Physicians and the Health Care Technology Industry*, 283 JAMA 391, 393 (2000).

Journal 2000 Examines data from several studies evaluating conflicts of interest triggered by gifts given to physicians by the pharmaceutical industry. Concludes that the efficacy of professional society guidelines to control such conflicts is questionable and there should be more systematic policies to address these concerns. References Opinion 8.061. Wazana, *Physicians and the*

Pharmaceutical Industry: Is a Gift Ever Just a Gift? 283 JAMA 373, 380 (2000).

Journal 1999 Focuses on the purposes and broad applicability of the Medicare antikickback law. Describes how the law pertains to prescription drug and medical device manufacturers. Provides suggestions for antikickback law reform. Quotes Opinion 8.061. Bulleit & Krause, *Kickbacks, Courtesies, or Cost-Effectiveness?: Application of the Medicare Antikickback Law to the Marketing and Promotional Practices of Drug and Medical Device Manufacturers*, 54 Food & Drug L. J. 279, 296 (1999).

Journal 1999 Discusses the impact *Daubert v. Merrell Dow Pharmaceuticals, Inc.* has had on scientific expert testimony. Explains that the scientific approach of dealing with bias may be inappropriate for maintaining scientific objectivity in litigation. Provides a strategy to deal with conflicts of interest in this context. Quotes Opinions 9.07. Cites Opinion 8.061. Patterson, *Conflicts of Interest in Scientific Expert Testimony*, 40 Wm. & Mary L. Rev. 1313, 1330, 1332, 1335, 1371 (1999).

Journal 1998 Discusses the conflict of interest posed by managed care organizations offering financial incentives to physicians. Explains that the duty to disclose and professionalism are not adequate protections against conflicts of interest. Suggests that financial incentives should be carefully circumscribed and that managed care organizations should focus primarily on quality of care. References Opinion 8.061. Emanuel & Goldman, *Protecting Patient Welfare in Managed Care: Six Safeguards*, 23 J. Health Pol. Pol'y & L. 635, 641 (1998).

Journal 1998 Examines the transition from paper medical records to electronic medical records. Identifies issues of confidentiality and privacy that arise as a result of the move to electronic medical records. Concludes that federal protection is needed to safeguard personal medical information. Quotes Principle IV and Opinions 5.07 and 5.075. Cites Opinion 8.061. Tsai, *Cheaper and Better: The Congressional Administrative Simplification Mandate Facilitates the Transition to Electronic Medical Records*, 19 J. Legal Med. 549, 570, 581 (1998).

Journal 1997 Discusses the process for marketing new drugs, medical devices, or biologics. Considers issues such as whether insurers or payers will cover these products, how much each will cost, and whether marketing programs comply with government regulations. References Opinion 8.061. Reiss, *Commentary on Payment and Reimbursement Issues Affecting the Marketing of Drugs, Medical Devices, and Biologics, with Emphasis on the Anti-Kickback Statute and Stark II*, 52 Food & Drug L. J. 99, 107 (1997).

Journal 1997 Explores the extent to which pharmaceutical drug samples are taken by physicians or other medical staff for personal use. Concludes that this practice is common and raises pertinent ethical issues. Quotes Opinion 8.061. Westfall, McCabe, & Nicholas, *Personal Use of Drug Samples by Physicians and Office Staff*, 278 JAMA 141, 142 (1997).

Journal 1994 Discusses the role of professional societies in establishing ethical guidelines for physicians in the context of using medical innovations and new technologies. Observes that these standards must be supplemented by additional external measures or incentives in order to be most effective. Cites Opinions 1.01, 1.02, 8.061, 9.04, and 9.131. Orentlicher, *The Influence of a Professional Organization on Physician Behavior*, 57 Alb. L. Rev. 583, 592, 593, 594, 595, 596 (1994).

Journal 1993 Examines how the Food and Drug Administration (FDA) regulates marketing of new medical devices and its authority to do so. Describes how these regulations differ from those governing drugs. References Opinion 8.061. Dennis, *Promotion of Devices: An Extension of FDA Drug Regulation or a New Frontier?*, 48 Food & Drug L. J. 87 (1993).

Journal 1992 Surveys federal and state antikickback and antireferral statutes pertaining to drug and device marketing activities. Considers the effectiveness of regulatory safe harbors. Quotes Opinion 6.04 [now Opinion 8.06]. References Opinion 8.061. Kirschenbaum & Kuhlik, *Federal and State Laws Affecting Discounts, Rebates, and Other Marketing Practices for Drugs and Devices*, 47 Food & Drug L. J. 533, 560 (1992).

Journal 1992 Discusses the extent of the Food and Drug Administration's (FDA) authority to regulate oral sales promotion of pharmaceuticals. Explores the debate over the extent of the FDA's power to regulate. References Opinion 8.061. Noah, *Death of a Salesman: To What Extent Can the FDA Regulate the Promotional Statements of Pharmaceutical Sales Representatives?*, 47 Food & Drug L. J. 309, 316 (1992).

Journal 1992 Reviews concerns about commercial involvement in and funding of continuing medical education. Discusses CME requirements, accumulation of CME credits, and changes in standards governing commercial sponsorship. References Opinions 8.061 and 9.011. Wentz, Osteen, & Cannon, *Continuing Medical Education: Unabated Debate*, 268 JAMA 1118 (1992).

Journal 1991 Examines legal, ethical, and economic concerns surrounding pharmaceutical company promotions. Concludes that pharmaceutical freebies can serve a positive role in health care if adequately regulated. Quotes Opinions 8.061 and 8.08. Note, *The Economic Wisdom of Regulating Pharmaceutical "Freebies,"* 1991 Duke L.J. 206, 216, 233, 234 (1991).

Journal 1991 Discusses commercial support of continuing medical education. Explains ethical guidelines for accepting such assistance and how those guidelines have changed. References Opinions 8.061 and 9.011. Wentz, Osteen, & Gannon, *Refocusing Support and Direction*, 266 JAMA 953 (1991).

Clarification of Opinion 8.061, "Gifts to Physicians from Industry"

Scope

Opinion 8.061, "Gifts to Physicians from Industry," is intended to provide ethical guidance to physicians. Other parties involved in the health care sector, including the pharmaceutical, devices, and medical equipment industries and related entities or business partners, should view the guidelines as indicative of standards of conduct for the medical profession. Ultimately, it is the responsibility of individual physicians to minimize conflicts of interest that may be at odds with the best interest of patients and to access the necessary information to inform medical recommendations.

The guidelines apply to all forms of gifts, whether they are offered in person, through intermediaries, or through the Internet. Similarly, limitations on subsidies for educational activities should apply regardless of the setting in which, or the medium through which, the educational activity is offered.

General Questions

(a) **Do the guidelines apply only to pharmaceutical, device, and equipment manufacturers?**

"Industry" includes all "proprietary health-related entities that might create a conflict of interest."

Guideline 1

Any gifts accepted by physicians individually should primarily entail a benefit to patients and should not be of substantial value. Accordingly, textbooks, modest meals, and other gifts are appropriate if they serve a genuine educational function. Cash payments should not be accepted. The use of drug samples for personal or family use is permissible as long as these practices do not interfere with patient access to drug samples. It would not be acceptable for non-retired physicians to request free pharmaceuticals for personal use or for use by family members.

(a) **May physicians accept gram stain test kits, stethoscopes, or other diagnostic equipment?**

Diagnostic equipment primarily benefits the patient. Hence, such gifts are permissible as long as they are not of substantial value. In considering the value of the gift, the relevant measure is not the cost to the company of providing the gift. Rather, the relevant measure is the cost to the physician if the physician purchased the gift on the open market.

(b) **May companies invite physicians to a dinner with a speaker and donate $100 to a charity or medical school on behalf of the physician?**

There are positive aspects to the proposal. The donations would be used for a worthy cause, and the physicians would receive important information about patient care. There is a direct personal benefit to the physician as well, however. An organization that is important to the physician–and one that the physician might have ordinarily felt obligated to make a contribution to–receives financial support as a result of the physician's decision to attend the meeting. On balance, physicians should make their own judgment about these inducements. If the charity is predetermined without the physician's input, there would seem to be little problem with the arrangement.

(c) **May contributions to a professional society's general fund be accepted from industry?**

The guidelines are designed to deal with gifts from industry which affect, or could appear to affect, the judgment of individual practicing physicians. In general, a professional society should make its own judgment about gifts from industry to the society itself.

(d) **When companies invite physicians to a dinner with a speaker, what are the relevant guidelines?**

First, the dinner must be a modest meal. Second, the guideline does allow gifts that primarily benefit patients and that are not of substantial value. Accordingly, textbooks and other gifts that primarily benefit patient care and that have a value to the physician in the general range of $100 are permissible. When educational meetings occur in conjunction with a social event such as a meal, the educational component must have independent value, such as a presentation by an authoritative speaker other than a sales representative of the company. Also, the meal should be a modest one similar to what a physician routinely might have when dining at his or her own expense. In an office or hospital encounter with a company representative, it is permissible to accept a meal of nominal value, such as a sandwich or snack.

(e) **May physicians accept vouchers that reimburse them for uncompensated care they have provided?**

No. Such a voucher would result directly in increased income for the physician.

(f) **May physicians accumulate "points" by attending several educational or promotional meetings and then choose a gift from a catalogue of education options?**

This guideline permits gifts only if they are not of substantial value. If accumulation of points would result in physicians receiving a substantial gift by combining insubstantial gifts over a relatively short period of time, it would be inappropriate.

(g) **May physicians accept gift certificates for educational materials when attending promotional or educational events?**

The Council views gift certificates as a grey area which is not per se prohibited by the guidelines. Medical textbooks are explicitly approved as gifts under the guidelines. A gift certificate for educational materials, ie, for the selection by the physician from an exclusively medical textbook catalogue, would not seem to be materially different. The issue is whether the gift certificate gives the recipient such control as to make the certificate similar to cash. As with charitable donations, preselection by the sponsor removes any question. It is up to the individual physician to make the final judgment.

(h) **May physicians accept drug samples or other free pharmaceuticals for personal use or use by family members?**

The Council's guidelines permit personal or family use of free pharmaceuticals (i) in emergencies and other cases where the immediate use of a drug is indicated, (ii) on a trial basis to assess tolerance, and (iii) for the treatment of acute conditions requiring short courses of inexpensive therapy, as permitted by Opinion 8.19, "Self-Treatment or Treatment of Immediate Family Members." It would not be acceptable for physicians to accept free pharmaceuticals for the long-term treatment of chronic conditions.

(i) **May companies invite physicians to a dinner with a speaker and offer them a large number of gifts from which to choose one?**

In general, the greater the freedom of choice given to the physician, the more the offer seems like cash. A large number of gifts presented to physicians who attend a dinner would therefore be inappropriate.

There is no precise way of deciding an appropriate upper limit on the amount of choice that is acceptable. However, it is important that a specific limit be chosen to ensure clarity in the guidelines. A limit of eight has been chosen because it permits flexibility but prevents undue freedom of choice. Each of the choices must have a value to the physicians of no more than $100.

(j) **May physicians charge for their time with industry representatives or otherwise receive material compensation for participation in a detail visit?**

Guideline 1 states that gifts in the form of cash payments should not be accepted. Also, Guideline 6 makes clear that, in the context of the industry-physician relationship, only physicians who provide genuine services may receive reasonable compensation. When considering the time a physician spends with an industry representative, it is the representative who offers a service, namely the presentation of information. The physician is a beneficiary of the service. Overall, these guidelines do not view that physicians should be compensated for the time spent participating in educational activities, nor for time spent receiving detail information from an industry representative.

Guideline 2

Individual gifts of minimal value are permissible as long as the gifts are related to the physician's work (eg, pens and notepads).

(a) **May physicians, individually or through their practice group, accept electronic equipment, such as hand held devices or computers, intended to facilitate their ability to receive detail information electronically?**
Although Guideline 2 recognizes that gifts related to a physician's practice may be appropriate, it also makes clear that these gifts must remain of minimal value. It is not appropriate for physicians to accept expensive hardware or software equipment even though one purpose only may pertain to industry-related activities of a modest value.

Guideline 3

The Council on Ethical and Judicial Affairs defines a legitimate "conference" or "meeting" as any activity, held at an appropriate location, where (a) the gathering is primarily dedicated, in both time and effort, to promoting objective scientific and educational activities and discourse (one or more educational presentation(s) should be the highlight of the gathering), and (b) the main incentive for bringing attendees together is to further their knowledge on the topic(s) being presented. An appropriate disclosure of financial support or conflict of interest should be made.

Guideline 4

Subsidies to underwrite the costs of continuing medical education conferences or professional meetings can contribute to the improvement of patient care and therefore are permissible. Since the giving of a subsidy directly to a physician by a company's sales representative may create a relationship which could influence the use of the company's products, any subsidy should be accepted by the conference's sponsor who in turn can use the money to reduce the conference's registration fee. Payments to defray the costs of a conference should not be accepted directly from the company by the physicians attending the conference.

(a) **Are conference subsidies from the educational division of a company covered by the guidelines?**
Yes. When the Council says "any subsidy," it would not matter whether the subsidy comes from the sales division, the educational division, or some other section of the company.

(b) **May a company or its intermediary send physicians a check or voucher to offset the registration fee at a specific conference or a conference of the physician's choice?**
Physicians should not directly accept checks or certificates which would be used to offset registration fees. The gift of a reduced registration should be made across the board and through the accredited sponsor.

Guideline 5

Subsidies from industry should not be accepted directly or indirectly to pay for the costs of travel, lodging, or other personal expenses of physicians attending conferences or meetings, nor should subsidies be accepted to compensate for the physicians' time. Subsidies for hospitality should not be accepted outside of modest meals or social events held as a part of a conference or meeting. It is appropriate for faculty at conferences or meetings to accept reasonable honoraria and to accept reimbursement for reasonable travel, lodging, and meal expenses. It is also appropriate for consultants who provide genuine services to receive reasonable compensation and to accept reimbursement for reasonable travel, lodging, and meal expenses. Token consulting or advisory arrangements cannot be used to justify the compensation of physicians for their time or their travel, lodging, and other out-of-pocket expenses.

(a) **If a company invites physicians to visit its facilities for a tour or to become educated about one of its products, may the company pay travel expenses and honoraria?**
This question has come up in the context of a rehabilitation facility that wants physicians to know of its existence so that they may refer their patients to the facility. It has also come up in the context of surgical device or equipment manufacturers who want physicians to become familiar with their products.

In general, travel expenses should not be reimbursed, nor should honoraria be paid for the visiting physician's time since the presentations are analogous to a pharmaceutical company's educational or promotional meetings. The Council recognizes that medical devices, equipment, and other technologies may require, in some circumstances, special evaluation or training in proper usage which can not practicably be provided except on site. Medical specialties are in a better position to advise physicians regarding the appropriateness of reimbursement with regard to these trips. In cases where the company insists on such visits as a means of protection from liability for improper usage, physicians and their specialties should make the judgment. In no case would honoraria be appropriate and any travel expenses should be only those strictly necessary.

(b) **If the company invites physicians to visit its facilities for review and comment on a product, to discuss their independent research projects, or to explore the potential for collaborative research, may the company pay travel expenses and an honorarium?**
If the physician is providing genuine services, reasonable compensation for time and travel expenses can be given. However, token advisory or consulting arrangements cannot be used to justify compensation.

(c) **May a company hold a sweepstakes for physicians in which five entrants receive a trip to the Virgin Islands or airfare to the medical meeting of their choice?**
No. The use of a sweepstakes or raffle to deliver a gift does not affect the permissibility of the gift. Since the sweepstakes is not open to the public,

the guidelines apply in full force.

(d) **If a company convenes a group of physicians to recruit clinical investigators or convenes a group of clinical investigators for a meeting to discuss their results, may the company pay for their travel expenses?**
Expenses may be paid if the meetings serve a genuine research purpose. One guide to their propriety would be whether the National Institute of Health (NIH) conducts similar meetings when it sponsors multi-center clinical trials. When travel subsidies are acceptable, the guidelines emphasize that they be used to pay only for "reasonable" expenses. The reasonableness of expenses would depend on a number of considerations. For example, meetings are likely to be problematic if overseas locations are used for exclusively domestic investigators. It would be inappropriate to pay for recreation or entertainment beyond the kind of modest hospitality described in this guideline.

(e) **How can a physician tell whether there is a "genuine research purpose?"**
A number of factors can be considered. Signs that a genuine research purpose exists include the facts that there are (1) a valid study protocol, (2) recruitment of physicians with appropriate qualifications or expertise, and (3) recruitment of an appropriate number of physicians in light of the number of study participants needed for statistical evaluation.

(f) **May a company compensate physicians for their time and travel expenses when they participate in focus groups?**
Yes. As long as the focus groups serve a genuine and exclusive research purpose and are not used for promotional purposes, physicians may be compensated for time and travel expenses. The number of physicians used in a particular focus group or in multiple focus groups should be an appropriate size to accomplish the research purpose, but no larger.

(g) **Do the restrictions on travel, lodging, and meals apply to educational programs run by medical schools, professional societies, or other accredited organizations which are funded by industry, or do they apply only to programs developed and run by industry?**
The restrictions apply to all conferences or meetings which are funded by industry. The Council drew no distinction on the basis of the organizer of the conference or meeting. The Council felt that the gift of travel expenses is too substantial even when the conference is run by a non-industry sponsor. (Industry includes all "proprietary health-related entities that might create a conflict of interest.")

(h) **May company funds be used for travel expenses and honoraria for bona fide faculty at educational meetings?**
This guideline draws a distinction between attendees and faculty. As was stated, "[i]t is appropriate for faculty at conferences or meetings to accept reasonable honoraria and to accept reimbursement for reasonable travel, lodging, and meal expenses."

Companies need to be mindful of the guidelines of the Accreditation Council on Continuing Medical Education. According to those guidelines, "[f]unds from a commercial source should be in the form of an educational grant made payable to the CME sponsor for the support of programming."

(i) **May travel expenses be reimbursed for physicians presenting a poster or a "free paper" at a scientific conference?**
Reimbursement may be accepted only by bona fide faculty. The presentation of a poster or a free paper does not by itself qualify a person as a member of the conference faculty for purposes of these guidelines.

(j) **When a professional association schedules a long-range planning meeting, is it appropriate for industry to subsidize the travel expenses of the meeting participants?**
The guidelines are designed to deal with gifts from industry which affect, or could appear to affect, the judgment of individual practicing physicians. In general, a professional society should make its own judgment about gifts from industry to the society itself.

(k) **May continuing medical education conferences be held in the Bahamas, Europe, or South America?**
There are no restrictions on the location of conferences as long as the attendees are paying their own travel expenses.

(l) **May travel expenses be accepted by physicians who are being trained as speakers or faculty for educational conferences and meetings?**
In general, no. If a physician is presenting as an independent expert at a CME event, both the training and its reimbursement raise questions about independence. In addition, the training is a gift because the physician's role is generally more analogous to that of an attendee than a participant. Speaker training sessions can be distinguished from meetings (See 5d) with leading researchers, sponsored by a company, designed primarily for an exchange of information about important developments or treatments, including the sponsor's own research, for which reimbursement for travel may be appropriate.

(m) **What kinds of social events during conferences and meetings may be subsidized by industry?**
Social events should satisfy three criteria. First, the value of the event to the physician should be modest. Second, the event should facilitate discussion among attendees and/or discussion between attendees and faculty. Third, the educational part of the conference should account for a substantial majority of the total time accounted for by the educational activities and social events together. Events that would be viewed (as in the succeeding question) as lavish or expensive should be avoided. But modest social activities that are not elaborate or unusual are permissible, eg, inexpensive boat rides, barbecues, entertainment that draws on the local performers. In general, any such events which are a part of the conference program should be open to all registrants.

(n) **May a company rent an expensive entertainment complex for a evening during a medical conference and invite the physicians attending the conference?**
No. The guidelines permit only modest hospitality.

(o) **If physicians attending a conference engage in interactive exchange, may their travel expenses be paid by industry?**
No. Mere interactive exchange would not constitute genuine consulting services.

(p) **If a company schedules a conference and provides meals for the attendees that fall within the guidelines, may the company also pay for the costs of the meals for spouses?**
If a meal falls within the guidelines, then the physician's spouse may be included.

(q) **May companies donate funds to sponsor a professional society's charity golf tournament?**
Yes. But it is sensible if physicians who play in the tournament make some contribution themselves to the event.

(r) **If a company invites a group of consultants to a meeting and a consultant brings a spouse, may the company pay the costs of lodging or meals of the spouse? Does it matter if the meal is part of the program for the consultants?**
Since the costs of having a spouse share a hotel room or join a modest meal are nominal, it is permissible for the company to subsidize those costs. However, if the total subsidies become substantial, then they become unacceptable.

Guideline 6
Scholarship or other special funds to permit medical students, residents, and fellows to attend carefully selected educational conferences may be permissible as long as the selection of students, residents, or fellows who will receive the funds is made by the academic or training institution. Carefully selected educational conferences are generally defined as the major educational, scientific, or policy-making meetings of national, regional, or specialty medical associations.

(a) **When a company subsidizes the travel expenses of residents to an appropriately selected conference, may the residents receive the subsidy directly from the company?**
Funds for scholarships or other special funds should be given to the academic departments or the accredited sponsor of the conference. The disbursement of funds can then be made by the departments or the conference sponsor.

(b) **What is meant by "carefully selected educational conferences?"**
The intent of Guideline 6 is to ensure that financial hardship does not

prevent students, residents, and fellows from attending major educational conferences. For example, we did not want to deny cardiology fellows the opportunity to attend the annual scientific meeting of the American College of Cardiology or orthopedic surgery residents the opportunity to attend the annual scientific meeting of the American Academy of Orthopedic Surgeons. However, it was not the intent of the guideline to permit reimbursement of travel expenses in other circumstances, such as when conferences or symposia are designed specifically for students, residents, or fellows.

Accordingly, "carefully selected educational conferences" should be interpreted as follows: funds may be used for the reasonable travel and lodging expenses of students, residents, and fellows to attend the major educational, scientific, or policy-making meetings of national, regional, or specialty medical associations.

The Council recognizes that there may be some exceptional conferences for all physicians or even for just students, residents, or fellows that do not fall within this definition of carefully selected educational conferences but that meet the spirit of Guideline 6. Accordingly, the Council will consider proposals for travel and lodging subsidies for such conferences on a case-by-case basis and grant approval to those that meet the spirit of the guidelines.

Guideline 7

No gifts should be accepted if there are strings attached. For example, physicians should not accept gifts if they are given in relation to the physician's prescribing practices. In addition, when companies underwrite medical conferences or lectures other than their own, responsibility for and control over the selection of content, faculty, educational methods, and materials should belong to the organizers of the conferences or lectures.

(a) **May companies send their top prescribers, purchasers, or referrers on cruises?**
No. There can be no link between prescribing or referring patterns and gifts. In addition, travel expenses, including cruises, are not permissible.

(b) **May the funding company itself develop the complete educational program that is sponsored by an accredited continuing medical education sponsor?**
No. The funding company may finance the development of the program through its grant to the sponsor, but the accredited sponsor must have responsibility and control over the content and faculty of conferences, meetings, or lectures. Neither the funding company nor an independent consulting firm should develop the complete educational program for approval by the accredited sponsor.

(c) **How much input may a funding company have in the development of a conference, meeting, or lectures?**

214

The guidelines of the Accreditation Council on Continuing Medical Education on commercial support of continuing medical education address this question.

Issued 1992.

Updated December 2000 and June 2002, (*Food and Drug Law Journal*, 2001;56(1):27-40).

8.062 Sale of Non-Health-Related Goods from Physicians' Offices

The sale of non-health-related goods by physicians presents a conflict of interest and threatens to erode the primary obligation of physicians to serve the interests of their patients before their own. Furthermore, this activity risks placing undue pressure on the patient and risks demeaning the practice of medicine.

Physicians should not sell non-health-related goods from their offices or other treatment settings, with the exception noted below.

Physicians may sell low-cost non-health-related goods from their offices for the benefit of community organizations, provided that (1) the goods in question are low-cost; (2) the physician takes no share in profit from their sale; (3) such sales are not a regular part of the physician's business; (4) sales are conducted in a dignified manner; and (5) sales are conducted in such a way as to assure that patients are not pressured into making purchases. (I, II)

Issued June 1998 based on the report "Sale of Non-Health-Related Goods from Physicians' Offices," adopted December 1997. (JAMA 1998 Aug 12;280(6):563.)

Journal 2002 Examines the ethical aspects of e-medicine. Concludes that, although e-medicine has benefits, physicians must understand its impact on the physician-patient relationship. Cites Opinions 8.062 and 8.063. Berg, *Ethics and E-Medicine*, 46 St. Louis U. L.J. 61, 66 (2002).

8.063 Sale of Health-Related Products from Physicians' Offices

"Health-related products" are any products that, according to the manufacturer or distributor, benefit health. "Selling" refers to the activity of dispensing items that are provided from the physician's office in exchange for money and also includes the activity of endorsing a product that the patient may order or purchase elsewhere that results in direct remuneration for the physician. This Opinion does not apply to the sale of prescription items which is already addressed in Opinion 8.06, "Prescribing and Dispensing Drugs and Devices."

Physicians who engage in in-office sales practices should be aware of the related guidelines presented in Opinion 8.062, "Sale of Non-Health-Related Goods from Physicians' Offices;" Opinion 8.06, "Prescribing and Dispensing Drugs and Devices;" Opinion 8.032, "Conflicts of Interest: Health Facility Ownership by a Physician;" Opinion 3.01, "Nonscientific Practitioners;" Opinion 8.20, "Invalid Medical Treatment;" as well as the reports from which these opinions are extracted.

In-office sale of health-related products by physicians presents a financial conflict of interest, risks placing undue pressure on the patient, and threatens to erode patient trust and undermine the primary obligation of physicians to serve the interests of their patients before their own.

(1) Physicians who choose to sell health-related products from their offices should not sell any health-related products whose claims of benefit lack scientific validity. When judging the efficacy of a product, physicians should rely on peer-reviewed literature and other unbiased scientific sources that review evidence in a sound, systematic, and reliable fashion.

(2) Because of the risk of patient exploitation and the potential to demean the profession of medicine, physicians who choose to sell health-related products from their offices must take steps to minimize their financial conflicts of interest. The following guidelines apply:

   (a) In general, physicians should limit sales to products that serve the immediate and pressing needs of their patients. For example, if traveling to the closest pharmacy would in some way jeopardize the welfare of the patient (eg, forcing a patient with a broken leg to travel to a local pharmacy for crutches), then it may be appropriate to provide the product from the physician's office. These conditions are explained in more detail in the Council's Opinion 8.06, "Prescribing and Dispensing Drugs and Devices," and are analogous to situations that constitute exceptions to the permissibility of self-referral.

   (b) Physicians may distribute other health-related products to their patients free of charge or at cost, in order to make useful products readily available to their patients. When health-related products are offered free or at cost, it helps to ensure removal of the elements of personal gain and financial conflicts of interest that may interfere, or appear to interfere, with the physician's independent medical judgment.

(3) Physicians must disclose fully the nature of their financial arrangement with a manufacturer or supplier to sell health-related products. Disclosure includes informing patients of financial interests as well as about the availability of the product or other equivalent products elsewhere. Disclosure can be accomplished through face-to-face communication or by posting an easily understandable written notification in a prominent location that is accessible by all patients in the office. In addition, physicians should, upon request, provide patients with understandable literature that relies on scientific standards in addressing the risks, benefits, and limits of knowledge regarding the health-related product.

(4) Physicians should not participate in exclusive distributorships of health-related products which are available only through physicians' offices. Physicians should encourage manufacturers to make products of established benefit more fairly and more widely accessible to patients than exclusive distribution mechanisms allow. (II)

Issued December 1999 based on the report "Sale of Health-Related Products from Physicians' Offices," adopted June 1999.

Journal 2002 Examines the ethical aspects of e-medicine. Concludes that, although e-medicine has benefits, physicians must understand its impact on the physician-patient relationship. Cites Opinions 8.062 and 8.063. Berg, *Ethics and E-Medicine*, 46 St. Louis U. L.J. 61, 66 (2002).

Clarification of Opinions 8.062, Sale of Non-Health-Related Goods from Physicians' Offices, and 8.063, Sale of Health-Related Goods from Physicians' Offices

Do the guidelines discussing the sale of health-related products (8.063) and the sale of non-health-related goods (8.062) apply to physicians' practice Web-sites?

Yes. The physician who provides or sells products to patients must follow the above guidelines regardless of whether the products are provided in the physician's office or through a practice Web-site.

Adopted December 2000 as "Addendum III: Council on Ethical and Judicial Affairs Clarification on Sale of Products from Physicians' Offices (E-8.062 and E-8.063)."

8.07   "Gifts to Physicians: Offers of Indemnity," issued June 1992, was deleted in June 2002 and combined with Opinion 6.04, "Fee Splitting: Drug or Device Prescription Rebates" and Opinion 8.06, "Drugs and Devices: Prescribing" into the current Opinion 8.06, "Prescribing and Dispensing Drugs and Devices."

8.08   Informed Consent

The patient's right of self-decision can be effectively exercised only if the patient possesses enough information to enable an intelligent choice. The patient should make his or her own determination on treatment. The physician's obligation is to present the medical facts accurately to the patient or to the individual responsible for the patient's care and to make recommendations for management in accordance with good medical practice. The physician has an ethical obligation to help the patient make choices from among the therapeutic alternatives consistent with good medical practice. Informed consent is a basic social policy for which exceptions are permitted: (1) where the patient is unconscious or otherwise incapable of consenting and harm from failure to treat is imminent or (2) when risk disclosure poses such a serious psychological threat of detriment to the patient as to be medically contraindicated. Social policy does not accept the paternalistic view that the physician may remain silent because divulgence might prompt the patient to forego needed therapy. Rational, informed patients should not be expected to act uniformly, even under similar circumstances, in agreeing to or refusing treatment. (I, II, III, IV, V)

Issued March 1981.

7th Cir. 2002 Prosecutors appealed order enjoining enforcement of informed consent provisions of Indiana abortion statute on the grounds that they unconstitutionally created an undue burden. Court of Appeals reversed and held injunction was an abuse of discretion. The court found the statute was substantively identical to a law upheld in previous decisions. Further, the court held that the state was entitled to have the law evaluated on the basis of actual experience. Dissenting judge quoted Opinion 8.08 regarding need for patient to be capable of giving informed consent. *A Woman's Choice-East Side Women's Clinic v. Newman,* 305 F.3d 684, 716.

Alaska 2002 Patient brought malpractice and informed consent claims against physician. In part, patient alleged physician's failure to appropriately advise her regarding her abdominal pain after surgery led to permanent injuries. Trial court entered judgment for physician. On appeal, Alaska

Supreme Court remanded the informed consent claim, holding that the jury instruction should have reflected a "reasonable patient" standard. Quotes Opinion 8.08. *Marsingill v. O'Malley, 58 P.3d 495, 499, 504-05.*

Ga. App. 2000 Plaintiff alleged failure on the part of a dentist to inform him of the risks of root canal in a malpractice action. The appeals court noted that state case law did not recognize the informed consent doctrine. In evaluating this precedent, the court quoted Opinion 8.08 and Fundamental Element (1) [now Opinion 10.01]. The court stated that the AMA *Code of Medical Ethics* should be understood to reflect the standard of care of the medical profession on the issue of informed consent. While the court ruled in favor of the dentist, it prospectively recognized the doctrine of informed consent. *Ketchup v. Howard, 247 Ga. App. 54, 543 S.E.2d 371, 376, 377.*

Ind. 1992 Plaintiffs filed suit against physician after medical review panel found no evidence that physician committed malpractice in performing a bladder suspension and cryosurgery that resulted in plaintiff's cervix adhering to wall of her vagina. The trial court granted summary judgment for the defendant but appellate court reversed in part holding that the informed consent claim did not require expert medical testimony. The state supreme court affirmed the summary judgment, determining that the reasonably prudent physician standard applied in informed consent cases. In support of its decision, the court quoted Opinion 8.08, regarding informed consent. The court also held that expert medical testimony was required for plaintiff's informed consent claim because the standard of care for the procedure preformed was not common knowledge for lay persons. *Culbertson v. Mernitz, 602 N.E.2d 98, 103, 106.*

Ind. App. 1999 Patient brought malpractice suit against surgeon, claiming that he would not have consented to surgery if the surgeon had disclosed that he would perform only a fusion for the patient's back, rather than the recommended procedure. The trial court granted summary judgment. The appellate court reversed, and held that a plaintiff is not required to introduce expert testimony to establish the standard of care or the causation elements in an informed consent action when lay people can understand that a failure to meet the standard of care occurred. The court cited *Culbertson v. Mernitz*, 602 N.E.2d 98 (Ind. 1992), where the Indiana Supreme Court quoted Opinion 8.08, regarding informed consent. *Bowman v. Beghin, 713 N.E.2d 913, 916.*

N.J. 1999 Patient sued surgeon for lack of informed consent and malpractice on grounds that the surgeon decided to treat patient's hip fracture with bed rest rather than utilizing other alternatives. The trial court held that the patient could not sustain a claim for lack of informed consent. The New Jersey Supreme Court held that the informed consent requirement extends to non-invasive procedures. The court quoted Opinion 8.08 regarding a patient's right to be fully informed of medically reasonable treatments. *Matthies v. Mastromonaco, 160 N.J. 26, 733 A.2d 456, 463.*

W. Va. 1995 West Virginia Board of Medicine received a complaint from patient that physician was using depossession treatment. The hearing examiner in part found that there had been a lack of informed consent for such treatment. The Board changed the examiner's report and added sanctions. In doing so, it quoted Opinion 8.08. On appeal, the circuit court reversed, finding the Board's order arbitrary and an abuse of discretion. The appellate court agreed that the Board abused its discretion, but remanded the case for consideration of the issue of informed consent for depossession treatment. *Modi v. West Virginia Board of Medicine, 465 S.E.2d 230, 236.*

Journal 2003 Discusses whether, and how, legal rights may be waived. Concludes that, in addressing these questions, emphasis should be placed on concepts of autonomy and voluntariness. Cites Opinion 8.08. Berg, *Understanding Waiver*, 40 Hous. L. Rev. 281, 329 (2003).

Journal 2003 Argues that affirmative measures should be taken by the Air Force to ensure access to abortion services. Concludes that regulatory changes will reduce barriers to access. Quotes Opinion 10.01. Cites Opinion 8.08. Wilde, *Air Force Women's Access to Abortion Services and the Erosion of 10 U.S.C. § 1093*, 9 Wm. & Mary J. Women & L. 351, 371 (2003).

Journal 2002 Examines how managed care has adversely affected information disclosure in the physician-patient relationship. Concludes that, unless courts expand applicability of principles of informed consent, patient self-determination and autonomy will continue to be undermined. Quotes Principle VIII and Opinions 8.03, 8.053, 8.054, and 8.08. Morris, *Dissing Disclosure: Just What the Doctor Ordered*, 44 Ariz. L. Rev. 313, 344, 349, 362, 363, 366 (2002).

Journal 2002 Considers the dilemma of informed consent in the context of prescribing psychotropic medication to patients with mental illness and mental retardation. Recognizes the need for substituted decisionmaking in certain situations. Concludes that legislation would help address this issue. Quotes Preamble, Principles I, III, IV, VIII, and IX, and Opinion 8.08. O'Sullivan & Borcherding, *Informed Consent for Medication in Persons with Mental Retardation and Mental Illness*, 12 Health Matrix 63, 75, 86, 87, 88 (2002).

Journal 2002 Analyzes the role of prognostication in physician-patient communication. Concludes that the patient-physician model of shared decision-making offers the best hope for reestablishing prognostication. Quotes Principles Ch. I, Art. I, Sec. 2 and 4 (1846) [now Principle IV and Opinions 8.12 and 10.01]. Cites Opinion 8.08. Rich, *Prognostication in Clinical Medicine: Prophecy or Professional Responsibility? 23 J. Legal Med.* 297, 299, 318, 327 (2002).

Journal 2000 Examines physician value neutrality (PVN). Defines PVN as providing a foundation to suggest physicians must keep their values—religious, political, or otherwise—out of the patient-physician relationship. Concludes it is not clear how values can be removed from the patient-physician relationship without removing the very thing PVN supporters are trying to protect, the intrinsic value of persons. References Opinions 2.01, 2.02, 8.032, 8.05, 8.08, and 8.132. Beckwith & Peppin, *Physician Value Neutrality: A Critique, 28 J. L. Med. & Ethics* 67, 72-73 (2000).

Journal 2000 Explores the United States Supreme Court's use of the First Amendment's viewpoint neutrality mandate. Concludes that viewpoint discrimination should be applied to limit government censorship of private speech in nonpublic forums and selective subsidy programs. Quotes Opinion 8.08. Casarez, *Public Forums, Selective Subsidies, and Shifting Standards of Viewpoint Discrimination, 64 Alb. L. Rev.* 501, 558 (2000).

Journal 2000 Considers the objective of the informed consent doctrine. Concludes that, in practice, the doctrine falls short of its intended purpose. Quotes Opinion 8.08. Kurtz, *The Law of Informed Consent: From "Doctor is Right" to "Patient has Rights," 50 Syracuse L. Rev.* 1243, 1245 (2000).

Journal 2000 Describes the fiduciary aspects of the physician-patient relationship. Explores the conflicts that may occur between physicians and pregnant women in the health care setting. Proposes legal strategies to address these conflicts. Quotes Opinions 8.08 and 10.01. References Opinion 8.13. Oberman, *Mothers and Doctors' Orders: Unmasking the Doctor's Fiduciary Role in Maternal-Fetal Conflicts, 94 Nw. U. L. Rev.* 451, 456, 462, 493 (2000).

Journal 2000 Examines issues relating to parental consent to circumcision. Identifies legal and ethical requirements for consent when medical professionals are treating adult patients. Analyzes the implications of those requirements for routine circumcision of infant males. Concludes that only when the male is an adult and capable of making decisions can circumcision be ethically and legally performed. Quotes Opinion 8.08. References Opinions 8.03 and 9.011. Svoboda, Van Howe, & Dwyer, *Informed Consent for Neonatal Circumcision: An Ethical and Legal Conundrum, 17 J. Contemp. Health L. & Pol'y* 61, 67, 73, 82 (2000).

Journal 2000 Discusses traditional medical ethics and the physician's duty to benefit patients. Concludes that, in the twenty-first century, physicians will no longer be expected to determine on their own what will benefit their patients. Quotes Principle II and Opinion 8.08. Veatch, *Doctor Does Not Know Best: Why in the New Century Physicians Must Stop Trying to Benefit Patients, 25 J. Med. & Phil.* 701, 710, 711 (2000).

Journal 2000 Discusses the development and history of the ethical doctrine of informed consent. Examines the current state of the law in Pennsylvania and concludes it does not adequately fulfill the goals of ethical and legal doctrines. Quotes Principle IV and Opinion 10.01. References Opinion 8.08. Warren, *Pennsylvania Medical Informed Consent Law: A Call to Protect Patient Autonomy Rights By Abandoning the Battery Approach, 38 Duq. L. Rev.* 917, 925 (2000).

Journal 1999 Observes that, under statute and common law, the doctrine of informed consent in Pennsylvania does not apply in situations involving nonsurgical procedures. Argues that state law should be expanded to include a duty to obtain informed consent in these situations. Quotes Opinion 8.08. Durst, *Cutting Through Pennsylvania's Medical Informed Consent Statute: A Reasonable Interpretation Abolishing the Surgical Requirement, 104 Dick. L. Rev.* 197, 225 (1999).

Journal 1998 Discusses legal aspects of physician-assisted suicide. Identifies acceptable end-of-life choices and compares them to physician-assisted suicide. Points out that physician-assisted suicide has the potential for abuse and that safeguards have not been implemented to protect people from that risk. Quotes Opinion 2.211. Cites Opinions 2.20 and 8.08. Mitchell, *Physician-Assisted Suicide: A Survey of the Issues Surrounding Legalization, 74 N. D. L. Rev.* 341, 349 (1998).

Journal 1998 Discusses current abortion malpractice claims. Describes three general types of malpractice causes of action. Argues that specialized procreative torts should be implemented to adequately protect a woman's procreative autonomy. Quotes Opinion 8.08. Northern, *Procreative Torts: Enhancing the Common-Law Protection for Reproductive Autonomy*, 1998 U. Ill. L. Rev. 489, 525 (1998).

Journal 1998 Explains the connection and differences between bioethics and the law. States that the distinction between ethics and law is that ethics places additional emphasis on moral ideals. References Opinions 8.08 and 8.115. Sullivan & Reynolds, *Where Law and Bioethics Meet . . . and Where They Don't*, 75 U. Det. Mercy L. Rev. 607, 612 (1998).

Journal 1997 Examines the evolution of the Indiana health care system. Discusses developments in Indiana jurisprudence regarding the physician-patient relationship. Explores various challenges facing the relationship and recognizes the need for legal rules to help address these challenges. Quotes Opinion 8.08. Cites Opinions 2.20, 9.06, and 9.12. Kinney & Selby, *History and Jurisprudence of the Physician-Patient Relationship in Indiana*, 30 Ind. L. Rev. 263, 269, 272, 276 (1997).

Journal 1997 Explores the meaning of cardiopulmonary resuscitation and legal issues involving DNR orders. Considers problems created by DNR orders in operating rooms in light of patients' rights. Concludes that hospitals must adopt clear policies for their surgical teams to follow. Quotes Opinion 8.08. References Opinion 2.22. Lonchyna, *To Resuscitate or Not . . . In the Operating Room: The Need for Hospital Policies for Surgeons Regarding DNR Orders*, 6 Annals Health L. 209, 215, 217 (1997).

Journal 1996 Examines the constitutional implications of government-subsidized speech. Proposes two key characterization questions that should be answered when undertaking legal analysis. Observes, among other things, that potential ethical conflicts may exist when governmental subsidies are utilized to control the discourse between physicians and their patients. Quotes Opinion 8.08. Post, *Subsidized Speech*, 106 Yale L. J. 151, 173 (1996).

Journal 1996 Discusses new abortion legislation in Utah. Notes that patient consent must be obtained in accordance with AMA ethical standards, requiring physicians to provide all relevant data. Concludes that new laws require more detailed and comprehensive information be given to women. Quotes Opinion 8.08. Schnibbe, *Recent Legislative Developments in Utah Law: Family Law*, 1996 Utah L. Rev. 1335, 1394 (1996).

Journal 1996 Considers the ethical requirement for physicians to receive informed consent from patients before beginning treatment. Reviews the case of *Jacobson v. Massachusetts*, discussing its impact on informed consent and vaccination policy in the United States. Quotes Fundamental Elements (2). References Opinion 8.08. Severyn, *Jacobson v. Massachusetts: Impact on Informed Consent and Vaccine Policy*, 5 J. Pharmacy & L. 249, 253, 274 (1996).

Journal 1995 Observes that physicians are unable to obtain informed consent because they can not guess which treatment alternatives will best serve an individual patient's interests. Suggests that this situation would be improved if patients were paired with physicians who share their personal values. Quotes Opinion 8.08. Veatch, *Abandoning Informed Consent*, 25 Hastings Center Rep. 5, 6 (March/April 1995).

Journal 1994 Discusses how physicians historically have taken too much license with patients' bodies and placed greater value on longevity than on quality of life. Suggests that greater emphasis should be given to physician disclosure obligations in order to improve the quality of patient consent. Quotes Opinion 8.07 (1981) [now Opinion 8.08]. Katz, *Informed Consent: Must It Remain a Fairy Tale?*, 10 J. Contemp. Health L. & Pol'y 69, 80 (1994).

Journal 1994 Reviews the evolution of the physician-patient relationship, with attention to patient autonomy. Examines the changing health care delivery environment. Quotes Preamble, Principles I, II, III, IV, V, and VI, Fundamental Elements (1) and (2), and Opinions 1.02 and 8.07 (1981) [now Opinion 8.08]. Cites Opinion 1.01. Szczygiel, *Beyond Informed Consent*, 21 Ohio N.U.L. Rev. 171, 217, 218, 220, 225, 226, 256 (1994).

Journal 1993 Considers how patient self-determination may be affected by cardiopulmonary resuscitation and Do-Not-Resuscitate policies. Opposes a "futility" exception to informed consent as being violative of a physician's fiduciary duties to patients. Cites Opinion 8.07 (1986) [now Opinion 8.08]. References Opinion 2.22. Boozang, *Death Wish: Resuscitating Self-Determination for the Critically Ill*, 35 Ariz. L. Rev. 23, 24, 28, 52 (1993).

Journal 1993 Discusses physicians' duty to disclose medical treatment alternatives to patients that are not readily available. Proposes that based on the historical development and legal requirements of the informed consent doctrine, physicians should be required to inform patients of nonreadily available alternatives or face liability for breach of such obligation. Quotes Principles I, II, III, IV, and V and Opinion 8.08. Note, *Informed Choice: Physicians' Duty to Disclose Nonreadily Available Alternatives*, 43 Case W. Res. L. Rev. 491, 491, 498-499, 508, 509 (1993).

Journal 1993 Examines the case of *Rust v. Sullivan*, in which the Supreme Court sustained regulations barring abortion counseling and referral at federally-funded clinics. Criticizes the Court's deference to the executive branch and its failure to classify the regulations as violative of constitutional rights to free speech. Quotes Opinion 8.08. Note, *Rust on the Constitution: Politics and Gag Rules*, 37 How. L.J. 83, 96 (1993).

Journal 1993 Critiques the Supreme Court's decision in *Rust v. Sullivan*, which upheld regulations prohibiting employees of Title X-funded clinics from discussing abortions with patients. Advocates an affirmative government obligation to provide abortion counseling to Title X patients. Cites Opinion 8.08. Roberts, *Rust v. Sullivan and the Control of Knowledge*, 61 Geo. Wash. L. Rev. 587, 641 (1993).

Journal 1993 Discusses legal attempts to control reproduction by HIV-positive women. Suggests that controls will not achieve the goal of lessening children's suffering, but will discourage HIV-positive women from seeking health care services. Quotes Opinion 8.08. Sangree, *Control of Childbearing by HIV-Positive Women: Some Responses to Emerging Legal Policies*, 41 Buff. L. Rev. 309, 362 (1993).

Journal 1992 Examines the constitutionality of certain restrictions on speech in federally funded programs. Advocates greater first amendment protections in these situations. Quotes Opinion 8.08. Cole, *Beyond Unconstitutional Conditions: Charting Spheres of Neutrality in Government-Funded Speech*, 67 N.Y.U. L. Rev. 675, 744 (1992).

Journal 1992 Discusses the problem of protecting the privacy and confidentiality of public figures in light of contemporary tabloid journalism. Argues that current tort law does not adequately address this problem and advocates a new cause of action based on breach of confidentiality. Quotes Opinion 8.08. Harvey, *Confidentiality: A Measured Response to the Failure of Privacy*, 140 Univ. Pa. L. Rev. 2385, 2454 (1992).

Journal 1992 Analyzes the case of *Rust v. Sullivan* in which the US Supreme Court let stand regulations restricting abortion counseling in federally funded clinics. Concludes that *Rust* limits this right by expanding government powers. Cites Opinion 8.08. Note, *Constitutional Law—Judicial Deference—Supreme Court Will Defer to "Reasonable" Abortion Restrictions*, 14 Univ. Ark. Little Rock 557, 573 (1992).

Journal 1992 Discusses limitations on abortion counseling in federally funded clinics in light of the US Supreme Court decision in *Rust v. Sullivan*. Concludes that the *Rust* decision improperly limits freedom of speech. Cites Opinion 8.08. Note, *The Policy Against Federal Funding for Abortions Extends Into the Realm of Free Speech After Rust v. Sullivan*, 19 Pepperdine L. Rev. 637, 681 (1992).

Journal 1991 Discusses the manner in which a changing economy and an evolving health care system require society to expand its understanding of the physician-patient relationship. Concludes that open patient-physician discussion about available medical services and costs may become part of the standard of care. References Opinions 8.08 and 8.12. Morreim, *Economic Disclosure and Economic Advocacy: New Duties in the Medical Standard of Care*, 12 J. Legal Med. 275, 306 (1991).

Journal 1991 Considers how administrative restrictions on abortion counseling in Title X-funded clinics were affected by the Supreme Court's decision in *Rust v. Sullivan*. Concludes that *Rust* expands the powers of administrative agencies and narrows first amendment free speech rights and fifth amendment due process rights. Cites Opinion 8.08. Note, *Administrative Agencies Get Their Way Over Constitutional Rights in Rust v. Sullivan*, 28 Willamette L. Rev. 173, 193 (1991).

Journal 1991 Examines legal, ethical, and economic concerns surrounding pharmaceutical company promotions. Concludes that pharmaceutical freebies can serve a positive role in health care if adequately regulated. Quotes Opinions 8.061 and 8.08. Note, *The Economic Wisdom of Regulating Pharmaceutical "Freebies,"* 1991 Duke L.J. 206, 216, 233, 234 (1991).

Journal 1990 Examines Minnesota's "Crack Baby" law as a response to the increasing problem of drug abuse. Concludes that Minnesota's "Crack Baby" law endangers basic constitutional rights of women. Quotes Opinion 8.07 (1986) [now Opinion 8.08]. Johnson, *Minnesota's "Crack Baby" Law: Weapon of War or Link in a Chain?*, 8 Law & Ineq. 485, 494, 495, 496 (1990).

Journal 1983 Discusses both moral and legal dilemmas in the use of placebos in treating patients. Concludes that, while arguments against placebo therapy are noble, a complete ban of placebo therapy is impractical and undesirable. Quotes Opinions 8.07 (1982) [now Opinion 8.08] and 8.11 (1982) [now Opinion 8.12]. Kapp, *Placebo Therapy and the Law: Prescribe With Care*, 8 Am. J. Law & Med. 371, 391 (1983).

8.081 Surrogate Decision Making

Competent adults may formulate, in advance, preferences regarding a course of treatment in the event that injury or illness causes severe impairment or loss of decision-making capacity. These preferences should be followed by the health care team out of respect for patient autonomy. Patients may establish an advance directive by documenting their treatment preferences and goals or by designating a proxy to make health care decisions on their behalf.

If an incompetent patient is to receive medical treatment, a reasonable effort should be made to identify the presence of an advance directive. When such a patient lacks a documented advance directive, or when reasonable efforts have failed to uncover such documentation, physicians should defer to state law to identify a surrogate decision maker. In the absence of state law specifying either appropriate surrogate decision makers or a process to identify them, the patient's family should become the surrogate decision maker. Family includes persons with whom the patient is closely associated such as close friends or unmarried living partners. In the case when there is no family, but there are persons who have some relevant knowledge of the patient, such persons should participate in the decision-making process. In all other instances, a physician may wish to utilize an ethics committee to aid in identifying a surrogate decision maker or to facilitate sound decision making.

When there is evidence of the patient's preferences and values, decisions concerning the patient's care should be made by substituted judgment. This entails considering the patient's advance directive (if any), the patient's values about life and how it should be lived, how the patient constructed his or her identity or life story, and the patient's attitudes towards sickness, suffering, and certain medical procedures.

In some instances, a patient with diminished or impaired decision-making capacity can participate in various aspects of health care decision making. The attending physician should promote the autonomy of such individuals by involving them to a degree commensurate with their capabilities.

If there is no reasonable basis on which to interpret how a patient would have decided, the decision should be based on the best interests of the patient, or the outcome that would best promote the patient's well-being. Factors that should be considered when weighing the harms and benefits of various treatment options include the pain and suffering associated with treatment, the degree of and potential for benefit, and any impairments that may result from treatment. Any quality of life considerations should be measured as the worth to the individual whose course of treatment is in question, and not as a measure of social worth. One way to ensure that a decision using the best interest standard is not inappropriately influenced by the surrogate's own values is to determine the course of treatment that most reasonable persons would choose for themselves in similar circumstances.

Physicians should recognize the proxy or surrogate as an extension of the patient, entitled to the same respect as the competent patient. Physicians should provide advice, guidance, and support; explain that decisions should be based on substituted judgment when possible and otherwise on the best interest principle; and offer relevant medical information as well as medical opinions in a timely manner. In addition to the physician, other hospital staff or ethics committees are often helpful to providing support for the decision makers.

In general, physicians should respect decisions made by the appropriately designated surrogate on the basis of sound substituted judgment reasoning or the best interest standard. In cases where there is a dispute among family members, physicians should work to resolve the conflict through mediation. Physicians or an ethics committee should try to uncover the reasons that underlie the disagreement and present information that will facilitate decision making. When a physician believes that a decision is clearly not what the patient would have decided or could not be reasonably judged to be within the patient's best interests, the dispute should be referred to an ethics committee before resorting to the courts.

Physicians should encourage their patients to document their treatment preferences or to appoint a health care proxy with whom they can discuss their values regarding health care and treatment. Because documented advance directives are often not available in emergency situations, physicians should emphasize to patients the importance of discussing treatment preferences with individuals who are likely to act as their surrogates. (I, III, VIII)

Issued December 2001 based on the report "Surrogate Decision Making," adopted June 2001.

8.085   Waiver of Informed Consent for Research in Emergency Situations

The current state of emergency medicine and research has resulted in the application of standard treatments that often have not been scientifically evaluated for safety and effectiveness and may render unsatisfactory outcomes. Given the insufficiency of standard treatment alternatives, it is appropriate, in certain situations and with special safeguards, to provide experimental treatments without obtaining the informed consent of the subject. However, in order to protect the rights and welfare of the subjects, several conditions must be met:

(1) This type of research is limited to emergency, life-threatening situations, and may involve only experimental treatments that are ready for trials involving human subjects.

(2) The subject must lack the capacity to give informed consent for participation in the research.

(3) The window of opportunity for intervention must be so narrow as to make obtaining surrogate consent unfeasible.

(4) Obtaining prospective informed consent for the protocol must not be feasible (ie, the life threatening emergency situation could not have been anticipated).

(5) The experimental treatment must have a realistic probability of benefit equal to or greater than standard care.

(6) The risks associated with the research should be reasonable in light of the critical nature of the conditions and the risks associated with standard treatment.

(7) Where informed consent is waived, subjects or their representatives must be informed as soon as possible about inclusion in the study and asked to consent to further participation. Subjects, or their representatives, may choose to discontinue participation at any time after being fully informed about the possible consequences. Additionally, if the patient dies while participating in the research protocol, the patient's family or representative must be informed that the patient was involved in an experimental protocol.

(8) Community input should be sought prior to approval of the protocol, and public disclosure should be made of study results. Fair randomization of research subjects should be given thorough consideration. Moreover, an independent data monitoring board should be established to oversee the ongoing trial. (I, V)

Issued December 1997 based on the report "Waiver of Informed Consent for Research in Emergency Situations," adopted June 1997.

8.087 Medical Student Involvement in Patient Care

(1) Patients and the public benefit from the integrated care that is provided by health care teams that include medical students. Patients should be informed of the identity and training status of individuals involved in their care and all health care professionals share the responsibility for properly identifying themselves. Students and their supervisors should refrain from using terms that may be confusing when describing the training status of students.

(2) Patients are free to choose from whom they receive treatment. When medical students are involved in the care of patients, health care professionals should relate the benefits of medical student participation to patients and should ensure that they are willing to permit such participation. Generally, attending physicians are best suited to fulfill this responsibility.

(3) In instances where the patient will be temporarily incapacitated (eg, anesthetized) and where student involvement is anticipated, involvement should be discussed before the procedure is undertaken whenever possible. Similarly, in instances where a patient may not have the capacity to make decisions, student involvement should be discussed with the surrogate decision-maker involved in the care of the patient whenever possible. (V, VII)

Issued June 2001 based on the report "Medical Student Involvement in Patient Care," adopted December 2000 (J Clin Ethics. 2001; 12 :111-15).

8.09   Laboratory Services

(1) A physician should not misrepresent or aid in the misrepresentation of laboratory services performed and supervised by a non-physician as the physician's professional services. Such situations could involve a laboratory owned by a physician who directs and manages its financial and business affairs with no professional medical services being provided; laboratory work being performed by technicians and directly supervised by a medical technologist with no participation by the physician; or the physician's name being used in connection with the laboratory so as to create the appearance that it is owned, operated, and supervised by a physician when this is not so.

(2) If a laboratory is owned, operated, and supervised by a non-physician in accordance with state law and performs tests exclusively for physicians who receive the results and make their own medical interpretations, the following considerations would apply:

> The physician's ethical responsibility is to provide patients with high quality services. This includes services that the physician performs personally and those that are delegated to others. A physician should not utilize the services of any laboratory, irrespective of whether it is operated by a physician or non-physician, unless she or he has the utmost confidence in the quality of its services. A physician must always assume personal responsibility for the best interests of his or her patients. Medical judgment based upon inferior laboratory work is likewise inferior. Medical considerations, not cost, must be paramount when the physician chooses a laboratory. The physician who disregards quality as the primary criterion or who chooses a laboratory solely because it provides low-cost laboratory services on which the patient is charged a profit, is not acting in the best interests of the patient. However, if reliable, quality laboratory services are available at lower cost, the patient should have the benefit of the savings. As a professional, the physician is entitled to fair compensation for his or her services. A physician should not charge a markup, commission, or profit on the services rendered by others. A markup is an excessive charge that exploits patients if it is nothing more than a tacked on amount for a service already provided and accounted for by the laboratory. A physician may make an acquisition charge or processing charge. The patient should be notified of any such charge in advance. (I, II, III, IV, V)

Issued prior to April 1977.

Updated June 1994.

8.095   Reporting Clinical Test Results: General Guidelines

To alleviate patients' anxieties, physicians should report clinical test results to patients within a reasonable time frame. Since many variables contribute to the urgency of a particular situation, physicians should use their best professional judgment when determining what length of time is reasonable for the particular situation at hand. Anticipated delays should be explained to patients at the time of testing.

Physicians should adopt a consistent reporting policy that accommodates the demands of their practice while at the same time being considerate of patients' anxieties. The reporting policy should be disclosed to patients, for instance when tests are administered, so patients know what to expect. Reporting policies should take into consideration under what circumstances (eg, all results, only abnormal results) and by whom (eg, the laboratory or the physician) test results are appropriately reported to the patient. Any anticipated inconsistencies should be disclosed to patients as soon as they are discovered.

Physicians should provide test results in language understandable to the patient and in the manner deemed most appropriate by the physician. Any information gathered from test results that would be necessary for patients to make intelligent medical decisions and give informed consent on future medical treatments must be disclosed to them.

Physicians should take all appropriate precautions to ensure the confidentiality of test results. Such precautions may include, but are not limited to, not leaving test results on an answering machine, on voice mail, or with a third party unless previously given permission to do so by the patient, not delivering test results via electronic mail, and not sending test results through the mail in any form other than a sealed envelope. (II, IV, V)

Issued December 1998 based on the report "Reporting Clinical Test Results: General Guidelines," adopted June 1998.

8.10 Lien Laws

In states where there are lien laws, a physician may file a lien as a means of assuring payment of his or her fee provided the fee is fixed in amount and not contingent on the amount of settlement of the patient's claim against a third party. (I, VI)

Issued prior to April 1977.

8.11 Neglect of Patient

Physicians are free to choose whom they will serve. The physician should, however, respond to the best of his or her ability in cases of emergency where first aid treatment is essential. Once having undertaken a case, the physician should not neglect the patient. (I, VI)

Issued prior to April 1977.

Updated June 1996.

Ariz. 1965 Physician appealed denial of medical license which was based on alleged violations of local medical society rules and Principles 3, 5, and 10 (1957) [now Principles III and VII, and Opinions 3.01, 8.11, and 9.06]. Alleged violations included treating a patient without first obtaining a prior treating physician's permission, inadequate patient care, performing operations without hospital privileges, and signing the medical record of a deceased patient who had been treated by interns. The court held that the evidence failed to show any clear violation of the Principles and that a local medical society had no right to prescribe a code of ethics for state licensing purposes. *Arizona State Bd. of Medical Examiners v. Clark*, 97 Ariz. 205, 398 P.2d 908, 914-915, 915 n.3.

Ariz. App. 1980 Malpractice suit against a paid on call physician for refusal to treat decedent resulting in delay in treatment. The court quoted Principle 5 (1957) [now Principle VI and Opinion 8.11] as establishing an ethical duty to provide emergency care. However, court distinguished any such ethical obligation from its holding that physician had a contractual duty to treat emergency patients to the best of his ability. *Hiser v. Randolph*, 126 Ariz. 608, 617 P.2d 774, 776 n.1, 777, 778.

Cal. App. 1978 Surviving spouse sued physicians who were on emergency surgical call panel for malpractice where patient died during surgery. Although defendants claimed immunity under state Good Samaritan statute, the court held the statute inapplicable since the legislative purpose was to encourage physicians to render care on an irregular basis to unattended persons discovered by chance at the scene of an emergency. In so holding, the court noted that Principle 5 (1957) [now Principle VI and Opinions 8.11 and 9.06] imposed an ethical duty to render emergency medical care. *Colby v. Schwartz*, 78 Cal. App. 3d 885, 144 Cal. Rptr. 624, 627 n.2.

Ill. App. 1997 Physician was found to be in civil contempt for violating a covenant not to compete by performing administrative functions from his home office. The trial court ordered the physician to desist from practicing medicine within the restricted area. The appellate court, in reversing, found that although the language of the agreement was ambiguous, it could be construed to prohibit the physician from practicing medicine. However, the court found that the practice of medicine does not include activities which are administrative or managerial in nature. Further, the court, quoting from Opinion 8.11, found that physicians have a legal and ethical duty to care for their patients, and may not neglect patients once they begin treatment. The court held that a finding of contempt for violating an agreement not to compete cannot be supported where physicians do not examine patients, but merely address medically related questions by phone. *Bloomington Urological Associates v. Scaglia*, 292 Ill. App. 3d, 793, 686 N.E. 2d 389, 394.

Ky. App. 1989 Malpractice suit was initiated against physician for failure to treat plaintiff's brother where defendant had repeatedly rebuffed plaintiff's request for emergency assistance and told him to get in line or sign in. Plaintiff removed his brother to another hospital where he subsequently died of heart attack. Plaintiff argued that defendant was under a duty to treat based upon, inter alia, the AMA Code of Ethics [apparently Principle VI and Opinion 8.11]. The court rejected the argument, finding that a breach of ethical standards may establish grounds for professional discipline, but not a civil cause of action, and held that defendant was under no legal duty to treat. *Noble v. Sartori*, 1989 Ky. App. LEXIS 67.

Ohio Att'y Gen. 1999 State attorney general concluded that physicians who render opinions regarding the necessity of medical services for health insuring corporations are not engaged in the practice of medicine. Additionally, physicians who render opinions regarding medical necessity for appeals of adverse determinations do not fall under the regulatory, investigatory, or enforcement authority of the Ohio State Medical Board. Quoting Opinions 8.03, 8.11, and 8.13, the attorney general stated that physicians have an ethical duty to provide appropriate treatment for patients. *Ohio Att'y Gen. Op. No. 99-044, 1999 WL 692623.*

Journal 1999 Discusses potential conflicts between a criminal defense attorney's religious beliefs and representation of the client. Explores theories that would allow an attorney to put religious beliefs over the client's interest. Offers analogies within the physician-patient relationship. Concludes that a defense attorney is bound by duty and must set aside conflicting religious beliefs. Quotes Principle VI and Opinions 8.11, 9.06, and 9.12. Reza, *Religion and the Public Defender*, 26 Fordham Urb. L. J. 1051, 1062, 1063 (1999).

Journal 1998 Explains when a surrogate is required to make health care decisions. Discusses limitations of a surrogate's authority. Emphasizes that the health care provider must recognize that ultimate decision-making regarding care first belongs to the patient, and then to the surrogate. Quotes Opinion 2.035. Cites Opinion 8.11. References Opinion 2.22. O'Neill, *Surrogate Health Care Decisions for Adults in Illinois—Answers to the Legal Questions That Health Care Providers Face on a Daily Basis*, 29 Loy. Univ. Chi. L. J. 411, 445, 448 (1998).

Journal 1995 Argues that nonabandonment should be a core physician obligation. Suggests that if nonabandonment is better incorporated into medical ethics, medicine will become more humanized and responsive to everyday physician-patient problems. Quotes Opinion 8.10 (1986) [now Opinion 8.11]. Quill & Cassel, *Nonabandonment: A Central Obligation for Physicians*, 10 *Trends in Health Care, Law & Ethics* 25, 27 (Winter/Spring 1995).

Journal 1995 Offers relevant historical perspectives and provides comprehensive ethical and legal discussion of physician-assisted suicide and euthanasia. Highlights important legislative developments, including the Oregon Death with Dignity Act, and analyzes significant judicial opinions. Quotes Principles III, IV, and VI and Opinions 2.21 and 9.12. Cites Opinions 2.20 and 8.11. Stone & Winslade, *Physician-Assisted Suicide and Euthanasia in the United States: Legal and Ethical Observations*, 16 J. Legal Med. 481, 483, 490, 497, 498, 499 (1995).

Journal 1993 Explores the idea of reverse informed consent, which would impose a duty on patients to inform health care professionals of their infectious status. Concludes that such a duty is justified. Quotes Principles IV and VI and Opinions 8.11 and 9.131. Oddi, *Reverse Informed Consent: The Unreasonably Dangerous Patient*, 46 Vand. L. Rev. 1417, 1449, 1463, 1465, 1479 (1993).

Journal 1988 Discusses the question of whether health professionals are obligated to subject themselves to the risks that attend treating patients with communicable diseases, particularly AIDS. Examines the ethical pronouncements and codes of the nursing and medical professions in this respect, noting that the most recent statements of professional values imply the existence of an obligation to treat HIV-infectious patients. Quotes Opinion 8.10 (1986) [now Opinion 8.11] and Principle VI. Cites Opinion 9.11 (1986) [now Opinion 9.12]. Freedman, *Health Professions, Codes, and the Right to Refuse to Treat HIV-Infectious Patients*, 18 Hastings Center Rep. 20 (Supp.), 23, 24 (April/May 1988).

Journal 1987 Concludes that a policy or practice of active voluntary euthanasia is not desirable, linking a moral prohibition against active voluntary euthanasia to the moral prohibition against physicians actively participating in capital punishment. In place of any practice of active voluntary euthanasia, recommends increased use of hospices, greater emphasis on training physicians to care for the dying patient, and further research aimed at producing symptomatic relief in dying patients. Cites Opinions 2.06, 8.10 (1986) [now Opinion 8.11], and 9.06. Shewmon, *Active Voluntary Euthanasia: A Needless Pandora's Box*, 3 Issues in Law and Med. 219, 220, 222, 243 (1987).

Journal 1986 Examines common law and statutory law applicable to patient dumping, and emphasizes the antidumping provisions of COBRA. Weaknesses in this federal legislative scheme are highlighted and recommendations for strengthening the statute and maximizing access to emergency medical care are offered. Quotes Principle VI and Opinion 8.10 (1986) [now Opinion 8.11]. Note, *Preventing Patient Dumping: Sharpening the COBRA's Fangs*, 61 N. Y. U. L. Rev. 1186, 1189-90 (1986).

8.115 Termination of the Physician-Patient Relationship

Physicians have an obligation to support continuity of care for their patients. While physicians have the option of withdrawing from a case, they cannot do so without giving notice to the patient, the relatives, or responsible friends sufficiently long in advance of withdrawal to permit another medical attendant to be secured. (I, VI)

Issued June 1996 (formerly included in Opinion 8.11, "Neglect of Patients").

Mass. Super. 1993 Plaintiff sought to enjoin defendant-physician from contacting patients that defendant treated while employed with plaintiff. The court denied the injunction, noting that under Opinion 8.11 [now Opinion 8.115] defendant has a duty to notify his patients before withdrawing from a case and an injunction would force defendant to choose between violating professional ethics or violating a court order. *Plastic Surgical Servs. of New England, P.C. v. Hall*, 1993 WL 818637.

Journal 1998 Explains the connection and differences between bioethics and the law. States that the distinction between ethics and law is that ethics places additional emphasis on moral ideals. References Opinions 8.08 and 8.115. Sullivan & Reynolds, *Where Law and Bioethics Meet . . . and Where They Don't*, 75 U. Det. Mercy L. Rev. 607, 612 (1998).

Journal 1997 Compares past ethical opinions to current opinions and notes the differences. Comments on the forces that have changed medical ethics through the years. Notes differing theories on the future course of medical ethics. Quotes Fundamental Elements (Preamble) and Opinions 5.05, 5.057, 7.01, 8.12, 9.12, and 9.131. Cites Fundamental Elements (5) and Opinions 8.115 and 8.13. Buchanan, *Medical Ethics at the Millennium: A Brief Retrospective*, 26 *Colo. Law. 141, 142, 143, 144, 145 (1997)*.

8.12 Patient Information

It is a fundamental ethical requirement that a physician should at all times deal honestly and openly with patients. Patients have a right to know their past and present medical status and to be free of any mistaken beliefs concerning their conditions. Situations occasionally occur in which a patient suffers significant medical complications that may have resulted from the physician's mistake or judgment. In these situations, the physician is ethically required to inform the patient of all the facts necessary to ensure understanding of what has occurred. Only through full disclosure is a patient able to make informed decisions regarding future medical care.

Ethical responsibility includes informing patients of changes in their diagnoses resulting from retrospective review of test results or any other information. This obligation holds even though the patient's medical treatment or therapeutic options may not be altered by the new information.

Concern regarding legal liability which might result following truthful disclosure should not affect the physician's honesty with a patient. (I, II, III, IV)

Issued March 1981.

Updated June 1994.

Minn. 1970 Defendant-physician appealed order to answer interrogatories, claiming that a medical malpractice plaintiff is prohibited from compelling expert testimony from a defendant to prove a charge of malpractice without calling other medical witnesses. In holding that a defendant could be compelled to provide expert medical opinion in response to interrogatories, the court quoted Principle 1 (1957) [now Principle II and Opinion 8.12] for the proposition that physicians owe a duty of disclosure to their patients. *Anderson v. Florence, 288 Minn. 351, 181 N.W.2d 873, 880, 880 n.7.*

Journal 2002 Discusses therapeutic jurisprudence and the importance of trust in the structure of health care law. Concludes that understanding trust provides tools to formulate responses to new ethical, legal, and policy challenges. Quotes Principle Ch. I, Art. I, Sec. 4 (1847) [now Principle II and Opinion 8.12]. Hall, *Law, Medicine, and Trust, 55 Stan. L. Rev. 463, 471 (2002)*.

Journal 2002 Advocates in favor of disclosure of information regarding a physician's clinical experience when obtaining informed consent. Concludes that the physician's experience is material and patients who inquire should be given this information. Quotes Principle Ch. I, Art. I, Sec. 4 (1847) [now Principle II and Opinion 8.12]. Iheukwumere, *Doctor, are You Experienced? The Relevance of Disclosure of Physician Experience to a Valid Informed Consent, 18 J. Contemp. Health L. & Pol'y 373, 376-77 (2002)*.

Journal 2002 Examines various interpretations of JCAHO standards regarding informing patients about medical errors. Concludes that further clarification is needed regarding reportable events. Quotes Opinion 8.12. LeGros & Pinkall, *The New JCAHO Patient Safety Standards and the Disclosure of Unanticipated Outcomes, 35 J. Health L. 189, 203 (2002)*.

Journal 2002 Analyzes the role of prognostication in physician-patient communication. Concludes that the patient-physician model of shared decision-making offers the best hope for reestablishing prognostication. Quotes Principles Ch. I, Art. I, Sec. 2 and 4 (1846) [now Principle IV and Opinions 8.12 and 10.01]. Cites Opinion 8.08. Rich, *Prognostication in Clinical Medicine: Prophecy or Professional Responsibility? 23 J. Legal Med. 297, 299, 318, 327 (2002)*.

Journal 2001 Discusses whether or not the medical profession needs a policy on honesty. Reviews ethical codes and concludes they fail to offer physicians with meaningful guidance about what constitutes "the truth" and when and how to disclose it. Quotes Principle II and Opinions 8.12 and 10.01. DeVita, *Honestly, Do We Need a Policy on Truth?* 11 Kennedy Inst. Ethics J. 157, 158 (2001).

Journal 2001 Examines the duty of physicians and medical students to disclose physician mistakes. Concludes that students develop professionally by recognizing personal ethical standards and determining how to manage conflicting priorities. Quotes Opinion 8.12. Wusthoff, *Medical Mistakes and Disclosure: The Role of the Medical Student*, 286 J.A.M.A. 1080, 1080 (2001).

Journal 2000 Examines the lost chance doctrine in medical malpractice cases. Reviews Texas law by evaluating the cases of *Kramer v. Lewisville Mem'l Hosp.* and *Park Place Hosp. v. Estate of Milo*. Examines the distinction between affirmative acts and omissions. Discusses the limitations and pitfalls of both cases. Quotes Opinion 8.12. Perdue & Binion, *A License to Kill: The Unintended (?) Consequence of Milo on Kramer*, 41 S. Tex. L. Rev. 293, 309 (2000).

Journal 1997 Compares past ethical opinions to current opinions and notes the differences. Comments on the forces that have changed medical ethics through the years. Notes differing theories on the future course of medical ethics. Quotes Fundamental Elements (Preamble) and Opinions 5.05, 5.057, 7.01, 8.12, 9.12, and 9.131. Cites Fundamental Elements (5) and Opinions 8.115 and 8.13. Buchanan, *Medical Ethics at the Millennium: A Brief Retrospective*, 26 Colo. Law. 141, 142, 143, 144, 145 (1997).

Journal 1996 Presents clinical problem-solving scenarios. Notes the AMA's instruction that physicians deal openly and honestly with patients. Considers the physician's role as educator and counselor. Opines that physicians must ensure that patients have the ability to make informed decisions. Quotes Opinion 8.12. Sirmon & Kreisberg, *The Invisible Patient*, 334 New Eng. J. Med. 908, 910, 911 (1996).

Journal 1991 Discusses the manner in which a changing economy and an evolving health care system require society to expand its understanding of the physician-patient relationship. Concludes that open physician-patient discussion about available medical services and costs may become part of the standard of care. References Opinions 8.08 and 8.12. Morreim, *Economic Disclosure and Economic Advocacy: New Duties in the Medical Standard of Care*, 12 J. Legal Med. 275, 306 (1991).

Journal 1983 Discusses both moral and legal dilemmas in the use of placebos in treating patients. Concludes that, while arguments against placebo therapy are noble, a complete ban of placebo therapy is impractical and undesirable. Quotes Opinions 8.07 (1982) [now Opinion 8.08] and 8.11 (1982) [now Opinion 8.12]. Kapp, *Placebo Therapy and the Law: Prescribe With Care*, 8 Am. J. Law & Med. 371, 391 (1983).

8.121 Ethical Responsibility to Study and Prevent Error and Harm

In the context of health care, an error is an unintended act or omission, or a flawed system or plan, that harms or has the potential to harm a patient. Patient safety can be enhanced by studying the circumstances surrounding health care errors. This can best be achieved through a legally protected review process, which is essential for reducing health care errors and preventing patient harm.

(1) Because they are uniquely positioned to have a comprehensive view of the care patients receive, physicians must strive to ensure patient safety and should play a central role in identifying, reducing, and preventing health care errors. This responsibility exists even in the absence of a patient-physician relationship.

(2) Physicians should participate in the development of reporting mechanisms that emphasize education and systems change, thereby providing a substantive opportunity for all members of the health care team to learn.

Specifically, physicians should work with other relevant health care professionals to:

(a) Establish and participate fully in an effective, confidential, and protected error-reporting mechanism

(b) Develop means for objective review and analysis of reports regarding errors, and to conduct appropriate investigations into the causes of harm to a patient

(c) Ensure that the investigation of causes of harm, and the review and study of error reports result in preventive measures that are conveyed to all relevant individuals

(d) Identify and promptly report impaired and/or incompetent colleagues so that rehabilitation, retraining or disciplinary action can occur in order to prevent harm to patients

(3) Physicians must offer professional and compassionate concern toward patients who have been harmed, regardless of whether the harm was caused by a health care error. An expression of concern need not be an admission of responsibility. When patient harm has been caused by an error, physicians should offer a general explanation regarding the nature of the error and the measures being taken to prevent similar occurrences in the future. Such communication is fundamental to the trust that underlies the patient-physician relationship, and may help reduce the risk of liability.

(4) Physicians have a responsibility to provide for continuity of care to patients who may have been harmed during the course of their health care. If, because of the harm suffered under the care of a physician, a patient loses trust in that physician, the obligation may best be fulfilled by facilitating the transfer of the patient to the care of another physician.

(5) Physicians should seek changes to the current legal system to ensure that all errors in health care can be safely and securely reported and studied as a learning experience for all participants in the health care system, without threat of discoverability, legal liability, or punitive action. (I, II, III, IV, VIII)

Issued December 2003 based on the report "Ethical Responsibility to Study and Prevent Error and Harm in the Provision of Health Care," adopted June 2003.

8.13   The previous Opinion 8.13, "Referral of Patients: Disclosure of Limitations," was changed to Opinion 8.132, "Referral of Patients: Disclosure of Limitations," in June 1996.

8.13   Managed Care

The expansion of managed care has brought a variety of changes to medicine including new and different reimbursement systems for physicians with complex referral restrictions and benefits packages for patients. Some of these changes have raised concerns that a physician's ability to practice ethical medicine will be adversely affected by the modifications in the system. In response to these concerns, the following points were developed to provide physicians with general guidelines that will assist them in fulfilling their ethical responsibilities to patients given the changes heralded by managed care.

(1) The duty of patient advocacy is a fundamental element of the patient-physician relationship that should not be altered by the system of health care delivery. Physicians must continue to place the interests of their patients first.

(2) When health care plans place restrictions on the care that physicians in the plan may provide to their patients, physicians should insist that the following principles be followed:

(a) Any broad allocation guidelines that restrict care and choices—which go beyond the cost/benefit judgments made by physicians as a part of their normal professional responsibilities—should be established at a policy-making level so that individual physicians are not asked to engage in bedside rationing.

(b) Regardless of any allocation guidelines or gatekeeper directives, physicians must advocate for any care they believe will materially benefit their patients.

(c) Physicians should be given an active role in contributing their expertise to any allocation process and should advocate for guidelines that are sensitive to differences among patients. Health care plans should create structures similar to hospital medical staffs that allow physicians to have meaningful input into the plan's development of allocation guidelines. Guidelines for allocating health care should be reviewed on a regular basis and updated to reflect advances in medical knowledge and changes in relative costs.

(d) Adequate appellate mechanisms for both patients and physicians should be in place to address disputes regarding medically necessary care. In some circumstances, physicians have an obligation to initiate appeals on behalf of their patients. Cases may arise in which a health plan has an allocation guideline that is generally fair but in particular circumstances results in unfair denials of care, ie, denial of care that, in the physician's judgment, would materially benefit the patient. In such cases, the physician's duty as patient advocate requires that the physician challenge the denial and argue for the provision of treatment in the specific case. Cases may also arise when a health plan has an allocation guideline that is generally unfair in its operations. In such cases, the physician's duty as patient advocate requires not only a challenge to any denials of treatment from the guideline but also advocacy at the health plan's policy-making level to seek an elimination or modification of the guideline. Physicians should assist patients who wish to seek additional, appropriate care outside the plan when the physician believes the care is in the patient's best interests.

(e) Health care plans must adhere to the requirement of informed consent that patients be given full disclosure of material information. Full disclosure requires that health care plans inform potential subscribers of limitations or restrictions on the benefits package when they are considering entering the plan.

(f) Physicians also should continue to promote full disclosure to patients enrolled in health care plans. The physician's obligation to disclose treatment alternatives to patients is not altered by any limitations in the coverage provided by the patient's health care plan. Full disclosure includes informing patients of all of their treatment options, even those that may not be covered under the terms of the health care plan. Patients may then determine whether an appeal is appropriate, or whether they wish to seek care outside the plan for treatment alternatives that are not covered.

(g) Physicians should not participate in any plan that encourages or requires care below minimum professional standards.

(3) When physicians are employed or reimbursed by health care plans that offer financial incentives to limit care, serious potential conflicts are created between the physicians' personal financial interests and the needs of their patients. Efforts to contain health care costs should not place patient welfare at risk. Thus, physicians should accept only those financial incentives that promote the cost-effective delivery of health care and not the withholding of medically necessary care.

(a) Physicians should insist that any incentives to limit care must be disclosed fully to patients by plan administrators upon enrollment and at least annually thereafter.

(b) Physicians should advocate that limits be placed on the magnitude of fee withholds, bonuses, and other financial incentives to limit care and that incentive payments be calculated according to the performance of a sizable group of physicians rather than on an individual basis.

(c) Physicians should advocate that health care plans or other groups develop financial incentives based on quality of care. Such incentives should complement those based on the quantity of services used.

(4) Physicians should encourage both that patients be aware of the benefits and limitations of their health care coverage and that they exercise their autonomy by public participation in the formulation of benefits packages and by prudent selection of health care coverage that best suits their needs. (I, II, III, V)

Issued June 1996 based on the report "Ethical Issues in Managed Care," adopted June 1994 (JAMA. 1995; 273: 330-35).

Updated June 2002.

D. N. J. 1999 Patient sued her managed care organization alleging that she suffered injuries due to failure to obtain timely approval for a non-member physician to perform her back surgery. The plaintiff apparently relied on Opinion 8.13 to show that the defendant had a duty to advocate for her in seeking prompt approval for her surgery. The court, however, stated that the plaintiff's reference to the Opinion failed to establish such a duty because the Code of Medical Ethics does not have the force of law. *Pryzbowski v. US Health Care, Inc., 64 F. Supp. 2d 361, 370.*

S.D.N.Y. 1997 Employee brought suit against a health maintenance organization (HMO) under contract with her employer to provide health benefits. The suit alleged various theories of liability ranging from breach of implied contract to breach of fiduciary duties. Employee sought redress pursuant to the civil enforcement provisions of the Employee Retirement Income Security Act of 1974 (ERISA). The court granted HMO's motion to dismiss all claims except for the breach of fiduciary duty stemming from HMO's alleged policy of restricting the disclosure of non-covered treatments. The court quoted report of AMA Council on Ethical and Judicial Affairs [now

Opinion 8.13] in holding that physicians have an ethical duty to fully disclose treatment options to patients regardless of whether treatment occurs in a managed care environment. *Weiss v. Cigna Healthcare, Inc., 972 F. Supp. 748, 751-52.*

Ohio Att'y Gen. 1999 State attorney general concluded that physicians who render opinions regarding the necessity of medical services for health insuring corporations are not engaged in the practice of medicine. Additionally, physicians who render opinions regarding medical necessity for appeals of adverse determinations do not fall under the regulatory, investigatory, or enforcement authority of the Ohio State Medical Board. Quoting Opinions 8.03, 8.11, and 8.13, the attorney general stated that physicians have an ethical duty to provide appropriate treatment for patients. *Ohio Att'y Gen. Op. No. 99-044, 1999 WL 692623.*

Journal 2002 Observes that changes in the health professions challenge certain assumptions about professional ethics. Concludes that these long-standing assumptions must be re-examined. Cites Opinion 2.161. References Opinion 8.13. Kelley, *The Meanings of Professional Life: Teaching Across the Health Professions, 27 J. Med. & Phil. 475, 485, 490, 491 (2002).*

Journal 2002 Considers whether physicians should be required to disclose information regarding financial incentives received from patients' HMOs. Concludes that physicians should not be required to disclose these incentives. References Opinion 8.13. Reuland, *Health Maintenance Organizations and Physician Financial Incentive Plans: Should Physician Disclosure be Mandatory? 27 Iowa J. Corp. L. 293, 312 (2002).*

Journal 2002 Examines whether managed care organizations should be obligated to disclose physician financial incentives that may limit patient care. Concludes that mandatory disclosure is in the best interest of patients and physicians. Quotes Opinions 2.03 and 8.13. Talesh, *Breaking the Learned Helplessness of Patients: Why MCOs Should be Required to Disclose Financial Incentives, 26 Law & Psychol. Rev. 49, 60-61, 63 (2002).*

Journal 2001 Examines issues relating to health care cost containment. Concludes that, if physicians are to meet the goals assigned to them in a cost-constrained health care system, then professional standards must be reevaluated and modified to afford meaningful guidance for clinical decision-making in the face of health care spending controls. Quotes Opinions 2.03, 2.09, 2.095, 8.032, and 9.04. Cites Opinions 8.02, 8.021, 8.051, and 8.13. Agrawal, *Resuscitating Professionalism: Self-Regulation in the Medical Marketplace, 66 Mo. L. Rev. 341, 354, 355, 360, 361, 378, 388 (2001).*

Journal 2001 Examines the doctrine of informed consent with respect to nontraditional issues, such as a physician's duty to disclose personal information. Concludes there must be a balance that will accommodate the needs of both the patient and the physician. References Opinion 8.13. Hanson, *Informed Consent and the Scope of a Physician's Duty of Disclosure, 77 N.D. L. Rev. 71, 89, 91 (2001).*

Journal 2001 Discusses the prohibition on non-lawyer ownership of legal service providers. Considers how ethical rules and standards governing physicians have been directed toward preserving independent judgment. Concludes that ethical conflicts created by abandoning the prohibition on non-lawyer ownership of legal service providers may be managed by following the medical ethics model. Quotes Principle VI and Opinions 2.03, 2.09, 8.02, 8.021, 8.03, 8.05, 8.051, 8.054, 8.13, and 8.132. Harris & Foran, *The Ethics of Middle-Class Access to Legal Services and What We Can Learn from the Medical Profession's Shift to a Corporate Paradigm, 70 Fordham L. Rev. 775, 817, 821, 822, 823, 824 (2001).*

Journal 2000 Discusses and evaluates different systems for addressing consumer concerns about managed health care. Asserts that current legal systems for identifying and resolving consumer concerns are not understood by most consumers and are not accessible by many, especially the uninsured. Concludes that several immediate steps are realistic for moving toward reform. Cites Principle VI. References Opinions 8.13 and 9.065. Kinney, *Tapping and Resolving Consumer Concerns About Health Care, 26 Am. J. Law & Med. 335, 337, 375 (2000).*

Journal 2000 Reviews the case of *Corporate Health Insurance, Inc. v. Texas Dept. of Insurance* and discusses its impact on HMO liability in Texas. Considers the conflicts of interest managed care imposes upon physicians. Concludes that, without national amendments to the scope of ERISA, HMOs are not compelled to provide quality health care. References Opinion 8.13. Lockhart, *The Safest Care is to Deny Care: Implications of Corporate Health Insurance, Inc. v. Texas Department of Insurance on HMO Liability in Texas, 41 S. Tex. L. Rev. 621, 628, 634 (2000).*

Journal 2000 Describes the fiduciary aspects of the physician-patient relationship. Explores the conflicts that may occur between physicians and pregnant women in the health care setting. Proposes legal strategies to address these conflicts. Quotes Opinions 8.08 and 10.01. References Opinion 8.13. Oberman, *Mothers and Doctors' Orders: Unmasking the Doctor's Fiduciary Role in Maternal-Fetal Conflicts*, 94 Nw. U. L. Rev. 451, 456, 462, 493 (2000).

Journal 1999 Describes the gag clause debate in managed care and analyzes the types of incentives that might limit physician-patient communication. Concludes that, to protect patient access to information about treatment options and their health plans, antigag legislation must be coupled with a thorough examination of the extent to which financial incentives will be permitted to impact managed health care delivery. Quotes Opinion 8.13. Krause, *The Brief Life of the Gag Clause: Why Antigag Clause Legislation Isn't Enough*, 67 Tenn. L. Rev. 1, 4, 43 (1999).

Journal 1999 Describes the development of managed care organizations. Examines professional associations' statements regarding managed care organizations. Argues that physicians and managed care organizations should be viewed as economically disciplined, moral co-fiduciaries for patients. References Opinions 8.13. McCullough, *A Basic Concept in the Clinical Ethics of Managed Care: Physicians and Institutions as Economically Disciplined Moral Co-Fiduciaries of Populations of Patients*, 24 J. Med. Phil. 77, 82-83, 87, 89, 91, 96 (1999).

Journal 1999 Explores the increased push toward mandatory disclosure laws regarding financial incentives imposed by managed care organizations. Discusses current laws and ethical guidelines. Emphasizes that efforts to mandate disclosure force physicians to focus on the effects of imposed incentives and the essence of the physician-patient relationship. References Opinions 8.032, 8.13, and 8.132. Miller & Sage, *Disclosing Physician Financial Incentives*, 281 JAMA 1424, 1425 (1999).

Journal 1999 Discusses the need for physicians to advocate on behalf of patients' rights in the context of health care delivery. Evaluates the nature and scope of the physician's role as advocate, noting that physicians cannot be expected to engage in attorney-like advocacy. Quotes Principles IV and VI, Fundamental Elements (2), (4), and (6) [now Opinion 10.01], Patient Responsibilities 5 [now Opinion 10.02], and Opinions 2.03, 2.07, 2.09, 2.16, 2.19, 3.06, 4.01, 4.04, 6.01, 7.02, 8.02, 8.03, 8.13, 8.132, 9.06, 9.07, and 9.131. Cites Opinions 5.05, 5.09, 7.01, 8.135, and 9.02. Sage, *Physicians as Advocates*, 35 Hous. L. Rev. 1529, 1537, 1541, 1542, 1552-53, 1554, 1556, 1557, 1559, 1561-62, 1564, 1571, 1574, 1576, 1580 (1999).

Journal 1999 Discusses the push to mandate disclosure in managed care programs. Explains the dangers of disclosing too much information. Provides objectives and goals for disclosure. Quotes Opinion 8.051. References Opinions 8.032 and 8.13. Sage, *Regulating Through Information: Disclosure Laws and American Health Care*, 99 Colum. L. Rev. 1701, 1753, 1758, 1760 (1999).

Journal 1999 Argues that the benefits of managed care organizations are outweighed by the resulting changes in the physician's role as advocate. Characterizes the traditional notion of physician advocacy. States that recent changes in the law regarding communication in managed care organizations have shifted the matter more toward patient self-advocacy. Quotes Opinion 8.13. Spielman, *Managed Care Regulation and the Physician-Advocate*, 47 Drake L. Rev. 713, 717, 719 (1999).

Journal 1999 Discusses financial incentives offered to physicians by managed care organizations. Argues that evidence of financial incentives should be admissible in medical malpractice cases. Quotes Opinion 8.13. References Opinion 8.132. Sugarman & Yarashus, *Admissibility of Managed Care Financial Incentives in Medical Malpractice Cases*, 34 Tort & Ins. L. J. 735, 743, 746, 759 (1999).

Journal 1999 Explores the impact managed care organizations have had on health care. Explains that patients may not understand restrictions and incentives imposed by their managed care organizations when entering the program. Argues that such information should be disclosed at various times during the period of plan coverage. Cites Opinions 2.03, 8.03, 8.032, 8.051, 8.13 and 8.132. Wolf, *Toward a Systemic Theory of Informed Consent in Managed Care*, 35 Hous. L. Rev. 1631, 1641, 1658, 1661, 1662, 1679 (1999).

Journal 1998 Analyzes Hall's book *Making Medical Spending Decisions: The Law, Ethics and Economics of Rationing Mechanisms*. Discusses cost-based rationing for medical services and physician bedside rationing. Concludes that patients should be informed in advance when their physician may receive financial incentives for withholding care. Quotes Opinion 8.13. Agrawal, *Chicago Hope Meets the Chicago School*, 96 Mich. L. Rev. 1793, 1804 (1998).

Journal 1998 Discusses changes in the health care system. Explains why patients need more power in the managed care system. Suggests that patients should use class action suits as a method to assert power over managed care organizations. References Opinions 8.13 and 8.132. Cerminara, *The Class Action Suit As a Method of Patient Empowerment in the Managed Care Setting*, 24 Am. J. Law & Med. 7, 16, 17, 23 (1998).

Journal 1998 Discusses conflicts of interest in the physician-patient relationship arising out of use of financial incentives by managed care organizations. Considers how such conflicts are dealt with in the attorney-client relationship. Suggests that a financial incentive should be legally denounced if it unreasonably interferes with a physician's duty to properly care for and treat patients. Quotes Preamble, Fundamental Elements (1) [now Opinion 10.01] and Opinions 4.04, 5.01, 8.03, 8.13, and 9.06. Cites Fundamental Elements (4) [now Opinion 10.01] and Opinions 2.07, 2.08, and 2.132. Hall, *Third-Party Payor Conflicts of Interest in Managed Care: A Proposal for Regulation Based on the Model Rules of Professional Conduct*, 29 Seton Hall L. Rev. 95, 96, 107, 108, 109, 110, 111, 112, 134, 135, 136 (1998).

Journal 1998 Asserts that managed care organizations assume fiduciary obligations by exercising discretionary control over the administration of an ERISA plan. Argues that ERISA requires managed care organizations and physicians to disclose financial incentives intended to influence physician decision-making. References Opinions 8.13 and 8.132. Johnson, *ERISA Doctor in the House? The Duty to Disclose Physician Incentives to Limit Health Care*, 82 Minn. L. Rev. 1631, 1639, 1649, 1655 (1998).

Journal 1998 Discusses changes in the health care system. Analyzes conflicts of interest arising from the practice of capitation. Argues that physicians should refuse to sign contracts with health care plans offering incentives that may present a temptation to under-treat patients. References Opinion 8.13. Kassirer, *Managing Care—Should We Adopt a New Ethic?*, 339 New Eng. J. Med. 397 (1998).

Journal 1998 Expresses concern about the impact of managed care cost-containment practices on the physician-patient relationship. Advocates the need for disclosure of information about these practices to patients. Evaluates and recommends a Maryland law that requires such disclosure. Cites Opinion 8.13. Khanna, Silverman, & Schwartz, *Disclosure of Operating Practices By Managed-Care Organizations to Consumers of Healthcare: Obligations of Informed Consent*, 9 J. Clinical Ethics 291, 293, 296 (1998).

Journal 1998 Discusses quality and safety concerns arising under managed care systems. Explores benefits and detriments of the proposed patients' bill of rights. Advocates legislation to provide safeguards from cost-containment mechanisms utilized by managed care programs. Quotes Opinion 8.13. Misocky, *The Patients' Bill of Rights: Managed Care Under Siege*, 15 J. Contemp. Health L. & Pol'y 57, 73 (1998).

Journal 1998 Explores clinical freedom and the Hippocratic Oath. Discusses issues of patient trust and confidence. Suggests that a sense of confidence will not be present if managerial priorities are dominant factors in resource allocation. References Opinion 8.13. Newdick, *Public Health Ethics and Clinical Freedom*, 14 J. Contemp. Health L. & Pol'y 335, 336, 339, 356, 359, 361 (1998).

Journal 1998 Discusses communication conflicts between physicians and managed care organizations. Describes legal responses to gag provisions imposed by managed care organizations. Assesses the impact of gag practices on physician-patient communication. Quotes Opinion 8.13. Spielman, *After the Gag Episode: Physician Communication in Managed Care Organizations*, 22 Seton Hall Legis. J. 437, 453, 461, 463 (1998).

Journal 1998 Argues that health maintenance organizations (HMOs) do not have an incentive to act reasonably because they are not held accountable under tort law. Points out that the duty to act reasonably is imposed on most of society in order to deter negligence. Advocates imposing the same duty on HMOs. References Opinion 8.13. Wertheimer, *Ockham's Scalpel: A Return to a Reasonableness Standard*, 43 Vill. L. Rev. 321, 327 (1998).

Journal 1997 Discusses the quality of neurological care and the ethical conflicts that are created by the drive to contain costs. Focuses on quality management and cost-containment programs and the conflicts created when neurologists attempt to reconcile the interests of patients and society. References Opinions 8.032 and 8.13. Bernat, *Quality of Neurological Care: Balancing Cost Control and Ethics*, 54 Arch. Neurol. 1341, 1343, 1345 (1997).

Journal 1997 Compares past ethical opinions to current opinions and notes the differences. Comments on the forces that have changed medical ethics through the years. Notes differing theories on the future course of medical ethics. Quotes Fundamental Elements (Preamble) and Opinions 5.05, 5.057, 7.01, 8.12, 9.12, and 9.131. Cites Fundamental Elements (5) and Opinions

8.115 and 8.13. Buchanan, *Medical Ethics at the Millennium: A Brief Retrospective*, 26 Colo. Law. 141, 142, 143, 144, 145 (1997).

Journal 1997 Examines the use of gag clauses in the managed care setting. Explores the conflict of interest between physicians' loyalty to HMOs and their duty to patients. Questions whether patients can give informed consent based on inadequate information. Emphasizes the need for more comprehensive regulation. Quotes Opinion 8.13. Comment, *Physician Gag Clauses—The Hypocrisy of the Hippocratic Oath*, 21 So. Ill. U. L. J. 313, 318, 320 (1997).

Journal 1997 Reviews the conflict between the economics of managed care and physicians' ethical obligations to patients. Questions whether a patient may give informed consent to treatment without knowledge of all available alternatives. Offers a proposal for disclosure of managed care cost-containment mechanisms and incentives to patients. Quotes Opinion 8.13. Hall, *A Theory of Economic Informed Consent*, 31 Ga. L. Rev. 511, 521, 524-25 (1997).

Journal 1997 Posits that cost-containment schemes in managed care systems have eroded the fiduciary duty physicians owe patients. Notes that MCOs are prohibiting patients from trusting and relying on physicians. Concludes that patients must seek quality assurance from sources other than their physicians. Quotes Opinions 2.03, 2.09, and 8.13. Jacobi, *Patients at a Loss: Protecting Health Care Consumers through Data Driven Quality Assurance*, 45 U. Kan. L. Rev. 705, 720, 721, 759 (1997).

Journal 1997 Explores the responsibilities imposed on physicians by managed care and capitation. Notes that physicians are called on to act as gatekeepers, controlling access to specialty services and tests. Considers whether primary care physicians in capitated groups are satisfied with the quality of care they provide. References Opinion 8.13. Kerr, Hays, Mittman, Siu, Leake, & Brook, *Primary Care Physicians' Satisfaction with Quality of Care in California Capitated Medical Groups*, 278 JAMA 308, 312 (1997).

Journal 1997 Discusses the practice of physician deselection by managed care organizations. Suggests that deselection harms the physician-patient relationship and creates a conflict of interest. Argues that solutions to deselection should consider effects on the patient rather than on the physician. Quotes Principle III. Cites Principle I and Opinions 8.05 and 8.13. Liner, *Physician Deselection: The Dynamics of a New Threat to the Physician-Patient Relationship*, 23 Am. J. Law & Med. 511, 513, 527 (1997).

Journal 1997 Examines national health care reform and managed care. Notes that state regulatory policies in this context evidence common concerns. Suggests ways in which the government can promote patient and physician rights. References Opinion 8.13. Miller, *Managed Care Regulation: In the Laboratory of the States*, 278 JAMA 1102, 1104, 1108-09 (1997).

Journal 1997 Discusses physician frustration with managed care plans caused by gag clauses and cost-containment mechanisms. Reviews the development of managed care organizations and federal attempts at limiting the use of gag clauses. Concludes that gag clauses are inherently flawed and compromise quality health care. Quotes Principles II and V, Fundamental Elements (1), and Opinion 8.13. Note, *Physicians, Bound and Gagged: Federal Attempts to Combat Managed Care's Use of Gag Clauses*, 21 Seton Hall Legis. J. 567, 601-02 (1997).

Journal 1997 Describes gag provisions in managed care contracts. Explains the context in which gag provisions may undermine the physician-patient relationship, as well as the conflicts of interest they may create. Proposes legislation to address these problems. Quotes Opinion 8.13. Note, *Stop Gagging Physicians!*, 7 Health Matrix 187, 193, 200, 208-09 (1997).

Journal 1997 Examines the need for change in interpretation of state laws under the saving clause of the Employment Retirement Income Security Act. Discusses any willing provider laws and concludes that they should receive saving clause protection. References Opinion 8.13. Pittman, *Any Willing Provider Laws and ERISA's Saving Clause: A New Solution for an Old Problem*, 64 Tenn. L. Rev. 409, 416 (1997).

Journal 1997 Discusses the need for balance between business ethics and medical ethics in the context of managed care. Explores two models for integrating ethics and managed care. Proposes the adoption of a collective responsibility model to improve quality of care. Quotes Principles I, II, III, IV, and V. Cites Preamble. References Opinion 8.13. Regan, *Regulating the Business of Medicine: Models for Integrating Ethics and Managed Care*, 30 Colum. J.L. & Soc. Probs. 635, 651, 656, 657 (1997).

Journal 1997 Examines utilization review in the managed care context. Discusses a survey of third-party utilization review firms, noting practices that advance and undermine adherence to important professional norms. Quotes Opinion 9.031. References Opinion 8.13. Schlesinger, Gray, & Perreira, *Medical Professionalism under Managed Care: The Pros and Cons of Utilization Review*, 16 Health Affairs 106, 119, 120, 124 (1997).

Journal 1996 Discusses the use of practice guidelines to improve medical care quality and to aid in decreasing health care costs. Evaluates pertinent ethical considerations. Concludes that, when used appropriately, guidelines have clinical value. References Opinion 8.13. Berger & Rosner, *The Ethics of Practice Guidelines*, 156 Arch. Intern. Med. 2051, 2053, 2056 (1996).

Journal 1996 Considers the economic implications for physicians brought about by the change from traditional fee-for-service care to capitation. Discusses capitation payments in the American health care system. Alludes to pertinent ethical issues. References Opinion 8.13. Bodenheimer & Grumbach, *Capitation or Decapitation: Keeping Your Head in Changing Times*, 276 JAMA 1025, 1031 (1996).

Journal 1996 Examines the business of health care and the ethical implications of managed care. Describes incentives that affect the delivery of health care. Suggests that a redistribution of excess revenues would help both patients and nonprofit hospitals co-exist with managed care. Quotes Opinion 8.13. Bond, *Diverse and Perverse Incentives In Managed Care: Where Will the Pendulum Stop?*, 1 Widener L. Symp. J. 141, 151, 154 (1996).

Journal 1996 Discusses the trend toward health care reform. Focuses on benefits and problems posed by managed mental health care. Posits that the moral problems of managed mental health care, including quality concerns, are curable. Concludes that managed mental health care may prove superior to fee-for-service care. References Opinion 8.13. Boyle, *Managed Care in Mental Health: A Cure, or a Cure Worse Than the Disease?*, 40 St. Louis U. L. J. 437, 448 (1996).

Journal 1996 Discusses the threat managed health care poses to patients and physicians. Explores direct incentives given to physicians by managed care organizations and the impact these incentives have on physician behavior. Proposes possible methods for dealing with the problems that such incentives create. References Opinion 8.13. Greely, *Direct Financial Incentives in Managed Care: Unanswered Questions*, 6 Health Matrix 53, 81 (1996).

Journal 1996 Discusses the change from fee-for-service health care financing to managed care. Notes that cost-containment mechanisms modify physicians' behaviors and patients' access to health care. Emphasizes that physicians must remain committed to following ethical guidelines. References Opinion 8.13. Hammes & Webster, *Professional Ethics and Managed Care in Dermatology*, 132 Arch. Dermatol. 1070, 1072, 1073 (1996).

Journal 1996 Discusses workers' compensation and the medical care provided to injured employees. Examines the effect of managed care on workers' compensation. Advocates focusing on prevention of injuries and quality of care. References Opinion 8.13. Hashimoto, *The Future Role of Managed Care and Capitation in Workers' Compensation*, XXII Am. J. Law & Med. 233, 258, 259 (1996).

Journal 1996 Considers challenges to the psychiatrist-patient relationship that are triggered by managed care cost-containment methodologies. Offers guidance to psychiatrists for addressing these challenges. References Opinions 2.095, 8.13, and 8.132. Hoge, *APA Resource Document: I. The Professional Responsibilities of Psychiatrists in Evolving Health Care Systems*, 24 Bull. Am. Acad. Psychiatry Law 393, 405 (1996).

Journal 1996 Discusses the problems managed care raises within the framework of the physician-patient relationship. Considers issues specific to psychiatry. Advocates legal regulation to improve upon and bring structural change to managed care systems. Cites Opinion 8.13. Hoge, *APA Resource Document: II. Regulatory Guidelines for Protecting the Interests of Psychiatric Patients in Emerging Health Care Systems*, 24 Bull. Am. Acad. Psychiatry Law 407, 412, 418 (1996).

Journal 1996 Considers procedural issues relative to patient protection in the context of capitated health care plans. Examines regulations governing capitated health plans and consumer protection issues. Offers suggestions regarding policy making, rate setting, dispute resolution, and judicial review. References Opinion 8.13. Kinney, *Procedural Protections for Patients in Capitated Health Plans*, XXII Am. J. Law & Med. 301, 319-20 (1996).

Journal 1996 Explains the conflict between managed care, which focuses on controlling costs, and traditional health care values, which focus on patient autonomy. Proposes a solution to this conflict requiring that patients incur certain economic consequences in obtaining health care and that managed care organizations disclose resource management techniques. References Opinion 8.13. Morreim, *Diverse and Perverse Incentives of Managed Care: Bringing Patients into*

Alignment, 1 Widener L. Symp. J. 89, 129 (1996).

Journal 1996 Discusses efforts to reduce health care costs. Considers whether personal financial incentives given to physicians decreases level of care given to patients. Suggests that, while financial incentives may create ethical concerns, they serve an important function by containing costs. Concludes that efforts to eliminate them completely are misguided. References Opinion 8.13. Orentlicher, *Paying Physicians More to Do Less: Financial Incentives to Limit Care*, 30 U. Rich. L. Rev. 155, 167 (1996).

In June 1996, Opinion 8.13, "Referral of Patients: Disclosure of Limitations," was renumbered as Opinion 8.132, "Referral of Patients: Disclosure of Limitations."

8.132 Referral of Patients: Disclosure of Limitations

When a physician agrees to provide treatment, he or she thereby enters into a contractual relationship and assumes an ethical obligation to treat the patient to the best of his or her ability. Some health care plans contracts generally restrict the participating physician's scope of referral to medical specialists, diagnostic laboratories, and hospitals that have contractual arrangements with the health plan. Some plans also restrict the circumstances under which referrals may be made to contracting medical specialists. If the health care plan does not permit referral to a non-contracting medical specialist or to a diagnostic or treatment facility when the physician believes that the patient's condition requires such services, the physician should so inform the patient so that the patient may decide whether to accept the outside referral at his or her own expense or confine herself or himself to services available within the health care plan. In determining whether treatment or diagnosis requires referral to outside specialty services, the physician should be guided by standards of good medical practice.

Physicians must not deny their patients access to appropriate medical services based upon the promise of personal financial reward, or the avoidance of financial penalties. Because patients must have the necessary information to make informed decisions about their care, physicians have an obligation to assure the disclosure of medically appropriate treatment alternatives, regardless of cost.

Physicians must assure disclosure of any financial inducements that may tend to limit the diagnostic and therapeutic alternatives that are offered to patients or that may tend to limit patients' overall access to care. Physicians may satisfy this obligation by assuring that the health care plan makes adequate disclosure to enrolled patients. Physicians should also promote an effective program of peer review to monitor and evaluate the quality of the patient care services within their practice setting. (II, IV)

Issued June 1986.

Updated June 1994 based on the report "Financial Incentives to Limit Care: Ethical Implications for HMOs and IPAs," adopted June 1990; updated June 2002.

III. App. 1999 Administrator of estate brought suit against physician and health maintenance organization. The suit alleged medical negligence and breach of a fiduciary duty to deceased for the physician's failure to disclose contract with the HMO that created incentives to minimize diagnostic tests and specialist referrals. The court quoted Opinion 8.132, stating that, while a violation of professional ethics does not in itself establish a breach of the legal standard of care, it is relevant in determining whether such a breach occurred. *Neade v. Portes, 303 Ill.App.3d 799, 710 N.E. 2d 418, 427*.

Journal 2002 Explores how courts have attempted to provide relief when managed care organizations cause harm. Concludes that the judiciary has evidenced respect for the legislative process in this context. Quotes Opinion 8.132. Spector, *Managed Healthcare Liability Issues, 32 Cumb. L. Rev. 311, 335-36 (2002)*.

Journal 2001 Discusses the prohibition on non-lawyer ownership of legal service providers. Considers how ethical rules and standards governing physicians have been directed toward preserving independent judgment. Concludes that ethical conflicts created by abandoning the prohibition on non-lawyer ownership of legal service providers may be managed by following the medical ethics model. Quotes Principle VI and Opinions 2.03, 2.09, 8.02, 8.021, 8.03, 8.05, 8.051, 8.054, 8.13, and 8.132. Harris & Foran, *The Ethics of Middle-Class Access to Legal Services and What We Can Learn from the Medical Profession's Shift to a Corporate Paradigm, 70 Fordham L. Rev. 775, 817, 821, 822, 823, 824 (2001)*.

Journal 2001 Examines the changing duties of health care providers to disclose managed care financial incentives to patients. Concludes that managed care organizations, not physicians, should be obligated to make such disclosures. Quotes Opinion 8.132. Kurfirst, *The Duty to Disclose HMO Physician Incentives, 13 (3) Health Law. 18, 18, 22 (2001)*.

Journal 2001 Examines patient attitudes toward physician compensation models. Concludes that most wealthier, well-educated, caucasian patients are the least satisfied with capitation. References Opinion 8.132. Pereira & Pearson, *Patient Attitudes toward Physician Financial Incentives, 161 Arch. Intern. Med. 1313, 1316, 1317 (2001)*.

Journal 2001 Examines the concept of fiduciary duty in the managed care context. Considers potential liability of health plans and providers for breach of this duty. Reviews the United States Supreme Court decision in *Pegram v. Herdrich*. Concludes that Pegram left many unanswered questions concerning ERISA's fiduciary requirements for health plans and providers. Quotes Opinion 8.132. Rosoff, *Breach of Fiduciary Duty Lawsuits Against MCOs, 22 J. Legal Med. 55, 65 (2001)*.

Journal 2000 Examines physician value neutrality (PVN). Defines PVN as providing a foundation to suggest physicians must keep their values—religious, political, or otherwise—out of the patient-physician relationship. Concludes it is not clear how values can be removed from the patient-physician relationship without removing the very thing PVN supporters are trying to protect, the intrinsic value of persons. References Opinions 2.01, 2.02, 8.032, 8.05, 8.08, and 8.132. Beckwith & Peppin, *Physician Value Neutrality: A Critique, 28 J. L. Med. & Ethics 67, 72-73 (2000)*.

Journal 2000 Examines the fiduciary nature of the physician-patient relationship. Explores crucial policy implications of the *Neade v. Portes* decision. Concludes that policy makers, not courts, should address whether physician involvement in managed care plans fundamentally implies a profit motive. Quotes Opinion 8.132. Potter, *Failure to Disclose HMO Incentives and the Breach of Fiduciary Duty: Is a New Cause of Action Against Physicians the Best Solution?, 34 USF. L. Rev. 733, 753 (2000)*.

Journal 1999 Considers the viability of a legal cause of action for negligent referral in the physician-patient relationship. Examines differences between the legal and medical professions and discusses variations in the applicable standards of care. Cites Opinion 8.132. Martin, *Legal Malpractice: Negligent Referral as a Cause of Action, 29 Cumb. L. Rev. 679, 686 (1999)*.

Journal 1999 Explores the increased push toward mandatory disclosure laws regarding financial incentives imposed by managed care organizations. Discusses current laws and ethical guidelines. Emphasizes that efforts to mandate disclosure force physicians to focus on the effects of imposed incentives and the essence of the physician-patient relationship. References Opinions 8.032, 8.13, and 8.132. Miller & Sage, *Disclosing Physician Financial Incentives, 281 JAMA 1424, 1425 (1999)*.

Journal 1999 Discusses the need for physicians to advocate on behalf of patients' rights in the context of health care delivery. Evaluates the nature and scope of the physician's role as advocate, noting that physicians cannot be expected to engage in attorney-like advocacy. Quotes Principles

IV and VI, Fundamental Elements (2), (4), and (6) [now Opinion 10.01], Patient Responsibilities 5 [now Opinion 10.02], and Opinions 2.03, 2.07, 2.09, 2.16, 2.19, 3.06, 4.01, 4.04, 6.01, 7.02, 8.02, 8.03, 8.13, 8.132, 9.06, 9.07, and 9.131. Cites Opinions 5.05, 5.09, 7.01, 8.135, and 9.02. Sage, *Physicians as Advocates*, 35 Hous. L. Rev. 1529, 1537, 1541, 1542, 1552-53, 1554, 1556, 1557, 1559, 1561-62, 1564, 1571, 1574, 1576, 1580 (1999).

Journal 1999 Discusses financial incentives offered to physicians by managed care organizations. Argues that evidence of financial incentives should be admissible in medical malpractice cases. Quotes Opinion 8.13. References Opinion 8.132. Sugarman & Yarashus, *Admissibility of Managed Care Financial Incentives in Medical Malpractice Cases*, 34 Tort & Ins. L. J. 735, 743, 746, 759 (1999).

Journal 1999 Explores the impact managed care organizations have had on health care. Explains that patients may not understand restrictions and incentives imposed by their managed care organizations when entering the program. Argues that such information should be disclosed at various times during the period of plan coverage. Cites Opinions 2.03, 8.03, 8.032, 8.051, 8.13 and 8.132. Wolf, *Toward a Systemic Theory of Informed Consent in Managed Care*, 35 Hous. L. Rev. 1631, 1641, 1658, 1661, 1662, 1679 (1999).

Journal 1998 Discusses changes in the health care system. Explains why patients need more power in the managed care system. Suggests that patients should use class action suits as a method to assert power over managed care organizations. References Opinions 8.13 and 8.132. Cerminara, *The Class Action Suit As a Method of Patient Empowerment in the Managed Care Setting*, 24 Am. J. Law & Med. 7, 16, 17, 23 (1998).

Journal 1998 Asserts that managed care organizations assume fiduciary obligations by exercising discretionary control over the administration of an ERISA plan. Argues that ERISA requires managed care organizations and physicians to disclose financial incentives intended to influence physician decision-making. References Opinions 8.13 and 8.132. Johnson, *ERISA Doctor in the House? The Duty to Disclose Physician Incentives to Limit Health Care*, 82 Minn. L. Rev. 1631, 1639, 1649, 1655 (1998).

Journal 1996 Considers challenges to the psychiatrist-patient relationship that are triggered by managed care cost-containment methodologies. Offers guidance to psychiatrists for addressing these challenges. References Opinions 2.095, 8.13, and 8.132. Hoge, *APA Resource Document: I. The Professional Responsibilities of Psychiatrists in Evolving Health Care Systems*, 24 Bull. Am. Acad. Psychiatry Law 393, 405 (1996).

Journal 1990 Examines various cost control mechanisms utilized by prepaid health plans and other managed care programs and considers the impact of such mechanisms on clinical decision making. Emphasis is placed on the possible existence of conflicts of interest on the part of health care providers in this context. Quotes Opinions 8.03 and 8.13 [now Opinion 8.132]. Hirshfeld, *Defining Full and Fair Disclosure in Managed Care Contracts*, 60 The Citation 67, 70 (1990).

The previous Opinion 8.135, "Managed Care Cost Containment Involving Prescription Drugs," issued June 1996, was replaced by the current Opinion 8.135, "Cost Containment Involving Prescription Drugs in Health Care Plans."

8.135 Cost Containment Involving Prescription Drugs in Health Care Plans

When health care plans, whether publicly or privately financed, establish drug formulary systems, physicians are obligated to advocate for formularies that meet the medical needs of their patients.

(1) Physicians should maintain awareness of plan decisions about drug selection by staying informed, where appropriate, about pharmacy and therapeutics (P&T) committee actions and by ongoing personal review of formulary composition. P&T committee members should include independent physician representatives. Mechanisms should be established for ongoing peer review of formulary policy. Physicians who perceive inappro-

priate influences on formulary development should notify the proper regulatory authorities.

(2) When scientifically based evidence is available, physicians are ethically required to advocate for changes to the formulary that would benefit the patient. Physicians also should advocate for exceptions to the formulary on a case-by-case basis when justified by the health care needs of particular patients. Mechanisms to appeal formulary exclusions should be established. Other cost-containment mechanisms, including prescription caps and prior authorization, should not unduly burden physicians or patients in accessing optimal drug therapy. Quality improvement rather than cost containment should be the primary determinant for formulary exclusions. In order to be cost efficient, however, physicians should select the lowest cost medication of equal efficacy for their patients.

(3) Physicians should advocate that limits be placed on the extent to which health care plans use incentives or pressures to lower prescription drug costs. Financial incentives are permissible when they promote cost-effectiveness, not when they require withholding medically necessary care. Physicians should not be made to feel that they jeopardize their compensation or participation in a health care plan if they prescribe drugs that are necessary for their patients but that may also be costly. There should be limits on the magnitude of financial incentives, which should be calculated according to the practices of a sizeable group of physicians rather than on an individual basis, and incentives based on quality of care rather than cost of care should be used. Prescriptions should not be changed without the physician's knowledge and authorization. This affords the physician the opportunity to discuss the change with the patient.

(4) Physicians should encourage health care plans to develop mechanisms to educate and assist physicians in cost-effective prescribing practices, including the availability of clinical pharmacists. Such initiatives are preferable to financial incentives or pressures by health care plans or hospitals, which can be ethically problematic.

(5) Physicians should advocate that methods to limit prescription drug costs within health care plans in which they participate be disclosed to patients. In particular, they should encourage health care plans to inform patients upon enrollment concerning:
   (i)   the existence of formularies
   (ii) provisions for cases in which the physician prescribes a drug that is not included in the formulary
   (iii) incentives or other mechanisms used to encourage formulary compliance by physicians
   (iv) relationships with pharmaceutical benefit management companies or pharmaceutical companies that could influence the composition of the formulary

If physicians exhaust all avenues to secure a formulary exception for a significantly advantageous drug, they are still obligated to disclose the option of the more beneficial drug to the patient, so that the patient can consider whether to obtain the medication out-of-plan. Under circumstances in which the health care program will not subsidize the drug, physicians should help patients by identifying alternative forms of financial assistance, such as those available through pharmaceutical companies' assistance programs. (III)

Issued June 1996 based on the report "Managed Care Cost Containment Involving Prescription Drugs," adopted June 1995 (*Food and Drug Law Journal*. 1998; 53: 25-34); updated June 2002.

Cal. App. 2002 State agency appealed a writ of mandamus requiring it to approve managed care plan's proposed amendment to discontinue coverage of sexual dysfunction prescription drugs. Agency based its authority to disapprove on a statute empowering it to regulate health plan prescription drug coverage. California Court of Appeals affirmed. The court held that the agency exceeded its statutory authority. References Opinion 8.135 regarding managed care drug formulary systems. *Kaiser Foundation Health Plan, Inc. v. Zingale*, 99 Cal. App. 4th 1018, 121 Cal. Rptr. 2d 741, 746.

Journal 2000 Describes the American formulary system and the economic efficiencies that can be realized when physicians comply. Describes how the formulary system fits into and underlies health care electronic data interchange. Concludes that congressional action is needed to fully extend the formulary system to Medicaid programs in all fifty states. References Opinion 8.135. Buckles, *Electronic Formulary Management and Medicaid: Maximizing Economic Efficiency and Quality of Care in the Age of Electronic Prescribing*, 11 U. Fla. J. L. & Pub. Pol'y 179, 182-83 (2000).

Journal 1999 Discusses the need for physicians to advocate on behalf of patients' rights in the context of health care delivery. Evaluates the nature and scope of the physician's role as advocate, noting that physicians cannot be expected to engage in attorney-like advocacy. Quotes Principles IV and VI, Fundamental Elements (2), (4), and (6) [now Opinion 10.01], Patient Responsibilities 5 [now Opinion 10.02], and Opinions 2.03, 2.07, 2.09, 2.16, 2.19, 3.06, 4.01, 4.04, 6.01, 7.02, 8.02, 8.03, 8.13, 8.132, 9.06, 9.07, and 9.131. Cites Opinions 5.05, 5.09, 7.01, 8.135, and 9.02. Sage, *Physicians as Advocates*, 35 Hous. L. Rev. 1529, 1537, 1541, 1542, 1552-53, 1554, 1556, 1557, 1559, 1561-62, 1564, 1571, 1574, 1576, 1580 (1999).

8.137   The previous Opinion 8.137, "Restrictions on Disclosure in Managed Care Contracts," issued June 1997, was deleted in June 2000 and combined with Opinion 8.053, "Restrictions on Disclosure in Managed Care Contracts."

8.14   Sexual Misconduct in the Practice of Medicine

Sexual contact that occurs concurrent with the patient-physician relationship constitutes sexual misconduct. Sexual or romantic interactions between physicians and patients detract from the goals of the physician-patient relationship, may exploit the vulnerability of the patient, may obscure the physician's objective judgment concerning the patient's health care, and ultimately may be detrimental to the patient's well-being.

If a physician has reason to believe that non-sexual contact with a patient may be perceived as or may lead to sexual contact, then he or she should avoid the non-sexual contact. At a minimum, a physician's ethical duties include terminating the physician-patient relationship before initiating a dating, romantic, or sexual relationship with a patient.

Sexual or romantic relationships between a physician and a former patient may be unduly influenced by the previous physician-patient relationship. Sexual or romantic relationships with former patients are unethical if the physician uses or exploits trust, knowledge, emotions, or influence derived from the previous professional relationship. (I, II, IV)

Issued December 1989.

Updated March 1992 based on the report "Sexual Misconduct in the Practice of Medicine," adopted December 1990 (JAMA. 1991; 266: 2741-45).

S. D. N.Y. 1999 Physician brought a 42 U.S.C. § 1983 claim seeking to enjoin the State Board from revoking his license to practice medicine. The charges against the physician included allegations of engaging in sexual relations with patients. The Board quoted Opinion 8.14 as a basis for its conclusion that engaging in sexual relations with patients is an ethical violation. The court held that, in order to enjoin the Board, the physician had to show a substantial likelihood of success on the merits. Further, the court found that abstention was appropriate because the physician's case was pending administrative appeal. Finally, the court held that the statute that prohibited the stay of a license revocation pending appeal complied with due process. *Selkin v. State Board for Professional Medical Conduct*, 63 F. Supp. 2d 397, 399-400.

Cal. 1995 Patient sued ultrasound technician, who sexually assaulted her, and hospital for professional negligence, battery, and intentional and negligent infliction of emotional distress. In differentiating between the physician-patient relationship and the technician-patient relationship, the court cited AMA Council on Ethical and Judicial Affairs, Sexual Misconduct in the Practice of Medicine, 266 JAMA 2741 (1991) [now Opinion 8.14]. Finding that the technician's acts did not arise from any events or conditions of his employment, the court held that the hospital was not liable under respondeat superior. *Lisa M. v. Henry Mayo Newhall Memorial Hosp.*, 12 Cal. 4th 291, 907 P.2d 358, 48 Cal. Rptr. 2d 510, 517.

Cal. App. 1992 Physician who had sexual relationship with patient brought a mandamus action challenging discipline imposed by Medical Board. The court concluded that a sexual relationship between physician and patient was alone an insufficient basis for discipline. An expert witness, referring to Opinion 8.14, testified that it is unethical for a physician to have a sexual relationship with a patient. However, focusing on the applicable state statute, the court found the relationship must affect the functions and duties of a physician to be a basis for discipline. *Gromis v. Medical Board*, 8 Cal. App. 4th 589, 10 Cal. Rptr. 2d 452, 455 n.3, reh'g denied, 1992 Cal. App. LEXIS 1047, and review denied, 1992 Cal. LEXIS 5101.

Md. App. 2003 Physician appealed decision upholding State Board's order to revoke his medical license for unprofessional conduct. The physician engaged in consensual sexual relationships with several of his patients at places and times other than when medical care was given. Appeals court affirmed the Board's ruling and held that the conduct occurred within the practice of medicine. Quotes Opinion 8.14. *Finucan v. Maryland State Board of Physicians Quality Assurance*, 151 Md. App. 399, 827 A.2d 176, 181-82.

Md. App. 1992 Patient's husband sought damages from defendant psychiatrist because of the sexual relationship initiated during treatment of the patient by the defendant. Although the court held that the plaintiff in this case could not recover damages in tort for disruption of a marriage, it cited favorably Opinion 8.14 (1989) for its declaration that "sexual misconduct in the practice of medicine" is unethical. *Homer v. Long*, 90 Md. App. 1, 3 n.1 , 599 A.2d 1193, 1193 n.1.

Mass. App. 2003 Patient appealed summary judgment in suit against physician's estate for harm caused by their two-year consensual sexual affair. Once the affair began, the physician stopped treating the patient. The patient alleged malpractice, breach of fiduciary duty, intentional infliction of emotional distress, and unfair or deceptive practices. Appellate court upheld summary judgment. In analyzing the fiduciary duty claim, the court quoted Opinion 8.14. *Korper v. Weinstein*, 57 Mass. App. 433, 783 N.E.2d 877, 881, n. 9.

N.Y. 2002 Surgical resident sexually assaulted patient while she was in recovery room. Patient sued hospital for negligence and vicarious liability. Trial court denied hospital's motion for summary judgment, but intermediate appellate court granted motion. New York Court of Appeals modified the ruling. It held that patient's vicarious liability claim failed because the misconduct was not in furtherance of hospital business or in the scope of the resident's employment. The court found, however, a sufficient basis for a negligence claim. References Opinion 8.14. *N.X. v. Cabrini Medical Center*, 97 N.Y 2d 247, 765 N.E 2d 844, 847, n.2, 739 N.Y.S.2d 348.

N.Y. Sup. 1998 Physician was convicted of sodomizing a patient and falsifying her records. He appealed in part on grounds that the prosecutor had introduced evidence regarding his sexual relationship with another patient in violation of a pre-trial ruling. The court reversed the convictions and remanded the case for a new trial. The dissent cited Opinion 8.14, stating that the physician's sexual relationship with another patient violated ethical standards. Furthermore, the dissent argued that evidence of such a relationship was relevant to the case at hand. *People v. Griffin, 242 A.D.2d 70, 671 N.Y.S. 2d 34, 39.*

Ohio 1991 State medical board revoked license of physician who had consensual sexual relations with his patient. The court upheld the board's ruling that this violated Principles I, II and IV. Dissenting judge, citing AMA Council on Ethical and Judicial Affairs, Sexual Misconduct in the Practice of Medicine, 266 JAMA 2741 [now Opinion 8.14], argued that until 1991, the AMA did not clearly deem sexual contact with a patient unethical. *Pons v. Ohio State Medical Bd., 66 Ohio St. 3d 619, 623, 625, 614 N.E.2d 748, 752, 753.*

Journal 2003 Highlights the inadequacies of Washington tort law with respect to holding employers of sexually exploitative therapists accountable. Concludes that courts should premise employer liability on the foreseeability of transference. References Opinion 8.14. Allen, *The Foreseeability of Transference: Extending Employer Liability Under Washington Law for Therapist Sexual Exploitation of Patients, 78 Wash. L. Rev. 525, 531 (2003).*

Journal 2001 Explores changes in common law and statutory law that have promoted the marginalization of chastity. Considers rules governing the professions. Concludes with a legal agenda intended to help restore the social value of chastity. References Opinion 8.14. Rodes, *On Law and Chastity, 76 Notre Dame L. Rev. 643, 675 (2001).*

Journal 2000 Evaluates consensual sexual relationships between patients and physicians. Emphasis is placed on whether, and in what situation, a sexual relationship may constitute medical malpractice. Concludes that people should learn to take responsibility for their actions and that certain limitations should be placed on recovery for malpractice. References Opinion 8.14. Puglise, *"Calling Dr. Love": The Physician-Patient Sexual Relationship as Grounds for Medical Malpractice – Society Pays While the Doctor and Patient Play, 14 J. L. & Health 321, 324-25, 349 (2000).*

Journal 1999 Examines countertransference in professional relationships. Observes how the resulting power imbalance may give rise to the potential for sexual exploitation. Concludes by offering strategies for identifying and addressing emotional interference in the lawyer/client relationship. Cites Opinion 8.14. Silver, *Love, Hate, and Other Emotional Interference in the Lawyer/Client Relationship, 6 Clinical L. Rev. 259, 266 (1999).*

Journal 1998 Provides policy reasons why attorney-client sexual relations should be prohibited. Urges states to codify rules precluding such conduct during representation. Explains that such rules would pass constitutional scrutiny. Cites Opinion 8.14. Awad, *Attorney-Client Sexual Relations, 22 J. Legal. Prof. 131, 190 (1998).*

Journal 1998 Discusses types of discipline taken against physicians for sexual offenses. Points out that some physicians still may be permitted to practice medicine despite the commission of sexual misconduct. Proposes ways that might increase the chance that sex-related offenses will be reported. Quotes Opinion 8.14. Dehlendorf & Wolfe, *Physicians Disciplined for Sex-Related Offenses, 279 JAMA. 1883 (1998).*

Journal 1997 Examines the balance needed between clinical objectivity and physician-patient bonding. Discusses personal boundaries and methods of coping with transgressions by both physicians and patients. Advocates a focus on communication with patients to allow physicians to maintain both an empathetic and objective relationship. References Opinion 8.14. Farber, Novack, & O'Brien, *Love, Boundaries, and the Physician-Patient Relationship, 157 Arch. Intern. Med. 2291, 2292, 2293, 2294 (1997).*

Journal 1996 Discusses the ethical implications of sexual misconduct in the medical field. Examines the current civil and criminal tools used to curb physician-patient misconduct. Notes the inadequacy of physician reporting. Proposes a statutory approach to discipline physicians who abuse their fiduciary duties. Quotes Principle II. References Opinion 8.14. Note, *Sexual Conduct Within the Physician-Patient Relationship: A Statutory Framework for Disciplining this Breach of Fiduciary Duty, 1 Widener L. Symp. J. 501, 507 (1996).*

Journal 1994 Explores the negative consequences of physician-patient sexual relationships. Suggests that sexual contact be prohibited during the physician-patient relationship and for a period of time thereafter. Quotes Opinion 8.14. Appelbaum, Jorgenson, & Sutherland, *Sexual Relationships Between Physicians and Patients*, 154 Arch. Intern. Med. 2561, 2561 (1994).

Journal 1993 Examines the potential problems created by attorney-client sexual relations and the need for ethical guidelines. Examines ethical rules being debated in various states and proposes a model rule. References Opinion 8.14. Davis & Grimaldi, *Sexual Confusion: Attorney-Client Sex and the Need for a Clear Ethical Rule*, 7 Notre Dame J. Law, Ethics, & Pub. Pol. 57, 61 (1993).

Journal 1993 Discusses family privacy rights and considers the meaning of justice, self respect, and the fundamental principles of physician ethics. Concludes that physicians have an ethical duty to intervene in domestic violence so long as such intervention does not breach confidentiality or violate patient autonomy. Quotes Principle IV and Opinion 5.05. References Opinions 8.14 and 9.131. Jecker, *Privacy Beliefs and the Violent Family: Extending the Ethical Argument for Physician Intervention*, 269 JAMA 776, 778, 779 (1993).

Journal 1993 Discusses the potential impact on health care practitioners of the AMA's prohibition against sexual relations between physicians and patients. Focuses on how the prohibition will influence disciplinary actions. Cites Opinion 8.14. Johnson, *Judicial Review of Disciplinary Action for Sexual Misconduct in the Practice of Medicine*, 270 JAMA 1596 (1993).

Journal 1993 Discusses potential problems caused by attorney-client sexual relations and examines various means to check such conduct. Proposes a new rule that would prohibit attorney-client sexual relations. References Opinion 8.14. Livingston, *When Libido Subverts Credo: Regulation of Attorney-Client Sexual Relations*, 62 Fordham L. Rev. 5, 55 (1993).

Journal 1993 Discusses the problems physicians may encounter by exposing the errant colleague, such as harm to the reporting physician's reputation and the fear of litigation. States that problems involving physician competency and unethical behavior should be investigated, and that physicians should take personal responsibility for reporting problems they observe. References Principle II and Opinions 8.14 and 9.031. Morreim, *Am I My Brother's Warden? Responding to the Unethical or Incompetent Colleague*, 23 Hastings Center Rep. 19, 23 (May/June 1993).

Journal 1993 Discusses the medical profession's ethical prohibition on physician-patient sexual contact. Concludes that legislatures and courts should give greater weight to the ethical code when defining standards of conduct for physician-patient sexual contact. Quotes Opinion 8.14. Note, *Physician-Patient Sexual Contact: The Battle Between the State and the Medical Profession*, 50 Wash. & Lee L. Rev. 1725, 1725-26, 1734, 1752 (1993).

Journal 1992 Discusses the problem of sex in the attorney-client relationship and compares this to that of the physician-patient. Proposes an explicit ban on sexual involvement between attorneys and their clients and advocates promulgation of a "bright line" rule. References Opinion 8.14. Goldberg, *Sex and the Attorney-Client Relationship: An Argument for a Prophylactic Rule*, 26 Akron L. Rev. 45 (1992).

Journal 1992 Examines the similarities and differences between the physician-patient and lawyer-client relationships regarding the problems associated with sexual relations. Advocates a rebuttable presumption that sexual contact between attorneys and clients is wrongful. Cites Opinion 8.14. Gutheil, Jorgenson, & Sutherland, *Prohibiting Lawyer-Client Sex*, 20 Bull. Am. Acad. Psychiatry Law 365 (1992).

Journal 1992 Finds that state medical boards increasingly rely upon psychiatric testimony in cases of alleged sexual abuse by physicians. Proposes that states adopt clear standards governing the admissibility of psychiatric testimony in administrative hearings. Quotes Opinion 8.14. Hyams, *Expert Psychiatric Evidence in Sexual Misconduct Cases Before State Medical Boards*, XVIII Am. J. Law & Med. 171, 173, 174 (1992).

8.145 Sexual or Romantic Relations between Physicians and Key Third Parties

Patients are often accompanied by third parties who play an integral role in the patient-physician relationship. The physician interacts and communicates with these individuals and often is in a position to offer them information, advice, and emotional support. The more deeply involved the individual is in the clinical encounter and in medical decision making, the more troubling sexual or romantic contact with the physician would be. This is especially true for the individual whose decisions directly impact on the health and welfare of the patient. Key third parties include, but are not limited to, spouses or partners, parents, guardians, and proxies.

Physicians should refrain from sexual or romantic interactions with key third parties when it is based on the use or exploitation of trust, knowledge, influence, or emotions derived from a professional relationship. The following factors should be considered when considering whether a relationship is appropriate: the nature of the patient's medical problem, the length of the professional relationship, the degree of the third party's emotional dependence on the physician, and the importance of the clinical encounter to the third party and the patient. (I, II)

Issued December 1998 based on the report "Sexual or Romantic Relations between Physicians and Key Third Parties," adopted June 1998.

8.15   Substance Abuse

It is unethical for a physician to practice medicine while under the influence of a controlled substance, alcohol, or other chemical agents which impair the ability to practice medicine. (I)

Issued December 1986.

Journal 1994 Discusses the issue of whom physicians must serve first: themselves, their patients, insurers, or society. Focuses on risks arising out of provider economic arrangements and risks arising out of other individual physician characteristics. Quotes Opinions 8.03 and 9.13. Cites Opinion 8.15. Bobinski, *Autonomy and Privacy: Protecting Patients from Their Physicians*, 55 U. Pitt. L. Rev. 291, 302, 313 (1994).

8.16   Substitution of Surgeon without Patient's Knowledge or Consent

A surgeon who allows a substitute to operate on his or her patient without the patient's knowledge and consent is deceitful. The patient is entitled to choose his or her own physician and should be permitted to acquiesce to or refuse the substitution.

The surgeon's obligation to the patient requires the surgeon to perform the surgical operation: (1) within the scope of authority granted by the consent to the operation; (2) in accordance with the terms of the contractual relationship; (3) with complete disclosure of facts relevant to the need and the performance of the operation; and (4) utilizing best skill.

It should be noted that it is the operating surgeon to whom the patient grants consent to perform the operation. The patient is entitled to the services of the particular surgeon with whom he or she contracts. The operating surgeon, in accepting the patient, is obligated to utilize his or her personal talents in the performance of the operation to the extent required by the agreement creating the physician-patient relationship. The surgeon cannot properly delegate to another the duties which he or she is required to perform personally.

Under the normal and customary arrangement with patients, and with reference to the usual form of consent to operation, the operating surgeon is obligated to perform the operation but may be assisted by residents or other surgeons. With the consent of the patient, it is not unethical for the operating surgeon to delegate the performance of certain aspects of the operation to the assistant provided this is done under the surgeon's participatory supervision, ie, the surgeon must scrub. If a resident or other physician is to perform the operation under non-participatory supervision, it is necessary to make a full disclosure of this fact to the patient, and this should be evidenced by an appropriate statement contained in the consent. Under these circumstances, it is the resident or other physician who becomes the operating surgeon. (I, II, IV, V)

Issued prior to April 1977.

Updated June 1994.

Ala. 1985 Patient sued physicians alleging fraud and conspiracy to commit fraud. The court clarified its previous holding in the case (461 So. 2d 775) that a new trial was ordered only on fraud and conspiracy to commit fraud theories. The court also noted that the trier of fact would need to decide whether the Current Opinions of the Judicial Council of the American Medical Association pamphlet was properly excluded under the learned treatise doctrine and whether, if properly authenticated, it might be admissible at a new trial as to the issue of whether ghost surgery, condemned by Opinion 8.12 (1984) [now Opinion 8.16], constitutes fraud. *McMurray v. Johnson, 481 So. 2d 887, 889.*

Md. App. 1999 Patient sued hospital and the surgeon named in consent form for negligence and breach of contract. The plaintiff claimed that the defendants breached their contract when a resident performed surgery, rather than the surgeon authorized by the plaintiff. The trial court dismissed the breach of contract claim and entered judgment upon the jury verdict for the defendants. The appeals court cited Opinion 8.12 (1982) [now Opinion 8.16], stating that it is unethical and deceitful for another surgeon to perform an operation without the patient's knowledge or consent. *Belin v. Dingle, 127 Md. App. 68, 732 A.2d 301, 302-03, 307.*

N.J. 1983 Patient who consented to surgery by one surgeon, but was actually operated on by another, sued both surgeons. Pursuant to state law, patient submitted case to malpractice panel which found no basis to patient's claims and jury returned verdict for defendant surgeons. In holding that failure to permit plaintiff to show possible bias of panel doctor and to impeach the testimony constituted reversible error, the court quoted Opinion 8.12 (1982) [now Opinion 8.16] indicating that substitution of one surgeon for another without patient consent is a deceit and deviates from standard medical care, constituting the violation of a legal obligation as well as a tenet of the medical profession. *Perna v. Pirozzi, 92 N.J. 446, 457 A.2d 431, 434, 440, n.3.*

N.J. Super. 1991 Two physicians were sued by a patient claiming that one of the physician-surgeons had committed "ghost surgery" battery. The court acknowledged the rule in *Perna v. Pirozzi,* 92 N.J. 446, 457 A.2d 431 (1983). The court there, taking judicial notice of the standard of care set out by Opinion 8.12 (1982) [now Opinion 8.16], held that an intent to injure is not required to establish battery when a medical procedure is performed by a "substitute" physician. However, the court here held that the plaintiff had failed to establish by competent medical opinion that one of the physicians was an unauthorized operating surgeon. Furthermore, the court stated that to hold otherwise would create a punitive damage claim based on a patient's lay opinion concerning the proper role of an authorized surgeon in team surgery. *Monturi v. Englewood Hosp., 246 N.J. Super. 547, 552, 588 A.2d 408, 410, 411.*

N.J. Super. 1982 In a medical malpractice suit against a surgeon for negligence and for allowing a different surgeon to operate on plaintiff without plaintiff's express consent, the court noted Opinions and Reports of the Judicial Council Sec. 1, Para. 5 (1969) [now Opinion 8.16] as quoted in 209 J.A.M.A. 947-48 (1969) that it is fraudulent and deceitful for a surgeon to allow another surgeon to operate on a patient without that patient's consent. The court ultimately concluded that the doctrine of informed consent is a theory of professional liability independent from malpractice, and thus was not relevant to the case at bar. *Perna v. Pirozzi, 182 N.J. Super. 510, 442 A.2d 1016, 1019, rev'd, 92 N.J. 446, 457 A.2d 431 (1983).*

Okla. App. 1974 Owner of a bull sued veterinarian for malpractice and failure to disclose possible adverse reactions to penicillin. The appellate court held that the veterinarian was liable for damages to the plaintiff resulting from the death of the bull. In so holding, the court noted Opinions and Reports of the Judicial Council Sec. 1, Para. 5 (1969) [now Opinion 8.16] which, inter alia, requires a surgeon to make a complete disclosure of all facts relevant to the operation to be performed. *Hull v. Tate, No. 46443 (Okla. Ct. App. April 16, 1974) (LEXIS, States library, Okla. file), rev'd, No. 46443 (Okla. Sup. Ct. Oct. 29, 1974) (LEXIS, States library, Okla. file).*

Pa. Super. 1998 Parents of child who died during a catheterization procedure sued the pediatrician, cardiologist, and the hospital on various theories including battery. In referring to an earlier decision, the court quoted Opinion 8.12 (1982) [now Opinion 8.16], in support of a patient's right to consent to a specific physician to perform a medical procedure. The court held that the jury should have decided whether the parents consented for the pediatrician instead of the cardiologist, to perform the procedure. *Taylor v. Albert Einstein Medical Ctr., 723 A.2d 1027, 1036.*

Pa. Super. 1996 Physician told patient he would perform necessary surgery. As a result of the surgery, patient developed a drop foot which would drag whenever he walked. The patient later discovered that his treating physician did not appear for or participate in his surgery. When the hospital was unable to reach the physician, it contacted his office where another physician instructed the hospital to perform the surgery with a third physician. All of this was done without patient's consent and was not disclosed after recovery. Patient sued the physician for failure to perform the surgery and for directing or permitting a third party to perform the surgery. The court quoted from Opinion 8.12 (1982) [now Opinion 8.16] which provides that the patient is entitled to choose his or her physician and should be permitted to acquiesce in or refuse to accept any substitutions. *Grabowski v. Quigley, 454 Pa. Super. 27, 684 A.2d 610, 617.*

Journal 1996 Considers how practice guidelines may be used in malpractice litigation as inculpatory or exculpatory evidence. Concludes that use of guidelines as inculpatory evidence should not be eliminated until there is evidence of undesirable effects. Quotes Opinion 8.16. Hyams, Shapiro, & Brennan, *Medical Practice Guidelines in Malpractice Litigation: An Early Retrospective, 21 J. Health Pol. Pol'y & L. 289, 298 (1996).*

Journal 1996 Discusses tort liability in cases of substitution of surgeons without patient consent. Explores whether substitutions are a battery thereby allowing recovery, regardless of outcome. Concludes that ghost surgery should not automatically constitute a battery but that courts should allow recovery for infliction of emotional distress stemming from the substitution. Quotes Opinion 8.12 (1982) [now Opinion 8.16]. Lundmark, *Surgery by an Unauthorized Surgeon as a Battery, 10 J. L. & Health 287, 293 (1996).*

8.17   Use of Restraints

All individuals have a fundamental right to be free from unreasonable bodily restraint. Physical and chemical restraints should therefore be used only in the best interest of the patient and in accordance with the following guidelines:

(1) The use of restraints, except in emergencies, may be implemented only upon the explicit order of a physician, in conformance with reasonable professional judgment.

(2) Judgment should be exercised in issuing pro re nata (PRN) orders for the use of physical or chemical restraints, and the implementation of such orders should be frequently reviewed and documented by the physician.

(3) The use of restraints should not be punitive, nor should they be used for convenience or as an alternative to reasonable staffing.

(4) Restraints should be used only in accordance with appropriate clinical indications.

(5) As with all therapeutic interventions, informed consent by the patient or surrogate decision maker is a key element in the application of physical and chemical restraints, and should be incorporated into institutional policy.

(6) In certain limited situations, it may be appropriate to restrain a patient involuntarily. For example, restraints may be needed for the safety of the patient or others in the area. When restraints are used involuntarily, the restraints should be removed when they are no longer needed. (I, IV)

Issued March 1992 based on the report "Guidelines for the Use of Restraints in Long Term Care Facilities," adopted June 1989.

8.18   Informing Families of a Patient's Death

Disclosing the death of a patient to the patient's family is a duty which goes to the very heart of the patient-physician relationship and should not be readily delegated to others by the attending physician. The emotional needs of the family and the integrity of the physician-patient relationship must at all times be given foremost consideration.

Physicians in residency training may be asked to participate in the communication of information about a patient's death, if that request is commensurate with the physician's prior training or experience and previous close personal relationship with the family.

It would not be appropriate for the attending physician or resident to request that a medical student notify family members of a patient's death. Medical students should be trained in issues of death and dying, and should be encouraged to accompany attending physicians when news of a patient's death is conveyed to the family members. (I, IV)

Issued March 1992 based on the report "Informing Families of a Patient's Death: Guidelines for the Involvement of Medical Students," adopted December 1989.

Updated June 1994.

Journal 1995 Examines four essential principles of bioethics–patient autonomy, nonmaleficence, beneficence, and justice–and describes the application of these in clinical settings according to bioethical norms and AMA opinions. Concludes that such an approach promotes compassionate medical caregiving and that laws should reflect these values. Quotes Opinions 2.01 and 8.18. References Opinion 2.211. Cohen, *Toward a Bioethics of Compassion*, 28 Ind. L. Rev. 667, 673, 681-82, 683 (1995).

8.181   Performing Procedures on the Newly Deceased for Training Purposes

Physicians should work to develop institutional policies that address the practice of performing procedures on the newly deceased for purposes of training. Any such policy should ensure that the interests of all the parties involved are respected under established and clear ethical guidelines. Such policies should consider rights of patients and their families, benefits to trainees and society, as well as potential harm to the ethical sensitivities of trainees, and risks to staff, the institution, and the profession associated with performing procedures on the newly deceased without consent. The following considerations should be addressed before medical trainees perform procedures on the newly deceased:

(1) The teaching of life-saving skills should be the culmination of a structured training sequence, rather than relying on random opportunities. Training should be performed under close supervision, in a manner and environment that takes into account the wishes and values of all involved parties.

(2) Physicians should inquire whether the deceased individual had expressed preferences regarding handling of the body or procedures performed after death. In the absence of previously expressed preferences, physicians should obtain permission from the family before performing such procedures. When reasonable efforts to discover previously expressed preferences of the deceased or to find someone with authority to grant permission for the procedure have failed, physicians must not perform procedures for training purposes on the newly deceased patient.

In the event post-mortem procedures are undertaken on the newly deceased, they must be recorded in the medical record. (I, V)

Issued December 2001, based on the report, "Performing Procedures on the Newly Deceased for Training Purposes," adopted June 2001, (*Acad. Med.* 2002; 77:1212-1216).

Journal 2003 Analyzes the effect of Virginia law and court decisions on administrative law. Discusses one provision of law that incorporates the AMA's nonbinding ban on nonconsensual use of newly dead patients as training subjects. References Opinion 8.181. Kibler, *Administrative Law*, 38 U. Rich. L. Rev. 39, 47 (2003).

8.19 Self-Treatment or Treatment of Immediate Family Members

Physicians generally should not treat themselves or members of their immediate families. Professional objectivity may be compromised when an immediate family member or the physician is the patient; the physician's personal feelings may unduly influence his or her professional medical judgment, thereby interfering with the care being delivered. Physicians may fail to probe sensitive areas when taking the medical history or may fail to perform intimate parts of the physical examination. Similarly, patients may feel uncomfortable disclosing sensitive information or undergoing an intimate examination when the physician is an immediate family member. This discomfort is particularly the case when the patient is a minor child, and sensitive or intimate care should especially be avoided for such patients. When treating themselves or immediate family members, physicians may be inclined to treat problems that are beyond their expertise or training. If tensions develop in a physician's professional relationship with a family member, perhaps as a result of a negative medical outcome, such difficulties may be carried over into the family member's personal relationship with the physician.

Concerns regarding patient autonomy and informed consent are also relevant when physicians attempt to treat members of their immediate family. Family members may be reluctant to state their preference for another physician or decline a recommendation for fear of offending the physician. In particular, minor children will generally not feel free to refuse care from their parents. Likewise, physicians may feel obligated to provide care to immediate family members even if they feel uncomfortable providing care.

It would not always be inappropriate to undertake self-treatment or treatment of immediate family members. In emergency settings or isolated settings where there is no other qualified physician available, physicians should not hesitate to treat themselves or family members until another physician becomes available. In addition, while physicians should not serve as a primary or regular care provider for immediate family members, there are situations in which routine care is acceptable for short-term, minor problems.

Except in emergencies, it is not appropriate for physicians to write prescriptions for controlled substances for themselves or immediate family members. (I, II, IV)

Issued June 1993.

8.20   Invalid Medical Treatment

The following general guidelines are offered to serve physicians when they are called upon to decide among treatments:
(1) Treatments which have no medical indication and offer no possible benefit to the patient should not be used (Opinion 2.035, "Futile Care").
(2) Treatments which have been determined scientifically to be invalid should not be used (Opinion 3.01, "Nonscientific Practitioners").
(3) Among the treatments that are scientifically valid, medically indicated, and offer a reasonable chance of benefit for patients, some are regulated or prohibited by law; physicians should comply with these laws. If physicians disagree with such laws, they should seek to change them.
(4) Among the various treatments that are scientifically valid, medically indicated, legal, and offer a reasonable chance of benefit for patients, the decision of which treatment to use should be made between the physician and patient. (I, III, IV)

Issued June 1998 based on the report "Invalid Medical Treatment," adopted December 1997.

8.21   Use of Chaperones During Physical Exams

From the standpoint of ethics and prudence, the protocol of having chaperones available on a consistent basis for patient examinations is recommended. Physicians aim to respect the patient's dignity and to make a positive effort to secure a comfortable and considerate atmosphere for the patient; such actions include the provision of appropriate gowns, private facilities for undressing, sensitive use of draping, and clear explanations on various components of the physical examination. A policy that patients are free to make a request for a chaperone should be established in each health care setting. This policy should be communicated to patients, either by means of a well-displayed notice or preferably through a conversation initiated by the intake nurse or the physician. The request by a patient to have a chaperone should be honored.

An authorized health professional should serve as a chaperone whenever possible. In their practices, physicians should establish clear expectations about respecting patient privacy and confidentiality to which chaperones must adhere.

If a chaperone is to be provided, a separate opportunity for private conversation between the patient and the physician should be allowed. The physician should keep inquiries and history-taking, especially those of a sensitive nature, to a minimum during the course of the chaperoned examination. (I, IV)

Issued December 1998 based on the report "Use of Chaperones During Physical Exams," adopted June 1998.

9.00 Opinions on Professional Rights and Responsibilities

9.01 Accreditation

Physicians who engage in activities that involve the accreditation, approval, or certification of institutions, facilities, and programs that provide patient care or medical education or certify the attainment of specialized professional competence have the ethical responsibility to apply standards that are relevant, fair, reasonable, and nondiscriminatory. The accreditation of institutions and facilities that provide patient care should be based upon standards that focus upon the quality of patient care achieved. Standards used in the accreditation of patient care and medical education, or the certification of specialized professional attainment should not be adopted or used as a means of economic regulation. (II, IV, VII)

Issued December 1982.

9.011 Continuing Medical Education

Physicians should strive to further their medical education throughout their careers, for only by participating in continuing medical education (CME) can they continue to serve patients to the best of their abilities and live up to professional standards of excellence. Fulfillment of mandatory state CME requirements does not necessarily fulfill the physician's ethical obligation to maintain his or her medical expertise.

Attendees. Guidelines for physicians attending a CME conference or activity are as follows:
(1) The physician choosing among CME activities should assess their educational value and select only those activities which are of high quality and appropriate for the physician's educational needs. When selecting formal CME activities, the physician should, at a minimum, choose only those activities that (a) are offered by sponsors accredited by the Accreditation Council for Continuing Medical Education (ACCME), the American Academy of Family Physicians (AAFP), or a state medical society; (b) contain information on subjects relevant to the physician's needs; (c) are responsibly conducted by qualified faculty; (d) conform to Opinion 8.061, "Gifts to Physicians from Industry."

(2) The educational value of the CME conference or activity must be the primary consideration in the physician's decision to attend or participate. Though amenities unrelated to the educational purpose of the activity may play a role in the physician's decision to participate, this role should be secondary to the educational content of the conference.

(3) Physicians should claim credit commensurate with only the actual time spent attending a CME activity or in studying a CME enduring material.

(4) Attending promotional activities put on by industry or their designees is not unethical as long as the conference conforms to Opinion 8.061, "Gifts to Physicians from Industry," and is clearly identified as promotional to all participants.

Faculty. Guidelines for physicians serving as presenters, moderators, or other faculty at a CME conference are as follows:

(1) Physicians serving as presenters, moderators, or other faculty at a CME conference should ensure that (a) research findings and therapeutic recommendations are based on scientifically accurate, up-to-date information and are presented in a balanced, objective manner; (b) the content of their presentation is not modified or influenced by representatives of industry or other financial contributors, and they do not employ materials whose content is shaped by industry. Faculty may, however, use scientific data generated from industry-sponsored research, and they may also accept technical assistance from industry in preparing slides or other presentation materials, as long as this assistance is of only nominal monetary value and the company has no input in the actual content of the material.

(2) When invited to present at non-CME activities that are primarily promotional, faculty should avoid participation unless the activity is clearly identified as promotional in its program announcements and other advertising.

(3) All conflicts of interest or biases, such as a financial connection to a particular commercial firm or product, should be disclosed by faculty members to the activity's sponsor and to the audience. Faculty may accept reasonable honoraria and reimbursement for expenses in accordance with Opinion 8.061, "Gifts to Physicians from Industry."

Sponsors. Guidelines for physicians involved in the sponsorship of CME activities are as follows:

(1) Physicians involved in the sponsorship of CME activities should ensure that (a) the program is balanced, with faculty members presenting a broad range of scientifically supportable viewpoints related to the topic at hand; (b) representatives of industry or other financial contributors do not exert control over the choice of moderators, presenters, or other faculty, or modify the content of faculty presentations. Funding from industry or others may be accepted in accordance with Opinion 8.061, "Gifts to Physicians from Industry."

(2) Sponsors should not promote CME activities in a way that encourages attendees to violate the guidelines of the Council on Ethical and Judicial Affairs, including Opinion 8.061, "Gifts to Physicians from Industry," or the principles established for the AMA's Physician Recognition Award.

CME activities should be developed and promoted consistent with guideline 2 for Attendees.

(3) Any non-CME activity that is primarily promotional must be identified as such to faculty and participants, both in its advertising and at the conference itself.

(4) The entity presenting the program should not profit unfairly or charge a fee which is excessive for the content and length of the program.

(5) The program, content, duration, and ancillary activities should be consistent with the ideals of the AMA CME program. (I, V)

Issued December 1993.

Updated June 1996.

Journal 2000 Examines legal and ethical issues bearing upon pain management. Asserts that health care professionals have a legal and ethical duty to relieve pain and suffering of patients whenever possible. Suggests that this duty is legally enforceable. Quotes Principle V and Opinions 2.20 and 9.011. Rich, *A Prescription for the Pain: The Emerging Standard of Care for Pain Management*, 26 Wm. Mitchell L. Rev. 1, 35-36, 85 (2000).

Journal 2000 Examines issues relating to parental consent to circumcision. Identifies legal and ethical requirements for consent when medical professionals are treating adult patients. Analyzes the implications of those requirements for routine circumcision of infant males. Concludes that only when the male is an adult and capable of making decisions can circumcision be ethically and legally performed. Quotes Opinion 8.08. References Opinions 8.03 and 9.011. Svoboda, Van Howe, & Dwyer, *Informed Consent for Neonatal Circumcision: An Ethical and Legal Conundrum*, 17 J. Contemp. Health L. & Pol'y 61, 67, 73, 82 (2000).

Journal 2000 Examines the practice of gift-giving by the health care technology industry as incentives in the context of continuing medical education activities. Concludes that industry-wide standards must be developed governing interactions between physicians and representatives of health care technology industry companies. Cites Opinions 8.061 and 9.011. Tenery, *Interactions Between Physicians and the Health Care Technology Industry*, 283 JAMA 391, 393 (2000).

Journal 1992 Reviews concerns about commercial involvement in and funding of continuing medical education. Discusses CME requirements, accumulation of CME credits, and changes in standards governing commercial sponsorship. References Opinions 8.061 and 9.011. Wentz, Osteen, & Cannon, *Continuing Medical Education: Unabated Debate*, 268 JAMA 1118 (1992).

Journal 1991 Discusses commercial support of continuing medical education. Explains ethical guidelines for accepting such assistance and how those guidelines have changed. References Opinions 8.061 and 9.011. Wentz, Osteen, & Gannon, *Refocusing Support and Direction*, 266 JAMA 953 (1991).

9.012 Physicians' Political Communications with Patients and Their Families

Physicians enjoy the rights and privileges of free political speech shared by all Americans. It is laudable for physicians to run for political office; to lobby for political positions, parties or candidates; and in every other way to exercise the full scope of their political rights as citizens. These rights may be exercised individually or through involvement with organizations such as professional societies and political action committees.

In addition, physicians have a responsibility to work for the reform of, and to press for the proper administration of, laws that are related to health care. Physicians should keep themselves well-informed as to current political questions regarding needed and proposed changes to laws concerning such issues as access to health care, quality of health care services, scope of medical research, and promotion of public health.

It is natural that in fulfilling these political responsibilities, physicians will express their views to patients or their families. However, communications by telephone or other modalities with patients and their families about political matters must be conducted with the utmost sensitivity to patients' vulnerability and desire for privacy. Conversations about political matters are not appropriate at times when patients or families are emotionally pressured by significant medical circumstances. Physicians are best able to judge both the intrusiveness of the discussion and the patient's level of comfort. In general, when conversation with the patient or family concerning social, civic, or recreational matters is acceptable, discussion of items of political import may be appropriate.

Under no circumstances should physicians allow their differences with patients or their families about political matters to interfere with the delivery of high-quality professional care. (I, VII)

Issued June 1999 based on the report "Physicians' Political Communications with Patients and Their Families," adopted December 1998.

9.02   The previous Opinion 9.02, "Agreements Restricting the Practice of Medicine," was deleted in June 1998 and replaced with the current Opinion 9.02, "Restrictive Covenants and the Practice of Medicine."

9.02   Restrictive Covenants and the Practice of Medicine

Covenants-not-to-compete restrict competition, disrupt continuity of care, and potentially deprive the public of medical services. The Council on Ethical and Judicial Affairs discourages any agreement which restricts the right of a physician to practice medicine for a specified period of time or in a specified area upon termination of an employment, partnership, or corporate agreement. Restrictive covenants are unethical if they are excessive in geographic scope or duration in the circumstances presented, or if they fail to make reasonable accommodation of patients' choice of physician. (VI, VII)

Issued prior to April 1977.

Updated June 1994 and June 1998.

N.D. Ill. 1996 A corporation which provided hair transplants brought suit against a physician group under contract to provide medical services to the corporation. The complaint alleged that the defendants had breached the contract in bad faith by attempting to start their own company, by hiring staff members away, and by threatening to enforce noncompetition covenants in their contracts should any physicians attempt to remain with the corporation. The court referred to Opinion 9.02 as explicitly discouraging the use of restrictive covenants in contracts with physicians. Additionally, with apparent reference to Opinion 7.03, the court noted that defendants had not sent notices advising patients of the departure of physicians from the corporation, or of the departing physicians' new practice locations. *Cleveland Hair Clinic, Inc. v. Puig, 968 F. Supp. 1227, 1246.*

Ariz. 1999 Medical practice sought to enforce a restrictive covenant with defendant-physician. The trial court denied the plaintiff's request for a preliminary injunction and found that the restrictive covenant was unenforceable. The Arizona Supreme Court held that covenants not to compete between physicians will be strictly construed for reasonableness. Under this analysis, the court found that the restrictive covenant was unreasonable, over-broad, and unenforceable. The court quoted Opinions 9.02 and 9.06, recognizing that the AMA discourages restrictive covenants and supports free choice and competition. *Valley Medical Specialists v. Farber*, 194 Ariz. 363, 982 P.2d 1277, 1282.

Ariz. App. 1989 Plaintiff, an orthopaedic surgeon formerly employed by defendant, appealed a lower court's grant of a preliminary injunction which enforced the restrictive covenant in plaintiff's employment contract with defendant. Plaintiff asserted that Opinion 9.02 discouraged the use of such restrictive covenants and thus the covenant at issue should be declared per se unenforceable. The appellate court declined to make that declaration, noting that not all restrictive covenants are contrary to public policy and that the lower court had appropriately modified the terms of the covenant. *Phoenix Orthopaedic Surgeons, Ltd. v. Peairs*, 164 Ariz. 54, 60, 790 P.2d 752, 758.

Ga. 1988 Following termination of employment contract between the employer, a provider of psychiatric services, and a physician, the employer filed suit seeking an injunction to enforce a covenant not to compete. Supreme court, without opinion, upheld trial court's order granting an injunction. Dissenting judge, quoting Opinion 9.02 (1986) reasoned that restrictive covenants in such physician employment agreements are "illegal per se as against public policy irrespective of whether the covenant is reasonable." *Shankman v. Coastal Psychiatric Assocs.*, 258 Ga. 294, 295, 368 S.E.2d 753, 754 (dissent).

Ill. App. 2002 Ophthalmologist terminated employment contract with an eye clinic and intentionally practiced in an area prohibited by a noncompetition clause in the contract. The Illinois Appellate Court, while noting that under Opinion 9.02 (1986) noncompetition agreements are "discouraged," held that such agreements are enforceable in the medical profession in Illinois. *Prairie Eye Center v. Butler*, 329 Ill. App. 3d 293, 768 N.E.2d 414, 420.

Ill. App. 2000 Physician challenged trial court's decision upholding non-compete clause in the physician's employment contract with a health care provider. The appellate court reversed the decision, quoting Opinions 9.02 (1986) and 9.06 (1982). The court stated that the AMA disfavors the use of any restrictive employment or partnership agreements among physicians and emphasized the fact that such agreements are not in the public interest. The court also noted that patients might suffer if such agreements are upheld. *Carter-Shields v. Alton Health Institute*, 317 Ill. App. 3d 260, 739 N.E.2d 569, 576-77, vacated 201 Ill. 2d 441, 777 N.E.2d 948 (2002).

Ind. App. 1987 Medical corporation sued physician who was former employee at will pursuant to covenant not to compete in employment contract seeking an injunction or liquidated damages. Court upheld covenant against physician's claim that enforcement was inappropriate where he had been terminated without good cause. Concurring judge, citing Opinion 9.02 (1986), expressed view that such covenants should be unenforceable as against public policy. *Gomez v. Chua Medical Corp.*, 510 N.E.2d 191, 197.

Kan. App. 1985 Members of a medical partnership sought an injunction to enforce a covenant not to compete against defendant-physician, a former partner. Defendant asserted that the covenant was void as against public policy relying on Opinion 9.02 (1984). The court however ruled that the covenant was reasonable as defined by precedent and that it was bound to follow this precedent as opposed to the American Medical Association's position regarding such covenants. Defendant further argued enforcement of the covenant was precluded because the partnership had violated ethical norms, apparently referring to Opinions 6.03 and 6.04 (1984) [now Opinions 6.02 and 6.03] which were part of partnership contract. The court held defendant was estopped from complaining about the partnership's actions due to his own conduct. *Axtell Clinic v. Cranston*, No. 56,745 (Kan. Ct. App. June 20, 1985) (LEXIS, States Library, Ka. file).

Minn. 1983 Dispute arose between physician and clinic concerning covenant not to compete contained in employment contract entered into by physician after commencement of employment. Physician challenged enforceability of covenant due to lack of consideration to support it. The court agreed with physician and denied enforcement. In so ruling court did not reach issue of whether such covenants, in the context of medical practice, are against public policy. The court however noted that under Opinion 9.01 (1982) [now Opinion 9.02] the American

Medical Association discourages such restrictive covenants. *Freeman v. Duluth Clinic, 334 N.W.2d 626, 631.*

N.J. 1978 Plaintiff and defendant, both physicians, had entered into an employment contract which included in its terms a restrictive covenant provision. When defendant failed to abide by the covenant upon termination of the employment contract, plaintiff sued to enforce the covenant. In affirming the lower court's decision to enforce the restrictive covenant, the appellate court quoted Current Opinion 4.63 (1977) [now Opinion 9.02] and stated that, although it hesitated to give weight to the rules of private organizations, even if it followed the Opinion the decision to uphold the covenant would be proper. *Karlin v. Weinberg, 77 N.J. 408, 390 A.2d 1161, 1168 n.6.*

N.J. Super. 1977 Plaintiff, a dermatologist who had previously employed defendant-dermatologist, sued to enforce a post-employment restrictive covenant signed by defendant. In holding the covenant enforceable, the court noted Opinion 4.63 (1977) [now Opinion 9.02] which at the time stated there was "no ethical proscription" against entering into a restrictive covenant if its terms are reasonable. Note that Opinion 9.02 now "discourages" such restrictive agreements. *Karlin v. Weinberg, 148 N.J. Super. 243, 372 A.2d 616, 618, aff'd, 77 N.J. 408, 390 A.2d 1161 (1978).*

Ohio App. 1991 Medical corporation sought an injunction to enforce a covenant not to compete against defendant-physician. The lower court granted summary judgment based on a referee's report which concluded that, under Principle VI and Opinions 6.11, 9.02, and 9.06 (1989) restrictive covenants were *per se* unenforceable as a matter of public policy. While recognizing a strong public interest in allowing open access to health care, the appellate court in reversing held that Opinion 9.02, which applied specifically to restrictive covenants, only "discouraged" such covenants. *Ohio Urology, Inc. v. Poll, 72 Ohio. App. 446, 450, 451, 594 N.E.2d 1027, 1030, 1031.*

Journal 2003 Discusses conflicting Illinois case law regarding medical restrictive covenants. Concludes the Illinois Supreme Court should validate medical restrictive covenants that protect a business interest. Quotes Opinion 9.02. Gimbel & Zaremski, *Medical Restrictive Covenants in Illinois: At the Crossroads of Carter-Shields and Prairie Eye Center, 12 Annals Health L. 1, 12 (2003).*

Journal 2003 Highlights the legal and ethical concerns surrounding use of noncompetition clauses. Concludes that physicians should carefully evaluate these clauses given their likely enforceability. Quotes Opinions 9.02, 9.06, 10.01, and 10.015. Loeser, *The Legal, Ethical, and Practical Implications of Noncompetition Clauses: What Physicians Should Know Before They Sign, 31 J.L. Med. & Ethics 283, 286, 287, 290 (2003).*

Journal 2000 Examines strikingly different approaches to enforcement of reasonable contractual restraints on competition in the medical and legal fields. Observes that most recent cases find the public harm caused by noncompetition agreements to be generally insufficient to deny enforcement. Quotes Opinion 9.02. Wilcox, *Enforcing Lawyer Non-Competition Agreements While Maintaining the Profession: The Role of Conflict of Interest Principles, 84 Minn. L. Rev. 915, 966 (2000).*

Journal 1999 Discusses the need for physicians to advocate on behalf of patients' rights in the context of health care delivery. Evaluates the nature and scope of the physician's role as advocate, noting that physicians cannot be expected to engage in attorney-like advocacy. Quotes Principles IV and VI, Fundamental Elements (2), (4), and (6) [now Opinion 10.01], Patient Responsibilities 5 [now Opinion 10.02], and Opinions 2.03, 2.07, 2.09, 2.16, 2.19, 3.06, 4.01, 4.04, 6.01, 7.02, 8.02, 8.03, 8.13, 8.132, 9.06, 9.07, and 9.131. Cites Opinions 5.05, 5.09, 7.01, 8.135, and 9.02. Sage, *Physicians as Advocates, 35 Hous. L. Rev. 1529, 1537, 1541, 1542, 1552-53, 1554, 1556, 1557, 1559, 1561-62, 1564, 1571, 1574, 1576, 1580 (1999).*

Journal 1998 Discusses the ramifications of physician license revocation for failing to pay child support. Points out that patients stand to lose access to trusted physicians and confidence in the health care system. Concludes that children need the most protection and that patients will have an easier time finding another physician than children will have finding another means for support. Quotes Opinion 5.05. Cites Opinions 9.02 and 9.06. Noyes, *Higher Penalties for Failing to Pay Child Support: A Look at Medical License Revocation, 19 J. Legal Med. 127, 138 (1998).*

Journal 1997 Examines noncompetition clauses in the medical field. Reviews policy concerns and historical and common-law analyses of agreements not to compete. Posits that, the more commercialized the medical profession becomes, the more noncompetition clauses infringe upon the physician-patient relationship and patients' rights. Quotes Opinions 9.02 and 9.06. Cites

Preamble and Opinion 6.11. Comment, *Noncompetition Clauses in Physician Employment Contracts in Oregon*, 76 Or. L. Rev. 195, 204-06 (1997).

Journal 1997 Examines the judicial assessment of restrictive covenants within the legal and medical fields. Observes that courts tend to uphold physician, but not attorney, restrictive covenants. Concludes that covenants in medical practice should be treated in a manner similar to those in legal practice. Opinion 9.02. Levy, *Because Judges Went to Law School, Not Medical School: Restrictive Covenants in the Practices of Law and Medicine*, 30 J. Health & Hosp. L. 89, 92, 101 (1997).

Journal 1995 Analyzes South Carolina judicial treatment of covenants not to compete and liquidated damages provisions. Considers approaches in other jurisdictions and proposes guidelines for drafting contractual agreements. Quotes Opinion 9.06. Cites Opinion 9.01 (1982) [now Opinion 9.02]. Note, *Covenants Not to Compete and Liquidated Damages Clauses: Diagnosis and Treatment for Physicians*, 46 S.C. L. Rev. 505, 514 (1995)

Journal 1991 Considers the question of whether physicians should provide medical treatment to those who come to them for second opinions. Concludes that each physician must individually decide whether to treat these patients. Quotes Opinions 6.11, 9.06, and 9.12. Cites Opinion 9.02. Ile, *Should Physicians Treat Patients Who Seek Second Opinions?*, 266 JAMA 273, 274 (1991).

Journal 1982 Discusses the legal status of restrictive covenants in employment contracts against the background of the AMA's position discouraging such agreements as not serving the public interest. Observes that courts generally have upheld restrictive covenants if the limits are reasonable. Cites Opinion 9.01 (1982) [now Opinion 9.02]. Cooper, *Restrictive Covenants*, 248 JAMA 3091, 3091 (1982).

9.021 Covenants-Not-to-Compete for Physicians-in-Training

It is unethical for a teaching institution to seek a non-competition guarantee in return for fulfilling its educational obligations. Physicians-in-training (residents in programs approved by the Accreditation Council for Graduate Medical Education [ACGME], fellows in ACGME-approved fellowship programs, and fellows in programs approved by one of the American Board of Medical Specialties specialty boards) should not be asked to sign covenants-not-to-compete as a condition of their entry into any residency or fellowship program. (III, IV, VI)

Issued December 1997 based on the report "Covenants-Not-to-Compete for Physicians-in-Training," adopted June 1997 (JAMA. 1997; 278: 530).

9.025 Collective Action and Patient Advocacy

Collective action should not be conducted in a manner that jeopardizes the health and interests of patients. Formal unionization of physicians and physicians-in-training may tie physicians' interests to the interests of workers who may not share physicians' primary and overriding commitment to patients and the public health. Physicians should not form workplace alliances with those who do not share these ethical priorities.

Strikes reduce access to care, eliminate or delay necessary care, and interfere with continuity of care. Each of these consequences is contrary to the physician's ethic. Physicians should refrain from the use of the strike as a bargaining tactic.

There are some measures of collective action that may not impinge on essential patient care. Collective activities aimed at ultimately improving patient care may be warranted in some circumstances, even if they create inconvenience for the management.

Physicians and physicians-in-training should take full advantage of the tools of collective action through which to press for needed reforms. Informational campaigns, non-disruptive public demonstrations, lobbying and publicity campaigns, and collective negotiation are among the options available which do not limit services to patients.

Physicians' collective activities should be in conformance with the law. (I, III)

Issued December 1998 based on the report "Collective Action and Patient Advocacy," adopted June 1998.

Journal 1999 Considers the growing interest on the part of physicians to unionize and engage in collective bargaining. Discusses how legislatures and the courts may affect the evolution of physician unions. Analyzes potential benefits and detriments of unionization. References Opinion 9.025. Phan, *Physician Unionization: The Impact on the Medical Profession, 20 J. Legal Med. 115, 136, 137 (1999).*

9.03 Civil Rights and Professional Responsibility

Opportunities in medical society activities or membership, medical education and training, employment, and all other aspects of professional endeavors should not be denied to any duly licensed physician because of race, color, religion, creed, ethnic affiliation, national origin, sex, sexual orientation, age, or handicap. (IV)

Issued prior to April 1977.

Updated June 1994.

Journal 1996 Examines possible legal avenues for addressing claims of employment discrimination based upon sexual orientation. Concludes that lesbians and gay men need greater employment protection and an explicit statutory cause of action. Quotes Opinion 9.03. Gilmore, *Employment Protection for Lesbians and Gay Men, 6 L. & Sex. 83, 95 (1996).*

9.031 Reporting Impaired, Incompetent, or Unethical Colleagues

Physicians have an ethical obligation to report impaired, incompetent, and unethical colleagues in accordance with the legal requirements in each state and assisted by the following guidelines:

Impairment. Impairment should be reported to the hospital's in-house impairment program, if available. Otherwise, either the chief of an appropriate clinical service or the chief of the hospital staff should be alerted. Reports may also be made directly to an external impaired physician program. Practicing physicians who do not have hospital privileges should be reported directly to an impaired physician program, such as those run by medical societies, when appropriate. If none of these steps would facilitate the entrance of the impaired physician into an impairment program, then the impaired physician should be reported directly to the state licensing board.

Incompetence. Initial reports of incompetence should be made to the appropriate clinical authority who would be empowered to assess the potential impact on patient welfare and to facilitate remedial action. The hospital peer review body should be notified where appropriate. Incompetence which poses an immediate threat to the health of patients should be reported directly to the state licensing board. Incompetence by physicians without a hospital affiliation should be reported to the local or state medical society and/or the state licensing or disciplinary board.

Unethical conduct. With the exception of incompetence or impairment, unethical behavior should be reported in accordance with the following guidelines.

Unethical conduct that threatens patient care or welfare should be reported to the appropriate authority for a particular clinical service. Unethical behavior which violates state licensing provisions should be reported to the state licensing board or impaired physician programs, when appropriate. Unethical conduct which violates criminal statutes must be reported to the appropriate law enforcement authorities. All other unethical conduct should be reported to the local or state medical society.

Where the inappropriate behavior of a physician continues despite the initial report(s), the reporting physician should report to a higher or additional authority. The person or body receiving the initial report should notify the reporting physician when appropriate action has been taken. Physicians who receive reports of inappropriate behavior have an ethical duty to critically and objectively evaluate the reported information and to assure that identified deficiencies are either remedied or further reported to a higher or additional authority. Anonymous reports should receive appropriate review and confidential investigation. Physicians who are under scrutiny or charge should be protected by the rules of confidentiality until such charges are proven or until the physician is exonerated. (II)

Issued March 1992 based on the report "Reporting Impaired, Incompetent, or Unethical Colleagues," adopted December 1991 (J Miss St Med Assoc. 1992; 33: 176-77).

Updated June 1994 and June 1996.

Ga. App. 1998 An emergency room physician sued another physician who examined a patient one day after the plaintiff, for libel and unfair business practices stemming from letters the second physician wrote regarding the emergency room physician's treatment of the patient. The court affirmed the trial court's grant of summary judgment on grounds that the concerns addressed in the letters were protected by a conditional privilege and that the plaintiff had not proved that the defendant wrote the letters with malice. The court quoted Opinion 9.031, as imposing a duty to report the plaintiff's treatment of the patient. Furthermore, the court noted that according to the Opinion, the defendant was neither required to address the problem with the offending physician first, nor required to confine her concerns to peer review groups. *Dominy v. Shumpert, 235 Ga. App. 500, 510 S.E.2d 81, 85-86.*

Mich. App. 1968 Physician was properly dismissed from hospital staff for violating Principle 4 (1957) [now Principle II and Opinion 9.031] when on numerous occasions physician vilified other physicians, swore and screamed in the hospital, and quarreled with staff and hospital visitors. *Anderson v. Bd. of Trustees of Caro Community Hosp., 10 Mich. App. 348, 159 N.W.2d 347, 348-50.*

Journal 1993 Discusses the problems physicians may encounter by exposing an errant colleague, such as harm to the reporting physician's reputation and the fear of litigation. States that problems involving physician competency and unethical behavior should be investigated, and that physicians should take personal responsibility for reporting problems they observe. References Principle II and Opinions 8.14 and 9.031. Morreim, *Am I My Brother's Warden? Responding to the Unethical or Incompetent Colleague*, 23 Hastings Center Rep. 19, 23 (May/June 1993).

9.032 Reporting Adverse Drug or Device Events

A physician who suspects the occurrence of an adverse reaction to a drug or medical device has an obligation to communicate that information to the broader medical community, (eg, through submitting a report or letter to a medical journal or informing the manufacturer of the suspect drug or device). In the case of a serious adverse event, the event should be reported to the Food and Drug Administration (FDA). Spontaneous reports of adverse events are irreplaceable as a source of valuable information about drugs and medical devices, particularly their rare or delayed effects, as well as their safety in vulnerable patient populations. Although premarketing and mandated postmarketing studies provide basic safeguards for the public health, they suffer from inherent deficiencies that limit their ability to detect rare or unexpected consequences of drug or medical device use. Physicians who prescribe and monitor the use of drugs and medical devices constitute the group best able to observe and communicate information about resulting adverse events.

Serious adverse events, such as those resulting in death, hospitalization, or medical or surgical intervention, are the most important to report and are the only adverse events for which the FDA desires a report. Certainty, or even reasonable likelihood, of a causal relationship between the drug or medical device and the serious adverse event will rarely exist and is not required before reporting the event to the FDA. Suspicion of such a relationship is sufficient to give rise to an obligation to participate in the reporting system. (I, V, VII)

Issued June 1993 based on the report "Reporting Adverse Drug and Medical Device Events," adopted June 1993.

Updated June 1994 (*Food & Drug L. J.* 1994; 49: 359-66).

Journal 2002 Challenges the general use of special informed consent disclosure rules in experimental therapy. Discusses the lack of a bright-line distinction between standard and experimental interventions. Concludes that focus should be placed on the distinctiveness of experimentation. Quotes Opinion 2.07. References Opinion 9.032. Noah, *Informed Consent and the Elusive Dichotomy Between Standard and Experimental Therapy*, 28 Am. J.L. & Med. 361, 394, 395 (2002).

Journal 2000 Describes possible solutions designed to improve post-approval regulation of prescription drugs so that fewer patients will suffer from adverse drug reactions. Concludes that the FDA along with physicians and clinical researchers should rethink the existing approach to monitoring of unexpected side effects. Quotes Principle V and Opinion 9.032. Cites Opinion 5.05. Noah, *Adverse Drug Reactions: Harnessing Experimental Data to Promote Patient Welfare*, 49 Cath. U. L. Rev. 449, 477, 497-98 (2000).

Journal 2000 Evaluates the regulatory framework governing prescription drugs. Considers problems faced by elderly patients when taking FDA-approved medications. Concludes that, in order to optimize patient safety, the existing regulatory system must undergo important structural changes. Quotes Principle V and Opinion 9.032. Noah & Brushwood, *Adverse Drug Reactions in Elderly Patients: Alternative Approaches to Postmarket Surveillance*, 33 J. Health L. 383, 400, 445 (2000).

Journal 1999 Discusses the duty of manufacturers to discover potential adverse drug interactions with new drugs. Suggests that a manufacturer's duty to warn about adverse drug interactions may be the future subject of products liability lawsuits. References Opinion 9.032. McCormick, *Pharmaceutical Manufacturer's Duty to Warn of Adverse Drug Interactions*, 66 Def. Couns. J. 59, 61 (1999).

Journal 1993 Explains MedWatch, an FDA program designed to facilitate the reporting of adverse events associated with the use of FDA-approved drugs and medical devices. Emphasizes that physicians are best able to provide such information. Quotes Opinion 9.032. Rheinstein, *MedWatch: The FDA Medical Products Reporting Program*, 48 Am. Fam. Physician 636, 636 (1993).

9.035 Gender Discrimination in the Medical Profession

Physician leaders in medical schools and other medical institutions should take immediate steps to increase the number of women in leadership positions as such positions become open. There is already a large enough pool of female physicians to provide strong candidates for such positions. Also, adjustments should be made to ensure that all physicians are equitably compensated for their work. Women and men in the same specialty with the same experience and doing the same work should be paid the same compensation.

Physicians in the workplace should actively develop the following: (1) retraining or other programs which facilitate the re-entry of physicians who take time away from their careers to have a family; (2) on-site child care services for dependent children; and (3) policies providing job security for physicians who are temporarily not in practice due to pregnancy or family obligations.

Physicians in the academic medical setting should strive to promote the following: (1) extension of tenure decisions through "stop the clock" programs, relaxation of the seven year rule, or part-time appointments that would give faculty members longer to achieve standards for promotion and tenure; (2) more reasonable guidelines regarding the appropriate quantity and timing of published material needed for promotion or tenure that would emphasize quality over quantity and that would encourage the pursuit of careers based on individual talent rather than tenure standards that undervalue teaching ability and overvalue research; and (3) fair distribution of teaching, clinical, research, administrative responsibilities, and access to tenure tracks between men and women. Also, physicians in academic institutions should consider formally structuring the mentoring process, possibly matching students or faculty with advisors through a fair and visible system.

Where such policies do not exist or have not been followed, all medical workplaces and institutions should create strict policies to deal with sexual harassment. Grievance committees should have broad representation of both sexes and other groups. Such committees should have the power to enforce harassment policies and be accessible to those persons they are meant to serve.

Grantors of research funds and editors of scientific or medical journals should consider blind peer review of grant proposals and articles for publication to help prevent bias. However, grantors and editors will be able to consider the author's identity and give it appropriate weight. (II, VII)

Issued June 1994 based on the report "Gender Discrimination in the Medical Profession," adopted June 1993 (*Women's Health Issues*. 1994; 4: 1-11).

Journal 2000 Reports on a study conducted to evaluate issues relating to the advancement of women through the ranks of surgery and academic medicine. Concludes that many of the obstacles women face in this context appear to be based upon subtle, even unconscious, societal attitudes and behaviors. References Opinion 9.035. Colletti, Mulholland, & Sonnad, *Perceived Obstacles to Career Success for Women in Academic Surgery*, 135 Arch. Surg. 972, 976 (2000).

Journal 1996 Considers the pharmaceutical industry's failure to test products on female subjects. Comments on the potential for harm. Notes legal difficulties women experience when attempting to prove a drug was not adequately tested. Posits that litigation can affect the behavior of pharmaceutical companies. References Opinion 9.035. Comment, *Tort Reform to Ensure the Inclusion of Fertile Women in Early Phases of Commercial Drug Research*, 3 U. Chi. L. Sch. Roundtable 355, 359 (1996).

9.037   Signing Bonuses to Attract Graduates of US Medical Schools

Signing bonuses or compensation should not be offered or denied to a resident based on the country where the resident attended or graduated from medical school. (II, III, IV, VI)

Issued June 2000 based on the report "Signing Bonuses to Attract Graduates of US Medical Schools," adopted December 1999.

9.04   Discipline and Medicine

Incompetence, corruption, or dishonest or unethical conduct on the part of members of the medical profession is reprehensible. In addition to posing a real or potential threat to patients, such conduct undermines the public's confidence in the profession. A physician should expose, without fear or loss of favor, incompetent or corrupt, dishonest, or unethical conduct on the part of members of the profession. Questions of such conduct should be reported and reviewed in accordance with Opinion 9.031, "Reporting Impaired, Incompetent, or Unethical Colleagues."

Violation of governmental laws may subject the physician to civil or criminal liability. Expulsion from membership is the maximum penalty that may be imposed by a medical society upon a physician who violates the ethical standards involving a breach of moral duty or principle. However, medical societies have a civic and professional obligation to report to the appropriate governmental body or state board of medical examiners credible evidence that may come to their attention involving the alleged criminal conduct of any physician relating to the practice of medicine.

Although a physician charged with allegedly illegal conduct may be acquitted or exonerated in civil or criminal proceedings, this does not discharge a medical society from its obligation to initiate a disciplinary proceeding against a member with reference to the same conduct where there is credible evidence tending to establish unethical conduct.

The Council cannot pass judgment in advance on a situation that may later come before it on appeal. The Council cannot be an attorney for a society or a member thereof and later judge in the same factual situation. The local medical society has the initial obligation of determining all the facts and whether or not disciplinary action is indicated. Questions asking for a review of a proposed course of action or an evaluation of an existing factual situation should be presented to the appropriate official of the physician's local society. (II, III, VII)

Issued prior to April 1977.

Updated June 1994.

Cal. App. 1956 Physician-petitioner sought mandamus against local medical association whose bylaws provided for the expulsion of any member who violated the Principles. Petitioner had been expelled under the provision and the expulsion was affirmed by the American Medical Association's Judicial Council. The initial grounds for expulsion was alleged violation of Principles Ch. III, Art. IV, Sec.4 (1947) [now Opinions 9.04 and 9.07] for disparaging statements regarding another physician in a report used in judicial proceedings. In holding that application of the provision to petitioner was contrary to public policy, the court noted that the physician's statements had been made at the request of a civil litigant and enjoyed a statutory testimonial privilege. Further, the court found that the American Medical Association's right to formulate ethical principles did not extend to defining the duties of witnesses. Expulsion was also based on petitioner's critical comments about other physicians overheard by their patients in violation of Principles Ch. III, Art. IV, Sec.1 (1947) [now Principle II and Opinion 9.04]. The court found application of this Principle under the circumstances reasonable and not contrary to public policy. *Bernstein v. Alameda-Contra Costa Medical Ass'n, 139 Cal. App. 2d 241, 293 P.2d 862, 863, 863 nn.1, 2, 865 nn.4, 6, 866, 866 n.8, 867.*

Ohio 1980 A physician, charged with violating the state medical licensing statute by distributing controlled substances without a proper license and writing prescriptions for narcotics in the name of one person when they were intended for another, challenged the state medical board's decision to suspend his license and place him on two years probation. Under the statute, a physician could be disciplined for various activities including violation of any provision of a code of ethics of a national professional organization such as the American Medical Association. The board found in part that the physician's actions violated Principles 4 and 7 (1957) [now Principles II and III and Opinions 8.06 and 9.04]. The trial court reversed, holding that the board had insufficient evidence for its decision, and the court of appeals affirmed. On appeal, the supreme court held that expert testimony was not required at a hearing before a medical licensing board because they were experts and could determine for themselves whether the Principles had been violated. *Arlen v. State, 61 Ohio St. 2d 168, 399 N.E.2d 1251, 1252, 1253-54.*

Journal 2001 Examines issues relating to health care cost containment. Concludes that, if physicians are to meet the goals assigned to them in a cost-constrained health care system, then professional standards must be reevaluated and modified to afford meaningful guidance for clinical decision-making in the face of health care spending controls. Quotes Opinions 2.03, 2.09, 2.095, 8.032, and 9.04. Cites Opinions 8.02, 8.021, 8.051, and 8.13. Agrawal, *Resuscitating Professionalism: Self-Regulation in the Medical Marketplace*, 66 Mo. L. Rev. 341, 354, 355, 360, 361, 378, 388 (2001).

Journal 1994 Discusses the role of professional societies in establishing ethical guidelines for physicians in the context of using medical innovations and new technologies. Observes that these standards must be supplemented by additional external measures or incentives in order to be most effective. Cites Opinions 1.01, 1.02, 8.061, 9.04, and 9.131. Orentlicher, *The Influence of a Professional Organization on Physician Behavior*, 57 Alb. L. Rev. 583, 592, 593, 594, 595, 596 (1994).

9.045   Physicians with Disruptive Behavior

This Opinion is limited to the conduct of individual physicians and does not refer to physicians acting as a collective, which is considered separately in Opinion 9.025, "Collective Action and Patient Advocacy."

(1) Personal conduct, whether verbal or physical, that negatively affects or that potentially may negatively affect patient care constitutes disruptive behavior. (This includes but is not limited to conduct that interferes with one's ability to work with other members of the health care team.) However, criticism that is offered in good faith with the aim of improving patient care should not be construed as disruptive behavior.

(2) Each medical staff should develop and adopt bylaw provisions or policies

for intervening in situations where a physician's behavior is identified as disruptive. The medical staff bylaw provisions or policies should contain procedural safeguards that protect due process. Physicians exhibiting disruptive behavior should be referred to a medical staff wellness—or equivalent—committee.

(3) In developing policies that address physicians with disruptive behavior, attention should be paid to the following elements:

(a) Clearly stating principal objectives in terms that ensure high standards of patient care and promote a professional practice and work environment.

(b) Describing the behavior or types of behavior that will prompt intervention.

(c) Providing a channel through which disruptive behavior can be reported and appropriately recorded. A single incident may not be sufficient for action, but each individual report may help identify a pattern that requires intervention.

(d) Establishing a process to review or verify reports of disruptive behavior.

(e) Establishing a process to notify a physician whose behavior is disruptive that a report has been made, and providing the physician with an opportunity to respond to the report.

(f) Including means of monitoring whether a physician's disruptive conduct improves after intervention.

(g) Providing for evaluative and corrective actions that are commensurate with the behavior, such as self-correction and structured rehabilitation. Suspension of responsibilities or privileges should be a mechanism of final resort. Additionally, institutions should consider whether the reporting requirements of Opinion 9.031, "Reporting Impaired, Incompetent, or Unethical Colleagues," apply in particular cases.

(h) Identifying which individuals will be involved in the various stages of the process, from reviewing reports to notifying physicians and monitoring conduct after intervention.

(i) Providing clear guidelines for the protection of confidentiality.

(j) Ensuring that individuals who report physicians with disruptive behavior are duly protected. (I, II, VIII)

Issued December 2000 based on the report "Physicians with Disruptive Behavior," adopted June 2000.

9.05   Due Process

The basic principles of a fair and objective hearing should always be accorded to the physician or medical student whose professional conduct is being reviewed. The fundamental aspects of a fair hearing are a listing of specific charges, adequate notice of the right of a hearing, the opportunity to be present and to rebut the evidence, and the opportunity to present a defense. These principles apply when the hearing body is a medical society tribunal, medical staff committee, or other similar body composed of peers. The composition of committees sitting in judgment of medical students, residents, or fellows should include a significant number of persons at a similar level of training.

These principles of fair play apply in all disciplinary hearings and in any other type of hearing in which the reputation, professional status, or livelihood of the physician or medical student may be negatively impacted.

All physicians and medical students are urged to observe diligently these fundamental safeguards of due process whenever they are called upon to serve on a committee which will pass judgment on a peer. All medical societies and institutions are urged to review their constitutions and bylaws and/or policies to make sure that these instruments provide for such procedural safeguards. (II, III, VII)

Issued prior to April 1977.

Updated June 1994.

Ill. App. 1979 Physician sued professional association of orthopaedic surgeons after it denied his application for membership. Plaintiff claimed he was not fully informed of the basis of denial, received no notice or opportunity to attend the hearing in which his application was considered, and was neither allowed to hear adverse evidence nor present a defense. Since the association's by-laws required adherence to the Principles, including Opinion 6.18 (1977) [now Opinion 9.05], which demanded that due process be afforded a physician whose conduct is being reviewed, plaintiff alleged that the association had violated its own procedures in the application process. The court held that the applicant did not have a right to have his application considered according to the association's bylaws and could not obtain judicial review without a showing of economic necessity. *Treister v. American Academy of Orthopaedic Surgeons*, 78 Ill. App. 3d 746, 396 N.E.2d 1225, 1228, 1232, 1238.

Va. App. 2003 Physician appealed Board of Medicine's license probation order for unprofessional conduct. Board found the physician's pattern of inappropriate advances towards medical students violated medical ethical standards. Appellate court reversed, holding that the evidence was insufficient to support Board's finding, since the ethical standards by which the physician should be adjudicated were not established by competent evidence. Quotes Opinions 3.08 and 9.05. *Goad v. Virginia Board of Medicine*, 40 Va. App. 621, 580 S.E.2d 494, 498, n.7, 499, n.9.

Journal 1984 Discusses litigation by physicians in situations where medical staff privileges have been denied, curtailed, or revoked. Offers an analysis of the relevant legal theories and practice considerations that form part of hospital privilege antitrust litigation but concludes that litigation based on the Sherman Act—the predominant antitrust legislative scheme—in this context generally has been unsuccessful due to stringent requirements of proof. Cites Opinion 9.04 (1982) [now Opinion 9.05]. Tabor, *The Battle for Hospital Privileges*, 251 JAMA 1602, 1602 (1984).

Journal 1983 Describes special problems that may confront family physicians in the context of applying for hospital privileges. Offers a recommended approach to the application process which encourages physicians to document areas of residency training, become familiar with the hospital policies, guidelines, and procedures involved in applying for privileges, and solicit the support of staff physicians. Quotes Opinion 9.04 (1981) [now Opinion 9.05]. Pugno, *Hospital Privileges for Family Physicians: Rights, Rationale, and Resources*, 17 J. Fam. Practice 77, 79 (1983).

9.055   Disputes between Medical Supervisors and Trainees

Clear policies for handling complaints from medical students, resident physicians, and other staff should be established. These policies should include adequate provisions for protecting the confidentiality of complainants whenever possible. Confidentiality of complainants should be protected when doing so does not hinder the subject's ability to respond to the complaint. Access to employment and evaluation files should be carefully monitored to remove the possibility of tampering. Resident physicians should be permitted access to their employment files and also the right to copy the contents thereof, within the provisions of applicable federal and state laws.

Medical students, resident physicians, and other staff should refuse to participate in patient care ordered by their supervisors in those rare cases in which they believe the orders reflect serious errors in clinical or ethical judgment, or physician impairment, that could result in a threat of imminent harm to the patient or to others. In these rare cases, the complainant may withdraw from the care ordered by the supervisor, provided withdrawal does not itself threaten the patient's immediate welfare. The complainant should communicate his or her concerns to the physician issuing the orders and, if necessary, to the appropriate persons for mediating such disputes. Mechanisms for resolving these disputes, which require immediate resolution, should be in place. Third-party mediators of such disputes may include the chief of staff of the involved service, the chief resident, a designated member of the institutional grievance committee, or, in large institutions, an institutional ombudsperson largely outside of the established hospital staff hierarchy.

Retaliatory or punitive actions against those who raise complaints are unethical and are a legitimate cause for filing a grievance with the appropriate institutional committee. (II, III, VII)

Issued June 1994 based on the report "Disputes Between Medical Supervisors and Trainees," adopted December 1993 (JAMA. 1994; 272: 1861-1865).

Journal 1997 Discusses professionalism among attorneys. Emphasizes the need for individual accountability. Concludes that the rules of professional conduct should be modified to hold lawyers responsible for their actions. Quotes Opinion 9.055. Rice, *The Superior Orders Defense in Legal Ethics: Sending the Wrong Message to Young Lawyers*, 32 Wake Forest L. Rev. 887, 908-09 (1997).

Journal 1995 Examines the rights of health care professionals to refuse to participate in patient care on the basis of conscientious objection. Suggests steps that health care facilities may take when dealing with health care professionals who object to participating in patient care. Quotes Principles I and VI and Opinions 1.02, 2.035, and 9.055. Dellinger & Vickery, *When Staff Object to Participating In Care*, 28 J. Health & Hospital Law 269, 272, 276 (1995).

9.06   Free Choice

Free choice of physicians is the right of every individual. One may select and change at will one's physicians, or one may choose a medical care plan such as that provided by a closed panel or group practice or health maintenance or service organization. The individual's freedom to select a preferred system of health care and free competition among physicians and alternative systems of care are prerequisites of ethical practice and optimal patient care.

In choosing to subscribe to a health maintenance or service organization or in choosing or accepting treatment in a particular hospital, the patient is thereby accepting limitations upon free choice of medical services.

The need of an individual for emergency treatment in cases of accident or sudden illness may, as a practical matter, preclude free choice of a physician, particularly where there is loss of consciousness.

Although the concept of free choice assures that an individual can generally choose a physician, likewise a physician may decline to accept that individual as a patient. In selecting the physician of choice, the patient may sometimes be obliged to pay for medical services which might otherwise be paid by a third party. (VI)

Issued prior to April 1977.

E.D. N.Y. 1975 Medical laboratories sought injunction against city's award of exclusive contracts for Medicaid services. The court granted a preliminary injunction and held that the laboratories had a substantial probability of success on the merits of the claim that Medicaid recipients would be deprived of statutory right of free choice of providers. In balancing the equities, the court also noted that the contracts would create an ethical dilemma for physicians who are required to provide patients with free choice of ancillary services under Opinions and Reports of the Judicial Council Sec. 1, Paras. 6 and 14 (1971) [now Opinions 8.03, 8.06, and 9.06]. *Bay Ridge Diagnostic Laboratory, Inc. v. Dumpson*, 400 F. Supp. 1104, 1109-10.

Ariz. 1999 Medical practice sought to enforce a restrictive covenant with defendant-physician. The trial court denied the plaintiff's request for a preliminary injunction and found that the restrictive covenant was unenforceable. The Arizona Supreme Court held that covenants not to compete between physicians will be strictly construed for reasonableness. Under this analysis, the court found that the restrictive covenant was unreasonable, over-broad, and unenforceable. The court quoted Opinions 9.02 and 9.06, recognizing that the AMA discourages restrictive covenants and supports free choice and competition. *Valley Medical Specialists v. Farber*, 194 Ariz. 363, 982 P.2d 1277, 1282.

Ariz. 1965 Physician appealed denial of medical license which was based on alleged violations of local medical society rules and Principles 3, 5, and 10 (1957) [now Principles III, VII, and Opinions 3.01, 8.11, and 9.06]. Alleged violations included treating a patient without first obtaining a prior treating physician's permission, inadequate patient care, performing operations without hospital privileges, and signing the medical record of a deceased patient who had been treated by interns. The court held that the evidence failed to show any clear violation of the Principles and that a local medical society had no right to prescribe a code of ethics for state licensing purposes. *Arizona State Bd. of Medical Examiners v. Clark*, 97 Ariz. 205, 398 P.2d 908, 914-915, 915 n.3.

Cal. App. 1978 Surviving spouse sued physicians who were on emergency surgical call panel for malpractice where patient died during surgery. Although defendants claimed immunity under state Good Samaritan statute, the court held the statute inapplicable since the legislative purpose was to encourage physicians to render care on an irregular basis to unattended persons discovered by chance at the scene of an emergency. In so holding, the court noted that Principle 5 (1957) [now Principle VI and Opinions 8.11 and 9.06] imposed an ethical duty to render emergency medical care. *Colby v. Schwartz*, 78 Cal. App. 3d 885, 144 Cal. Rptr. 624, 627 n.2.

Ill. App. 2000 Physician challenged trial court's decision upholding non-compete clause in the physician's employment contract with a health care provider. The appellate court reversed the decision, quoting Opinions 9.02 (1986) and 9.06 (1982). The court stated that the AMA disfavors the use of any restrictive employment or partnership agreements among physicians and emphasized the fact that such agreements are not in the public interest. The court also noted that patients might suffer if such agreements are upheld. *Carter-Shields v. Alton Health Institute*, 317 Ill. App. 3d 260, 739 N.E.2d 569, 576-77, vacated 201 Ill. 2d 441, 777 N.E.2d 948 (2002).

Ohio App. 1991 Medical corporation sought an injunction to enforce a covenant not to compete against defendant-physician. The lower court granted summary judgment based on a referee's report which concluded that, under Principle VI and Opinions 6.11, 9.02, and 9.06 (1989) restrictive covenants were *per se* unenforceable as a matter of public policy. While recognizing a strong public interest in allowing open access to health care, the appellate court in reversing held that Opinion 9.02, which applied specifically to restrictive covenants, only "discouraged" such covenants. *Ohio Urology, Inc. v. Poll*, 72 Ohio. App. 446, 450, 451, 594 N.E.2d 1027, 1030, 1031.

Wash. 1951 Plaintiff, a charitable, not-for-profit medical corporation, offered prepaid health care services to members and their families. Suit was filed against county medical society and others for damages and injunction for defendants' alleged efforts to monopolize prepaid medical care in area and unlawfully restrain competition by plaintiff and its physicians. Defendants alleged as affirmative defense that their efforts were designed to curb unethical prepaid contract practice by plaintiff. Court examined at length American Medical Association's position regarding contract practice including Principles Ch. III, Art. VI, Secs. 3 and 4 (1947) [now Principle VI and

Opinions 8.05 and 9.06] concluding nothing in plaintiff's practice violated the Association's ethical guidelines. Further, quoting Principles Ch. III, Art. III, Sec.1 (1947) [now Opinion 8.04] dealing with consultations, court noted that defendants' efforts impeded plaintiff's physicians from obtaining consultations. Court concluded that defendants' actions constituted unlawful, monopolistic behavior and issued an injunction, although it declined to award damages. *Group Health Coop. v. King County Medical Soc'y*, 39 Wash. 2d 586, 237 P.2d 737, 744, 750-51, 759-60.

Journal 2003 Highlights the legal and ethical concerns surrounding use of noncompetition clauses. Concludes that physicians should carefully evaluate these clauses given their likely enforceability. Quotes Opinions 9.02, 9.06, 10.01, and 10.015. Loeser, *The Legal, Ethical, and Practical Implications of Noncompetition Clauses: What Physicians Should Know Before They Sign*, 31 J.L. Med. & Ethics 283, 286, 287, 290 (2003).

Journal 1999 Discusses potential conflicts between a criminal defense attorney's religious beliefs and representation of the client. Explores theories that would allow an attorney to put religious beliefs over the client's interest. Offers analogies within the physician-patient relationship. Concludes that a defense attorney is bound by duty and must set aside conflicting religious beliefs. Quotes Principle VI and Opinions 8.11, 9.06, and 9.12. Reza, *Religion and the Public Defender*, 26 Fordham Urb. L. J. 1051, 1062, 1063 (1999).

Journal 1999 Discusses the need for physicians to advocate on behalf of patients' rights in the context of health care delivery. Evaluates the nature and scope of the physician's role as advocate, noting that physicians cannot be expected to engage in attorney-like advocacy. Quotes Principles IV and VI, Fundamental Elements (2), (4), and (6) [now Opinion 10.01], Patient Responsibilities 5 [now Opinion 10.02], and Opinions 2.03, 2.07, 2.09, 2.16, 2.19, 3.06, 4.01, 4.04, 6.01, 7.02, 8.02, 8.03, 8.13, 8.132, 9.06, 9.07, and 9.131. Cites Opinions 5.05, 5.09, 7.01, 8.135, and 9.02. Sage, *Physicians as Advocates*, 35 Hous. L. Rev. 1529, 1537, 1541, 1542, 1552-53, 1554, 1556, 1557, 1559, 1561-62, 1564, 1571, 1574, 1576, 1580 (1999).

Journal 1998 Discusses conflicts of interest in the physician-patient relationship arising out of use of financial incentives by managed care organizations. Considers how such conflicts are dealt with in the attorney-client relationship. Suggests that a financial incentive should be legally denounced if it unreasonably interferes with a physician's duty to properly care for and treat patients. Quotes Preamble, Fundamental Elements (1) [now Opinion 10.01] and Opinions 4.04, 5.01, 8.03, 8.13, and 9.06. Cites Fundamental Elements (4) [now Opinion 10.01] and Opinions 2.07, 2.08, and 2.132. Hall, *Third-Party Payor Conflicts of Interest in Managed Care: A Proposal for Regulation Based on the Model Rules of Professional Conduct*, 29 Seton Hall L. Rev. 95, 96, 107, 108, 109, 110, 111, 112, 134, 135, 136 (1998).

Journal 1998 Discusses the ramifications of physician license revocation for failing to pay child support. Points out that patients stand to lose access to trusted physicians and confidence in the health care system. Concludes that children need the most protection and that patients will have an easier time finding another physician than children will have finding another means for support. Quotes Opinion 5.05. Cites Opinions 9.02 and 9.06. Noyes, *Higher Penalties for Failing to Pay Child Support: A Look at Medical License Revocation*, 19 J. Legal Med. 127, 138 (1998).

Journal 1997 Examines noncompetition clauses in the medical field. Reviews policy concerns and historical and common-law analyses of agreements not to compete. Posits that, the more commercialized the medical profession becomes, the more noncompetition clauses infringe upon the physician-patient relationship and patients' rights. Quotes Opinions 9.02 and 9.06. Cites Preamble and Opinion 6.11. Comment, *Noncompetition Clauses in Physician Employment Contracts in Oregon*, 76 Or. L. Rev. 195, 204-06 (1997).

Journal 1997 Examines the evolution of the Indiana health care system. Discusses developments in Indiana jurisprudence regarding the physician-patient relationship. Explores various challenges facing the relationship and recognizes the need for legal rules to help address these challenges. Quotes Opinion 8.08. Cites Opinions 2.20, 9.06, and 9.12. Kinney & Selby, *History and Jurisprudence of the Physician-Patient Relationship in Indiana*, 30 Ind. L. Rev. 263, 269, 272, 276 (1997).

Journal 1995 Analyzes South Carolina judicial treatment of covenants not to compete and liquidated damages provisions. Considers approaches in other jurisdictions and proposes guidelines for drafting contractual agreements. Quotes Opinion 9.06. Cites Opinion 9.01 (1982) [now Opinion 9.02]. Note, *Covenants Not to Compete and Liquidated Damages Clauses: Diagnosis and Treatment for Physicians*, 46 S.C. L. Rev. 505, 514 (1995).

Journal 1991 Considers the question of whether physicians should provide medical treatment to those who come to them for second opinions. Concludes that each physician must individually decide whether to treat these patients. Quotes Opinions 6.11, 9.06, and 9.12. Cites Opinion 9.02. Ile, *Should Physicians Treat Patients Who Seek Second Opinions?*, 266 JAMA 273, 274 (1991).

Journal 1987 Concludes that a policy or practice of active voluntary euthanasia is not desirable, linking a moral prohibition against active voluntary euthanasia to the moral prohibition against physicians actively participating in capital punishment. In place of any practice of active voluntary euthanasia, recommends increased use of hospices, greater emphasis on training physicians to care for the dying patient, and further research aimed at producing symptomatic relief in dying patients. Cites Opinions 2.06, 8.10 (1986) [now Opinion 8.11], and 9.06. Shewmon, *Active Voluntary Euthanasia: A Needless Pandora's Box*, 3 Issues in Law and Med. 219, 220, 222, 243 (1987).

9.065 Caring for the Poor

Each physician has an obligation to share in providing care to the indigent. The measure of what constitutes an appropriate contribution may vary with circumstances such as community characteristics, geographic location, the nature of the physician's practice and specialty, and other conditions. All physicians should work to ensure that the needs of the poor in their communities are met. Caring for the poor should be a regular part of the physician's practice schedule.

In the poorest communities, it may not be possible to meet the needs of the indigent for physicians' services by relying solely on local physicians. The local physicians should be able to turn for assistance to their colleagues in prosperous communities, particularly those in close proximity.

Physicians are meeting their obligation, and are encouraged to continue to do so, in a number of ways such as seeing indigent patients in their offices at no cost or at reduced cost, serving at freestanding or hospital clinics that treat the poor, and participating in government programs that provide health care to the poor. Physicians can also volunteer their services at weekend clinics for the poor and at shelters for battered women or the homeless.

In addition to meeting their obligation to care for the indigent, physicians can devote their energy, knowledge, and prestige to designing and lobbying at all levels for better programs to provide care for the poor. (I, VII)

Issued June 1994 based on the report "Caring for the Poor," adopted December 1992 (JAMA. 1993; 269: 2533-37).

Journal 2000 Discusses and evaluates different systems for addressing consumer concerns about managed health care. Asserts that current legal systems for identifying and resolving consumer concerns are not understood by most consumers and are not accessible by many, especially the uninsured. Concludes that several immediate steps are realistic for moving toward reform. Cites Principle VI. References Opinions 8.13 and 9.065. Kinney, *Tapping and Resolving Consumer Concerns About Health Care*, 26 Am. J. Law & Med. 335, 337, 375 (2000).

Journal 2000 Evaluates recent Texas legislation that affords immunity to health care professionals who provide free health care services to the poor. Concludes that such legislation creates a dual standard of care, requiring indigent patients to forfeit their legal rights in exchange for health care. Quotes Opinion 10.01. References Opinion 9.065. Pulido, *Immunity of Volunteer Health Care Providers in Texas: Bartering Legal Rights for Free Medical Care*, 2 Scholar: St. Mary's L. Rev. Minority Issues 323, 330 (2000).

Journal 1999 Discusses regulatory concerns regarding genetic technology. Provides ideas on how society might regulate genetic enhancements. Argues that a variety of means of regulation need to be utilized to govern genetic technology. Quotes Opinion 2.11. Cites Opinion 9.065.

References Opinion 2.138. Mehlman, *How Will We Regulate Genetic Enhancement?*, 34 *Wake Forest L. Rev.* 671, 693-94, 695 (1999).

Journal 1997 Considers the current approach to health care in the United States. Examines financing mechanisms, and suggests that reform could be effected through a decentralized, community-based approach. Proposes use of volunteer systems in which medical personnel would care for certain patients free of charge or at reduced rates. Quotes Fundamental Elements (6). References Opinion 9.065. Solomon & Asaro, *Community-Based Health Care: A Legal and Policy Analysis*, 24 *Fordham Urb. L. J.* 235, 276-77 (1997).

Journal 1996 Describes the problem of lack of access to medical care by the indigent. Recognizes the commitment of the medical profession to providing care for indigent patients. Observes that state initiatives that provide physicians tort immunity in exchange for volunteer service can improve access to care by the indigent. Quotes Fundamental Elements (6). References Opinion 9.065. Comment, *Statutory Immunity for Volunteer Physicians: A Vehicle for Reaffirmation of the Doctor's Beneficent Duties—Absent the Rights Talk*, 1 *Widener L. Symp. J.* 425, 448, 449 (1996).

9.07 Medical Testimony

As a citizen and as a professional with special training and experience, the physician has an ethical obligation to assist in the administration of justice. If a patient who has a legal claim requests a physician's assistance, the physician should furnish medical evidence, with the patient's consent, in order to secure the patient's legal rights.

Medical experts should have recent and substantive experience in the area in which they testify and should limit testimony to their sphere of medical expertise. Medical witnesses should be adequately prepared and should testify honestly and truthfully to the best of their medical knowledge.

The medical witness must not become an advocate or a partisan in the legal proceeding. The medical witness should be adequately prepared and should testify honestly and truthfully. The attorney for the party who calls the physician as a witness should be informed of all favorable and unfavorable information developed by the physician's evaluation of the case. It is unethical for a physician to accept compensation that is contingent upon the outcome of litigation. (II, IV, V, VII)

Issued June 1986.

Updated June 1996 based on the report "Ethical Guidelines for Medical Experts," adopted December 1995.

M.D. Pa. 1947 Motion for new trial in malpractice action following verdict for defendant-physicians. Patient had been treated surgically for tube-ovarian abscess, had profuse post-operative bleeding, and died of infection secondary to ruptured ectopic pregnancy. Plaintiff moved for a new trial on grounds that an officer of a local medical society persuaded plaintiff's expert not to testify. Although it denied the motion on other grounds, the court criticized the officer's conduct, noting that it was contrary to Principles Ch. 1, Sec. 7 (1947) [now Opinion 9.07], but refused to impute the impropriety to the defendants. *McHugh v. Audet, 72 F. Supp. 394, 404.*

Cal. App. 1956 Physician-petitioner sought mandamus against local medical association whose bylaws provided for the expulsion of any member who violated the Principles. Petitioner had been expelled under the provision and the expulsion was affirmed by the American Medical Association's Judicial Council. The initial grounds for expulsion was alleged violation of Principles, Ch. III, Art. IV, Sec. 4 (1947) [now Opinions 9.04 and 9.07] for disparaging statements regarding another physician in a report used in judicial proceedings. In holding that application of the provision to petitioner was contrary to public policy, the court noted that the physician's statements had been made at the request of a civil litigant and enjoyed a statutory testimonial privilege. Further, the court found that the American Medical Association's right to formulate ethical principles did not extend to defining the duties of witnesses. Expulsion was also based on petitioner's critical comments about other physicians overheard by their patients in violation of Principles, Ch. III, Art. IV, Sec. 1 (1947) [now Principle II and Opinion 9.04]. The court found application of this Principle under the circumstances reasonable and not contrary to public policy. *Bernstein v. Alameda-Contra Costa Medical Ass'n, 139 Cal. App. 2d 241, 293 P.2d 862, 863, 863 nn.1, 2, 865 nn.4, 6, 866, 866 n.8, 867.*

N. J. 1995 Plaintiffs sued physician and manufacturer claiming that DPT shot administered to their daughter caused her to suffer seizures. Plaintiffs consulted pediatric neurologists, none of whom found a connection between the DPT vaccine and seizures. Court concluded that the videotaped depositions of two of the neurologists could be introduced by defendants because plaintiffs had waived all patient-physician privileges on this issue by bringing suit and because the neurologists did not examine the child in anticipation of litigation. The court cited Opinion 9.07 to support view that physicians have an obligation to assist in the administration of justice. *Stigliano v. Connaught Labs., Inc., 140 N.J. 305, 658 A.2d 715, 720-21.*

Wash. 1994 In a medical malpractice action against her former physician, plaintiff waived her physician-patient privilege with all physicians who had provided her care or treatment. In an ex parte interview, plaintiff's treating physician opined that defendant's conduct was not negligent. The defense listed the treating physician as an expert witness and plaintiff objected. The court concluded that waiver of the physician-patient privilege extends to all knowledge of the plaintiff's physicians. In holding that a patient cannot insist on physician confidentiality after bringing a civil proceeding, the court quoted Opinion 9.07. *Carson v. Fine, 123 Wash. 2d 206, 867 P.2d 610, 618.*

Journal 2003 Uses public policy arguments to support a preponderance standard for medical license revocations in situations involving false testimony by a medical expert witness. Concludes that medical licensing boards can more effectively protect the public by using a preponderance standard. Quotes Principles II, III, and IV, and Opinions 1.02 and 9.07. Widmer, *South Dakota Should Follow Public Policy and Switch to the Preponderance Standard for Medical License Revocation After In Re the Medical License of Dr. Reuben Setliff, M.D., 48 S.D. L. Rev. 388, 396-97, 402 (2003).*

Journal 2002 Examines the role and responsibilities of forensic bioethicists. Concludes that a professional code of conduct and other internal guidelines are needed to ensure professionalism in forensic bioethics. Quotes Opinion 9.07. Spielman, *Professionalism in Forensic Bioethics, 30 J.L. Med. & Ethics 420, 425, 427, 436 (2002).*

Journal 2000 Considers the rules governing expert testimony. Explores professional ethical standards affecting expert witnesses and concludes that codes of ethics have not succeeded in eliminating biased expert testimony. Recommends creation of an organization to assist courts in obtaining reliable expert witness testimony. Quotes Principle III and Opinion 6.01. Cites Principles I, II, and V and Opinions 1.02 and 9.07. Murphy, *Expert Witnesses at Trial: Where are the Ethics? 14 Geo. J. Legal Ethics 217, 231-32 (2000).*

Journal 1999 Describes historical and present views regarding medical diagnosis. Discusses pressures physicians face that may affect the diagnostic process. Suggests that legal institutions can reduce these pressures, which will enhance the physician-patient therapeutic relationship. Quotes Principle II and Opinion 9.07. Noah, *Pigeonholing Illness: Medical Diagnosis as a Legal Construct, 50 Hastings L. J. 241, 301, 302 (1999).*

Journal 1999 Discusses the impact *Daubert v. Merrell Dow Pharmaceuticals, Inc.* has had on scientific expert testimony. Explains that the scientific approach of dealing with bias may be inappropriate for maintaining scientific objectivity in litigation. Provides a strategy to deal with conflicts of interest in this context. Quotes Opinions 9.07. Cites Opinion 8.061. Patterson, *Conflicts of Interest in Scientific Expert Testimony, 40 Wm. & Mary L. Rev. 1313, 1330, 1332, 1335, 1371 (1999).*

Journal 1999 Discusses the need for physicians to advocate on behalf of patients' rights in the context of health care delivery. Evaluates the nature and scope of the physician's role as advocate, noting that physicians cannot be expected to engage in attorney-like advocacy. Quotes Principles IV and VI, Fundamental Elements (2), (4), and (6) [now Opinion 10.01], Patient Responsibilities 5 [now Opinion 10.02], and Opinions 2.03, 2.07, 2.09, 2.16, 2.19, 3.06, 4.01, 4.04, 6.01, 7.02, 8.02, 8.03, 8.13, 8.132, 9.06, 9.07, and 9.131. Cites Opinions 5.05, 5.09, 7.01, 8.135, and 9.02. Sage, *Physicians as Advocates, 35 Hous. L. Rev. 1529, 1537, 1541, 1542, 1552-53, 1554, 1556, 1557, 1559, 1561-62, 1564, 1571, 1574, 1576, 1580 (1999).*

Journal 1998 Examines mechanisms of oversight for expert witness testimony by medical, legal, legislative, and regulatory agencies. Points out that the amount of malpractice litigation will increase the need for medical expert witnesses. Concludes that improvements in this context must uphold principles of due process and be acceptable to the medical and legal communities. Cites Opinions 6.01, 8.04, and 9.07. McAbee, *Improper Expert Medical Testimony: Existing and Proposed Mechanisms of Oversight,* 19 J. Legal Med. 257, 265 (1998).

Journal 1997 Reports on a study of physician attitudes regarding expert witnesses. Notes that a majority of physicians believe that medical expert testimony should be subject to peer review and, when appropriate, medical licensing board discipline. Quotes Principles II and VI, and Opinion 9.07. Eitel, Hegeman, & Evans, *Medicine on Trial: Physicians' Attitudes about Expert Medical Witnesses,* 18 J. Legal Med. 345, 355, 358 (1997).

Journal 1997 Discusses the practice of ex parte communications between treating physicians and their patients' legal adversaries without informing the patient or obtaining consent. Examines harms that may occur in these situations. Argues that Oklahoma needs to prohibit treating physicians from communicating ex parte with their patients' legal adversaries. Quotes Opinions 5.05, 5.07, 5.08, 8.02, 8.03, and 9.07. Cites Opinion 7.02. McNaughton & McNaughton, *Divided Loyalty: The Dilemma of the Treating Physician Advocate,* 22 Okla. City U. L. Rev. 1051, 1052, 1054, 1056, 1058, 1059, 1062 (1997).

Journal 1994 Establishes guidelines for members of the American Academy of Pediatrics who are expert witnesses in medical liability cases. Emphasizes knowledge of the area of medicine involved, impartial testimony, evaluations based on generally accepted standards, and the duty to distinguish between malpractice and maloccurrence. Quotes Opinion 9.07. Cohn, Berger, Holzman, Lockhart, Reuben, Robertson, & Selbst, *Guidelines for Expert Witness Testimony in Medical Liability Cases,* 94 Pediatrics 755, 756 (1994).

Journal 1993 Discusses controversies surrounding how medical-legal consulting services and expert witnesses may be compensated. Examines relevant ethical guidelines in evaluating whether it is acceptable for a physician to be paid a flat fee for expert services rendered on behalf of a consulting business that receives a contingent fee. Quotes Opinion 9.07. Devlin, *Medical-Legal Consulting Services and Expert Witnesses: Payment Controversies,* 9 Medical Practice Management 141 (Nov./Dec. 1993).

Journal 1990 Considers the proper role of the expert witness in the realm of toxic tort litigation. Examines evidentiary rules regarding the admission of scientific evidence and considers various ways to solve testimonial problems. Quotes Opinion 9.07. Bernstein, *Out of the Frying Pan and Into the Fire: The Expert Witness Problem in Toxic Tort Litigation,* 10 Rev. Litigation 117, 143 (1990).

Journal 1990 Examines conflicting court decisions that have addressed the appropriateness of medical-legal consulting services and their use of contingent fee arrangements. Concludes by discussing the need for a less troublesome solution to the problems plaintiffs face in malpractice and personal injury cases. Quotes Opinion 6.01. Cites Opinions 6.12 (1989) [now Opinion 6.05] and 9.07. Dillon, *Contingent Fees and Medical-Legal Consulting Services: Economical or Unethical?,* 11 J. Legal Med. 93, 101, 111 (1990).

9.08   New Medical Procedures

In the ethical tradition expressed by Hippocrates and continuously affirmed thereafter, the role of the physician has been that of a healer who serves patients, a teacher who imparts knowledge of skills and techniques to colleagues, and a student who constantly seeks to keep abreast of new medical knowledge.

Physicians have an obligation to share their knowledge and skills and to report the results of clinical and laboratory research. Both positive and negative studies should be included even though they may not support the author's hypothesis. This tradition enhances patient care, leads to the early evaluation of new technologies, and permits the rapid dissemination of improved techniques.

The intentional withholding of new medical knowledge, skills, and techniques from colleagues for reasons of personal gain is detrimental to the medical profession and to society and is to be condemned.

Prompt presentation before scientific organizations and timely publication of clinical and laboratory research in scientific journals are essential elements in the foundation of good medical care. (I, II, V, VII)

Issued December 1984.

Updated June 1994.

Journal 2002 Evaluates the application of biomedical knowledge in clinical practice. Concludes that serious inadequacies exist in the current practice of evidence-based medicine. Quotes Principle V and Opinion 9.08. References Opinion 9.095. Noah, *Medicine's Epistemology: Mapping the Haphazard Diffusion of Knowledge in the Biomedical Community*, 44 Ariz. L. Rev. 373, 404, 447, 448 (2002).

Journal 2000 Discusses patent law and policy. Examines whether or not those who practice medicine should be excused from patent laws because of the conflict that medical procedure patents create with respect to the practice of medicine. Concludes that Congress should repeal section 287(c) of the Patent Act. Quotes Principle V and Opinions 9.08 and 9.09. Cites Opinion 8.03. References Opinion 10.01. Ho, *Patents, Patients, and Public Policy: An Incomplete Intersection at 35 U.S.C. § 287(c)*, 33 U.C. Davis L. Rev. 601, 603, 623, 624, 625, 631 (2000).

Journal 2000 Discusses the issues affecting the patentability of surgical procedures. Notes the ethical considerations involved in patenting surgical procedures versus surgical devices. Suggests each patent regime should strike a balance by weighing all the ethical factors considered important to society. Quotes Opinion 9.09. References Opinion 9.08 and Opinion 9.095. Martin, *Patentability of Methods of Medical Treatment: A Comparative Study*, 82 J. Pat. & Trademark Off. Soc'y 381, 383-84, 388, 423 (2000).

Journal 1999 Discusses congressional amendment of the United States patent code, which relieved health care providers from liability for medical procedure patent infringement. Explores the debate surrounding medical procedure patents and concludes that the enforcability of such patents should be reevaluated. Quotes Opinions 9.08 and 9.09. Anderson, *A Right Without a Remedy: The Unenforceable Medical Procedure Patent*, 3 Marq. Intell. Prop. L. Rev. 117, 132, 140 (1999).

Journal 1999 Describes historical and ethical considerations regarding medical patents. Points out that patenting medical procedures adversely affects the reputation of physicians in the eyes of the public. Argues that new laws need to be enacted to prevent abuse of the medical patent system. Quotes Opinion 9.08. Packer, *Ethics and Medical Patents*, 117 Arch. Ophthalmol. 824, 825 (1999).

Journal 1998 Rejects arguments to ban or permit unrestricted patenting of medical and surgical procedures. Explores arguments for and against patenting of medical and surgical procedures. Proposes a compromise position. Quotes Opinions 9.08 and 9.095. Wear, Coles, Szczygiel, McEvoy, & Pegels, *Patenting Medical and Surgical Techniques: An Ethical-Legal Analysis*, 23 J. Med. Phil. 75, 76, 87 (1998).

Journal 1997 Explores the debate enveloping the patenting of medical procedures. Examines the beneficial and detrimental aspects of a ban on medical patents and pertinent ethical and economical factors. Suggests that allowing patents exacts too great a toll on society and science. Quotes Opinion 9.08. References Opinion 9.095. Judge, *Issues Surrounding the Patenting of Medical Procedures*, 13 Santa Clara Computer & High Tech. L. J. 181, 202-03 (1997).

Journal 1997 Examines the controversy surrounding the patenting of medical procedures. Concludes that patenting medical procedures has a negative effect on the physician-patient relationship and the medical profession. Quotes Opinion 9.095. References Opinions 9.08 and 9.09. Note, *Patenting Medical Procedures: A Search for a Compromise Between Ethics and Economics*, 18 Cardozo L. Rev. 1527, 1544, 1547, 1554 (1997).

Journal 1996 Examines the current status of medical procedure patents and discusses the statutory and case law requirements for obtaining a patent. Considers the ethical implications of patenting medical procedures. Argues against a legislative ban on such patents. Quotes Opinions 9.08, 9.09, and 9.095. Garris, *The Case for Patenting Medical Procedures*, XXII Am. J. Law & Med. 85, 93, 94-95 (1996).

Journal 1996 Explores the current rules for patenting medical procedures. Discusses the AMA's position that medical procedure patents are unethical. Concludes that a failure to grant patents will deter the development of new medical procedures. Erroneously quotes Opinion 9.08 (see Opinion 9.095). Lafferty, *Statutory and Ethical Barriers in the Patenting of Medical and Surgical Procedures*, 29 J. Marshall L. Rev. 891, 912 (1996).

Journal 1995 Explores the debates and commentaries regarding patenting medical instruments and processes. Concludes that current patent law fails to address the ethical concerns of physicians and their patients. Quotes Principles of Medical Ethics §10 (1971) [now Principle VII] and Principle §2 (1971) [now Opinion 9.095] and Opinions 9.08 and 9.09. Reisman, *Physicians and Surgeons as Inventors: Reconciling Medical Process Patents and Medical Ethics*, 10 High Tech. L. J. 355, 356, 368-70, 385 (1995).

9.09 Patent for Surgical or Diagnostic Instrument

A physician may patent a surgical or diagnostic instrument he or she has discovered or developed. The laws governing patents are based on the sound doctrine that one is entitled to protect one's discovery. (V, VII)

Issued prior to April 1977.

Journal 2000 Discusses patent law and policy. Examines whether or not those who practice medicine should be excused from patent laws because of the conflict that medical procedure patents create with respect to the practice of medicine. Concludes that Congress should repeal section 287(c) of the Patent Act. Quotes Principle V and Opinions 9.08 and 9.09. Cites Opinion 8.03. References Opinion 10.01. Ho, *Patents, Patients, and Public Policy: An Incomplete Intersection at 35 U.S.C. § 287(c)*, 33 U.C. Davis L. Rev. 601, 603, 623, 624, 625, 631 (2000).

Journal 2000 Discusses the issues affecting the patentability of surgical procedures. Notes the ethical considerations involved in patenting surgical procedures versus surgical devices. Suggests each patent regime should strike a balance by weighing all the ethical factors considered important to society. Quotes Opinion 9.09. References Opinion 9.08 and Opinion 9.095. Martin, *Patentability of Methods of Medical Treatment: A Comparative Study*, 82 J. Pat. & Trademark Off. Soc'y 381, 383-84, 388, 423 (2000).

Journal 1999 Discusses congressional amendment of the United States patent code, which relieved health care providers from liability for medical procedure patent infringement. Explores the debate surrounding medical procedure patents and concludes that the enforcability of such patents should be reevaluated. Quotes Opinions 9.08 and 9.09. Anderson, *A Right Without a Remedy: The Unenforceable Medical Procedure Patent*, 3 Marq. Intell. Prop. L. Rev. 117, 132, 140 (1999).

Journal 1997 Examines the controversy surrounding the patenting of medical procedures. Concludes that patenting medical procedures has a negative effect on the physician-patient relationship and the medical profession. Quotes Opinion 9.095. References Opinions 9.08 and 9.09. Note, *Patenting Medical Procedures: A Search for a Compromise Between Ethics and Economics*, 18 Cardozo L. Rev. 1527, 1544, 1547, 1554 (1997).

Journal 1996 Examines the current status of medical procedure patents and discusses the statutory and case law requirements for obtaining a patent. Considers the ethical implications of patenting medical procedures. Argues against a legislative ban on such patents. Quotes Opinions 9.08, 9.09, and 9.095. Garris, *The Case for Patenting Medical Procedures*, XXII Am. J. Law & Med. 85, 93, 94-95 (1996).

Journal 1995 Explores the debates and commentaries regarding patenting medical instruments and processes. Concludes that current patent law fails to address the ethical concerns of physicians and their patients. Quotes Principles of Medical Ethic §10 (1971) [now Principle VII] and Principle §2 (1971) [now Opinion 9.095] and Opinions 9.08 and 9.09. Reisman, *Physicians and Surgeons as Inventors: Reconciling Medical Process Patents and Medical Ethics*, 10 High Tech. L. J. 355, 356, 368-70, 385 (1995).

Journal 1990 Explains how medical patents have developed into widely accepted legal instruments that receive broad respect from the courts. Questions the lack of Congressional expansion of patent protection in the field of biotechnology and suggests that Congress should begin expanding protection in this area. References Opinion 9.09. Noonan, *Patenting Medical Technology*, 11 J. Legal Med. 263, 268 (1990).

9.095 Patenting of Medical Procedures

A physician has the ethical responsibility not only to learn from but also to contribute to the total store of scientific knowledge when possible. Physicians should strive to advance medical science and make their advances known to patients, colleagues, and the public. This obligation provides not merely incentive but imperative to innovate and share the ensuing advances. The patenting of medical procedures poses substantial risks to the effective practice of medicine by limiting the availability of new procedures to patients and should be condemned on this basis. Accordingly, it is unethical for physicians to seek, secure, or enforce patents on medical procedures. (V, VII)

Issued June 1996 based on the report "Ethical Issues in the Patenting of Medical Procedures," adopted June 1995 (*Food & Drug L. J.* 1998; 53: 341-57).

Journal 2003 Examines financial conflicts of interest that arise in the context of university-based human research. Concludes that federal regulations should replace traditional models of self-regulation to meaningfully protect human subjects. References Opinion 9.095. Jordan, *Financial Conflicts of Interest in Human Subjects Research: Proposals for a More Effective Regulatory Scheme*, 60 Wash. & Lee L. Rev. 15, 23 (2003).

Journal 2002 Examines various concerns regarding gene patents and discusses other policy alternatives. Concludes that policymakers are exploring alternatives to ensure that gene patents will benefit society. Quotes Opinion 2.08. Cites Opinion 9.095. Andrews, *The Gene Patent Dilemma: Balancing Commercial Incentives with Health Needs*, 2 Hous. J. Health L. & Pol'y 65, 74, 104 (2002).

Journal 2002 Evaluates the application of biomedical knowledge in clinical practice. Concludes that serious inadequacies exist in the current practice of evidence-based medicine. Quotes Principle V and Opinion 9.08. References Opinion 9.095. Noah, *Medicine's Epistemology: Mapping the Haphazard Diffusion of Knowledge in the Biomedical Community*, 44 Ariz. L. Rev. 373, 404, 447, 448 (2002).

Journal 2000 Discusses the issues affecting the patentability of surgical procedures. Notes the ethical considerations involved in patenting surgical procedures versus surgical devices. Suggests each patent regime should strike a balance by weighing all the ethical factors considered important to society. Quotes Opinion 9.09. References Opinion 9.08 and Opinion 9.095. Martin, *Patentability of Methods of Medical Treatment: A Comparative Study*, 82 J. Pat. & Trademark Off. Soc'y 381, 383-84, 388, 423 (2000).

Journal 1998 Rejects arguments to ban or permit unrestricted patenting of medical and surgical procedures. Explores arguments for and against patenting of medical and surgical procedures. Proposes a compromise position. Quotes Opinions 9.08 and 9.095. Wear, Coles, Szczygiel, McEvoy, & Pegels, *Patenting Medical and Surgical Techniques: An Ethical-Legal Analysis*, 23 J. Med. Phil. 75, 76, 87 (1998).

Journal 1997 Explores the debate enveloping the patenting of medical procedures. Examines the beneficial and detrimental aspects of a ban on medical patents and pertinent ethical and economical factors. Suggests that allowing patents exacts too great a toll on society and science. Quotes Opinion 9.08. References Opinion 9.095. Judge, *Issues Surrounding the Patenting of Medical Procedures*, 13 Santa Clara Computer & High Tech. L. J. 181, 202-03 (1997).

Journal 1997 Considers the issues surrounding medical procedure patents. Reviews the adoption of federal legislation granting patent infringement immunity to physicians while performing medical or surgical procedures. Discusses the medical community's position favoring immunity. Concludes that such a law sets a dangerous precedent. References Opinion 9.095. Lee, *35 U.S.C. § 287(C)–The Physician Immunity Statute*, 79 J. Pat. & Trademark Off. Soc'y 701, 702-04 (1997).

Journal 1997 Examines the controversy surrounding the patenting of medical procedures. Concludes that patenting medical procedures has a negative effect on the physician-patient relationship and the medical profession. Quotes Opinion 9.095. References Opinions 9.08 and 9.09. Note, *Patenting Medical Procedures: A Search for a Compromise Between Ethics and Economics*, 18 *Cardozo L. Rev.* 1527, 1544, 1547, 1554 (1997).

Journal 1997 Discusses federal patent legislation that protects physicians from liability for patent infringements. Describes legal and medical opinions on the matter. Notes that the legislation was passed in response to concerns regarding health care costs and patients' interests. Proposes that Congress reconsider the legislation. References Opinion 9.095. Note, *The New Patent Infringement Liability Exception for Medical Procedures*, 23 *J. Legis.* 265, 268 (1997).

Journal 1996 Examines the current status of medical procedure patents and discusses the statutory and case law requirements for obtaining a patent. Considers the ethical implications of patenting medical procedures. Argues against a legislative ban on such patents. Quotes Opinions 9.08, 9.09, and 9.095. Garris, *The Case for Patenting Medical Procedures*, XXII *Am. J. Law & Med.* 85, 93, 94-95 (1996).

Journal 1996 Explores the current rules for patenting medical procedures. Discusses the AMA's position that medical procedure patents are unethical. Concludes that a failure to grant patents will deter the development of new medical procedures. Erroneously quotes Opinion 9.08 (see Opinion 9.095). Lafferty, *Statutory and Ethical Barriers in the Patenting of Medical and Surgical Procedures*, 29 *J. Marshall L. Rev.* 891, 912 (1996).

Journal 1996 Discusses possible effects of a 1996 legislative enactment that was designed to limit the remedies for infringements on patented medical activities. Describes the legislative history of this enactment and notes the AMA's position against patenting of medical and surgical procedures. References Opinion 9.095. Mossinghoff, *Remedies Under Patents on Medical and Surgical Procedures*, 78 *J. Pat. & Trademark Off. Soc'y* 789, 790 (1996).

Journal 1995 Explores the debates and commentaries regarding patenting medical instruments and processes. Concludes that current patent law fails to address the ethical concerns of physicians and their patients. Quotes Principles of Medical Ethics §10 (1971) [now Principle VII] and Principle §2 (1971) [now Opinion 9.095] and Opinions 9.08 and 9.09. Reisman, *Physicians and Surgeons as Inventors: Reconciling Medical Process Patents and Medical Ethics*, 10 *High Tech. L. J.* 355, 356, 368-70, 385 (1995).

9.10   Peer Review

Medical society ethics committees, hospital credentials and utilization committees, and other forms of peer review have been long established by organized medicine to scrutinize physicians' professional conduct. At least to some extent, each of these types of peer review can be said to impinge upon the absolute professional freedom of physicians. They are, nonetheless, recognized and accepted. They are necessary, and committees performing such work act ethically as long as principles of due process (Opinion 9.05, "Due Process") are observed. They balance the physician's right to exercise medical judgment freely with the obligation to do so wisely and temperately. (II, III, VII)

Issued prior to April 1977.

Updated June 1994.

9.11   The previous Opinion 9.11, "Physician Impairment," issued December 1986, was deleted in June 1994.

9.11 Ethics Committees in Health Care Institutions

The following guidelines have been developed to aid in the establishment and functioning of ethics committees in hospitals and other health care institutions that may choose to form such committees.

(1) Ethics committees in health care institutions should be educational and advisory in purpose. Generally, the function of the ethics committee should be to consider and assist in resolving unusual, complicated ethical problems involving issues that affect the care and treatment of patients within the health care institution. Recommendations of the ethics committee should impose no obligation for acceptance on the part of the institution, its governing board, medical staff, attending physician, or other persons. However, it should be expected that the recommendations of a dedicated ethics committee will receive serious consideration by decision makers.

(2) The size of the committee should be consistent with the needs of the institution but not so large as to be unwieldy. Committee members should be selected on the basis of their concern for the welfare of the sick and infirm, their interest in ethical matters, and their reputation in the community and among their peers for integrity and mature judgment. Experience as a member of hospital or medical society committees concerned with ethical conduct or quality assurance should be considered in selecting ethics committee members. Committee members should not have other responsibilities that are likely to prove incompatible with their duties as members of the ethics committee. Preferably, a majority of the committee should consist of physicians, nurses, and other health care providers. In hospitals, medical staff bylaws should delineate the functions of the committee, general qualifications for membership, and manner of selection of members, in accordance with these guidelines.

(3) The functions of the ethics committee should be confined exclusively to ethical matters. The *Code of Medical Ethics* of the American Medical Association is recommended for the guidance of ethics committees in making their own recommendations. The matters to be considered by the committee should consist of ethical subjects that a majority of its members may choose to discuss on its own initiative, matters referred to it by the executive committee of the organized medical staff or by the governing board of the institution, or appropriate requests from patients, families, or health care providers.

(4) In denominational health care institutions or those operated by religious orders, the recommendations of the ethics committee may be anticipated to be consistent with published religious tenets and principles. Where particular religious beliefs are to be taken into consideration in the committee's recommendations, this fact should be publicized to physicians, patients, and others concerned with the committee's recommendations.

(5) In its deliberations and communication of recommendations, the procedures followed by the ethics committee should comply with institutional and ethical policies for preserving the confidentiality of information regarding patients.

(6) Committee members should be prepared to meet on short notice and to render their recommendations in a timely and prompt fashion in accordance with the demands of the situation and the issues involved. (II, IV, VII)

Issued June 1994 based on the report "Guidelines for Ethics Committees in Health Care Institutions," adopted December 1984 (JAMA. 1985; 253: 2698-99).

Journal 2002 Discusses the role of clinical ethicists and their potential legal liability as a result of participating in case consultations. Concludes that clinical ethicists can limit their liability by acting primarily as mediators or facilitators. Quotes Opinion 9.11. Sontag, *Are Clinical Ethics Consultants in Danger? An Analysis of the Potential Legal Liability of Individual Clinical Ethicists, 151 U. Pa. L. Rev. 667, 679 (2002).*

9.115 Ethics Consultations

Ethics consultations may be called to clarify ethical issues without reference to a particular case, facilitate discussion of an ethical dilemma in a particular case, or resolve an ethical dispute. The consultation mechanism may be through an ethics committee, a subset of the committee, individual consultants, or consultation teams. The following guidelines are offered with respect to these services:

(1) All hospitals and other health care institutions should provide access to ethics consultation services. Health care facilities without ethics committees or consultation services should develop flexible, efficient mechanisms of ethics review that divide the burden of committee functioning among collaborating health care facilities.

(2) Institutions offering ethics consultation services must appreciate the complexity of the task, recognizing the potential for harm as well as benefit, and act responsibly. This includes true institutional support for the service.

(3) Ethics consultation services require a serious investment of time and effort by the individuals involved. Members should include either individuals with extensive formal training and experience in clinical ethics or individuals who have made a substantial commitment over several years to gain sufficient knowledge, skills, and understanding of the complexity of clinical ethics. A wide variety of background training is preferable, including such fields as philosophy, religion, medicine, and law.

(4) Explicit structural standards should be developed and consistently followed. These should include developing a clear description of the consultation service's role and determining which types of cases will be addressed, how the cases will be referred to the service, whether the service will provide recommendations or simply function as a forum for discussion, and whether recommendations are binding or advisory.

(5) Explicit procedural standards should be developed and consistently followed. These should include establishing who must be involved in the consultation process and how notification, informed consent, confidentiality and case write-ups will be handled.

(6) In general, patient and staff informed consent may be presumed for ethics consultation. However, patients and families should be given the opportunity, not to participate in discussions either formally, through the institu-

tional process, or informally.

(7) In those cases where the patient or family has chosen not to participate in the consultation process, the final recommendations of the consultant(s) should be tempered.

(8) In general, ethics consultation services, like social services, should be financed by the institution.

(9) A consultation service should be careful not to take on more than it can handle, ie, the complexity of the role should correspond to the level of sophistication of the service and the resources it has available. As a result, some services may offer only information and education, others a forum for discussion but not advice, others might serve a mediation role, and some might handle even administrative or organizational ethics issues. (IV, V)

Issued June 1998 based on the report "Ethics Consultations," adopted December 1997.

9.12 Patient-Physician Relationship: Respect for Law and Human Rights

The creation of the patient-physician relationship is contractual in nature. Generally, both the physician and the patient are free to enter into or decline the relationship. A physician may decline to undertake the care of a patient whose medical condition is not within the physician's current competence. However, physicians who offer their services to the public may not decline to accept patients because of race, color, religion, national origin, sexual orientation, or any other basis that would constitute invidious discrimination. Furthermore, physicians who are obligated under pre-existing contractual arrangements may not decline to accept patients as provided by those arrangements. (I, III, V, VI)

Issued July 1986.

Updated June 1994.

N.Y. Sup. 1993 Plaintiff brought malpractice action against attending physician, resident, and hospital alleging that they caused premature birth and cerebral palsy of twin daughters. Plaintiff, pregnant and complaining of abdominal pains, was admitted to hospital by attending physician. She was also examined by resident. Despite indication of polyhydramnios, an increase of amniotic fluid creating a risk of premature delivery, attending physician released plaintiff from hospital. Resident and hospital moved for summary judgment on grounds that neither had provided independent treatment for plaintiff. They also relied on the principle that if a hospital properly follows attending physician's orders, it cannot be held responsible for the physician's actions in caring for patients. The court affirmed denial of motion for summary judgment stating that a question of fact existed as to whether plaintiff's release from hospital was so contrary to normal practice that resident physician should have inquired into situation. Quoting Opinion 9.12, the dissent argued that the motion for summary judgment should be granted because the attending physician makes medical decisions regarding the patient and neither hospital nor its residents should interfere. *Somoza v. St. Vincent's Hosp. & Med. Ctr. of New York*, 192 A.D.2d 429, 596 N.Y.S.2d 789, 793.

Journal 2001 Discusses Internet auction technology and its application to health care services and products. Examines the medical industry's reaction to the emergence of surgery auction sites. Raises questions regarding the practice of online surgery auctions. Quotes Opinion 9.12. Caveney, *Going, Going, Gone … The Opportunities and Legal Pitfalls of Online Surgical Auctions*, 103 W. Va. L. Rev. 591, 607 (2001).

Journal 1999 Discusses potential conflicts between a criminal defense attorney's religious beliefs and representation of the client. Explores theories that would allow an attorney to put religious beliefs over the client's interest. Offers analogies within the physician-patient relationship. Concludes that a defense attorney is bound by duty and must set aside conflicting religious beliefs. Quotes Principle VI and Opinions 8.11, 9.06, and 9.12. Reza, *Religion and the Public Defender*, 26 Fordham Urb. L. J. 1051, 1062, 1063 (1999).

Journal 1998 Explores the increasing use of psychotherapy treatment via the Internet. Examines legal issues arising from Internet psychotherapy. Asserts that regulations need to be implemented to protect consumers. Quotes Opinion 9.12. Pergament, *Internet Psychotherapy: Current Status and Future Regulation*, 8 Health Matrix 233, 253 (1998).

Journal 1998 Discusses whether attorneys should be able to discriminate through the selection or handling of a client or potential client's case. Points out that standards for other professions prohibit discrimination. Concludes that attorneys should be prohibited from discriminating in selecting clients, but may use discretion regarding strategies to be used. Quotes Opinion 9.12. Stonefield, *Lawyer Discrimination Against Clients: Outright Rejection—No; Limitations on Issues and Arguments—Yes*, 20 W. New Eng. L. Rev. 103, 112 (1998).

Journal 1997 Compares past ethical opinions to current opinions and notes the differences. Comments on the forces that have changed medical ethics through the years. Notes differing theories on the future course of medical ethics. Quotes Fundamental Elements (Preamble) and Opinions 5.05, 5.057, 7.01, 8.12, 9.12, and 9.131. Cites Fundamental Elements (5) and Opinions 8.115 and 8.13. Buchanan, *Medical Ethics at the Millennium: A Brief Retrospective*, 26 Colo. Law. 141, 142, 143, 144, 145 (1997).

Journal 1997 Examines the evolution of the Indiana health care system. Discusses developments in Indiana jurisprudence regarding the physician-patient relationship. Explores various challenges facing the relationship and recognizes the need for legal rules to help address these challenges. Quotes Opinion 8.08. Cites Opinions 2.20, 9.06, and 9.12. Kinney & Selby, *History and Jurisprudence of the Physician-Patient Relationship in Indiana*, 30 Ind. L. Rev. 263, 269, 272, 276 (1997).

Journal 1995 Offers relevant historical perspectives and provides comprehensive ethical and legal discussion of physician-assisted suicide and euthanasia. Highlights important legislative developments, including the Oregon Death with Dignity Act, and analyzes significant judicial opinions. Quotes Principles III, IV, and VI and Opinions 2.21 and 9.12. Cites Opinions 2.20 and 8.11. Stone & Winslade, *Physician-Assisted Suicide and Euthanasia in the United States: Legal and Ethical Observations*, 16 J. Legal Med. 481, 483, 490, 497, 498, 499 (1995).

Journal 1994 Explores how the Americans with Disabilities Act has created, through federal civil rights mechanisms, a legal duty to treat HIV-infected patients. Discusses previous attempts to create a professional obligation to treat patients with AIDS. Quotes Principle VI and Opinion 9.131. Cites Opinion 9.12. Halevy & Brody, *Acquired Immunodeficiency Syndrome and the Americans with Disabilities Act: A Legal Duty to Treat*, 96 Am. J. Med. 282, 283, 284 (1994).

Journal 1993 Explores the traditional view that lawyers have unfettered discretion to select clients and New York's antidiscrimination disciplinary rule, statutes, and case law. Concludes that the legal profession should prohibit invidious or improper discrimination. Quotes Principle VI and Opinions 9.12 and 9.131. Begg, *Revoking the Lawyers' License to Discriminate in New York: The Demise of a Traditional Professional Prerogative*, 7 Geo. J. Legal Ethics 275, 298, 299 (1993).

Journal 1991 Considers the question of whether physicians should provide medical treatment to those who come to them for second opinions. Concludes that each physician must individually decide whether to treat these patients. Quotes Opinions 6.11, 9.06, and 9.12. Cites Opinion 9.02. Ile, *Should Physicians Treat Patients Who Seek Second Opinions?*, 266 JAMA 273, 274 (1991).

Journal 1991 Discusses the problem of noncompliant patients and whether a physician may deny treatment to these individuals. Concludes that physicians are not relieved of their duty to treat noncompliant patients, especially because these patients may not be able to adequately control their behavior. Cites Principle VI and Opinion 9.12. Orentlicher, *Denying Treatment to the Noncompliant Patient*, 265 JAMA 1579, 1581 (1991).

Journal 1988 Observes that the view of medicine as a profession committed to the sick conflicts with the apparent position of the AMA, that a physician is free to choose his or her patients. (See Principle VI). Concludes that physicians have a duty to treat AIDS patients and must be ready to assume certain levels of risk in fulfilling the duty. References Opinion 9.12. Emanuel, *Do Physicians Have an Obligation to Treat Patients With AIDS?*, 318 New Eng. J. Med. 1686, 1687 (1988).

Journal 1988 Discusses the question of whether health professionals are obligated to subject themselves to the risks that attend treating patients with communicable diseases, particularly AIDS. Examines the ethical pronouncements and codes of the nursing and medical professions in this respect, noting that the most recent statements of professional values imply the existence of an obligation to treat HIV-infectious patients. Quotes Opinion 8.10 (1986) [now Opinion 8.11] and Principle VI. Cites Opinion 9.11 (1986) [now Opinion 9.12]. Freedman, *Health Professions, Codes, and the Right to Refuse to Treat HIV-Infectious Patients*, 18 Hastings Center Rep. 20 (Supp.), 23, 24 (April/May 1988).

9.121 Racial Disparities in Health Care

Disparities in medical care based on immutable characteristics such as race must be avoided. Whether such disparities in health care are caused by treatment decisions, differences in income and education, sociocultural factors, or failures by the medical profession, they are unjustifiable and must be eliminated. Physicians should examine their own practices to ensure that racial prejudice does not affect clinical judgment in medical care. (I, IV)

Issued March 1992 based on the report "Black-White Disparities in Health Care," adopted December 1989 (JAMA. 1990; 263: 2344-46).

Updated June 1994.

Journal 2003 Addresses physician bias in health care. Concludes that existing legal responses to biased medical decisions are inadequate and further development is needed. Quotes Opinions 9.121 and 9.122. Crossley, *Infected Judgment: Legal Responses to Physician Bias*, 48 Vill. L. Rev. 195, 239, 297 (2003).

Journal 2002 Considers how to evaluate the performance of Medicare Managed Care Plans in serving ethnic minorities. Concludes that additional monitoring could help reduce existing disparities. References Opinion 9.121. Langwell & Moser, *Strategies for Medicare Health Plans Serving Racial and Ethnic Minorities*, 23 Health Care Financing Rev. 131, 134, 146 (2002).

Journal 2002 Examines how implicit cognitive biases of physicians may contribute to racial disparities in medical care. Considers legal safeguards that may address these disparities. Concludes that Congress must take affirmative steps to help remedy this problem. References Opinion 9.121. Shin, *Redressing Wounds: Finding a Legal Framework to Remedy Racial Disparities in Medical Care*, 90 Cal. L. Rev. 2047, 2056, 2057, 2100 (2002).

Journal 2001 Addresses racial and ethnic disparities in medical care. Concludes that the law plays a vital role in ending racial disparities in medical treatment through the enforcement of civil rights legislation. Quotes Opinion 9.121. Bowser, *Eliminating Racial and Ethnic Disparities in Medical Care*, 30 Brief 24, 25 (Summer 2001).

Journal 2001 Provides a comprehensive theoretical approach and policy recommendations to address racial profiling in health care. Concludes that medicine needs to rethink research and treatment in light of disparities based on race. Quotes Opinion 9.121. Bowser, *Racial Profiling in Health Care: An Institutional Analysis of Medical Treatment Disparities*, 7 Mich. J. Race & L. 79, 119 (2001).

Journal 2001 Explains the design and potential benefits of result-based compensation arrangements for health care. Concludes that a more reliable and efficient health care delivery system is fostered by such arrangements. Quotes Opinion 6.01. References Opinions 9.121 and 9.122. Hyman & Silver, *You Get What You Pay For: Result-Based Compensation for Health Care*, 58 Wash. & Lee L. Rev. 1427, 1459, 1460, 1461, 1481-82 (2001).

Journal 2001 Examines racial and ethic inequalities in health care. Explains civil rights enforcement strategies and limitations. Concludes by proposing a comprehensive systematic approach, including regulatory and market-based incentives, to decrease racial and ethnic disparities in health care. References Opinion 9.121. Watson, *Race, Ethnicity and Quality of Care: Inequalities and Incentives*, 27 Am. J. L. & Med. 203, 206 (2001).

Journal 1997 Considers the use of race and gender to assess health care status and medical needs. Discusses the lack of consideration that Asian American women receive in the health care agenda. Proposes an examination of factors such as race, gender, and class status to provide a better understanding of the health needs of this group. References Opinions 9.121 and 9.122. Ikemoto, *The Fuzzy Logic of Race and Gender in the Mismeasure of Asian American Women's Health Needs*, 65 U. Cin. L. Rev. 799, 800, 804, 810 (1997).

Journal 1994 Observes that health care reform proposals present significant challenges to the role and ethics of attending physicians. Emphasizes that reform proposals must set forth the role envisioned for physicians and must articulate an acceptable ethical framework within which physicians may fulfill that role. Quotes Opinions 4.04, 9.121, and 9.122. Cites Opinions 2.03, 2.09, 5.01, and 8.03. Wolf, *Health Care Reform and the Future of Physician Ethics*, 24 Hastings Center Rep. 28, 32, 40 (March/April 1994).

Journal 1993 Presents findings by the Council on Graduate Medical Education regarding access to health care. Recommends that more emphasis be placed on primary care, the physician workforce be redistributed to increase the number of physicians in rural and inner city areas, and that there be more racial and ethnic diversity in the medical profession. References Opinion 9.121. Rivo & Satcher, *Improving Access to Health Care Through Physician Workforce Reform*, 270 JAMA 1074, 1075 (1993).

Journal 1992 Discusses the impact of physicians' values on end-of-life decision making for patients. Examines how and why physician values may become dominant. References Opinions 2.20, 2.22, and 9.121. Orentlicher, *The Illusion of Patient Choice in End-Of-Life Decisions*, 267 JAMA 2101, 2102 (1992).

Journal 1991 Describes the attributes of women who self-report pelvic inflammatory disease (PID). Presents the results of a study that examined these attributes, noting that risk factors were consistent with prior studies. References Opinion 9.121. Aral, Mosher, & Cates, *Self-Reported Pelvic Inflammatory Disease in the United States, 1988*, 266 JAMA 2570, 2573 (1991).

Journal 1991 Compares the health conditions of blacks in South Africa with those in the United States. Concludes that policy changes to address the health problems of South African blacks are also needed in this country. References Opinion 9.121. Brooks, Smith, & Anderson, *Medical Apartheid: An American Perspective*, 266 JAMA 2746, 2748 (1991).

Journal 1991 Discusses the lack of health care among the poor and uninsured. Notes the traditional role of physician as advocate for the poor and prescribes a method by which physicians may act as spokespersons for underserved populations. References Opinion 9.121. Kleinman, *Health Care in Crisis: A Proposed Role for the Individual Physician as Advocate*, 265 JAMA 1991 (1991).

9.122 Gender Disparities in Health Care

A patient's gender plays an appropriate role in medical decision making when biological differences between the sexes are considered. However, some data suggest that gender bias may be playing a role in medical decision making. Social attitudes, including stereotypes, prejudices, and other evaluations based on gender role expectations, may play themselves out in a variety of subtle ways. Physicians must ensure that gender is not used inappropriately as a consideration in clinical decision making. Physicians should examine their practices and attitudes for influence of social or cultural biases which could be inadvertently affecting the delivery of medical care.

Research on health problems that affect both genders should include male and female subjects, and results of medical research done solely on males should not be generalized to females without evidence that results apply to both sexes. Medicine and society in general should ensure that resources for medical research should be distributed in a manner which promotes the health of both sexes to the greatest extent possible. (I, IV)

Issued March 1992 based on the report "Gender Disparities in Clinical Decision Making," adopted December 1990 (JAMA. 1991; 266: 559-62).

Updated June 1994.

Journal 2003 Addresses physician bias in health care. Concludes that existing legal responses to biased medical decisions are inadequate and further development is needed. Quotes Opinions 9.121 and 9.122. Crossley, *Infected Judgment: Legal Responses to Physician Bias*, 48 Vill. L. Rev. 195, 239, 297 (2003).

Journal 2002 Analyzes gender disparities in the context of access to health care, insurance, treatment, and outcomes. Concludes that women are likely to encounter an unconscious bias in treatment or in the design of health care systems. References Opinion 9.122. Bobinski & Epps, *Women, Poverty, Access to Health Care, and the Perils of Symbolic Reform*, 5 J. Gender, Race & Just. 233, 238 (2002).

Journal 2001 Explains the design and potential benefits of result-based compensation arrangements for health care. Concludes that a more reliable and efficient health care delivery system is fostered by such arrangements. Quotes Opinion 6.01. References Opinions 9.121 and 9.122. Hyman & Silver, *You Get What You Pay For: Result-Based Compensation for Health Care*, 58 Wash. & Lee L. Rev. 1427, 1459, 1460, 1461, 1481-82 (2001).

Journal 2001 Examines the affects of sex and race on asthma care. Concludes that, in a group of well-educated and insured asthma patients, consistency of care varied in relationship to a patient's race and sex. References Opinion 9.122. Krishnan, Diette, Skinner, Clark, Steinwachs, & Wu, *Race and Sex Differences in Consistency of Care With National Asthma Guidelines in Managed Care Organizations*, 161 Arch. Intern. Med. 1660, 1660 (2001).

Journal 2001 Examines the woman-child stereotype and its connection to feminist goals. Concludes that the stereotype presents serious social and legal implications. References Opinion 9.122. Preston, *Baby Spice: Lost Between Feminine and Feminist*, 9 Am. U. J. Gender Soc. Pol'y & L. 541, 590 (2001).

Journal 2000 Describes mandatory prelitigation panels under the Utah Health Care Malpractice Act. Considers constitutional challenges to such panels. Concludes that prelitigation panels are an impediment to resolution of medical malpractice claims and should be eliminated. References Opinion 9.122. Brann, *Utah's Medical Malpractice Prelitigation Panel: Exploring State Constitutional Arguments Against a Nonbinding Inadmissible Procedure*, 2000 Utah L. Rev. 359, 399-400 (2000).

Journal 2000 Discusses racial disparities in health care. Supports development of national strategies to eliminate racial inequities in medical care. Concludes that strong political leadership and effective interdisciplinary research are needed to achieve this important goal. References Opinion 9.122. Williams & Rucker, *Understanding and Addressing Racial Disparities in Health Care*, 21 Health Care Fin. Rev. 75, 88 (2000).

Journal 1999 Discusses a study that evaluated the impact of gender differences on outcomes of hospitalized patients treated for infection. Concludes that gender may not be predictive of mortality. References Opinion 9.122. Crabtree, Pelletier, Gleason, Pruett, & Sawyer, *Gender-Dependent Differences in Outcome after the Treatment of Infection in Hospitalized Patients*, 282 JAMA 2143, 2148 (1999).

Journal 1997 Considers the use of race and gender to assess health care status and medical needs. Discusses the lack of consideration that Asian American women receive in the health care agenda. Proposes an examination of factors such as race, gender, and class status to provide a better understanding of the health needs of this group. References Opinions 9.121 and 9.122. Ikemoto, *The Fuzzy Logic of Race and Gender in the Mismeasure of Asian American Women's Health Needs*, 65 U. Cin. L. Rev. 799, 800, 804, 810 (1997).

Journal 1996 Considers the impact the doctrine of informed consent may have on the rate at which hysterectomy operations are performed. Discusses how stereotypes affect the quality of medical treatment women receive. Focuses on how informed consent may benefit the health and autonomy of women. References Opinion 9.122. Napoli, *The Doctrine of Informed Consent and Women: The Achievement of Equal Value and Equal Exercise of Autonomy*, 4 J. Gender & L. 335, 336 (1996).

Journal 1994 Observes that health care reform proposals present significant challenges to the role and ethics of attending physicians. Emphasizes that reform proposals must set forth the role envisioned for physicians and must articulate an acceptable ethical framework within which physicians may fulfill that role. Quotes Opinions 4.04, 9.121, and 9.122. Cites Opinions 2.03, 2.09, 5.01, and 8.03. Wolf, *Health Care Reform and the Future of Physician Ethics*, 24 Hastings Center Rep. 28, 32, 40 (March/April 1994).

Journal 1993 Discusses the underrepresentation of women in clinical trials and its medical relevance. Examines the extent to which women are underrepresented. Considers barriers to their participation and proposes ways to include women in clinical investigations. References Opinion 9.122. Bennett, *Inclusion of Women in Clinical Trials—Policies for Population Subgroups*, 329 New Eng. J. Med. 288, 289 (1993).

Journal 1993 Explains how the role of women in clinical trials has evolved historically. Examines specific current concerns related to women's involvement in clinical studies and how these concerns might be resolved. References Opinion 9.122. Merkatz, *Women in Clinical Trials: An Introduction*, 48 Food & Drug L. J. 161, 163 (1993).

Journal 1992 Investigates the exclusion of women and minorities from medical research study groups. Concludes that this problem illustrates the extent to which bias is still present in contemporary medicine and science. References Opinion 9.122. Dresser, *Wanted: Single, White Male for Medical Research*, 22 Hastings Center Rep. 24, 28 (Jan./Feb. 1992).

Journal 1992 Presents the results of a gender study analyzing the differences in quality of care for elderly patients hospitalized with one of four diseases. Concludes that study results are positive but notes that concerns regarding gender discrimination are not entirely eliminated. References Opinion 9.122. Pearson, Kahn, Harrison, Rubenstein, Rogers, Brook, & Keeler, *Differences in Quality of Care for Hospitalized Elderly Men and Women*, 268 JAMA 1883 (1992).

Journal 1992 Analyzes the impact of gender and age on hospital admissions for acute asthma attacks. Presents results of a study that looked at age and gender as factors affecting admissions and length of hospital stay. Concludes that biological distinctions between the sexes may play a role in the disease. References Opinion 9.122. Skobeloff, Spivey, St. Clair, & Schoffstall, *The Influence of Age and Sex on Asthma Admissions*, 268 J.A.M.A. 3437, 3439, 3440 (1992).

9.123 Disrespect and Derogatory Conduct in the Patient-Physician Relationship

The relationship between patients and physicians is based on trust and should serve to promote patients' well-being while respecting their dignity and rights. Trust can be established and maintained only when there is mutual respect.

Derogatory language or actions on the part of physicians can cause psychological harm to those they target. Also, such language or actions can cause reluctance in members of targeted groups to seek or to trust medical care and thus create an environment that strains relationships among patients, physicians, and the health care team. Therefore, any such conduct is profoundly antithetical to the Principles of Medical Ethics.

Patients who use derogatory language or otherwise act in a prejudicial manner toward physicians, other health care professionals, or others in the health care setting, seriously undermine the integrity of the patient-physician relationship. Such behavior, if unmodified, may constitute sufficient justification for the physician to arrange for the transfer of care. (I, II, VI, IX)

Issued December 2003 based on the report "Disrespect and Derogatory Conduct in the Patient-Physician Relationship," adopted June 2003.

A physician who knows that he or she has an infectious disease, which if contracted by the patient would pose a significant risk to the patient, should not engage in any activity that creates a significant risk of transmission of that disease to the patient. The precautions taken to prevent the transmission of a contagious disease to a patient should be appropriate to the seriousness of the disease and must be particularly stringent in the case of a disease that is potentially fatal. (I, IV)

Issued August 1989.

Updated June 1996 and June 1999.

Md. 1993 Patients sued hospital and physician alleging that an operating surgeon has a duty to disclose his or her HIV-infected status. Quoting Opinions 9.13 and 9.131 (1992) for the proposition that a seropositive physician should not engage in activity that would create a risk of transmission of the disease to his or her patients, the court held that it could not say as a matter of law that an HIV-infected physician did not have a duty to warn patients of his condition or refrain from operating on them. *Faya v. Almaraz, 329 Md. 435, 449, 450, 620 A.2d 327, 334*.

Minn. App. 1993 Patients sued HIV-positive physician alleging negligent infliction of emotional distress. Trial court granted summary judgment holding that plaintiffs had failed to produce evidence sufficient to show "actual exposure" to the AIDS virus. The appellate court, in an unpublished opinion, held that the plaintiffs need only show that they were in the "zone of danger" of contracting HIV. The court referred to *Faya v. Almaraz, 329 Md. 435, 449, 620 A.2d 327, 334* (1993) which had quoted Opinions 9.13 and 9.131 for the proposition that a physician who has an infectious disease should not engage in any activity that creates a risk of transmission of that disease to the patient. *K.A.C. v. Benson, 1993 Minn. App. LEXIS 1201*.

N.J. Super. 1991 Physician's estate sued hospital alleging that it violated state law against discrimination by restricting the physician's surgery privileges and requiring him to inform patients of his HIV-infected status before performing invasive procedures. The defendant hospital was also alleged to have breached its duty to maintain confidentiality of his seropositive diagnosis. The court held that the hospital had not discriminated against the physician since the hospital had relied on ethical and professional standards, including a report of the Council on Ethical and Judicial Affairs of the AMA dealing with the issue of AIDS [now Opinions 9.13 and 9.131]. However, the hospital was held to have breached its fiduciary duty to maintain the confidentiality of the physician's medical records. Referring to *McIntosh v. Milano, 168 N.J. Super. 466, 403 A.2d 500* (1979) which had quoted AMA Principles of Medical Ethics sec. 9 (1957) [now Principle IV and Opinion 5.05] in applying the "duty to warn" exception, the court noted that the disclosure in this case went far beyond the medical personnel directly involved in the treatment of the physician and those patients entitled to informed consent. *Estate of Behringer v. Medical Ctr., 249 N.J. Super. 597, 614, 633, 592 A.2d 1251, 1259, 1268*.

Journal 2000 Explores issues involving HIV-infected physicians and patients. Examines ethical and policy considerations and the Americans with Disabilities Act. Concludes that infected patients have the right to be treated, but infected physicians are not always afforded equal protection. Quotes Opinions 9.13 and 9.131. Halevy, *AIDS, Surgery, and the Americans with Disabilities Act, 135 Arch. Surg. 51, 52, 53 (2000)*.

Journal 2000 Examines the effect of HIV/AIDS on the relationship between the general public and health care professionals (HCPs). Discusses the importance of creating an environment in which HIV-positive patients do not fear disclosing their HIV status. Discusses policies and guidelines that address methods to prevent transmission of HIV from HCPs to patients. Quotes Opinion 2.23. References Opinions 9.13 and 9.131. Rediger, *Living in a World with HIV: Balancing Privacy, Privilege and the Right to Know Between Patients and Health Care Professionals, 21 Hamline J. Pub. L. & Pol'y 443, 456-57, 461, 472 (2000)*.

Journal 1997 Opines that physicians infected with HIV have an ethical and legal duty to disclose their status to patients before beginning invasive procedures. Suggests that the doctrine of informed consent and medical ethics guidelines require disclosure. Disagrees with public policy arguments favoring nondisclosure. References Opinions 9.13 and 9.131. Iheukwumere, *HIV-Positive Medical Practitioners: Legal and Ethical Obligations to Disclose*, 71 St. John's L. Rev. 715, 732-34 (1997).

Journal 1996 Discusses the doctrine of informed consent and its purpose. Posits that, due to patients' rights of self-determination, and the deadly nature of AIDS, physicians are morally and legally obligated to disclose their HIV status to patients where risk of transmission exists. Quotes Opinion 9.13. Note, *Torts: Defining the Duty Imposed on Physicians by the Doctrine of Informed Consent*, 22 Wm. Mitchell L. Rev. 149, 160 (1996).

Journal 1994 Examines the scope of a physician's duty to reveal HIV status to a patient before performing invasive procedures. Discusses applicable case law and advocates use of comprehensive and objective scientific data in evaluating potential liability in cases where physicians fail to disclose HIV status to patients. Quotes Opinions 9.13 and 9.131. Beane, *AIDS Crisis and the Health Care Community: Public Concerns Triggering Questionable Private Rights of Action for Emotional Harms and Legislative Response*, 45 Mercer L. Rev. 633, 669 (1994).

Journal 1994 Discusses the issue of whom physicians must serve first: themselves, their patients, insurers, or society. Focuses on risks arising out of provider economic arrangements and risks arising out of other individual physician characteristics. Quotes Opinions 8.03 and 9.13. Cites Opinion 8.15. Bobinski, *Autonomy and Privacy: Protecting Patients from Their Physicians*, 55 U. Pitt. L. Rev. 291, 302, 313 (1994).

Journal 1994 Analyzes problems in proving emotional distress claims based on the fear of contracting AIDS, such as proof of exposure and injury, reasonableness of fear, and proof of negligence. Proposes that courts follow evidentiary and public policy standards developed in other phobia cases. Quotes Opinions 9.13 and 9.131. Comment, *AIDSphobia: Forcing Courts to Face New Areas of Compensation for Fear of a Deadly Disease*, 39 Vill. L. Rev. 241, 277 (1994).

Journal 1994 Examines the responsibilities of real estate brokers to disclose a seller's AIDS status in light of a potential buyer's right to know all material facts affecting property value. Concludes that a seller's AIDS status is a material fact that a real estate broker must disclose. Quotes Opinions 9.13 and 9.131. Hartog, *The Psychological Impact of AIDS on Real Property and a Real Estate Broker's Duty to Disclose*, 36 Ariz. L. Rev. 757, 772 (1994).

Journal 1993 Provides an overview of the doctrine of informed consent and evaluates the disclosure obligations of HIV-positive health care professionals. Concludes that in developing coherent guidelines for informed consent in this context, the best approach is to have a public determination of what level of risk is tolerable. Cites Opinion 9.13. Nodzenski, *HIV-Infected Health Care Professionals and Informed Consent*, 2 S. Cal. Interdisciplinary L. J. 299, 327 (1993).

9.131 HIV-Infected Patients and Physicians

A physician may not ethically refuse to treat a patient whose condition is within the physician's current realm of competence solely because the patient is seropositive for HIV. Persons who are seropositive should not be subjected to discrimination based on fear or prejudice.

When physicians are unable to provide the services required by an HIV-infected patient, they should make appropriate referrals to those physicians or facilities equipped to provide such services.

A physician who knows that he or she is seropositive should not engage in any activity that creates a significant risk of transmission of the disease to others. A physician who has HIV disease or who is seropositive should consult colleagues as to which activities the physician can pursue without creating a risk to patients. (I, II, IV)

Issued March 1992 based on the report "Ethical Issues in the Growing AIDS Crisis," adopted December 1987 (JAMA. 1988; 259: 1360-61).

Updated June 1996 and June 1998.

Md. 1993 Patients sued hospital and physician alleging that an operating surgeon has a duty to disclose his or her HIV-infected status. Quoting Opinions 9.13 and 9.131 (1992) for the proposition that a seropositive physician should not engage in activity that would create a risk of transmission of the disease to his or her patients, the court held that it could not say as a matter of law that an HIV-infected physician did not have a duty to warn patients of his condition or refrain from operating on them. *Faya v. Almaraz, 329 Md. 435, 449, 450, 620 A.2d 327, 334.*

Md. App. 1996 Members of patient's family sued physician, hospital, and laboratory for negligence in failing to inform the patient and his family of patient's human immunodeficiency virus (HIV) positive status. The patient was discharged from the hospital prior to receipt of test results. The patient's family provided home health care, and in so, doing came into contact with the patient's bodily secretions. The family all tested negative for HIV. The court noted that the common law duty of care owed by a health care provider to diagnose, evaluate, and treat a patient ordinarily flows only to the patient, not to third parties. However, courts have recognized a duty to third parties in limited circumstances, mostly involving situations in which the patient has, or is thought to have, a communicable disease or otherwise presents a clear danger to a specific person. The court noted, with apparent reference to Opinion 9.131, that the AMA has urged that infected physicians should not engage in activity that creates a risk of transmission and therefore physicians have a duty to disclose their HIV positive status prior to invasive surgery. However, in the instant case, the court held that no duty to inform third parties of a patient's HIV status could exist because such a duty would constitute a wholly unwarranted invasion of the patient's privacy. *Lemon v. Stewart, 111 Md. App. 511, 523, 682 A.2d 1177, 1182.*

Minn. App. 1993 Patients sued HIV-positive physician alleging negligent infliction of emotional distress. Trial court granted summary judgment holding that plaintiffs had failed to produce evidence sufficient to show "actual exposure" to the AIDS virus. The appellate court, in an unpublished opinion, held that the plaintiffs need only show that they were in the "zone of danger" of contracting HIV. The court referred to *Faya v. Almaraz, 329 Md. 435, 449, 620 A.2d 327, 334* (1993) which had quoted Opinions 9.13 and 9.131 for the proposition that a physician who has an infectious disease should not engage in any activity that creates a risk of transmission of that disease to the patient. *K.A.C. v. Benson, 1993 Minn. App. LEXIS 1201.*

N.J. Super. 1991 Physician's estate sued hospital alleging that it violated state law against discrimination by restricting the physician's surgery privileges and requiring him to inform patients of his HIV-infected status before performing invasive procedures. The defendant hospital was also alleged to have breached its duty to maintain confidentiality of his seropositive diagnosis. The court held that the hospital had not discriminated against the physician since the hospital had relied on ethical and professional standards, including a report of the Council on Ethical and Judicial Affairs of the AMA dealing with the issue of AIDS [now Opinions 9.13 and 9.131]. However, the hospital was held to have breached its fiduciary duty to maintain the confidentiality of the physician's medical records. Referring to *McIntosh v. Milano, 168 N.J. Super. 466, 403 A.2d 500* (1979) which had quoted AMA Principles of Medical Ethics sec. 9 (1957) [now Principle IV and Opinion 5.05] in applying the "duty to warn" exception, the court noted that the disclosure in this case went far beyond the medical personnel directly involved in the treatment of the physician and those patients entitled to informed consent. *Estate of Behringer v. Medical Ctr., 249 N.J. Super. 597, 614, 633, 592 A.2d 1251, 1259, 1268.*

N.Y. 1996 Two dentists were found guilty of unlawful discriminatory practice, in violation of the state Human Rights Law, for refusing to treat patients who were known or suspected of having human immunodeficiency virus (HIV). On appeal the court affirmed the verdict and noted that both the American Dental Association and the American Medical Association, in Opinion 9.131, have adopted the position that it is unethical to refuse to treat an HIV-positive patient solely because of that diagnosis. In clarifying its holding, the court noted that the decision does not interfere with the provider's ability to prescribe treatment or refer patients elsewhere, provided it is done for a legitimate nondiscriminatory reason. *Cahill v. Rosa, 89 N.Y.2d 14, 24, 674 N.E.2d 274, 278, 651 N.Y.S.2d 344, 348.*

Pa. Super. 1991 HIV-infected physician appealed order of lower court authorizing hospitals to disclose the physician's identity to the limited class of those patients whose contact with the physician involved intrusive procedures. Appellate court held that the hospitals met their burden of proving a compelling need under the state's confidentiality act. The court cited to AMA Council on Ethical and Judicial Affairs, Ethical Issues Involved in the Growing AIDS Crisis, 259 JAMA 1360, 1361 (March 4, 1988) [now Opinion 9.131] stating that medical professionals have an obligation to their patients to provide safe and adequate health care. *In re Milton S. Hershey*

Medical Ctr., 407 Pa. Super. 565, 575, 582 n.18, 595 A.2d 1290, 1295, 1300 n.18.

Journal 2002 Provides ethical arguments in favor of transplantation in HIV-patients. Concludes that preventing such transplants is unethical and discriminatory. References Opinions 2.16 and 9.131. Halpern, Ubel, & Caplan, *Solid-Organ Transplantation in HIV-Infected Patients*, 347 New Eng. J. Med. 284, 287 (2002).

Journal 2000 Explores issues involving HIV-infected physicians and patients. Examines ethical and policy considerations and the Americans with Disabilities Act. Concludes that infected patients have the right to be treated, but infected physicians are not always afforded equal protection. Quotes Opinions 9.13 and 9.131. Halevy, *AIDS, Surgery, and the Americans with Disabilities Act*, 135 Arch. Surg. 51, 52, 53 (2000).

Journal 2000 Explores issues associated with wrongful transmission of HIV-AIDS within the family. Proposes possible legal avenues for compensating injured spouses and children. Concludes the current law in the area must be critically evaluated. Quotes Opinion 9.131. LeDoux, *Interspousal Liability and the Wrongful Transmission of HIV-AIDS: An Argument for Broadening Legal Avenues for the Injured Spouse and Further Expanding Children's Rights to Sue Their Parents*, 34 New Eng. L. Rev. 392, 411 (2000).

Journal 2000 Examines the effect of HIV/AIDS on the relationship between the general public and health care professionals (HCPs). Discusses the importance of creating an environment in which HIV-positive patients do not fear disclosing their HIV status. Discusses policies and guidelines that address methods to prevent transmission of HIV from HCPs to patients. Quotes Opinion 2.23. References Opinions 9.13 and 9.131. Rediger, *Living in a World with HIV: Balancing Privacy, Privilege and the Right to Know Between Patients and Health Care Professionals*, 21 Hamline J. Pub. L. & Pol'y 443, 456-57, 461, 472 (2000).

Journal 2000 Examines current laws prohibiting discrimination in the context of access to health care, placing emphasis on people with HIV/AIDS. Considers the implications of *Bragdon v. Abbott*. Concludes that everyone should be entitled to health care in the absence of an acceptable justification for its denial. Quotes Preamble, Principle VI, and Opinion 9.131. Shepherd, *HIV, the ADA, and the Duty to Treat*, 37 Hous. L. Rev. 1055, 1061, 1083-84 (2000).

Journal 1999 Discusses the need for physicians to advocate on behalf of patients' rights in the context of health care delivery. Evaluates the nature and scope of the physician's role as advocate, noting that physicians cannot be expected to engage in attorney-like advocacy. Quotes Principles IV and VI, Fundamental Elements (2), (4), and (6) [now Opinion 10.01], Patient Responsibilities 5 [now Opinion 10.02], and Opinions 2.03, 2.07, 2.09, 2.16, 2.19, 3.06, 4.01, 4.04, 6.01, 7.02, 8.02, 8.03, 8.13, 8.132, 9.06, 9.07, and 9.131. Cites Opinions 5.05, 5.09, 7.01, 8.135, and 9.02. Sage, *Physicians as Advocates*, 35 Hous. L. Rev. 1529, 1537, 1541, 1542, 1552-53, 1554, 1556, 1557, 1559, 1561-62, 1564, 1571, 1574, 1576, 1580 (1999).

Journal 1999 Discusses whether health care professionals have the right to refuse to treat patients under common law and federal statutes and regulations. Explores the impact of the Americans with Disabilities Act and the United States Supreme Court decision in *Bragdon v. Abbott* on the duties of health care professionals in the context of providing treatment to HIV-positive patients. Quotes Principle VI and Opinions 2.23 and 9.131. White, *Health Care Professionals and Treatment of HIV-Positive Patients*, 20 J. Legal Med. 67, 86 (1999).

Journal 1998 Examines two lines of cases stemming from the Americans with Disabilities Act. Discusses cases where courts have permitted discrimination claims against HIV-infected health care professionals, but conversely, have rejected discrimination claims against HIV-positive patients. Concludes that the diverging approaches may be attributed to a nonreciprocal assumption of risk. Cites Opinion 9.131. Bobinski, *Patients and Providers in the Courts: Fractures in the Americans with Disabilities Act*, 61 Alb. L. Rev. 785, 790, 806 (1998).

Journal 1998 Discusses provider secrets that may increase treatment risks for patients. Encourages greater disclosure of information to patients, including a physician's experience and performance with a procedure. References Opinion 9.131. Furrow, *Doctor's Dirty Little Secrets: The Dark Side of Medical Privacy*, 37 Washburn L. Rev. 283, 290 (1998).

Journal 1998 Reflects on the *Bragdon v. Abbott* decision, which held that individuals infected with HIV are entitled to protection against discrimination under anti-discrimination law. Discusses HIV discrimination and application of the Americans with Disabilities Act to those infected with HIV. Cites Opinion 9.131. Parmet, *The Supreme Court Confronts HIV: Reflections on Bragdon v. Abbott*, 26 J. Law, Med. & Ethics 225 (1998).

Journal 1997 Compares past ethical opinions to current opinions and notes the differences. Comments on the forces that have changed medical ethics through the years. Notes differing theories on the future course of medical ethics. Quotes Fundamental Elements (Preamble) and Opinions 5.05, 5.057, 7.01, 8.12, 9.12, and 9.131. Cites Fundamental Elements (5) and Opinions 8.115 and 8.13. Buchanan, *Medical Ethics at the Millennium: A Brief Retrospective*, 26 Colo. Law. 141, 142, 143, 144, 145 (1997).

Journal 1997 Opines that physicians infected with HIV have an ethical and legal duty to disclose their status to patients before beginning invasive procedures. Suggests that the doctrine of informed consent and medical ethics guidelines require disclosure. Disagrees with public policy arguments favoring nondisclosure. References Opinions 9.13 and 9.131. Iheukwumere, *HIV-Positive Medical Practitioners: Legal and Ethical Obligations to Disclose*, 71 St. John's L. Rev. 715, 732-34 (1997).

Journal 1996 Considers the extent of discrimination against HIV-infected patients in the dental setting. Reviews approaches to solving the problem of discrimination in this context. Concludes that legal intervention may aid in ending non-treatment based on discrimination. Quotes Opinion 9.131. Burris, *Dental Discrimination Against the HIV-Infected: Empirical Data, Law and Public Policy*, 13 Yale J. On Reg. 1, 41 (1996).

Journal 1996 Considers the extreme risk to patients where physicians and surgeons infected with HIV perform invasive medical procedures. Advocates civil litigation and liability in situations where HIV-infected physicians refuse testing but perform invasive procedures on patients who are uninformed. References Opinion 9.131. Closen, *HIV-AIDS, Infected Surgeons and Dentists, and the Medical Profession's Betrayal of Its Responsibility to Patients*, 41 N.Y.L. Sch. L. Rev. 57, 65, 71-72, 129 (1996).

Journal 1996 Explores whether patients have a duty to disclose their HIV status to treating physicians. Suggests that recognizing such a duty may subject patients to a lower standard of care and provide a disincentive to be tested. Concludes that courts should not impose a duty to disclose on patients. Quotes Principle 9 (1957) [now Principle IV] and Opinion 9.131. DeNatale & Parrish, *Health Care Workers' Ability to Recover in Tort for Transmission or Fear of Transmission of HIV from a Patient*, 36 Santa Clara L. Rev. 751, 782-83, 787 (1996).

Journal 1995 Analyzes the secular approach to the duty to treat HIV-infected individuals and the duty to warn those who are sexual partners of, or who share needles with, people infected with HIV. Observes that the secular approach leaves these issues unresolved; but indicates that Jewish law compels physicians both to treat and to warn. Quotes Opinions 5.05 and 9.131. Shorr, *AIDS, Judaism, and the Limits of the Secular Society*, 20 Second Opinion 23, 24, 27 (1995).

Journal 1994 Examines the scope of a physician's duty to reveal HIV status to a patient before performing invasive procedures. Discusses applicable case law and advocates use of comprehensive and objective scientific data in evaluating potential liability in cases where physicians fail to disclose HIV status to patients. Quotes Opinions 9.13 and 9.131. Beane, *AIDS Crisis and the Health Care Community: Public Concerns Triggering Questionable Private Rights of Action for Emotional Harms and Legislative Response*, 45 Mercer L. Rev. 633, 669 (1994).

Journal 1994 Considers how the Americans with Disabilities Act (ADA) has affected health care providers. Illustrates various legal issues arising under the ADA by analyzing cases involving patients and health care providers with AIDS. Quotes Opinion 9.131. Benesch, *Disability Discrimination in the Health Care Workplace*, 9 Trends in Health Care, Law & Ethics 45, 46 (Summer 1994).

Journal 1994 Analyzes problems in proving emotional distress claims based on the fear of contracting AIDS, such as proof of exposure and injury, reasonableness of fear, and proof of negligence. Proposes that courts follow evidentiary and public policy standards developed in other phobia cases. Quotes Opinions 9.13 and 9.131. Comment, *AIDSphobia: Forcing Courts to Face New Areas of Compensation for Fear of a Deadly Disease*, 39 Vill. L. Rev. 241, 277 (1994).

Journal 1994 Explores how the Americans with Disabilities Act has created, through federal civil rights mechanisms, a legal duty to treat HIV-infected patients. Discusses previous attempts to create a professional obligation to treat patients with AIDS. Quotes Principle VI and Opinion 9.131. Cites Opinion 9.12. Halevy & Brody, *Acquired Immunodeficiency Syndrome and the Americans with Disabilities Act: A Legal Duty to Treat*, 96 Am. J. Med. 282, 283, 284 (1994).

Journal 1994 Examines the responsibilities of real estate brokers to disclose a seller's AIDS status in light of a potential buyer's right to know all material facts affecting property value. Concludes that a seller's AIDS status is a material fact that a real estate broker must disclose. Quotes Opinions 9.13 and 9.131. Hartog, *The Psychological Impact of AIDS on Real Property and a Real Estate Broker's Duty to Disclose*, 36 Ariz. L. Rev. 757, 772 (1994).

Journal 1994 Discusses obligation of HIV-infected health professionals to inform patients of their serological status. Discusses common law and regulatory developments that appear to favor patients' rights to know their health professional's serological status before consenting to treatment. Quotes Opinion 9.131. LeBlang, *Obligations of HIV-Infected Health Professionals to Inform Patients of Their Serological Status: Evolving Theories of Liability*, 27 J. Marshall L. Rev. 317, 318 (1994).

Journal 1994 Analyzes competing privacy and public health interests as they relate to HIV transmission in the dentist-patient relationship. Proposes a statute and possible dental association policies to minimize the risk of HIV transmission. Quotes Opinion 9.131. Note, *HIV and Dentistry*, 29 Val. U.L. Rev. 297, 317 (1994).

Journal 1994 Discusses the role of professional societies in establishing ethical guidelines for physicians in the context of using medical innovations and new technologies. Observes that these standards must be supplemented by additional external measures or incentives in order to be most effective. Cites Opinions 1.01, 1.02, 8.061, 9.04, and 9.131. Orentlicher, *The Influence of a Professional Organization on Physician Behavior*, 57 Alb. L. Rev. 583, 592, 593, 594, 595, 596 (1994).

Journal 1993 Explores the traditional view that lawyers have unfettered discretion to select clients and New York's antidiscrimination disciplinary rule, statutes, and case law. Concludes that the legal profession should prohibit invidious or improper discrimination. Quotes Principle VI and Opinions 9.12 and 9.131. Begg, *Revoking the Lawyers' License to Discriminate in New York: The Demise of a Traditional Professional Prerogative*, 7 Geo. J. Legal Ethics 275, 298, 299 (1993).

Journal 1993 Addresses both patient rights under California consent and confidentiality laws relating to AIDS and prohibitions on unreasonable searches and seizures under the US Constitution. Concludes that any health care worker who can document an exposure to blood or body fluids should have the option of compelling a nonconsenting patient to be tested for HIV. Quotes Principle VI and Opinion 9.131. Comment, *Nonconsensual HIV Testing in the Health Care Setting: The Case for Extending the Occupational Protections of California Proposition 96 to Health Care Workers*, 26 Loy. L.A. L. Rev. 1251, 1269 (1993).

Journal 1993 Discusses family privacy rights and considers the meaning of justice, self respect, and the fundamental principles of physician ethics. Concludes that physicians have an ethical duty to intervene in domestic violence so long as such intervention does not breach confidentiality or violate patient autonomy. Quotes Principle IV and Opinion 5.05. References Opinions 8.14 and 9.131. Jecker, *Privacy Beliefs and the Violent Family: Extending the Ethical Argument for Physician Intervention*, 269 J.A.M.A. 776, 778, 779 (1993).

Journal 1993 Examines the law regarding HIV testing for health care workers with particular emphasis on risk determination, mandatory testing, and duty to warn patients. Proposes that CDC guidelines be reformed to more closely match evolving common law. References Opinion 9.131. Johnson, *HIV Testing of Health Care Workers: Conflict Between the Common Law and the Centers for Disease Control*, 42 Am. Univ. L. Rev. 479, 518 (1993).

Journal 1993 Explores the idea of reverse informed consent, which would impose a duty on patients to inform health care professionals of their infectious status. Concludes that such a duty is justified. Quotes Principles IV and VI and Opinions 8.11 and 9.131. Oddi, *Reverse Informed Consent: The Unreasonably Dangerous Patient*, 46 Vand. L. Rev. 1417, 1449, 1463, 1465, 1479 (1993).

Journal 1992 Discusses the problem of discrimination based on HIV status, particularly among women and children. Examines medical and public health issues involving HIV. Cites Principle VII. References Opinion 9.131. Gittler & Rennart, *HIV Infection Among Women and Children and Antidiscrimination Laws: An Overview*, 77 Iowa L. Rev. 1313, 1363 (1992).

Journal 1992 Examines issues related to HIV-infected health care workers protecting patients from infection, including mandatory testing, disclosure to coworkers and supervisors, and the degree to which the practice of an HIV-infected health care worker should be modified. Concludes that courts likely will impose a requirement to disclose HIV-positive status to patients when there is a substantial risk of HIV transmission. Quotes Opinions 8.03 (1989) [now Opinion 8.032], and 8.07 (1989) [now Opinion 8.03]. References Opinion 9.131. Lieberman & Derse, *HIV-Positive Health Care Workers and the Obligation to Disclose: Do Patients Have a Right to Know?*, 13 J. Legal Med. 333, 353, 354 (1992).

Journal 1992 Claims that a number of teaching hospitals deny emergency care to the impoverished. Concludes that medical educators must instill more altruistic values in their students. References Opinion 9.131. Miles, *What Are We Teaching About Indigent Patients?*, 268 JAMA 2561, 2562 (1992).

Journal 1992 Argues that the ADA and other laws prohibiting discrimination will not alone solve discrimination against HIV-infected patients and the resulting lack of access to health care. Proposes additional steps to augment anti-discrimination laws including implementing protections for health care workers against accidental transmission and adequately funding health care needs of AIDS patients. References Opinion 9.131. Note, *The Americans With Disabilities Act: Magic Bullet or Band-Aid for Patients and Health Care Workers Infected With the Human Immunodeficiency Virus?*, 57 Brooklyn L. Rev. 1277, 1279, 1305 (1992).

Journal 1991 Considers important issues of HIV testing of patients and health care workers, prevention of HIV transmission, and costs that attend accidental transmission. Proposes that hospitals develop comprehensive policies to address these issues. Quotes Opinion 9.131. Brennan, *Transmission of the Human Immunodeficiency Virus in the Health Care Setting—Time for Action*, 324 New Eng. J. Med. 1504, 1505, 1506 (1991).

Journal 1991 Considers whether physicians have an obligation to provide medical care to HIV-infected patients. Examines various sources for such a duty, including a moral obligation not to discriminate and a social responsibility to provide access to health care. Quotes Opinion 9.131. Cites Principle VI. Daniels, *Duty to Treat or Right to Refuse?*, 21 Hastings Center Rep. 36, 37, 42 (March/April 1991).

Journal 1991 Looks at two mandatory AIDS testing schemes and whether they serve the public interest. Concludes that mandatory HIV testing does not further legitimate public health concerns, except in the area of sexual assault. Quotes Opinion 9.131. Eisenstat, *An Analysis of the Rationality of Mandatory Testing for the HIV Antibody: Balancing the Governmental Public Health Interests With the Individual's Privacy Interest*, 52 Univ. Pittsburgh L. Rev. 327, 347 (1991).

Journal 1991 Finds that a majority of dentists do not believe CDC report and feel that dentist-to-patient HIV transmission is unlikely. Also finds, however, that most dentists believe HIV-infected practitioners should modify their practice and that patients should be informed if their dentist is HIV-positive. References Opinion 9.131. Gerbert, Bleecker, Miyasaki, & Maguire, *Possible Health Care Professional-to-Patient HIV Transmission: Dentists' Reactions to a Centers for Disease Control Report*, 265 JAMA 1845, 1846, 1847 (1991).

Journal 1991 Examines the extent to which physicians provide primary care to AIDS patients and various barriers that stand in the way. Presents the results of a survey indicating that many physicians are responding professionally to the AIDS crisis but that attitudinal barriers block some physicians from providing care. References Opinion 9.131. Gerbert, Maguire, Bleecker, Coates, & McPhee, *Primary Care Physicians and AIDS: Attitudinal and Structural Barriers to Care*, 266 JAMA 2837, 2838 (1991).

Journal 1991 Examines why HIV-infected individuals have difficulty receiving medical care from private physicians. Presents a Virginia community's response to this problem, which is based on a voluntary rotating referral system using a pool of primary care physicians. References Opinion 9.131. Green, Haggerty, & Hale, *Community-Based Plan for Treating Human Immunodeficiency Virus-Infected Individuals Sponsored by Local Medical Societies and an Acquired Immunodeficiency Syndrome Service Organization*, 151 Arch. Intern. Med. 2061, 2064 (1991).

Journal 1991 Discusses the issue of HIV-infected surgeons in light of the New Jersey case decision in *Behringer v. Medical Center*. Summarizes the case and presents its implications. Considers future developments. References Opinions 8.032 and 9.131. Orentlicher, *HIV-Infected Surgeons: Behringer v. Medical Center*, 266 JAMA 1134, 1136 (1991).

Journal 1990 Suggests that hospitals should focus on infection control in general, rather than HIV transmission in particular. Concludes that HIV-infected health care workers should be allowed to continue working as long as they take prudent measures to avoid the risk of transmission. References Opinion 9.131. Barnes, Rango, Burke, & Chiarello, *The HIV-Infected Health Care Professional: Employment Policies and Public Health*, 18 Law, Med. & Health Care 311, 314, 315 (1990).

Journal 1990 Discusses ways in which physicians attempt to avoid malpractice liability, including use of written contracts and refusal to see certain types of patients. Concludes that this behavior is undesirable and that more positive steps can be taken to eliminate much of the tension between physicians, patients, and lawyers. Quotes Opinion 9.131. Comment, *Physician Retaliation: Can the Physician-Patient Relationship Be Protected?*, 94 Dickinson L. Rev. 965, 986 (1990).

Journal 1990 Analyzes the major issues involved in mandatory AIDS testing. Concludes that forced testing is inappropriate and that resources could be used better in other ways. References Opinion 9.131. Field, *Testing for AIDS: Uses and Abuses*, XVI Am. J. Law & Med. 34, 50 (1990).

Journal 1990 Examines patients' fears about AIDS, their knowledge about transmission of the disease, and their perceived risk of HIV transmission by health care workers. Recommends that physicians actively work to educate the public. References Opinion 9.131. Marshall, O'Keefe, Fisher, Caruso, & Surdukowski, *Patients' Fear of Contracting the Acquired Immune Deficiency Syndrome From Physicians*, 150 Arch. Intern. Med. 1501, 1505 (1990).

Journal 1990 Examines the risk of HIV transmission from surgeon to patient. Concludes that the risk of HIV transmission is extremely low. References Opinion 9.131. Mishu, Schaffner, Horan, Wood, Hutcheson, & McNabb, *A Surgeon With AIDS: Lack of Evidence of Transmission to Patients*, 264 JAMA 467 (1990).

Journal 1990 Considers the propriety of HIV testing for hospital patients prior to non-emergency surgery. Concludes that testing of patients should be permitted so long as it is not done with the intent, nor the effect, of discriminating against individual patients. Quotes Principle VI and Opinion 9.131. Naccasha, *The Permissibility of Routine AIDS Testing in the Health Care Context*, 5 Notre Dame J.L. Ethics & Pub. Pol'y, 223, 241 (1990).

Journal 1989 Discusses the legal and ethical challenges that AIDS poses for health care providers. Proposes that health care providers actively participate in preventing HIV infection, providing care for HIV-infected individuals, and fighting AIDS and its associated stigma. Quotes Principle VI and Opinion 9.131. Forrester, *AIDS: The Responsibility to Care*, 34 Vill. L. Rev. 799, 811 (1989).

9.132 Health Care Fraud and Abuse

The following guidelines encourage physicians to play a key role in identifying and preventing fraud:

(1) Physicians must renew their commitment to Principle II of the American Medical Association's Principles of Medical Ethics which states that "a physician shall deal honestly with patients and colleagues, and strive to expose those physicians deficient in character, competence, or who engage in fraud or deception."

(2) Physicians should make no intentional misrepresentations to increase the level of payment they receive or to secure non-covered health benefits for their patients. (II)

Issued June 1998 based on the report "Health Care Fraud and Abuse," adopted December 1997 (J. Okla. St. Med. Assoc. 1998; 91: 408-09).

Journal 2001 Explores the extent to which pediatricians should rely on their expertise when prescribing therapies and durable medical equipment for children with special health care needs. Emphasizes the importance of the pediatrician's role in this context and urges pediatricians to comply with pertinent AMA guidelines and relevant state and federal laws. Quotes Opinion 8.06. References Opinion 9.132. Sneed, May, & Stencel, *Physicians' Reliance on Specialists, Therapists, and Vendors When Prescribing Therapies and Durable Medical Equipment for Children with Special Health Care Needs*, 107 Pediatrics 1283, 1287, 1288, 1289 (2001).

10.00 Opinions on the Patient-Physician Relationship

10.01 Fundamental Elements of the Patient-Physician Relationship

From ancient times, physicians have recognized that the health and well-being of patients depends upon a collaborative effort between physician and patient. Patients share with physicians the responsibility for their own health care. The patient-physician relationship is of greatest benefit to patients when they bring medical problems to the attention of their physicians in a timely fashion, provide information about their medical condition to the best of their ability, and work with their physicians in a mutually respectful alliance. Physicians can best contribute to this alliance by serving as their patients' advocate and by fostering these rights:

(1) The patient has the right to receive information from physicians and to discuss the benefits, risks, and costs of appropriate treatment alternatives. Patients should receive guidance from their physicians as to the optimal course of action. Patients are also entitled to obtain copies or summaries of their medical records, to have their questions answered, to be advised of potential conflicts of interest that their physicians might have, and to receive independent professional opinions.

(2) The patient has the right to make decisions regarding the health care that is recommended by his or her physician. Accordingly, patients may accept or refuse any recommended medical treatment.

(3) The patient has the right to courtesy, respect, dignity, responsiveness, and timely attention to his or her needs.

(4) The patient has the right to confidentiality. The physician should not reveal confidential communications or information without the consent of the patient, unless provided for by law or by the need to protect the welfare of the individual or the public interest.

(5) The patient has the right to continuity of health care. The physician has an obligation to cooperate in the coordination of medically indicated care with other health care providers treating the patient. The physician may not discontinue treatment of a patient as long as further treatment is medically indicated, without giving the patient reasonable assistance and sufficient opportunity to make alternative arrangements for care.

(6) The patient has a basic right to have available adequate health care. Physicians, along with the rest of society, should continue to work toward this goal. Fulfillment of this right is dependent on society providing

resources so that no patient is deprived of necessary care because of an inability to pay for the care. Physicians should continue their traditional assumption of a part of the responsibility for the medical care of those who cannot afford essential health care. Physicians should advocate for patients in dealing with third parties when appropriate. (I, IV, V, VIII, IX)

Issued June 1992 based on the report "Fundamental Elements of the Patient-Physician Relationship," adopted June 1990 (*JAMA*. 1990; 262: 3/33).

Updated 1993.

Colo. App. 1999 Physician filed suit seeking reinstatement, compensatory damages, and an opportunity to respond to the reasons for termination. The defendants claimed that the contract with the physician provided for termination without cause. The trial court granted the defendants' motion for summary judgment. The appellate court affirmed, holding that the termination clause allowed either party to terminate the contract without cause. In a separate dissenting opinion, judge stated that termination without cause significantly impacts the physician-patient relationship and referenced Fundamental Element (5) [now Opinion 10.01], regarding the continuity of this relationship. *Grossman v. Columbine Medical Group, Inc.*, 1999 WL 1024015, 4-5.

Ga. App. 2000 Plaintiff alleged failure on the part of a dentist to inform him of the risks of root canal in a malpractice action. The appeals court noted that state case law did not recognize the informed consent doctrine. In evaluating this precedent, the court quoted Opinion 8.08 and Fundamental Element (1) [now Opinion 10.01]. The court stated that the AMA Code of Medical Ethics should be understood to reflect the standard of care of the medical profession on the issue of informed consent. While the court ruled in favor of the dentist, it prospectively recognized the doctrine of informed consent. *Ketchup v. Howard*, 247 Ga. App. 54, 543 S.E.2d 371, 376, 377.

Tenn. App. 1998 Plaintiff challenged the constitutionality of various sections of state abortion statute. Among the provisions at issue was one requiring that a woman be "orally informed by her attending physician" as to specified information regarding the abortion. The court stated that the information requirement and physician counseling provision did not unduly burden a woman's right to an abortion. Physicians who supported this portion of the statute quoted Fundamental Element (1) [now Opinion 10.01], regarding a physician's duty to counsel a patient about the best treatments available. *Planned Parenthood of Middle Tennessee v. Sundquist*, 1998 WL 467110, 33.

Journal 2003 Highlights the legal and ethical concerns surrounding use of noncompetition clauses. Concludes that physicians should carefully evaluate these clauses given their likely enforceability. Quotes Opinions 9.02, 9.06, 10.01, and 10.015. Loeser, *The Legal, Ethical, and Practical Implications of Noncompetition Clauses: What Physicians Should Know Before They Sign, 31 J.L. Med. & Ethics 283, 286, 287, 290 (2003).*

Journal 2003 Considers the legal, medical, and ethical issues of physician-patient confidentiality in disclosure of paternity. Concludes that a balancing test should be applied to making determinations regarding disclosure of paternity. Quotes Principles I, IV, and V, and Opinions 1.02, 5.055, and 10.01. Cites Principle II and Opinion 5.05. Richards & Wolf, *Medical Confidentiality and Disclosure of Paternity*, 48 S.D. L. Rev. 409, 411, 412, 413 (2003).

Journal 2003 Argues that affirmative measures should be taken by the Air Force to ensure access to abortion services. Concludes that regulatory changes will reduce barriers to access. Quotes Opinion 10.01. Cites Opinion 8.08. Wilde, *Air Force Women's Access to Abortion Services and the Erosion of 10 U.S.C. § 1093, 9 Wm. & Mary J. Women & L.* 351, 371 (2003).

Journal 2002 Argues for a more comprehensive approach in the management and treatment of intersex children. Emphasizes the importance of informed decisionmaking by parents and children. Quotes Opinion 10.01. Hermer, *Paradigms Revised: Intersex Children, Bioethics & the Law, 11 Annals Health L.* 195, 221 (2002).

Journal 2002 Discusses issues regarding regulation of elderly drivers. Concludes that mandating physicians to report unfit elderly patients will protect the public and help resolve ethical and legal dilemmas. Quotes Opinions 1.02, 2.24, 5.05, and 10.01. Kane, *Driving into the Sunset: A Proposal for Mandatory Reporting to the DMV by Physicians Treating Unsafe Elderly Drivers, 25 U. Haw. L. Rev.* 59, 59, 61, 62, 67, 69, 82, 83 (2002).

Journal 2002 Reviews how changes in the health care delivery system underscore the importance of information in patient empowerment. Concludes that patients should use information to take charge of their health care. Quotes Principle V and Opinion 10.02. Cites Opinion 10.01. Kane, *Information is the Key to Patient Empowerment*, 11 Annals Health L. 25, 29-30, 44 (2002).

Journal 2002 Considers the ethical and legal issues regarding breach of confidentiality in situations where a patient is pregnant and uses teratogenic substances. Concludes that a breach of confidentiality causes damage to the physician-patient relationship. Quotes Principle IV and Opinion 10.01. Plambeck, *Divided Loyalties: Legal and Bioethical Considerations of Physician-Pregnant Patient Confidentiality and Prenatal Drug Abuse*, 23 J. Legal Med. 1, 8, 25 (2002).

Journal 2002 Analyzes the role of prognostication in physician-patient communication. Concludes that the patient-physician model of shared decision-making offers the best hope for reestablishing prognostication. Quotes Principles Ch. I, Art. I, Sec. 2 and 4 (1846) [now Principle IV and Opinions 8.12 and 10.01]. Cites Opinion 8.08. Rich, *Prognostication in Clinical Medicine: Prophecy or Professional Responsibility?* 23 J. Legal Med. 297, 299, 318, 327 (2002).

Journal 2002 Discusses legal and medical policies that protect confidentiality in the physician-patient relationship. Concludes that reducing the current level of privacy protection would jeopardize health care. Quotes Preamble and Opinions 2.136, 5.05, and 10.01. References Principles VIII and IX. Sciarrino, *Ferguson v. City of Charleston: "The Doctor Will See You Now, Be Sure to Bring Your Privacy Rights in With You!"* 12 Temp. Pol. & Civ. Rts. L. Rev. 197, 213, 215, 220, 221, 222 (2002).

Journal 2001 Explores the ethical and legal dilemmas associated with doctors and lawyers providing advice over the internet. Concludes the law must ensure that cyberprofessionals comply with ethical and legal duties to their clients and their professions. Quotes Opinion 10.01. Deady, *Cyberadvice: The Ethical Implications of Giving Professional Advice over the Internet*, 14 Geo. J. Legal Ethics 891, 905 (2001).

Journal 2001 Discusses whether or not the medical profession needs a policy on honesty. Reviews ethical codes and concludes they fail to offer physicians with meaningful guidance about what constitutes "the truth" and when and how to disclose it. Quotes Principle II and Opinions 8.12 and 10.01. DeVita, *Honestly, Do We Need a Policy on Truth?* 11 Kennedy Inst. Ethics J. 157, 158 (2001).

Journal 2001 Discusses issues surrounding the privacy of genetic information. Considers the social, ethical, and legal responses to problems that arise in this context. Concludes with a unique view of privacy that would protect the right of individuals not to know genetic information about themselves. Quotes Principle IV and Opinion 10.01. Laurie, *Challenging Medical-Legal Norms: The Role of Autonomy, Confidentiality, and Privacy in Protecting Individual and Familial Group Rights in Genetic Information*, 22 J. Legal Med. 1, 24 (2001).

Journal 2001 Considers conflicts of interest in clinical research and other types of medical practice. Compares the way in which doctors and lawyers address conflicts of interest in professional practice. Concludes that physicians are unaware of the need to create a meaningful conflict-of-interest doctrine for medical practice. Quotes Preamble, Principle IV, and Opinions 2.07, 8.03, 8.031, and 10.01. Moore, *What Doctors Can Learn from Lawyers about Conflicts of Interest*, 81 B.U.L. Rev. 445, 447, 449-50 (2001).

Journal 2001 Compares ongoing efforts to control reproduction and to control drug abuse with a view toward finding more effective solutions in both areas. Concludes that a coherent approach will build stronger coalitions in support of drug policy reform and reproductive freedom. Quotes Opinion 10.01. Paltrow, *The War on Drugs and the War on Abortion: Some Initial Thoughts on the Connections, Intersections and the Effects*, 28 S.U. L. Rev. 201, 219 (2001).

Journal 2001 Considers how much information regarding the adverse effects of medication physicians should disclose to patients. Concludes that most patients want complete information. Quotes Opinion 10.01. Ziegler, Mosier, Buenaver, & Okuyemi, *How Much Information About Adverse Effects of Medication Do Patients Want From Physicians?*, 161 Arch. Intern. Med. 706, 710 (2001).

Journal 2000 Introduces the debate surrounding the benefits and dangers of diagnosing and treating patients over the Internet and explores the issue of how cybermedicine will change the traditional physician-patient relationship. Concludes cybermedicine is the future of medical care, and the physician-patient relationship will have to change to accommodate the predicted online medical boom. Quotes Opinion 10.01. Gelein, *Are Online Consultations a Prescription for Trouble?*

The Uncharted Waters of Cybermedicine, 66 Brook. L. Rev. 209, 239 (2000).

Journal 2000 Discusses patent law and policy. Examines whether or not those who practice medicine should be excused from patent laws because of the conflict that medical procedure patents create with respect to the practice of medicine. Concludes that Congress should repeal section 287(c) of the Patent Act. Quotes Principle V and Opinions 9.08 and 9.09. Cites Opinion 8.03. References Opinion 10.01. Ho, *Patents, Patients, and Public Policy: An Incomplete Intersection at 35 U.S.C. § 287(c)*, 33 U.C. Davis L. Rev. 601, 603, 623, 624, 625, 631 (2000).

Journal 2000 Describes the fiduciary aspects of the physician-patient relationship. Explores the conflicts that may occur between physicians and pregnant women in the health care setting. Proposes legal strategies to address these conflicts. Quotes Opinions 8.08 and 10.01. References Opinion 8.13. Oberman, *Mothers and Doctors' Orders: Unmasking the Doctor's Fiduciary Role in Maternal-Fetal Conflicts*, 94 Nw. U. L. Rev. 451, 456, 462, 493 (2000).

Journal 2000 Evaluates recent Texas legislation that affords immunity to health care professionals who provide free health care services to the poor. Concludes that such legislation creates a dual standard of care, requiring indigent patients to forfeit their legal rights in exchange for health care. Quotes Opinion 10.01. References Opinion 9.065. Pulido, *Immunity of Volunteer Health Care Providers in Texas: Bartering Legal Rights for Free Medical Care*, 2 Scholar: St. Mary's L. Rev. Minority Issues 323, 330 (2000).

Journal 2000 Considers the topic of physician liability for genetic malpractice. Explores how new genetic technologies may affect the medical and legal communities. Concludes by observing that the legal system is not prepared to address the wave of litigation that may grow out of emerging genetic technologies. Quotes Opinion 10.01. Reutenauer, *Medical Malpractice Liability in the Era of Genetic Susceptibility Testing*, 19 QLR 539, 571 (2000).

Journal 2000 Discusses managed care in terms of problems, responses, and accomplishments. Demonstrates how a physician union's collective bargaining process can benefit patients and physicians in addressing problems with managed care. Concludes that barriers preventing such unions should be removed. Quotes Principles VI and VII and Opinion 10.01. Rugg, *An Old Solution to a New Problem: Physician Unions Take the Edge Off Managed Care*, 34 Colum. J. L. & Soc. Probs. 1, 41 (2000).

Journal 2000 Examines ethical and legal issues regarding medical privacy. Discusses authorized and unauthorized uses of information contained in medical records and identifies who may access these records. Analyzes the ethical balance between patient privacy and societal benefits derived from sacrificing it. Concludes privacy is very important to maintaining a full and open physician-patient relationship. Quotes Opinion 10.01. Scott, *Is Too Much Privacy Bad for Your Health? An Introduction to the Law, Ethics, and HIPAA Rule on Medical Privacy*, 17 Ga. St. U. L. Rev. 481, 494 (2000).

Journal 2000 Discusses the development and history of the ethical doctrine of informed consent. Examines the current state of the law in Pennsylvania and concludes it does not adequately fulfill the goals of ethical and legal doctrines. Quotes Principle IV and Opinion 10.01. References Opinion 8.08. Warren, *Pennsylvania Medical Informed Consent Law: A Call to Protect Patient Autonomy Rights By Abandoning the Battery Approach*, 38 Duq. L. Rev. 917, 925 (2000).

Journal 1999 Examines reporting of AIDS and HIV under Texas law. Discusses limitations on a physician's ability to warn potentially at-risk third parties. Concludes that Texas law should be changed to place a duty upon physicians to notify at-risk third parties of a patient's HIV-positive status. Quotes Principle IV and Opinion 10.01. Acosta, *The Texas Communicable Disease Prevention and Control Act: Are We Offering Enough Protection to Those Who Need It Most?* 36 Hous. L. Rev. 1819, 1822, 1830, 1831 (1999).

Journal 1999 Discusses the need for physicians to advocate on behalf of patients' rights in the context of health care delivery. Evaluates the nature and scope of the physician's role as advocate, noting that physicians cannot be expected to engage in attorney-like advocacy. Quotes Principles IV and VI, Fundamental Elements (2), (4), and (6) [now Opinion 10.01], Patient Responsibilities 5 [now Opinion 10.02], and Opinions 2.03, 2.07, 2.09, 2.16, 2.19, 3.06, 4.01, 4.04, 6.01, 7.02, 8.02, 8.03, 8.13, 8.132, 9.06, 9.07, and 9.131. Cites Opinions 5.05, 5.09, 7.01, 8.135, and 9.02. Sage, *Physicians as Advocates*, 35 Hous. L. Rev. 1529, 1537, 1541, 1542, 1552-53, 1554, 1556, 1557, 1559, 1561-62, 1564, 1571, 1574, 1576, 1580 (1999).

Journal 1998 Discusses conflicts of interest in the physician-patient relationship arising out of use of financial incentives by managed care organizations. Considers how such conflicts are dealt with in the attorney-client relationship. Suggests that a financial incentive should be legally denounced if it unreasonably interferes with a physician's duty to properly care for and treat patients. Quotes Preamble, Fundamental Elements (1) [now Opinion 10.01] and Opinions 4.04, 5.01, 8.03, 8.13, and 9.06. Cites Fundamental Elements (4) [now Opinion 10.01] and Opinions 2.07, 2.08, and 2.132. Hall, *Third-Party Payor Conflicts of Interest in Managed Care: A Proposal for Regulation Based on the Model Rules of Professional Conduct*, 29 Seton Hall L. Rev. 95, 96, 107, 108, 109, 110, 111, 112, 134, 135, 136 (1998).

Journal 1997 Compares past ethical opinions to current opinions and notes the differences. Comments on the forces that have changed medical ethics through the years. Notes differing theories on the future course of medical ethics. Quotes Fundamental Elements (Preamble) and Opinions 5.05, 5.057, 7.01, 8.12, 9.12, and 9.131. Cites Fundamental Elements (5) and Opinions 8.115 and 8.13. Buchanan, *Medical Ethics at the Millennium: A Brief Retrospective*, 26 Colo. Law. 141, 142, 143, 144, 145 (1997).

Journal 1997 Reviews ethical issues raised by genetic research. Explores the duty a physician may have to reveal the genetic diseases found in patients to their relatives. Considers case law and statutory law, and concludes that a limited duty to disclose exists. Quotes Fundamental Elements (4). Deftos, *Genomic Torts: The Law of the Future—The Duty of Physicians to Disclose the Presence of a Genetic Disease to the Relatives of Their Patients with the Disease*, 32 USF. L. Rev. 105, 130 (1997).

Journal 1997 Discusses physician frustration with managed care plans caused by gag clauses and cost-containment mechanisms. Reviews the development of managed care organizations and federal attempts at limiting the use of gag clauses. Concludes that gag clauses are inherently flawed and compromise quality health care. Quotes Principles II and V, Fundamental Elements (1), and Opinion 8.13. Note, *Physicians, Bound and Gagged: Federal Attempts to Combat Managed Care's Use of Gag Clauses*, 21 Seton Hall Legis. J. 567, 601-02 (1997).

Journal 1997 Considers the current approach to health care in the United States. Examines financing mechanisms, and suggests that reform could be effected through a decentralized, community-based approach. Proposes use of volunteer systems in which medical personnel would care for certain patients free of charge or at reduced rates. Quotes Fundamental Elements (6). References Opinion 9.065. Solomon & Asaro, *Community-Based Health Care: A Legal and Policy Analysis*, 24 Fordham Urb. L. J. 235, 276-77 (1997).

Journal 1996 Describes the problem of lack of access to medical care by the indigent. Recognizes the commitment of the medical profession to providing care for indigent patients. Observes that state initiatives that provide physicians tort immunity in exchange for volunteer service can improve access to care by the indigent. Quotes Fundamental Elements (6). References Opinion 9.065. Comment, *Statutory Immunity for Volunteer Physicians: A Vehicle for Reaffirmation of the Doctor's Beneficent Duties—Absent the Rights Talk*, 1 Widener L. Symp. J. 425, 448, 449 (1996).

Journal 1996 Considers the ethical requirement for physicians to receive informed consent from patients before beginning treatment. Reviews the case of *Jacobson v. Massachusetts*, discussing its impact on informed consent and vaccination policy in the United States. Quotes Fundamental Elements (2). References Opinion 8.08. Severyn, *Jacobson v. Massachusetts: Impact on Informed Consent and Vaccine Policy*, 5 J. Pharmacy & L. 249, 253, 274 (1996).

Journal 1996 Examines medically futile treatment in light of legislative enactments in Virginia and Maryland. Observes that the futility debate arises when requests for life-prolonging treatment are viewed as medically inappropriate by health care providers. Concludes that, while the ethical integrity of the medical profession justifies some legal recognition of futility, such recognition must be limited by respect for patient autonomy. References Fundamental Elements (5). Shiner, *Medical Futility: A Futile Concept?*, 53 Wash. & Lee L. Rev. 803, 834 (1996).

Journal 1995 Examines the impact of health care reform on physician-patient relationships. Discusses how reform may threaten the physician's fiduciary duty of loyalty by forcing physicians to make rationing decisions and giving physicians financial incentives to limit use of health care resources. Quotes Fundamental Elements (5) [now Opinion 10.01]. Cites Opinion 5.05. Orentlicher, *Health Care Reform and the Patient-Physician Relationship*, 5 Health Matrix 141, 143, 148 (1995).

Journal 1994 Considers whether an exception should be made to physician-patient confidentiality that would allow a physician to reveal parental medical history to a child. Concludes that such an exception would not completely erode physician-patient confidentiality. Quotes Principles IV,

Fundamental Elements (4), and Opinion 5.05. Cites Principle I and Fundamental Elements (1). Friedland, *Physician-Patient Confidentiality: Time to Re-Examine a Venerable Concept in Light of Contemporary Society and Advances in Medicine*, 15 J. Legal Med. 249, 257, 264, 276 (1994).

Journal 1994 Explores the ethical issues involved in a multidisciplinary team working with children in legal proceedings. Focuses on the relationships between professionals and the conflicts that arise regarding disclosure of confidential information and forced disclosure of non-privileged information. Quotes Principles III, IV, Fundamental Elements (4) and Opinions 1.02 (1992) and 5.07 (1992) [now Opinion 5.05]. Cites Opinions 2.02. Glynn, *Multidisciplinary Representation of Children: Conflicts Over Disclosures of Client Communications*, 27 J. Marshall L. Rev. 617, 625, 626, 630-32, 637, 639, 643 (1994).

Journal 1994 Discusses physician-patient confidentiality and the exception that permits breach of a patient's confidence if required by law. Argues that this is always a legitimate exception to the confidentiality rule. Quotes Principle IV and Fundamental Elements (4). McConnell, *Confidentiality and the Law*, 20 J. Med. Ethics 47, 47 (1994).

Journal 1994 Reviews the evolution of the physician-patient relationship, with attention to examines the changing health care delivery environment. Quotes Preamble, Principles I, II, III, IV, V, and VI, Fundamental Elements (1) and (2), and Opinions 1.02 and 8.07 (1981) [now Opinion 8.08]. Cites Opinion 1.01. Szczygiel, *Beyond Informed Consent*, 21 Ohio N.U.L. Rev. 171, 217, 218, 220, 225, 226, 256 (1994).

Journal 1994 Discusses the importance of confidentiality in the physician-patient relationship and under what circumstances patient information may be released. Examines unique considerations that apply when a physician provides medical care to a minor or an HIV-infected individual. Quotes Principle IV and Fundamental Elements (4). Weiner & Wettstein, *Confidentiality of Patient-Related Information*, 112 Arch. Ophthalmology 1032, 1033 (1994).

Journal 1993 Analyzes the implications of giving patients and their families an absolute right to control medical treatment. Argues that courts should refrain from ordering physicians to treat patients when physicians believe that treatment would be ineffective. Quotes Fundamental Elements (5) [now Opinion 10.01] and Opinions 2.11 (1982) [now Opinion 2.20] and 2.18 (1986) [now Opinion 2.20]. Comment, *Beyond Autonomy: Judicial Restraint and the Legal Limits Necessary to Uphold the Hippocratic Tradition and Preserve the Ethical Integrity of the Medical Profession*, 9 J. Contemp. Health L. & Pol'y 451, 467, 468 (1993).

10.015 The Patient-Physician Relationship

The practice of medicine, and its embodiment in the clinical encounter between a patient and a physician, is fundamentally a moral activity that arises from the imperative to care for patients and to alleviate suffering.

A patient-physician relationship exists when a physician serves a patient's medical needs, generally by mutual consent between physician and patient (or surrogate). In some instances the agreement is implied, such as in emergency care or when physicians provide services at the request of the treating physician. In rare instances, treatment without consent may be provided under court order (see Opinion 2.065, "Court-Initiated Medical Treatments in Criminal Cases"). Nevertheless, the physician's obligations to the patient remain intact.

The relationship between patient and physician is based on trust and gives rise to physicians' ethical obligations to place patients' welfare above their own self-interest and above obligations to other groups, and to advocate for their patients' welfare.

Within the patient-physician relationship, a physician is ethically required to use sound medical judgment, holding the best interests of the patient as paramount. (I, II, VI, VIII)

Issued December 2001 based on the report "The Patient-Physician Relationship," adopted June 2001.

Journal 2003 Highlights the legal and ethical concerns surrounding use of noncompetition clauses. Concludes that physicians should carefully evaluate these clauses given their likely enforceability. Quotes Opinions 9.02, 9.06, 10.01, and 10.015. Loeser, *The Legal, Ethical, and Practical Implications of Noncompetition Clauses: What Physicians Should Know Before They Sign, 31 J.L. Med. & Ethics 283, 286, 287, 290 (2003).*

Journal 2002 Examines sports-related concussions among football players. Considers the responsibilities of team physicians. Concludes that litigation will increase without treatment guidelines for concussion management. References Opinion 10.015. Hecht, *Legal and Ethical Aspects of Sports-Related Concussions: The Merril Hoge Story, 12 Seton Hall J. Sport L. 17, 42-43 (2002).*

10.017 Gifts from Patients

Gifts that patients offer to physicians are often an expression of appreciation and gratitude or a reflection of cultural tradition, and can enhance the patient-physician relationship.

Some gifts signal psychological needs that require the physician's attention. Some patients may attempt to influence care or to secure preferential treatment through the offering of gifts or cash. Acceptance of such gifts is likely to damage the integrity of the patient-physician relationship. Physicians should make clear that gifts given to secure preferential treatment compromise their obligation to provide services in a fair manner.

There are no definitive rules to determine when a physician should or should not accept a gift. No fixed value determines the appropriateness or inappropriateness of a gift from a patient; however, the gift's value relative to the patient's or the physician's means should not be disproportionately or inappropriately large. One criterion is whether the physician would be comfortable if acceptance of the gift were known to colleagues or the public.

Physicians should be cautious if patients discuss gifts in the context of a will. Such discussions must not influence the patient's medical care.

If, after a patient's death, a physician should learn that he or she has been bequeathed a gift, the physician should consider declining the gift if the physician believes that its acceptance would present a significant hardship (financial or emotional) to the family.

The interaction of these various factors is complex and requires the physician to consider them sensitively. (I, II)

Issued December 2003 based on the report "Gifts from Patients," adopted June 2003.

10.02 Patient Responsibilities

It has long been recognized that successful medical care requires an ongoing collaborative effort between patients and physicians. Physician and patient are bound in a partnership that requires both individuals to take an active role in the healing process. Such a partnership does not imply that both partners have identical responsibilities or equal power. While physicians have the responsibility to provide health care services to patients to the best of their ability, patients have the responsibility to communicate openly, to participate in decisions about the diagnostic and treatment recommendations, and to comply with the agreed-upon treatment program.

Like patients' rights, patients' responsibilities are derived from the principle of autonomy. The principle of patient autonomy holds that an individual's physical, emotional, and psychological integrity should be respected and upheld. This principle also recognizes the human capacity to self-govern and choose a course of action from among different alternative options. Autonomous, competent patients assert some control over the decisions which direct their health care. With that exercise of self-governance and free choice comes a number of responsibilities.

(1) Good communication is essential to a successful patient-physician relationship. To the extent possible, patients have a responsibility to be truthful and to express their concerns clearly to their physicians.

(2) Patients have a responsibility to provide a complete medical history, to the extent possible, including information about past illnesses, medications, hospitalizations, family history of illness, and other matters relating to present health.

(3) Patients have a responsibility to request information or clarification about their health status or treatment when they do not fully understand what has been described.

(4) Once patients and physicians agree upon the goals of therapy and a treatment plan, patients have a responsibility to cooperate with that treatment plan and to keep their agreed-upon appointments. Compliance with physician instructions is often essential to public and individual safety. Patients also have a responsibility to disclose whether previously agreed upon treatments are being followed and to indicate when they would like to reconsider the treatment plan.

(5) Patients generally have a responsibility to meet their financial obligations with regard to medical care or to discuss financial hardships with their physicians. Patients should be cognizant of the costs associated with using a limited resource like health care and try to use medical resources judiciously.

(6) Patients should discuss end-of-life decisions with their physicians and make their wishes known. Such a discussion might also include writing an advance directive.

(7) Patients should be committed to health maintenance through health-enhancing behavior. Illness can often be prevented by a healthy lifestyle, and patients should take personal responsibility when they are able to avert the development of disease.

(8) Patients should also have an active interest in the effects of their conduct on others and refrain from behavior that unreasonably places the health of others at risk. Patients should inquire as to the means and likelihood of infectious disease transmission and act upon that information which can best prevent further transmission.

(9) Participation in medical education is to the mutual benefit of patients and the health care system. Patients are encouraged to participate in medical education by accepting care, under appropriate supervision, from medical

students, residents, and other trainees. Consistent with the process of informed consent, the patient or the patient's surrogate decision maker is always free to refuse care from any member of the health care team.

(10) Patients should discuss organ donation with their physicians and, if donation is desired, make applicable provisions. Patients who are part of an organ allocation system and await needed transplant should not try to go outside of or manipulate the system. A fair system of allocation should be answered with public trust and an awareness of limited resources.

(11) Patients should not initiate or participate in fraudulent health care and should report illegal or unethical behavior by physicians and other providers to the appropriate medical societies, licensing boards, or law enforcement authorities. (I, IV, VI)

Issued June 1994 based on the report "Patient Responsibilities," adopted June 1993.

Updated June 1998, December 2000, and June 2001.

Journal 2002 Reviews how changes in the health care delivery system underscore the importance of information in patient empowerment. Concludes that patients should use information to take charge of their health care. Quotes Principle V and Opinion 10.02. Cites Opinion 10.01. Kane, *Information is the Key to Patient Empowerment*, 11 Annals Health L. 25, 29-30, 44 (2002).

Journal 2002 Discusses state regulation of health information and the Federal Health Privacy Rule, noting that it provides inadequate protection. Concludes state laws can bridge gaps in protection. Quotes Opinion 10.02. Pritts, *Altered States: State Health Privacy Laws and the Impact of the Federal Health Privacy Rules*, 2 Yale J. Health Pol'y, L. & Ethics 327, 351 (2002).

Journal 1999 Discusses the need for physicians to advocate on behalf of patients' rights in the context of health care delivery. Evaluates the nature and scope of the physician's role as advocate, noting that physicians cannot be expected to engage in attorney-like advocacy. Quotes Principles IV and VI, Fundamental Elements (2), (4), and (6) [now Opinion 10.01], Patient Responsibilities 5 [now Opinion 10.02], and Opinions 2.03, 2.07, 2.09, 2.16, 2.19, 3.06, 4.01, 4.04, 6.01, 7.02, 8.02, 8.03, 8.13, 8.132, 9.06, 9.07, and 9.131. Cites Opinions 5.05, 5.09, 7.01, 8.135, and 9.02. Sage, *Physicians as Advocates*, 35 Hous. L. Rev. 1529, 1537, 1541, 1542, 1552-53, 1554, 1556, 1557, 1559, 1561-62, 1564, 1571, 1574, 1576, 1580 (1999).

Journal 1994 Discusses notions of quality in health care, asking who is responsible to define *quality*, who is responsible to deliver it, and who is responsible for quality of care when it is unsatisfactory. Concludes that significant economic changes will require a reallocation of these responsibilities among patients, providers, and payers. References Patient Responsibilities (1), (4), and (5). Morreim, *Redefining Quality by Reassigning Responsibility*, 20 Am. J. Law & Med. 79, 103 (1994).

10.03 Patient-Physician Relationship in the Context of Work-Related and Independent Medical Examinations

When a physician is responsible for performing an isolated assessment of an individual's health or disability for an employer, business, or insurer, a limited patient-physician relationship should be considered to exist. Both "Industry Employed Physicians" (IEPs), who are employed by businesses or insurance companies for the purpose of conducting medical examinations, and "Independent Medical Examiners" (IMEs), who are independent contractors providing medical examinations within the realm of their specialty, may perform such medical examinations.

Despite their ties to a third party, the responsibilities of IEPs and IMEs are in some basic respects very similar to those of other physicians. IEPs and IMEs have the same obligations as physicians in other contexts to:

(1) Evaluate objectively the patient's health or disability. In order to maintain objectivity, IEPs and IMEs should not be influenced by the preferences of the patient-employee, employer, or insurance company when making a diagnosis during a work-related or independent medical examination.

(2) Maintain patient confidentiality as outlined by Opinion 5.09, "Industry Employed Physicians and Independent Medical Examiners."

(3) Disclose fully potential or perceived conflicts of interest. The physician should inform the patient about the terms of the agreement between himself or herself and the third party as well as the fact that he or she is acting as an agent of that entity. This should be done at the outset of the examination, before health information is gathered from the patient-employee. Before the physician proceeds with the exam, he or she should ensure to the extent possible that the patient understands the physician's unaltered ethical obligations, as well as the differences that exist between the physician's role in this context and the physician's traditional fiduciary role.

IEPs and IMEs are responsible for administering an objective medical evaluation but not for monitoring patients' health over time, treating patients, or fulfilling many other duties traditionally held by physicians. Consequently, a limited patient-physician relationship should be considered to exist during isolated assessments of an individual's health or disability for an employer, business, or insurer.

The physician has a responsibility to inform the patient about important health information or abnormalities that he or she discovers during the course of the examination. In addition, the physician should ensure to the extent possible that the patient understands the problem or diagnosis. Furthermore, when appropriate, the physician should suggest that the patient seek care from a qualified physician and, if requested, provide reasonable assistance in securing follow-up care. (I)

Issued December 1999 based on the report "Patient-Physician Relationship in the Context of Work-Related and Independent Medical Examinations," adopted June 1999.

Ariz. 2003 Employee appealed summary judgment and dismissal in malpractice action against a radiologist and x-ray company for failure to inform her of medical results that could have led to an earlier diagnosis of lung cancer. Employee was referred by her employer to the radiologist for a chest x-ray. The radiologist did not inform the employee of abnormalities noted in his report. Quoting Opinion 10.03, the appellate court held the physician had a duty to directly inform the employee of the results. The x-ray company was not liable however, since the radiologist was an independent contractor. *Stanley v. McCarver, 204 Ariz. 339, 63 P.3d 1076, 1081.*

N.J. 2001 Deceased patient's wife filed a medical malpractice action against a physician who conducted pre-employment screening. The physician failed to inform the deceased about a condition he discovered during the physical. The New Jersey Supreme Court reversed the lower courts and held that a physician under contract with a third party to perform pre-employment physicals has a non-delegable duty to inform the patient of any potentially serious medical conditions. The court quoted Opinion 10.03, expressing the view that, although this may not be a traditional physician-patient relationship, the physician still has a responsibility to inform the patient. *Reed v. Bojarski, 166 N.J.89, 764 A.2d 433, 444.*

(1) Physicians must keep their professional obligations to provide care to patients in accord with their prerogative to choose whether to enter into a patient-physician relationship.

(2) The following instances identify the limits on physicians' prerogative:

    (a) Physicians should respond to the best of their ability in cases of medical emergency (Opinion 8.11, "Neglect of Patient").

    (b) Physicians cannot refuse to care for patients based on race, gender, sexual orientation, or any other criteria that would constitute invidious discrimination (Opinion 9.12, "Patient-Physician Relationship: Respect for Law and Human Rights"), nor can they discriminate against patients with infectious diseases (Opinion 2.23, "HIV Testing").

    (c) Physicians may not refuse to care for patients when operating under a contractual arrangement that requires them to treat (Opinion 10.015, "The Patient-Physician Relationship"). Exceptions to this requirement may exist when patient care is ultimately compromised by the contractual arrangement.

(3) In situations not covered above, it may be ethically permissible for physicians to decline a potential patient when:

    (a) The treatment request is beyond the physician's current competence.

    (b) The treatment request is known to be scientifically invalid, has no medical indication, and offers no possible benefit to the patient (Opinion 8.20, "Invalid Medical Treatment").

    (c) A specific treatment sought by an individual is incompatible with the physician's personal, religious, or moral beliefs.

(4) Physicians, as professionals and members of society, should work to assure access to adequate health care (Opinion 10.01, "Fundamental Elements of the Patient-Physician Relationship").* Accordingly, physicians have an obligation to share in providing charity care (Opinion 9.065, "Caring for the Poor") but not to the degree that would seriously compromise the care provided to existing patients. When deciding whether to take on a new patient, physicians should consider the individual's need for medical service along with the needs of their current patients. Greater medical necessity of a service engenders a stronger obligation to treat. (I, VI, VIII, IX)

Issued December 2000 based on the report "Potential Patients, Ethical Considerations," adopted June 2000.

Updated December 2003.

* Considerations in determining an adequate level of health care are outlined in Opinion 2.095, "The Provision of Adequate Health Care."

American Medical Association
Relevant Bylaws

1.00 Membership

1.11 Active Constituent.

1.111 Admission. A person eligible for active constituent membership in the American Medical Association becomes a member of the AMA upon certification by the secretary of the constituent association to the Executive Vice President of the AMA, provided there is no disapproval by the Council on Ethical and Judicial Affairs. The Council may consider information pertaining to the character, ethics, professional status and professional activities of the applicant. The Council shall provide by rule for an appropriate hearing procedure to be provided to the applicant.

1.12 Active Direct.

1.121 Admission. Active direct members are admitted to membership upon application to the Executive Vice President of the American Medical Association, provided that there is no disapproval by the Council on Ethical and Judicial Affairs. The Council may consider information pertaining to the character, ethics, professional status and professional activities of the applicant. The Council shall provide by rule for an appropriate hearing procedure to be provided to the applicant.

1.1212 Objections. Objections to applicants for active direct membership must be received by the Executive Vice President of the American Medical Association within forty-five (45) days of receipt by the constituent association of the notice of the application for such membership. All objections will immediately be referred to the Council on Ethical and Judicial Affairs for prompt disposition pursuant to the rules of the Council on Ethical and Judicial Affairs.

1.13 Affiliate Members. Persons who belong to one of the following classes may become affiliate members:
a. Physicians in foreign countries who have attained distinction in medicine and who are members of their national medical society or such other medical organization as will verify their professional credentials.
b. American physicians located in foreign countries or in possessions of the United States who are engaged in medical missionary, educational or philanthropic endeavors.

c. Dentists who hold the degree of D.M.D. or D.D.S. who are members of the American Dental Association and their state and local dental societies.

d. Pharmacists who are active members of the American Pharmaceutical Association.

e. Teachers of medicine or of the sciences allied to medicine who are citizens of the United States and are ineligible for active membership.

f. Individuals engaged in scientific endeavors allied to medicine and others who have attained distinction in their fields of endeavor but who are not eligible for other categories of membership.

1.131   Admission. Membership is conferred by majority vote of the House of Delegates following nomination by the Council on Ethical and Judicial Affairs. Nominations for d, e, and f must also be approved by the appropriate component and constituent medical society. The election of affiliate members shall take place at a time recommended by the Committee on Rules and Credentials and approved by the House of Delegates.

1.15   International Members.

1.151   Admission. International members are admitted to membership upon application to the Executive Vice President of the American Medical Association, provided that the completed application is accompanied by the required documentation. The Council on Ethical and Judicial Affairs shall provide by rule for an appropriate hearing procedure to be provided to the applicant should denial of membership be based upon information pertaining to the applicant's character, ethical conduct or professional status.

1.20   Maintenance of Membership.
A member may hold only one type of membership in the American Medical Association at any one time. Membership may be retained only as long as the member complies with the provisions of the Constitution and Bylaws and Principles of Medical Ethics of the AMA.

1.40   Termination of Membership.
Upon official notification to the American Medical Association that an active constituent member is not in good standing in a constituent association, such member shall cease to be a member of the AMA, subject to the member's right of appeal as provided in 1.613.

1.60   Discipline.

1.61   Active Constituent Members.

1.611 The Council on Ethical and Judicial Affairs, after due notice and hearing may censure, suspend or expel an active constituent member from the American Medical Association for an infraction of the Constitution or these Bylaws, for a violation of the Principles of Medical Ethics, or for unethical or illegal conduct.

1.612 In addition to the disciplinary action referred to in 1.611, active constituent members may be subject to the following disciplinary actions:

1.6121 Actions under the constitution and bylaws of the component society and constituent association to which the member belongs.

1.6122 A request from the constituent association to which a member belongs for the AMA to take disciplinary action.

1.6123 A request by the AMA to the constituent association to which the member belongs to consent to disciplinary proceedings by the AMA.

1.613 Appeals.

1.6131 All disciplinary actions by a component society or a constituent association against a member may be appealed to the Council on Ethical and Judicial Affairs of the American Medical Association on questions of law and procedure only, but not on questions of fact.

1.62 All Other Members.

1.621 The Council on Ethical and Judicial Affairs, after due notice and hearing, may censure, suspend or expel any active direct, affiliate, honorary or international member of the AMA for an infraction of the Constitution or these Bylaws, for a violation of the Principles of Medical Ethics, or for unethical or illegal conduct.

2.00   House of Delegates

2.7162 Opinions and Reports of the Council on Ethical and Judicial Affairs. The Council on Ethical and Judicial Affairs issues opinions and reports. Opinions will be considered informational and filed. Motions are in order to extract an opinion, and request that the Council reconsider or withdraw the opinion. Reports may be adopted, not adopted or referred, and may be amended for clarification only with the concurrence of the Council.

6.00   Councils of the American Medical Association

6.01   Commencement of Term. Members of Councils of the American Medical Association who are elected by the House of Delegates pursuant to the provisions of these Bylaws shall assume office immediately upon their election. Members of Councils of the AMA who are appointed shall assume office as provided in the Bylaws.

6.011   Term of Resident/Fellow Physician or Medical Student Member. A resident/fellow physician or medical student member of a Council of the

AMA who graduates from a Liaison Committee on Medical Education or American Osteopathic Association accredited program, or completes an approved residency program within 90 days prior to an Annual Meeting shall be permitted to serve on the Council until the completion of the Annual Meeting. Service on a Council as a resident/fellow physician or medical student member shall not be counted in determining maximum Council tenure.

6.02   Rules and Regulations. Each Council shall select a Chair and Vice Chair or Chair-Elect and may adopt such rules and regulations as it deems necessary and appropriate for the conduct of its affairs, subject to approval by the Board of Trustees.

6.04   Reports and Referrals.

> **6.041   Information and Recommendations.** All Councils of the AMA have a continuing duty to provide information and to submit recommendations to the House of Delegates, through the Board of Trustees, on matters relating to the areas of responsibility assigned to them under the provisions of these Bylaws.

> **6.042   Method of Reporting.** Councils of the AMA, with the exception of the Councils on Ethical and Judicial Affairs and Legislation, shall submit their reports to the House of Delegates through the Board of Trustees. The Board of Trustees may make such non-binding recommendations regarding the reports to the Councils as it deems appropriate, prior to transmitting the reports to the House of Delegates without delay or modification by the Board. The Board may also submit written recommendations regarding the reports to the House of Delegates.

> **6.043   Method of Referral.** Referrals from the House of Delegates to a Council or Councils of the AMA shall be made through the Board of Trustees. The Board may, in addition, refer the matter to such other councils as it deems appropriate.

6.40   Council on Ethical and Judicial Affairs.

> **6.401   Authority.** The Council on Ethical and Judicial Affairs is the judicial authority of the American Medical Association and its decision shall be final.

> **6.402   Functions.** The functions of the Council on Ethical and Judicial Affairs are:

> > **6.4021** To interpret the Principles of Medical Ethics of the American Medical Association through the issuance of Opinions;

6.4022 To interpret the Constitution, Bylaws and rules of the Association;

6.4023 To investigate general ethical conditions and all matters pertaining to the relations of physicians to one another or to the public, and make recommendations to the House of Delegates or the constituent associations through the issuance of Reports or Opinions;

6.4024 To receive appeals filed by applicants who allege that they, because of sex, color, creed, race, religion, disability, ethnic origin, national origin, sexual orientation or age, or for any other reason unrelated to character or competence have been unfairly denied membership in a component and/or constituent association, to determine the facts in the case, and to report the findings to the House of Delegates. If the Council determines that the allegations are indeed true, it shall admonish, censure, or in the event of repeated violations, recommend to the House of Delegates that the constituent and/or component association involved be declared to be no longer a constituent and/or component member of the AMA;

6.4025 To request that the President appoint investigating juries to which it may refer complaints or evidence of unethical conduct which in its judgment are of greater than local concern. Such investigative juries, if probable cause for action be shown, shall submit formal charges to the President, who shall appoint a prosecutor to prosecute such charges against the accused before the Council on Ethical and Judicial Affairs in the name and on behalf of the AMA. The Council may acquit, admonish, suspend or expel the accused; and

6.4026 To approve applications and nominate candidates for affiliate membership as otherwise provided for in 1.131 of these Bylaws.

6.403 Original Jurisdiction. The Council on Ethical and Judicial Affairs shall have original jurisdiction in:

6.4031 All questions involving membership as provided in 1.111, 1.121, 1.131, 1.151, 1.611, and 1.62 of these Bylaws.

6.4032 All controversies arising under this Constitution and Bylaws and under the Principles of Medical Ethics to which the American Medical Association is a party.

6.4033 Controversies between two or more state associations or their members and between a constituent association and a component society or societies of another state association or associations or their members.

6.404 **Appellate Jurisdiction.** The Council on Ethical and Judicial Affairs shall have appellate jurisdiction in questions of law and procedure but not of fact in all cases which arise:

a. Between a constituent association and one or more of its component societies.

b. Between component societies of the same constituent association.

c. Between a member or members and the component society to which the member or members belong following an appeal to the member's constituent association.

d. Between a member and the component society or the constituent association to which the member belongs regarding disciplinary action taken against the member by the society or association.

e. Between members of different component societies of the same constituent association following a decision by the constituent association.

6.4041 **Appeal Mechanisms.** Notice of appeal shall be filed with the Council on Ethical and Judicial Affairs within thirty (30) days of the date of the decision by the component society or the constituent association and the appeal shall be perfected within sixty (60) days thereof; provided, however, that the Council on Ethical and Judicial Affairs, for what it considers good and sufficient cause, may grant an additional thirty (30) days for perfecting the appeal.

6.405 **Membership.** The Council on Ethical and Judicial Affairs shall consist of nine active members of the American Medical Association, including one resident/fellow physician member and one medical student member. Members elected to the Council on Ethical and Judicial Affairs shall resign all other positions held by them in the AMA upon their election to the Council. No member, while serving on the Council on Ethical and Judicial Affairs, shall be a delegate or an alternate delegate to the House of Delegates, or a General Officer of the AMA, or serve on any other council, committee or as representative to or Governing Council member of a Section of the AMA.

6.4051 **Limit on Medical Student Participation.** The medical student member of the Council shall have the right to participate fully in the work of the Council, including the right to make motions and vote on policy issues, elections, appointments, or nominations conducted by the Council, except that in disciplinary matters and in matters relating to membership the medical student member shall participate only if a medical student is the subject of the disciplinary matter or is the applicant for membership.

6.406 **Nomination and Election.** The full-term members of the Council shall be elected by the House of Delegates on nomination by the President-Elect who assumes the office of President at the conclusion of the meeting. State medical associations, national medical specialty societies, Sections of the AMA, and other organizations represented in the AMA House of

Delegates, and members of the Board of Trustees may submit the names and qualifications of candidates for consideration by the President-Elect.

6.407   Term. Members of the Council on Ethical and Judicial Affairs shall be elected by the House of Delegates for the following terms of office:

6.4071 The medical student member of the Council shall be elected for a term of two years. If the medical student member ceases to be enrolled in a Liaison Committee on Medical Education or American Osteopathic Association accredited program at any time prior to the expiration of the term for which the medical student member was elected, the service of such medical student member on the Council shall thereupon terminate, and the position shall be declared vacant.

6.4072 The resident/fellow physician member of the Council shall be elected for a term of three years provided that if the resident/fellow physician member ceases to be a participant in an approved training program at any time prior to the expiration of the term for which the resident/fel low physician member was elected, the service of such resident/fellow physician member on the Council shall thereupon terminate, and the position shall be declared vacant. The resident/fellow physician member shall have the right to vote in all matters in which the member participates under the rules of the Council.

6.4073 All other members of the Council shall be elected by the House of Delegates for a term of seven years, so arranged that at each Annual Convention the term of one member shall expire.

6.408   Tenure. Members of the Council on Ethical and Judicial Affairs may serve only one term, except that the resident/fellow physician member and the medical student member shall be eligible to serve for two terms. A member elected to serve an unexpired term shall not be regarded as having served a term unless such member has served at least half of the term.

6.409   Vacancies.

6.4091 Members Other than the Resident/Fellow Physician Member. Any vacancy among the members of the Council on Ethical and Judicial Affairs other than the resident/fellow physician member shall be filled at the next meeting of the House of Delegates. The new member shall be elected by the House of Delegates, on nomination by the President, for the remainder of the unexpired term.

6.4092 Resident/Fellow Physician Member. If the resident/fellow physician member of the Council is unable, for any reason, to complete the term for which he or she was elected, the remainder of the term shall be deemed to have expired. The successor shall be elected by the House of Delegates at the next Annual Meeting, on nomination by the

President, for a term to expire at the conclusion of the third Annual Meeting of the House of Delegates following the meeting at which the resident/fellow physician was elected.

Glossary of Terms

Council on Ethical and Judicial Affairs Opinions: Interpretations of the Principles of Medical Ethics on matters of (1) ethical principles or (2) social policy which involves issues of morality in the practice of medicine. Opinions establish standards of honorable conduct for physicians and cannot be amended by the House of Delegates. The Council may be requested by the House of Delegates to reconsider an opinion, but it is not required to do so. Unless withdrawn by the Council on Ethical and Judicial Affairs, Opinions of the AMA are published as Current Ethical Opinions in the AMA Policy Compendium and in the AMA *Code of Medical Ethics*.

Council on Ethical and Judicial Affairs Reports: Reports of the Council on Ethical and Judicial Affairs may be prepared in response to a resolution or on an issue of importance to physicians and may include recommendations for action by the House of Delegates. Recommendations in reports of the Council may be adopted, not adopted, or referred by the House of Delegates but cannot be amended without the concurrence of the Council. If adopted, the recommendations are included in the Policy Compendium.

Preface to the Rules of the Council on Ethical and Judicial Affairs

Professionalism generally is defined according to three key elements: the expertise that is acquired by a professional through specialized training; the committment to providing services of value to others; and self-regulation, which often leads to the establishment of a code of conduct. These characteristics, which engender public trust, clearly pertain to the medical profession and have been embodied in many of the activities of the American Medical Association since it was established in 1847.

The Council on Ethical and Judicial Affairs, and its predecessors, has been instrumental in defining the elements of medical professional integrity by establishing standards of ethical conduct and by encouraging physicians to uphold these standards. The Council's work also includes the review of physician misconduct on the basis of our AMA's *Principles of Medical Ethics* and possible action against membership in the A ssociation. These activities help fulfill the responsibility a profession holds in preserving professional integrity by establishing, as well as enforcing, standards of conduct. By conferring membership only upon those physicians who uphold the values of medical ethics and professionalism, the AMA assumes a leading role in demonstrating that the medical profession considers self-regulation a paramount responsibility.

General Rules of the Council on Ethical and Judicial Affairs

Rule I. Administration

A. **Meetings.** The Council on Ethical and Judicial Affairs will meet during the Annual and Interim Meetings of the American Medical Association. Other meetings of the Council may be called, on reasonable notice, by the Chair of the Council; or they shall be called, on reasonable notice, by the Executive Vice President of the American Medical Association on the written request of at least five members of the Council.

B. **Chair and Vice-Chair.** At the reorganization meeting of the Council which shall be held during each Annual Meeting of the AMA after election of members to the Council, the Council on Ethical and Judicial Affairs shall elect a chair and a vice-chair from among its members except that the resident physician and medical student members of the Council shall not be eligible to serve as chair or vice-chair. The chair and the vice-chair shall retain the right to vote on all matters. No member of the Council shall serve more than two consecutive years as chair or two consecutive years as vice-chair.

The chair and vice-chair to be so elected shall be elected on separate, secret ballots. The balloting and voting for chair shall be completed and a chair elected before the balloting and voting for the vice-chair begins. A majority vote of the entire Council shall be required to so elect either a chair or a vice-chair, with balloting and voting to be repeated, if necessary, until a member is elected to each position.

In the event that the position of chair becomes permanently vacant for any reason during the term of the then currently serving chair, the then currently serving vice-chair shall immediately assume the position of chair for the remainder of the term. A new vice-chair shall then be elected by secret ballot at the ensuing meeting of the Council to serve the remainder of the immediately preceding vice-chair's term. A majority vote of the entire Council, as then constituted, shall be required to so elect a vice-chair, with balloting and voting to be repeated, if necessary, until a member is elected vice-chair. The serving of the balance of a term as chair or vice-chair due to such a vacancy shall not be counted in determining whether a member of the Council has served more than two consecutive years as chair or two consecutive years as vice-chair.

In the event that the position of vice-chair becomes permanently vacant for any reason during the term of the then currently serving vice-chair, a new vice-chair shall be elected by secret ballot at the ensuing meeting of the Council to serve the remainder of the immediately preceding vice-chair's term. A majority vote of the entire Council, as then constituted, shall be required to so elect a vice-chair, with balloting and voting to be repeated, if necessary, until a member is elected vice-chair. The serving of the balance of a term as vice-chair due to such a vacancy shall not be counted in determining whether a member of the Council has served more than two consecutive years as vice-chair.

C. **Student Members.** The medical student member of the Council shall participate as a regular member in the interpretation of the Principles of Medical Ethics of the American Medical Association, the interpretation of the Constitution, Bylaws and rules of the Association, and the investigation of general ethical conditions and all matters pertaining to the relations of physicians to one another or to the public. The medical student member of the Council shall have the right to participate in disciplinary matters and in matters relating to membership only if a medical student is the subject of the disciplinary matter or is the applicant for membership.

D. **Quorum.** A majority of the members of the Council on Ethical and Judicial Affairs eligible to vote on a matter shall constitute a quorum and shall be required to adopt any action.

E. **Confidentiality.** All matters under consideration for adoption by the Council shall be treated as confidential until adopted by the Council.

Rule II. Applications for Membership

A. **Active Membership.** Applications for membership in the American Medical Association will be considered by the Council on Ethical and Judicial Affairs at any meeting upon presentation of the applications by the Executive Vice President of the Association.

B. **Affiliate Membership.** Applications for affiliate membership submitted by (1) physicians in foreign countries who have attained distinction in medicine and who are members of the national medical society or such other organization as will verify their professional credentials, (2) American physicians located in foreign countries or possessions of the United States and engaged in medical missionary, educational, or philanthropic endeavors, (3) dentists who hold the degree of DDS or DMD, who are members of the American Dental Association and their state and local dental societies, (4) pharmacists who are active members of the American Pharmaceutical Association, (5) teachers of medicine or of the sciences allied to medicine who are citizens of the United States and are ineligible for active or associate membership, or (6) individuals engaged in scientific endeavors allied to medicine and others who have attained distinction in their fields of endeavor who are not otherwise eligible for membership, may be considered at any meeting of the Council on presentation of the applications by the Executive Vice President of the Association. The Council will consider and approve only those applications which are accompanied by a statement of a responsible and qualified individual attesting to the requirements set forth above. (Employees of the AMA or any AMA affiliate or subsidiary may be eligible affiliate members under subsection (6). They must have five years of employment at the AMA, affiliate, or subsidiary and their distinction in their field of endeavor must be certified by an AMA Senior Vice President, or if the employee is a Senior Vice President, the Executive Vice President.)

C. **Refusal of Approval.** An applicant for membership in the American Medical Association whose application has not been approved by the Council on Ethical and Judicial Affairs will be promptly notified of such fact.

Rule III. Physicians Denied Membership in Component or Constituent Associations

Pursuant to 6.4024 of the Bylaws, any physician whose application for membership in a component and/or constituent association has allegedly been denied unfairly because of color, creed, race, religion, ethnic origin, national origin, or sex may appeal to the Council on Ethical and Judicial Affairs. The Council shall determine the facts in the case and report the findings to the House of Delegates. If the Council determines that the allegations are indeed true, it shall admonish, censure, or, in the event of repeated violations, recommend to the House of Delegates that the state association involved be declared to be no longer a constituent member of the American Medical Association.

Proceedings for such determination shall be initiated by a written statement. Such statement shall: (1) identify the parties to the case, (2) show that the appellant has exhausted remedies made available by the constitution and bylaws of the component society and the state association, and (3) include a concise factual resume of the case in sufficient detail to enable the Council to ascertain the facts. The appellant should also furnish such other information as may be requested by or helpful to the Council in determining the facts.

Rule IV. Original Controversies

Original proceedings before the Council on Ethical and Judicial Affairs shall be initiated by a written statement. Such statement shall include information (1) identifying the parties to the controversy, including membership affiliations, if applicable, and (2) explaining the nature of the controversy, setting forth the provisions of the Constitution, Bylaws, Rules, or Principles of Medical Ethics concerned.

Rule V. Appeals

Appellate proceedings before the Council on Ethical and Judicial Affairs shall be perfected by a written statement of appeal. Such statement shall include information (1) identifying the parties to the case and indicating membership affiliations when appropriate, (2) showing that the appellant has exhausted remedies made available by the constitution and bylaws of the component society and the state association, and (3) describing the error of law or procedure which is believed to have occurred during the proceedings. The statement shall also include a concise, factual resume of the case. Appellant shall submit with the statement the charges, complaints, findings, opinions, and decisions previously entered in the case.

Rule VI. Interpretation of the Constitution, Bylaws, Rules, and Principles of Medical Ethics of the American Medical Association

A. **Requests for Interpretation.** Requests for interpretation of the Constitution, Bylaws, Rules, or Principles of Medical Ethics of the Association shall be in writing and shall describe the matter to be interpreted in sufficient detail to enable the members of the Council on Ethical and Judicial Affairs to evaluate the request in all its aspects.

B. **Interpretations Initiated by the Council.** The Council on Ethical and Judicial Affairs on, its own motion, may render an opinion concerning the interpretation or application of the Constitution, Bylaws, Rules, or Principles of Medical Ethics of the Association and may, on its own motion, consider and decide the constitutionality and validity of all rules and regulations adopted by Councils and Committees of the Association pursuant to the Bylaws of the Association.

C. **Discretionary Power.** The Council on Ethical and Judicial Affairs may, in its own discretion, refuse to consider requests for interpretation of the Principles of Medical Ethics which in the opinion of the Council should be resolved by a component society or a state association. Requests for interpretation of the Principles of Medical Ethics which are not of national interest and relate to the observance of local customs and ideals may be readdressed to the component society or constituent association primarily responsible for knowledge of the requirements of such local customs and recognized ideals.

Rule VII. Jurisdiction

The Council on Ethical and Judicial Affairs may, on its own motion or on the motion of any party, determine the question of jurisdiction at any stage of the proceedings.

Rule VIII. Additional Statements and Record

After a statement has been submitted to the Council on Ethical and Judicial Affairs with the intention of initiating an action, all other parties in interest shall have the right to submit a statement on their behalf. Such statement shall be filed within thirty (30) days after the filing of the initiating statement unless additional time is granted by the Council.

The Council on Ethical and Judicial Affairs may thereafter require the parties to submit such transcripts of testimony, records, written statements supporting their contentions, or other material as the Council may deem necessary.

Rule IX. Hearings

A. **Notice of Hearings.** The Council may in its discretion determine whether a hearing is necessary or advisable. The Council will designate the time and place for all hearings, giving reasonable notice thereof to all parties.

B. **Attendance.** Attendance at hearings may be limited to the members of the Council on Ethical and Judicial Affairs, the staff, witnesses, if any, the parties, and counsel, who may speak in their behalf. Should any party to the controversy fail to appear, the Council may in its discretion continue, dismiss, or decide the matter.

C. **Evidence and Argument.** The Council on Ethical and Judicial Affairs will not be bound by technical rules of evidence usually employed in legal proceedings but may accept any evidence it deems appropriate and pertinent.

   In any appeal case, the review, if any, of the evidence will be limited to the evidence presented in the proceedings before the component society and constituent association or appropriate committee, board, or group thereof, provided, however, that in the event the Council is of the opinion such evidence is inadequate to determine the question of law or procedure presented, the Council, on its own motion or on the suggestion of any party, may require the production of additional evidence before the Council or refer the matter to the appropriate body for additional evidence.

   In matters other than appeal cases, the Council will grant the parties the right to present evidence to the extent the Council believes appropriate to the particular matter in controversy.

   In all hearings, the Council, within reasonable limitations, will allow oral argument.

D. **Record.** In hearings of original controversies, appeals, and in other proceedings, a transcript may be made at the discretion of the Council.

Rule X. Opinions

All opinions or decisions of the Council on Ethical and Judicial Affairs shall be in writing. Copies of the opinion or decision and the dissent, if any, will be filed as a part of the record and furnished to all the parties involved.

Rule XI. Filing and Copies

Ten (10) copies of all documents shall be submitted to the Secretary of the Council on Ethical and Judicial Affairs. One copy of each document shall be submitted at the same time to each of the other parties to the controversy.

Rule XII. AMA Membership Applications

A. **Bylaw Sections.** Section 1.121 of the AMA Bylaws provides that Active Direct members shall be admitted to membership upon application to the Executive Vice President of the AMA, provided that there is no disapproval by the AMA Council on Ethical and Judicial Affairs. Section

1.1212 of the AMA Bylaws provides that objections to applicants for Active Direct Membership will be referred to the Council for prompt disposition pursuant to the rules of the Council. Section 1.111 of the AMA Bylaws provides that Active Constituent members shall be admitted to membership upon certification by the secretary of the constituent association to the Executive Vice President of the AMA provided that there is no disapproval by the AMA Council on Ethical and Judicial Affairs.

B. **Initial Review.** In reviewing applications for AMA membership, the Council on Ethical and Judicial Affairs shall consider information contained in the application, information from other available sources and objections raised in response to notification of the state medical association or associations in the jurisdiction or jurisdictions in which the applicant practices. The Council may consider information pertaining to the character, ethics, professional status, and professional activities of the applicant. Any significant misstatements or omissions from the application shall constitute cause for denial of AMA membership. Once the Council or its staff receives a membership application, the Council shall retain jurisdiction to decide whether the applicant qualifies for AMA membership, notwithstanding an attempt by the applicant to withdraw the application.

C. **Initial Notice of Possible Denial.** Following review of the application for AMA membership and related information, the applicant shall be notified of any allegations, which if true, would justify denial of AMA membership. The applicant shall have thirty (30) days following receipt of the notice in which to file a written response. Failure of the applicant to respond within the thirty (30) day period waives any further consideration of the application. The Council on Ethical and Judicial Affairs shall consider any written response and determine whether additional information is needed to dispose of the matter in a fair and equitable manner.

D. **Subsequent Notice.** If additional information is needed to resolve disputed issues of fact or the Council on Ethical and Judicial Affairs finds cause for disapproving an application, the applicant shall be notified in writing of the disputed issues of fact or reasons for disapproval and shall have thirty (30) days following receipt of the notice to request a hearing. Failure to request a hearing within the thirty (30) day period waives any further consideration of the application.

E. **Notice of Hearing.** If the applicant submits a written request for a hearing, the Council on Ethical and Judicial Affairs shall notify the applicant of the date, place, and time of the hearing and shall provide the applicant with a copy of these rules. Notice shall also be sent to anyone who submitted written objections to AMA membership by the applicant, informing that person of the right, within seven (7) days after the date of the notice, to request to appear at their own expense to present evidence in support of the objections or refute evidence presented by the applicant. No objector shall have the right to cross-examine the applicant or any witnesses.

F. **Hearing Procedure.** The Council on Ethical and Judicial Affairs shall not be bound by technical legal rules of evidence and may accept any evidence or information deemed reliable or relevant. The applicant shall not be required to, but may be accompanied by legal counsel and either the applicant or legal counsel may cross-examine any witnesses who appear in opposition to the applicant's application for AMA membership.

G. **Transcript.** If a written transcript is made of the hearing, any party requesting a copy shall have it made available at his or her own expense.

H. **Decision.** The Council on Ethical and Judicial Affairs shall, within thirty (30) days after the hearing, notify the applicant and anyone who appeared at the hearing of its decision.

I. **Reapplication.** If the decision is to deny membership, the applicant may reapply for membership after one year following the date of the decision.

Rule XIII. Discipline

Section 1.20 of the Bylaws provides that a member may retain membership only as long as the provisions of the Constitution and Bylaws and Principles of Medical Ethics of the American Medical Association are complied with. Sections 1.621, 6.401, and 6.4022 of the Bylaws provide that the Council on Ethical and Judicial Affairs, after due notice and hearing, may censure, place on probation, suspend, or expel any active direct, associate, affiliate, or honorary member of the AMA for an infraction of the Constitution and Bylaws or for a violation of the Principles of Medical Ethics of the AMA. Section 1.611 provides that the Council on Ethical and Judicial Affairs, after due notice and hearing, may censure, suspend, or expel an active constituent association for an infraction of the Constitution and Bylaws or for a violation of the Principles of Medical Ethics of the AMA. In addition, the AMA may take disciplinary action with respect to an active constituent member's AMA membership (1) when a state medical association to which a member belongs requests the AMA to take such action; or (2) when, at the request of the AMA, a state association to which the member belongs consents to such action. Section 6.4025 of the Bylaws provides that the Council on Ethical and Judicial Affairs may request the President of the Association to appoint investigating juries to which the Council may refer complaints or evidences of unethical conduct which, in its judgment, are of greater than local concern. The following Rules of Procedure, respecting notice of charges and the conduct of hearings before the Council, are based upon these Sections of the Bylaws.

A. **Statement of Charges.** The statement of charges shall allege in writing an infraction of the AMA's Constitution or Bylaws or a violation of the Principles of Medical Ethics of the AMA.

B. **Notice.** A copy of the statement of charges shall be sent to the member by registered or certified mail.

C. **Answer.** The member shall have sixty (60) days after receipt of the notice to file a written answer. The Council on Ethical and Judicial Affairs shall consider any written response and determine whether additional information is needed to dispose of the matter in a fair and equitable manner. Failure of the member to respond within the sixty (60) day period shall constitute an admission of the allegations.

D. **Hearings.** Where additional information is needed to resolve disputed issues of fact or in cases where the Council on Ethical and Judicial Affairs finds cause for censuring, suspending, or expelling a member, the member shall be notified in writing of the disputed issues of fact or reasons for censure, suspension, or expulsion and shall have thirty (30) days following receipt of the notice to request a hearing. Failure to request a hearing within the thirty (30) day period waives the right to a hearing on the matter.

If the member submits a written request for a hearing, the Council on Ethical and Judicial Affairs shall notify the applicant of the date, place, and time of the hearing and shall provide the member with a copy of these rules. The member shall receive not less than thirty (30) days notice of the hearing. Notice shall also be sent to any state medical association to which an active constituent member belongs that has requested or consented to disciplinary action by the AMA; and such notice shall inform the state medical association of its right, within seven (7) days after the date of the notice, to request to appear at its own expense to present evidence in support of its allegation or refute evidence presented by the active constituent member, but the state medical association shall have no right to cross-examine the active constituent member or any witnesses.

The Council on Ethical and Judicial Affairs shall not be bound by technical legal rules of evidence and may accept any evidence or information deemed reliable or relevant. The General Counsel of the American Medical Association or her or his designee shall present the evidence against the member and may question the parties or their witnesses. The member shall not be required to, but may be accompanied by legal counsel and either the member or the member's legal counsel may cross-examine any witnesses who appear.

A written transcript shall be made of the hearing; any person requesting a copy shall have it made at his or her own expense.

E. **Decision**. The Council on Ethical and Judicial Affairs shall, within thirty (30) days after the hearing, notify the member of its decision and the reasons for any adverse decision. If the decision is to expel a member, he or she may reapply for membership after one year has elapsed from the date of the decision.

F. **Jurisdiction**. Upon issuance of the statement of charges to the respondent, the AMA shall retain jurisdiction to resolve the disciplinary process initiated by the statement of charges. The right of the AMA to discipline the respondent physician shall not be limited by the respondent physician's termination of or failure to renew membership in the AMA or a constituent organization.

Rules of the Council on Ethical and Judicial Affairs in Original Jurisdiction Cases

Preamble

6.4025 of the Bylaws provides that the Council on Ethical and Judicial Affairs may request the President of the Association to appoint investigating juries to which the Council may refer complaints or evidences of unethical conduct which, in its judgment, are of greater than local concern.

The following Rules of Procedure, respecting notice of charges, and the conduct of hearings before the Council on Ethical and Judicial Affairs are based upon this section of the Bylaws.

Investigating Jury

At the request of the Council on Ethical and Judicial Affairs, the President has appointed an investigating jury. Complaints or evidence of unethical conduct of greater than local concern will be submitted to this jury by the Council.

Institution of Proceedings

If after investigation a probable cause for action is shown, the investigating jury shall submit a statement of charges to the President. The President shall submit to the Council on Ethical and Judicial Affairs the statement of charges presented to him or her by the investigating jury for prosecution in the name and on behalf of the American Medical Association.

Statement of Charges

The statement of charges shall allege in writing an infraction of the AMA's Constitution or Bylaws or a violation of the Principles of Medical Ethics of the AMA. Exhibits may be attached.

Notice

A copy of the statement of charges shall be sent to the respondent physician by personal delivery or by registered or certified mail.

Answer

The respondent physician shall have thirty (30) days after personal delivery or mailing of the notice of statement of charges to file a written answer. If the respondent physician fails to file a written answer, the allegations shall be considered to be admitted.

Proceedings

The Chair of the Council on Ethical and Judicial Affairs shall designate one or more members of the Council to conduct a hearing on the statement of charges. This member or these members shall be known as the Hearing Officer.

Hearings shall be held at such reasonable time and place, designated by the Hearing Officer, as may be consistent with the nature of the proceedings and the convenience of the parties. The parties shall receive not less than fifteen (15) days of notice of the hearing.

The General Counsel of the American Medical Association or his or her designee shall prosecute the charges against the respondent physician.

Attendance at hearings may be limited to the members of the Council on Ethical and Judicial Affairs, the staff, witnesses, if any, the parties, and counsel who may speak in their behalf.

The Hearing Officer or his counsel may question the parties and their witnesses. The Hearing Officer shall not be bound by technical rules of evidence usually employed in legal proceedings but may accept any evidence deemed appropriate and pertinent.

Should any party to the controversy fail to appear at the hearing, the Hearing Officer may, in his or her discretion, continue, dismiss, or proceed with the hearing.

Findings and Conclusions

At the conclusion of the hearing, the Hearing Officer shall render a report in writing containing findings and conclusions and recommendations, if any. This report, together with a transcript of the proceedings, shall be submitted to the Council on Ethical and Judicial Affairs. A copy of the report shall be mailed to all parties of record.

Written Objections

Any party to the proceedings may submit written objections to the report to the Council on Ethical and Judicial Affairs. These objections must be submitted within twenty-one (21) days after the report has been submitted by the Hearing Officer to the Council on Ethical and Judicial Affairs.

Oral Argument

In addition to written objections, any party may request an opportunity to present oral arguments on its objections to the report of the Hearing Officer before the Council on Ethical and Judicial Affairs. This request must be made within twenty-one (21) days after the report has been submitted to the

Council. The granting of oral arguments shall be discretionary with the Council. If granted, the parties shall be notified by the Council of the place and date for such oral argument; all parties shall be given opportunity to be heard, and the time allotted to argument may be limited by the Council with due regard to the magnitude and complexities of the issues involved.

If any party fails to appear, the Council may continue or proceed with the oral argument.

Final Decision

The Council on Ethical and Judicial Affairs, including the member or members who serve as the Hearing Officer, shall render a final decision. A copy of that decision shall be mailed or otherwise served upon all parties.

Disciplinary Action

The Council on Ethical and Judicial Affairs shall have the authority to acquit, admonish, censure, or place on probation the accused physician or suspend or expel him or her from AMA membership as the facts may justify. This action shall be in accordance with the authority vested in the Council by 1.60, 6.401, and 6.402 of the Bylaws.

Transcript

A written transcript shall be made of the proceedings and of the oral argument before the Council on Ethical and Judicial Affairs.

If any party to the controversy requests a copy of the transcript, it shall be made available to the party at the party's expense.

Filing of Copies

Ten (10) copies of all pleadings and exhibits shall be submitted to AMA Headquarters to the Chairman of the Council on Ethical and Judicial Affairs. One copy of each document shall be submitted at the same time to each of the other parties to the controversy.

Index to Opinions

geographic priorities (transplants) - 2.16
managed care allocations, restrictions - 8.13
organ recipient selection - 2.16
organ transplants - 2.16, 2.169
racial disparities - 9.121
scarce, allocation - 2.03
society's role - 10.01
unnecessary services - 2.19, 4.04, 8.03, 8.032
xenotransplantation guidelines - 2.169
Health worker safety, *see* Occupational health
Healthy behaviors (patient responsibilities) - 10.02
Hearing rights, *see* Due process
Heart failure, do-not-resuscitate orders - 2.22
Hematopoietic stem cells, *see* Stem cells
Heredity, *see* Genetics
HIV, *see* Human immunodeficiency virus (HIV)
Home health care, conflict of interest - 8.035
Home infusion companies - 8.032
Homosexuality
artificial insemination for couples - 2.04
discrimination - 9.03, 9.12, 10.05
Honesty - Principle II
health care fraud and abuse - 9.132
patient information - 8.12
Hospice care - 2.211
Hospital privileges, *see* Medical staff
Hospitals and health facilities, *see also* Ethics
committees; Medical staff
accreditation - 9.01
admission fee - 4.01
billing for housestaff, student services - 4.03
compulsory assessments - 4.02
contractual relations with physicians - 4.06
divestment requirements, physician-owned
facilities - 8.032
ethics committees - 9.11
ethics consultations - 9.115
governing board and organized medical staff -
4.05
high-quality, low-priced facilities - 8.032
non-competition covenants for trainees - 9.021
peer review - 9.10
physician-owned facilities - 8.032
referrals, fee splitting - 6.03
referrals to in-hospital diagnostic and
therapeutic services - 8.032
reporting impairment, incompetence, unethical
conduct - 9.031
research review committees - 8.031
Housestaff, *see* Medical staff
Human cloning, *see* Cloning, human
Human genes, *see* Genes; Genomics; Genetics
Human genome, *see* Genome
Human immunodeficiency virus (HIV)
artificial insemination - 2.04, 2.05
confidentiality in autopsy reports - 5.057
infected patients - 9.131, 10.05
notification of third parties - 2.23
testing and refusal to be tested - 2.23
Human rights
respect for - 9.12
torture - 2.067

Human subjects
clinical investigation guidelines - 2.07
consent to experimental drugs or procedures,
2.07
DNA databanks in genomic research - 2.079
human cloning for research - 2.146
international research - 2.077
placebo controls - 2.075, 2.076
poor, disadvantaged - 2.071
selection, clinical trials - 2.071
surgical "placebo" controls - 2.076
unethical experiments - 2.30
Human tissue, commercial use - 2.08
Human umbilical cord blood, *see* Umbilical cord
blood

Illegal activities, *see* Fraud and abuse; Law
Immunization, medical record retention - 7.05
Impaired drivers, *see* Automobiles
Impaired physicians - 8.15, 9.031
In vitro fertilization, *see* Reproductive medicine
Incentives, financial, *see* Financial incentives and
interests
Incompetence, mental, *see* Mental competence
Incompetent colleagues - Principle II, 9.031
Independent medical examinations, *see* Physical
examinations
Indigent care - 9.065
fundamental elements - 10.01
physician obligations to those in need - 8.055
potential patients - 10.05
retainer practices - 8.055
Industry, *see* Drugs and devices
Infants
anencephalic, organ donors - 2.162
quality of life - 2.17
seriously ill newborns, treatment decisions -
2.215
Infectious diseases - 9.13, 10.05; *see also* Human
immunodeficiency virus (HIV)
patient responsibilities - 10.02
xenotransplantation guidelines - 2.169
Informed consent
artificial insemination - 2.04, 2.05
assisted reproductive technology - 2.055
carrier screening of genetic disorders - 2.137
circumstances detrimental to patients - 8.08
clinical investigation guidelines - 2.07
cloning to produce children - 2.147
commercial use of human tissue - 2.08
conflicts of interest in clinical trials - 8.0315
court-initiated treatment in criminal cases -
2.065
direct-to-consumer drug advertising - 5.015
DNA databanks in genomic research - 2.079
ethics consultations - 9.115
fetal research guidelines - 2.10
fetal tissue transplantation - 2.161
fetal umbilical cord blood - 2.165
filming patients - 5.045, 5.046
gene therapy - 2.11
genetic engineering, gene replacement - 2.13

signing bonuses - 9.037
Resource allocation, *see* Health resources
Respect, *see* Patient-physician relationship
Respiratory failure, do-not-resuscitate orders - 2.22
Restraints - 8.17
Restrictive covenants, *see* Contracts
Retainer practices - 8.055
Retirement - 7.03
Risk disclosure, *see* Informed consent
Romantic relations, *see* Sexual misconduct;
    Sexual relationships

Safety, impaired drivers - 2.24
Sale of practice, *see* Practice sales
Scarce resources, *see* Health resources
Scientific investigation, *see* Research
Scientific knowledge, advancement - Principle V
Screening, genetic, *see* Genetic testing
Second opinions - 8.04
Security, *see* Confidentiality
Self-referral - 8.032
    divestment requirements, physician-owned
        facilities - 8.032
    high-quality, low-priced facilities - 8.032
    home health care conflict of interest - 8.035
    home infusion or dialysis centers - 8.032
    in-hospital diagnostic and therapeutic services -
        8.032
    lab sharing and (clarification of opinion) - 8.032
    optical services - 8.032
    pharmacies - 8.032, 8.06
    physical therapists employed by physicians -
        8.032
Self-regulation, *see also* Physician colleagues
    AMA council's appellate function - 9.04
    disciplinary actions - 1.01, 2.055, 9.04, 9.05
    gifts to physicians from industry - 8.061
    peer review - 9.10
Self-treatment - 8.19
Semen, frozen, *see* Reproductive medicine
Sex-linked inheritable diseases - 2.04, 2.05
Sex selection, artificial insemination - 2.04, 2.05
Sexual harassment, *see* Sexual misconduct
Sexual misconduct - 8.14
    supervisors and trainees - 3.08
Sexual orientation - 9.03, 9.12, 10.05
Sexual relationships
    key third parties - 8.145
Sexually transmitted diseases (minors' care) - 5.055
Signing bonuses, *see* Financial incentives and
    interests
Social policy - 1.01, 2.00-2.30; *see also* Health
    resources; Policy making
Social worth - 2.03
Societies, medical, *see* Medical societies
Socioeconomic conditions, *see also* Indigent care
    policy making - 2.09, 2.095
    poor, disadvantaged persons as research subjects
        - 2.071
    provision of adequate care - 2.095
Somatic cell nuclear transfer technology - 2.146,
    2.147

Somatic cell therapy - 2.11
Specialties, medical
    court-initiated treatment in criminal cases - 2.065
    negotiating discounts - 8.052
Specialty societies, *see* Medical societies
Sperm donors, *see* Reproductive medicine
Sponsors, educational - 8.061, 9.011
Sports medicine - 3.06
Spouse abuse, *see* Abuse, domestic
Staff privileges, *see* Medical staff
Stem cells
    hematopoietic - 2.165
    human cloning for biomedical research - 2.146
Stock ownership, *see* Financial incentives and
    interests
Stop-loss, *see* Costs
Strikes - 9.025
Students, medical, *see also* Education
    disputes between supervisors and trainees -
        9.055
    hospital billing for services - 4.03
    informing family of patient's death - 8.18
    involvement in patient care - 8.087
    performing procedures on fellow students - 3.09
    refusal to participate in procedures on fellow
        students - 3.09
    self-identification to patients - 8.087
Subsidies (gifts from industry) - 8.061
Substance abuse - 8.15
    confidentiality in minors' care - 5.055
    impaired drivers - 2.24
    reporting impaired colleagues - 9.031
Substituted judgment, *see* Decision making
Suicide, physician-assisted - 2.211
Supervisors, *see* Education
Surgery
    assistants - 6.10
    co-management - 8.043
    delegation of tasks - 8.16
    patenting instruments - 9.09
    placebo controls - 2.076
    second opinions - 8.041
    substitution of surgeons - 8.16
Surrogate decision makers, *see* Decision making
Surrogate mothers, *see* Pregnancy

Teaching physicians, *see* Education; Faculty,
    medical
Teenagers, *see* Adolescents
Telecommunications
    advisory, referral services - 5.025
    diagnosis by - 5.025
    drug prescribing - 5.025
    electronic mail - 5.026, 5.027
    online health-related sites - 5.027
Telephones, advisory, referral services - 5.025
Tenure, *see* Faculty, medical
Terminally ill patients, *see also* Death
    advance directives - 2.225
    do-not-resuscitate orders - 2.22, 2.225
    euthanasia - 2.21
    futile care - 2.035, 2.037

Table of Cases

A Woman's Choice-East Side Women's Clinic v. Newman, 305 F.3d 684 (7th Cir. 2002) [8.08].

Aiken v. Business and Indus. Health Group, Inc., 886 F. Supp. 1565 (D. Kan. 1995) [I].

Allen v. Smith, 368 S.E.2d 924 (W. Va. 1988) [IV].

Amaral v. Saint Cloud Hospital, 598 N.W.2d 379 (Minn. 1999) [V].

American Medical Ass'n v. FTC, 638 F.2d 443, (2nd Cir. 1980), aff'd, 455 US 676 (1982) [5.02, 8.05].

American Medical Ass'n v. United States, 130 F.2d 233 (D.C. Cir. 1942), aff'd, 317 US 519 (1943) [8.05].

American Optometric Ass'n v. F.T.C., 626 F.2d 896 (D.C. Cir. 1980) [5.02].

Anderson v. Bd. of Trustees of Caro Community Hosp., 10 Mich. App. 348, 159 N.W.2d 347 (1968) [II; 9.031].

Anderson v. Florence, 288 Minn. 351, 181 N.W.2d 873 (1970) [II; 8.12].

Arizona State Bd. of Medical Examiners v. Clark, 97 Ariz. 205, 398 P.2d 908 (1965) [III, VII; 3.01, 8.11, 9.06].

Arlen v. State, 61 Ohio St. 2d 168, 399 N.E.2d 1251 (1980) [II, III; 8.06, 9.04].

Axtell Clinic v. Cranston, No. 56,745 (Kan. Ct. App. June 20, 1985) (LEXIS, States Library, Kan. file) [6.02, 6.03, 9.02].

Balian v. Board of Licensure in Medicine, 722 A.2d 364 (Me. 1999) [7.01, 7.02].

Bates v. State Bar of Ariz., 433 US 350 (1977) [5.02].

Bay Ridge Diagnostic Laboratory, Inc. v. Dumpson, 400 F. Supp. 1104 (E.D.N.Y. 1975) [8.03, 8.032, 8.06, 9.06].

Belin v. Dingle, 127 Md. App. 68, 732 A.2d 301 (1999) [8.16].

Berger v. Sonneland, 101 Wash. App. 141, 1 P.3d 1187 (2000) [IV].

Bernstein v. Alameda-Contra Costa Medical Ass'n, 139 Cal. App. 2d 241, 293 P.2d 862 (1st Dist. 1956) [II; 9.04, 9.07].

Best v. Taylor Machine Works, 179 Ill. 2d 367, 689 N.E. 2d 1057 (Ill. 1997) [IV; 5.05].

Biddle v. Warren General Hospital, 86 Ohio St. 3d 395, 715 N.E. 2d 518 (1999) [IV; 5.05].

Bloomington Urological Associates v. Scaglia, 292 Ill. App. 3d, 793, 686 N.E. 2d 389 (4th Dist. 1997) [8.11].

Boman v. Southeast Medical Services Group, 1998 WL 1182063 (Mass. Super. 1998) [6.02, 8.032].

Bouvia v. Superior Court, 179 Cal. App. 3d 1127, 225 Cal. Rptr. 297 (2d Dist. 1986) [2.20].

Bowman v. Beghin, 713 N.E.2d 913 (Ind. App. 1999) [8.08].

Brandt v. Medical Defense Assoc., 856 S.W.2d 667 (Mo. 1993) [IV; 5.05].

Bratt v. International Business Mach. Corp., 392 Mass. 508, 467 N.E.2d 126 (1984) [IV; 5.05, 5.09].

Brophy v. New England Sinai Hosp., Inc., 398 Mass. 417, 497 N.E.2d 626 (1986) [2.20].

Brown v. Bi-Lo, Inc, 354 S.C. 436, 581 S.E.2d 836 (2003) [IV].

Brown v. Warren, 858 So.2d 168 (Miss. App. 2003) [8.03, 8.05].

Bryant v. Hilst, 136 F.R.D. 487 (D. Kan. 1991) [IV; 5.05].

Bryson v. Tillinghast, 749 P.2d 110 (Okla. 1988) [IV; 5.05].

Cahill v. Rosa, 89 N.Y.2d 14, 24, 674 N.E.2d 274 651 N.Y.S.2d 344 (1996) [9.131].

Cal. Att'y Op. N. 98-104, 1998 WL 744399 [8.09].

Calvert v. Sharp, 748 F.2d 861, 863 (4th Cir. 1984), cert. denied, 471 US 1132 (1985) [VI].

Carson v. Fine, 123 Wash. 2d 206, 867 P.2d 610 (1994) [9.07].

Carter-Shields v. Alton Health Institute, 317 Ill. App. 3d 260, 739 N.E.2d 569 (5th Dist. 2000) vacated 201 Ill. 2d 441, 777 N.E.2d 948 (2002) [9.02, 9.06].

Castillo-Plaza v. Green, 655 So. 2d 197 (Fla. Dist. Ct. App. 1995) [II, IV; 5.05, 5.06, 5.08].

Chiropractic Coop. Ass'n v. AMA, 617 F. Supp. 264 (E.D. Mich. 1985), aff'd in part and rev'd in part, 867 F.2d 270 (6th Cir. 1989) [VI; 3.01, 3.04].

Chiropractic Coop. Ass'n v. AMA, 867 F.2d 270 (6th Cir. 1989) [VI; 3.01, 3.05, 3.04].

Chiropractic Coop. Ass'n v. AMA, 1986-2 Trade Cas. (CCH) & 67, 294 (E.D. Mich. 1986), aff'd in part and rev'd in part, 867 F.2d 270 (6th Cir. 1989) [VI; 3.01, 3.04].

Clayton v. Harkey, 826 So.2d 1283 (Miss. 2002) [8.03, 8.05].

Cleveland Hair Clinic, Inc. v. Puig, 968 F. Supp. 1227 (N.D. Ill. 1996) [7.03, 9.02].

Colby v. Schwartz, 78 Cal. App. 3d 885, 144 Cal. Rptr. 624 (2d Dist. 1978) [VI; 8.11, 9.06].

Compassion in Dying v. Washington, 79 F. 3d 790 (9th Cir. 1996), replacing, 49 F.3d 586 (9th Cir. 1995) [2.20, 2.21, 2.211].

Compassion in Dying v. Washington, 49 F.3d 586 (9th Cir. 1995), replaced, 79 F. 3d 790 (9th Cir. 1996) [2.211].

Conley v. Warren, 797 So. 2d 881 (Miss. 2001) [8.03, 8.05].

Corbett v. D'Alessandro, 487 So. 2d 368 (Fla. App. 1986) [IV; 2.20].

Corey v. Skelton, 834 So.2d 681 (Miss. 2003) [8.03, 8.05].

Couture v. Couture, 48 Ohio App. 3d 208, 549 N.E.2d 571 (1989) [2.20].

Crescenzo v. Crane, 350 N.J. Super. 531, 796 A.2d 283 (2002) [IV].

Crist v. Moffatt, 326 N.C. 326, 333, 389 S.E.2d 41 (1990) [IV; 5.05].

Cruzan v. Director, Missouri Department of Health, 497 US 261 (1990) [2.20].

Cruzan v. Harmon, 760 S.W.2d 408 (1988), aff'd, 497 US 261 (1990) [2.20].

Culbertson v. Mernitz, 602 N.E. 2d 98 (Ind. 1992) [8.08].

D.A.B v. Brown, 570 N.W. 2d 168 (Minn. App. 1997) [8.06].

Dade County Medical Ass'n v. Samartino, 213 So. 2d 627 (Fla. App. 1968) [5.02].

DeGrella v. Elston, 858 S.W.2d 698 (Ky. 1993) [2.20].

Delio v. Westchester County Medical Center, 134 Misc. 2d 206, 510 N.Y.S.2d 415 (Sup. Ct. 1986), rev'd, 129 A.D.2d 1, 516 N.Y.S.2d 677 (1987) [2.20].

Doe v. Roe, 93 Misc. 2d 201, 400 N.Y.S.2d 668 (Sup. Ct. 1977) [IV; 5.05].

Dominy v. Shumpert, 235 Ga. App. 500, 510 S.E.2d 81 (1998) [8.031].

Downey v. Weston, 451 Pa. 259, 301 A.2d 635 (1973) [IV; 5.05].

Dr. K. v. State Bd. of Physician Quality Assur., 98 Md. App. 103, 632 A.2d 453 (1993), cert. denied, 334 Md. 18, 637 A.2d 1191 (1994), and cert. denied, 115 S. Ct. 75, 130 L. Ed. 29 (1994) [II].

Dupree v. Malpractice Research, Inc., 179 Mich. App. 254, 445 N.W.2d 498 (1989) [6.01].

Duquette v. Superior Court, 161 Ariz. 269, 778 P.2d 634 (Ariz. Ct. App. 1989) [IV; 5.05].

Eli Lilly & Co. v. Marshall, 850 S.W.2d 155 (Tex. 1993) [V].

Emerich v. Philadelphia Center for Human Development, Inc., 554 Pa. 209, 720 A.2d 1032 (1999) [5.05].

Estate of Behringer v. Medical Ctr., 249 N.J. Super. 597, 592 A.2d 1251, 1268 (1991) [IV; 5.05, 9.13, 9.131].

Estate of Finkle, 90 Misc. 2d 550, 395 N.Y.S.2d 343 (Sur. Ct. 1977) [IV; 5.05, 7.04].

Estates of Morgan v. Fairfield Family Counseling Center, 77 Ohio St. 3d 284, 303, 673 N.E.2d 1311 (1997) [IV; 5.05].

Falcon v. Alaska Pub. Offices Comm'n, 570 P.2d 469 (Alaska 1977) [IV; 5.05].

Falcone v. Middlesex County Medical Soc'y, 62 N.J. Super. 184, 162 A.2d 324 (1960), aff'd, 34 N.J. 582, 170 A.2d 791 (1961) [VI; 3.01].

Faya v. Almaraz, 329 Md. 435, 620 A.2d 327 (1993) [9.13, 9.131].

Ferguson v. City of Charleston, 532 US 67, 121 S. Ct. 1281 (2001) [5.05].

Finucan v. Maryland State Board of Physicians Quality Assurance, 151 Md. App. 399, 827 A.2d 176 (2003) [8.14].

Fineman v. New Jersey Dept. of Human Servs., 272 N.J. Super. 606, 640 A.2d 1161 (App. Div. 1994), cert. denied, 138 N.J. 267, 649 A.2d 1287 (1994) [VI].

Forziati v. Board of Registration in Medicine, 333 Mass. 125, 128 N.E.2d 789 (1955) [II; 6.02].

Fosmire v. Nicoleau, 75 N.Y.2d 218, 551 N.E.2d 77, 551 N.Y.S.2d 876 (1990) [2.20].

Freeman v. Duluth Clinic, 334 N.W.2d 626 (Minn. 1983) [9.02].

Gadson v. Newman, 807 F. Supp. 1412 (C.D. Ill. 1992) [8.032].

Geisberger v. Willuhn, 72 Ill. App. 3d 435, 390 N.E.2d 945 (2d Dist. 1979) [IV; 5.05].

Gladieux v. Ohio State Medical Board, 1999 WL 770959 (Ohio App. 1999) [I, IV].

Goad v. Virginia Board of Medicine, 40 Va. App. 621, 580 S.E.2d 494 (2003) [3.08, 9.05].

Gomez v. Chua Medical Corp., 510 N.E.2d 191 (Ind. Ct. App. 1987) [9.02].

Grabowski v. Quigley, 454 Pa. Super. 27, 684 A.2d 610 (1996) [8.16].

Greenberg v. Miami Children's Hospital Research Institute, Inc., 264 F. Supp. 2d 1064 (S.D. Fla. 2003) [2.08].

Greisman v. Newcomb Hosp., 40 N.J. 389, 192 A.2d 817 (1963) [3.01].

Gromis v. Medical Board, 8 Cal. App. 4th 589, 10 Cal. Rptr. 2d 452 (1st Dist. 1992), reh'g denied, 1992 Cal. App. LEXIS 1047, and review denied, 1992 Cal. LEXIS 5101 [8.14].

Grossman v. Columbine Medical Group, Inc., 1999 WL 1024015 (Colo. App. 1999) [10.01].

Group Health Coop. v. King County Medical Soc'y, 39 Wash. 2d 586, 237 P.2d 737 (1951) [VI; 8.04, 8.05, 9.06].

Hague v. Williams, 37 N.J. 328, 181 A.2d 345 (1962) [IV; 5.05].

Hammonds v. Aetna Casualty & Sur. Co., 243 F. Supp. 793 (N.D. Ohio 1965) [IV; 5.08].

Harlan v. Lewis, 141 F.R.D. 107 (E.D. Ark. 1992) [5.05].

Health Sys. Agency v. Virginia State Bd. of Medicine, 424 F.Supp. 267 (E.D. Va. 1976) [5.02].

Heller v. Norcal Mutual Ins. Co., 8 Cal. 4th 30, 876 P.2d 999, 32 Cal. Rptr. 2d 200 (1994), cert. denied, 115 S. Ct. 669, 130 L. Ed. 2d 602 (1994) [5.05].

Hellman v. Board of Registration in Medicine, 404 Mass. 800, 537 N.E.2d 150 (1989) [IV].

Hiser v. Randolph, 126 Ariz. 608, 617 P.2d 774 (Ct. App. 1980) [VI; 8.11].

Homer v. Long, 90 Md. App. 1, 3 n.1, 599 A.2d 1193 (1992) [8.14].

Horn v. New York Times, 186 Misc. 2d 469, 719 N.Y.S. 2d 471 (Sup. Ct. 2000) [IV; 5.05, 5.09].

Horne v. Patton, 291 Ala. 701, 287 So. 2d 824 (1973) [IV; 5.05].

Hull v. Tate, No. 46443 (Okla. Ct. App. Apr. 16, 1974) (LEXIS States library, Okla. file), rev'd, No. 46443 (Okla. Sup. Ct. Oct. 29, 1974) (LEXIS, States library, Okla. file) [8.16].

In re AB, 196 Misc. 2d 940, 768 N.Y.S. 2d 256 (N.Y. Sup. 2003) [2.20, 2.215].

In re Capt. Wool, Inc., 1995 US Dist. LEXIS 20128 (E.D. Va. 1995) [8.032].

In re Conroy, 190 N.J. Super. 453, 464 A.2d 303 (1983), rev'd, 98 N.J. 321, 486 A.2d 1209 (1985) [2.17, 2.20].

In re Culbertson's Estate, 57 Misc. 2d 391, 292 N.Y.S.2d 806 (Surr. Ct. 1968) [7.01, 7.02, 7.03, 7.05].

In re Doe, 16 Phila. 229, 1987 Phila. Cty. Rptr. LEXIS 30 (1987) [2.20].

In re Doe, 411 Mass. 512, 583 N.E.2d 1263 (1992) [2.20].

In re Drabick, 200 Cal. App. 3d 185, 245 Cal. Rptr. 840 (6th Dist. 1988) [2.20].

In re Eli Lilly & Co., 142 F.R.D. 454 (S.D. Ind. 1992) [V].

In re Estate of Longeway, 133 Ill.2d 33, 549 N.E.2d 292 (1989) [2.20].

In re Farrell, 108 N.J. 335, 529 A.2d 404 (1987)
[2.20].

In re Fiori, 438 Pa. Super. 610, 652 A.2d 1350
(1995), app. granted, 655 A.2d 989 (Pa. 1995)
[2.20].

In re Gardner, 534 A.2d 947 (Me. 1987) [2.20].

In re Grant, 109 Wash. 2d 545, 747 P.2d 445
(1987) [2.20].

In re Jobes, 108 N.J. 394, 529 A.2d 434 (1987)
[2.20].

In re Lawrance, 579 N.E.2d 32 (Ind. 1991) [2.20].

In re Lifschutz, 2 Cal. 3d 415, 467 P.2d 557, 85 Cal.
Rptr. 829 (1970) [IV; 5.05].

In re Managed Care Litigation, 150 F. Supp. 2d 1330
(S.D. Fla. 2001) [8.053].

In re Milton S. Hershey Medical Ctr., 407 Pa. Super.
565, 595 A.2d 1290, 1295 (1991) [9.131].

In re Peter, 108 N.J. 365, 529 A.2d 419 (1987)
[2.20].

In re Prange, 166 Ill. App.3d 1091, 520 N.E.2d
946, vacated, 121 Ill. 2d 570, 527 N.E.2d 303
(1988) [2.20].

In re R.C., 775 P.2d 27 (Colo. 1989) [2.04, 2.05].

In re Rules Adoption, 224 N.J. Super. 252, 540 A.2d
212 (1988) [IV; 5.05].

In re Subpoena N. 22., Appeal of A.B., 709 A.2d
385 (Pa. Super. 1998) [5.05].

Johnson v. Blue Cross/Blue Shield, 677 F. Supp. 1112
(D.N.M. 1987) [VI; 3.01, 3.04].

Jones v. Fakehany, 261 Cal. App. 2d 298, 67 Cal.
Rptr. 810 (2d Dist. 1968) [5.02, 5.05, 6.08].

K.A.C. v. Benson, 1993 Minn. App. LEXIS 1201
(Minn. 1993) [9.13, 9.131].

Kaiser Foundation Health Plan, Inc. v. Zingale, 99
Cal. App. 4th 1018, 121 Cal. Rptr. 2d 741 (2002)
[8.135].

Karlin v. Weinberg, 148 N.J. Super. 243, 372 A.2d
616 (1977), aff'd, 77 N.J. 408, 390 A.2d 1161
(1978) [9.02].

Karlin v. Weinberg, 77 N.J. 408, 390 A.2d 1161
(1978) [9.02].

Kartell v. Blue Shield of Mass., Inc., 749 F.2d 922
(1st Cir. 1984), cert. denied, 471 US 1029 (1985)
[8.05].

Ketchup v. Howard, 247 Ga. App. 54, 543 S.E.2d
371 (2000) [8.08, 10.01].

Kirk v. Jefferson County Medical Soc'y, 577 S.W.2d
419 (Ky. Ct. App. 1978) [I, III].

Koefoot v. American College of Surgeons, 652 F.
Supp. 882 (N.D. Ill. 1986) [3.01].

Korper v. Weinstein, 57 Mass. App. 433, 783
N.E.2d 877 (2003) [8.14].

Krischer v. McIver, 697 So. 2d 97 (Fla. 1997)
[2.211].

Kunkel v. Walton, 179 Ill. 2d 519, 689 N.E. 2d
1047 (1997) [IV].

Kurdek v. West Orange Bd. of Educ., 222 N.J.
Super. 218, 536 A.2d 332 (1987) [IV; 5.05].

L.W. v. L.E. Phillips Career Dev. Ctr., 167 Wis. 2d
53, 482 N.W.2d 60 (1992) [2.20].

Lemon v. Stewart, 111 Md. App. 511, 523, 682
A.2d 1177 (Md. App. 1996) [9.131].

Lisa M. v. Henry Mays Newhall Memorial Hosp. 12
Cal. 4th 291, 907 P.2d 358, 48 Cal. Rptr. 510
(1995) [8.14].

Littleton v. Good Samaritan Hospital, 39 Ohio St. 3d
86, 529 N.E.2d 449 (1988) [IV; 5.05].

Loudon v. Mhyre, 110 Wash. 2d 675, 756 P.2d 138
(1988) [IV; 5.05].

Loui v. Board of Medical Examiners, 78 Haw. 21,
889 P.2d 705 (1995) [Preamble].

Lurch v. United States, 719 F.2d 333 (10th Cir. 1983),
cert. denied, 466 US 927 (1984) [8.03, 8.05].

Magan Medical Clinic v. California State Bd. of
Medical Examiners, 249 Cal. App. 2d 124, 57 Cal.
Rptr. 256 (2d Dist. 1967) [8.03, 8.032, 8.06].

Manion v. N.P.W. Medical Center of N.E. Pa., Inc.,
676 F.Supp. 585 (M.D. Pa. 1987) [IV; 5.05, 5.06,
5.07].

Marsingill v. O'Malley, 58 P.3d 495 (Alaska 2002)
[8.08].

Martin v. Baehler, 1993 Del. Super. LEXIS 199
(1993) [IV].

Maryland Att'y Gen. Op., 62 Op. Att'y Gen. 157 (1977) [IV; 2.02, 5.05].

Maryland Att'y Gen. Op. No. 89-022 (1989) [IV].

Maryland Att'y Gen. Op. No. 88-046, 73 Op. Att'y Gen. 162 (1988) [2.20].

Maryland Att'y Gen. Op. No. 86-030, 71 Op. Att'y. Gen. 407 (1986) [IV].

Matthies v. Mastromonaco, 160 N.J. 26, 733 A.2d 456 (1999) [8.08].

Maxey v. United States, 1989 US Dist. LEXIS 5827 (W.D. Ark. 1989) [VI].

McConnell v. Beverly Enterprises-Connecticut, Inc., 209 Conn. 692, 553 A.2d 596 (1989) [2.20].

McCormick v. England, 328 S.C. 627, 494 S.E. 2d 431 (Ct. App. 1997) [IV].

McHugh v. Audet, 72 F.Supp. 394 (M.D. Pa. 1947) [9.07].

McIntosh v. Milano, 168 N.J. Super. 466, 403 A.2d 500 (1979) [Preamble; I, IV; 5.05].

McMurray v. Johnson, 481 So. 2d 887 (Ala. 1985) [8.16].

Memphis Planned Parenhood v. Sundquist, 175 F.2d 456 (6th Cir. 1999) [2.015].

Mich. Att'y Gen. Opinion No. 5229, 1977-78 Att'y. Gen. Op. 234 (1977) [8.03, 8.032].

Mich. Att'y Gen. Opinion No. 5024, 1977-78 Att'y. Gen. Op. 299 (1978) [5.02].

Miller v. Meeks, 762 So. 2d 302 (Miss. 2000) [8.03, 8.05].

Missouri Att'y Gen. Op. N. 6 (July 8, 1982) (LEXIS, States Library, Mo. file) [8.06].

Modi v. West Virginia Board of Medicine, 465 S.E.2d 230 (W. Va. 1995) [8.08].

Montefiore Hosp. & Medical Center v. NLRB, 621 F.2d 510 (2d Cir. 1980) [VI].

Monturi v. Englewood Hosp., 246 N.J. Super. 547, 588 A.2d 408 (1991) [8.16].

Morrison v. Abramovice, 206 Cal. App. 3d 304, 309, 253 Cal. Rptr. 530, 533 (1988) [2.20].

Moses v. McWilliams, 379 Pa. Super. 150, 549 A.2d 950 (1988), appeal denied, 521 Pa. 630, 558 A.2d 532 (1989) [IV; 5.05, 5.07].

Ms. B. v. Montgomery County Emergency Service, Inc., 799 F. Supp. 534 (E.D. Pa. 1992) cert. denied, 114 S.Ct. 174 (1993) [5.05].

N.X. v. Cabrini Medical Center, 97 N.Y.2d 247, 765 N.E.2d 844, 739 N.Y.S.2d 348 (2002) [8.14].

Nash v. Wennar, 645 F.Supp. 238 (D. Vt. 1986) [I, IV; 8.05].

Neade v. Portes, 303 Ill. App. 3d 799, 710 N.E. 2d 418 (2d Dist. 1999) [8.132].

Nieto v. Kapoor, 268 F.3d 1208 (10th Cir. 2001) [I, IV]

Noble v. Sartori, 1989 Ky. App. LEXIS 67 (1989) [VI; 8.11].

Ohio Att'y Gen. Op. No. 99-044, 1999 WL 692 623 [8.03, 8.11, 8.13].

Ohio Urology, Inc. v. Poll, 72 Ohio. App. 446, 594 N.E.2d 1027 (1991) [VI; 6.11, 9.02, 9.06].

Ojeda v. Sharp Cabrillo Hosp., 8 Cal. App. 4th 1, 10 Cal. Rptr. 2d 230 (1992) [6.01].

Painter v. Abels, 998 P.2d 931 (Wyo. 2000) [2.07].

People v. Anyakora, 162 Misc. 2d 47, 616 N.Y.S.2d 149 (Sup. Ct. 1993) [VI].

People v. Griffin, 242 A.D.2d 70, 671 N.Y.S. 2d 34 (1998) [8.14].

People v. Kevorkian, 248 Mich. App. 373, 639 N.W.2d 291 (2001) [2.20, 2.21, 2.211].

People v. Stritzinger, 137 Cal. App. 3d 126, 186 Cal. Rptr. 750 (2d Dist. 1982), rev'd 34 Cal. 3d 505, 668 P.2d 738, 194 Cal. Rptr. 431 (1983) [IV; 2.02, 5.05].

Perna v. Pirozzi, 182 N.J. Super 510, 442 A.2d 1016 (1982), revd, 92 N.J. 446, 457 A.2d 431 (1983) [8.16].

Perna v. Pirozzi, 92 N.J. 446, 457 A.2d 431 (1983) [8.16].

Perreira v. State, 768 P.2d 1198 (Colo. 1989) [IV; 5.05].

Petrillo v. Syntex Laboratories, Inc., 148 Ill. App. 3d 581, 499 N.E.2d 952 (1st Dist. 1986), cert. denied, 483 US 1007 (1987) [II, IV; 5.05, 5.06, 5.07, 5.08].

Phoenix Orthopaedic Surgeons, Ltd. v. Peairs, 164 Ariz. 54, 790 P.2d 752 (Ct. App. 1989) [9.02].

Pierce v. Ortho Pharmaceutical Corp., 84 N.J. 58, 417 A.2d 505 (1980) [2.07].

Planned Parenthood League of Massachusetts, Inc. v. Attorney General, 424 Mass. 586, 677 N.E.2d 101, 107 (1997) [2.015].

Planned Parenthood of Central New Jersey v. Farmer, 165 N.J. 609, 762 A.2d 620 (2000) [2.015].

Planned Parenthood of Middle Tennessee v. Sundquist, 1998 WL 467110 (Tenn. App. 1998) [10.01].

Planned Parenthood v. Miller, 63 F.3d 1452 (8th Cir. 1995) [2.015].

Plastic Surgical Servs. of New England, P.C. v. Hall, 1993 WL 818637 (Mass. Super. 1993) [8.115].

Polo v. Gotchel, 225 N.J. Super. 429, 542 A.2d 947 (1987) [6.01].

Pons v. Ohio State Medical Bd., 66 Ohio St. 3d 619, 614 N.E.2d 748 (1993) [I, II, IV; 8.14].

Prairie Eye Center v. Butler, 329 Ill. App. 3d 293, 768 N.E.2d 414 (2002) [9.02].

Pryzbowski v. US Health Care, Inc., 64 F. Supp. 2d 361 (D.N.J. 1999) [8.13].

Quilico v. Kaplan, 749 F.2d 480 (7th Cir. 1984) [8.03, 8.05].

Rasmussen v. Fleming, 154 Ariz. 200, 741 P.2d 667 (Ct. App. 1986), aff'd in part and rev'd in part, 154 Ariz. 207, 741 P.2d 674 (1987) [2.20].

Rasmussen v. Fleming, 154 Ariz. 207, 741 P.2d 674 (1987) [2.20].

Reed v. Bojarski, 166 N.J.89, 764 A.2d 433 (2001) [10.03].

Reinninger v. Prestige Fabricators, Inc., 523 S.E. 2d 720 (N.C. App. 1999) [5.05].

Ritt v. Ritt, 98 N.J. Super. 590, 238 A.2d 196 (1967), rev'd, 52 N.J. 177, 244 A.2d 497 (1968) [IV; 5.05].

Rocca v. Southern Hills Counseling Center, Inc., 671 N.E. 2d 913 (Ind. App. 1996) [IV; 5.05].

Roe v. Wade, 410 US 113 (1973) [2.01].

Salt River Project v. Industrial Comm'n, 1992 Ariz. App. LEXIS 323, 129 Ariz. Adv. Rep. 39 (1992) [IV].

Sampson v. State, 31 P.3d 88 (Alaska 2001) [2.211].

San Juan-Torregosa v. Garcia, 80 S.W.3d 539 (Tenn. App. 2002) [2.20].

Scripps Clinic v. Superior Court, 108 Cal. App.4th 917, 134 Cal. Rptr. 2d 101 (2003) [VI, VIII].

Selkin v. State Board for Professional Medical Conduct, 63 F. Supp. 2d 397 (S.D.N.Y. 1999) [8.14].

Shankman v. Coastal Psychiatric Assoc., 258 Ga. 294, 368 S.E.2d 753 (1988) [9.02].

Singleton v. Norris, 319 F.3d 1018 (8th Cir. 2003) [2.06].

Singleton v. State, 437 S.E.2d 53 (S.C. 1993) [2.06].

Somoza v. St. Vincent's Hosp. & Medical Ctr. of New York, 192 A.D.2d 429, 596 N.Y.S.2d 789 (N.Y. App. Div. 1993) [9.12].

South Carolina Att'y Gen. Op. 1978 S.C. AG LEXIS 806 [7.01, 7.02, 7.03].

Sperry Rand Corp. v. Hill, 356 F.2d 181 (1st Cir.), cert. denied, 384 US 973 (1966) [5.02].

Spock v. Pocket Books, Inc., 48 Misc. 2d 812, 266 N.Y.S.2d 77 (Sup. Ct. 1965) [II; 5.02].

Springdale Diagnostic Clinic v. Northwest Physicians, 2003 Ark. App. LEXIS 697 (2003) [7.03].

Stanley v. McCarver, 204 Ariz. 339, 63 P.3d 1076 (2003) [10.03].

State ex. rel. Kitzmiller v. Henning, 437 S.E.2d 452 (W.Va. 1993) [IV; 5.05].

State ex. rel. Stufflebam v. Appelquist, 694 S.W.2d 882 (Mo. App. 1985) overuled by State ex. rel. Woytus v. Ryan, 776 S.W.2d 389 (Mo. 1989) [IV; 5.05].

State ex. rel. Woytus v. Ryan, 776 S.W.2d 389 (Mo. 1989) [IV; 5.05].

State v. Agacki, 226 Wis. 2d 349, 595 N.W. 2d 31 (1999) [5.05].

State v. AMA, 1981-2 Trade Cas. (CCH) & 64,195 (1981) [V, VI; 3.04, 3.07].

State v. Johnson, 968 S.W.2d 123 (Mo. 1998) [IV].

State v. Naramore, 25 Kan. App. 2d 302, 965 P.2d 211 (1998) [2.20, 2.22].

State v. Perry, 610 So. 2d 746 (La. 1992) [2.06].

Steele v. Hamilton County Cmty. Mental Health Bd., 90 Ohio St. 3d 176, 736 N.E.2d 10 (2000) [I].

Steeves v. United States, 294 F. Supp. 446 (D.S.C. 1968) [V; 8.04].

Steinberg v. Jensen, 186 Wis. 2d 237, 519 N.W.2d 753 (Ct. App. 1994), rev'd, 194 Wis. 2d 440, 534 N.W.2d 361 (1995) [IV; 5.05].

Steinberg v. Jensen, 194 Wis. 2d 440, 534 N.W.2d 361 (1995) [IV; 5.05].

Stempler v. Speidell, 100 N.J. 368, 495 A.2d 857 (1985), cert. denied, 483 US 1007 (1987) [IV; 5.05].

Stewart v. Midani, 525 F. Supp. 843 (N.D. Ga. 1981) [VI].

Stidham v. Clark, 74 S.W.3d 719 (Ky. 2002) [5.05].

Stigliano v. Connaught Labs., Inc., 140 N.J. 305, 658 A.2d 715 (1995) [9.07].

Sullivan v. Washington, 768 So. 2d 881 (Miss. 2000) [8.03, 8.05].

Swafford v. Harris, 967 S.W.2d 319 (Tenn. 1998) [6.01, 9.07].

Tarasoff v. Regents of Univ. of Cal., 17 Cal.3d 425, 551 P.2d 334, 131 Cal. Rptr. 14 (1976) [IV; 5.05].

Taylor v. Albert Einstein Medical Ctr., 723 A.2d 1027 (Pa. Super. 1998) [8.12, 8.16].

Thompson v. Sun City Community Hosp., Inc., 141 Ariz. 597, 688 P.2d 605 (1984) [VI].

Total Care Physicians v. O'Hara, 2002 Del. Super. LEXIS 493 (2002) [7.01, 7.03].

Treister v. American Academy of Orthopaedic Surgeons, 78 Ill. App. 3d 746, 396 N.E.2d 1225 (1st Dist. 1979) [9.05].

Trevino v. Ortega, 41 Tex. Sup. 907, 969 S.W.2d 950 (1998) [7.05].

United States v. Neufeld, 908 F. Supp. 491 (S.D. Ohio 1995) [3.04].

United States v. Weston, 134 F. Supp. 2d 115 (D.D.C. 2001) [2.06].

Utah Att'y Gen. Op. No. 77-294 (Feb. 15, 1978) [IV; 5.05].

Va. Att'y Gen. Op., 1994 Va. AG LEXIS 12 (1994) [2.06].

Va. Att'y Gen. Op., 1990 Va. AG LEXIS 63 (1990) [2.20].

Vacco v. Quill, 117 S. Ct. 2293, 138 L. Ed. 2d 834 (US 1997) [2.20, 2.211].

Valley Medical Specialists v. Farber, 194 Ariz. 363, 982 P.2d 1277 (1999) [9.02, 9.06].

Vassiliades v. Garfinckel's, Brooks Bros., 492 A.2d 580 (D.C. App. 1985) [IV; 5.05].

Washington v. Glucksberg, 117 S. Ct. 2258, 138 L. Ed. 2d 772 (US 1997) [2.211].

Webb v. Jarvis, 575 N.E.2d 992 (Ind. 1991) [Preamble].

Weiss v. Cigna Healthcare, Inc., 972 F. Supp. 748 (S.D.N.Y. 1997) [8.13].

Weiss v. York Hosp., 745 F.2d 786 (3d Cir. 1984), cert. denied, 470 US 1060 (1985) [3.01].

Wenninger v. Muesing, 307 Minn. 405, 240 N.W.2d 333 (1976) [IV; 5.05].

Wilk v. American Medical Association, 895 F.2d 352 (7th Cir. 1990) [3.01].

Wilk v. American Medical Association, 671 F.Supp. 1465 (N.D. Ill. 1987), aff'd, 895 F.2d 352 (7th Cir. 1990) [3.01].

Wilk v. American Medical Association, 735 F.2d 217 (7th Cir. 1983), cert. denied, 467 US 1210 (1984) [3.01].

Wilk v. American Medical Association, 719 F.2d 207 (7th Cir. 1983), Cert. denied, 467 US 1210 (1984) [3.01].

Wisconsin Att'y Gen. Op. 10-87 (Mar. 16, 1987), (LEXIS, States library, Wis. file) [IV; 2.02, 5.05].

Wood v. Upjohn Co., No. 6093-1-II (Wash. Ct. App. Sept. 4, 1984) (LEXIS, States library, Wash. file) [VI].

Wright v. Wasudev, 1994 Tenn. App. LEXIS 657 (1994) [IV; 5.05].

Yates v. El-Deiry, 160 Ill. App. 3d 198, 513 N.E.2d 519 (3d Dist. 1987) [IV; 5.05].

Table of Articles

Bard, *The Diagnosis is Anencephaly and the Parents Ask About Organ Donation: Now What? A Guide for Hospital Counsel and Ethics Committees*, 21 W. New Eng. L. Rev. 49, 62 (1999) [2.162].

Barnes, Rango, Burke, & Chiarello, *The HIV-Infected Health Care Professional: Employment Policies and Public Health*, 18 Law, Med. & Health Care 311, 314, 315 (1990) [9.131].

Baron, *Why Withdrawal of Life-Support for PVS Patients Is Not a Family Decision*, 19 Law, Med. & Health Care 73 (1991) [2.20].

Baron, Bergstresser, Brock, Cole, Dorfman, Johnson, Schnipper, Vorenberg, & Wanzer, *A Model State Act to Authorize and Regulate Physician-Assisted Suicide*, 33 Harv. J. Legis. 1, 2, 7 (1996) [2.20, 2.211].

Baum, *"To Comfort Always": Physician Participation in Executions*, 5 N.Y.U. J. Legis. & Pub. Pol'y 47, 56-57 (2001) [2.06].

Beane, *AIDS Crisis and the Health Care Community: Public Concerns Triggering Questionable Private Rights of Action for Emotional Harms and Legislative Response*, 45 Mercer L. Rev. 633, 669 (1994) [9.13, 9.131].

Beard, *The Impact of Changes in Health Care Provider Reimbursement Systems on the Recovery of Damages for Medical Expenses in Personal Injury Suits*, 21 Am. J. Trial Advoc. 453, 484 (1998) [6.11].

Beckwith & Peppin, *Physician Value Neutrality: A Critique*, 28 J. L. Med. & Ethics 67, 72-73 (2000) [2.01, 2.02, 8.032, 8.05, 8.08, 8.132].

Befort, *Pre-Employment Screening and Investigation: Navigating Between a Rock and a Hard Place*, 14 Hofstra Lab. L. J. 365, 391 (1997) [2.132].

Begg, *Revoking the Lawyers' License to Discriminate in New York: The Demise of a Traditional Professional Prerogative*, 7 Geo. J. Legal Ethics 275, 298, 299 (1993) [VI; 9.12, 9.131].

Bell, *Non-heart Beating Organ Donation: Old Procurement Strategy—New Ethical Problems*, 29 J. Med. Ethics 176, 181 (2003) [2.155, 2.162].

Bellacosa, *The Fusion of Medicine and Law for In Extremis Health and Medical Decisions: Does It Produce Energy and Light or Just Cosmic Debris?*, 18 Bull. Am. Acad. Psychiatry Law 5, 9 (1990) [2.20].

Benesch, *Disability Discrimination in the Health Care Workplace*, 9 Trends in Health Care, Law & Ethics 45, 46 (Summer 1994) [9.131].

Bennett, *Inclusion of Women in Clinical Trials—Policies for Population Subgroups*, 329 New Eng. J. Med. 288, 289 (1993) [9.122].

Bennett, *When Is Medical Treatment Futile?*, 9 Issues in Law & Med. 35, 39 (1993) [2.22].

Benson, *The Social Control of Human Biomedical Research: An Overview and Review of the Literature*, 29 Soc. Sci. Med. 1 (1989) [2.07].

Berg, *Ethics and E-Medicine*, 46 St. Louis U. L.J. 61, 66 (2002) [8.062, 8.063].

Berg, *Grave Secrets: Legal and Ethical Analysis of Postmortem Confidentiality*, 34 Conn. L. Rev. 81, 87, 117 (2001) [5.051, 7.02].

Berg, *Understanding Waiver*, 40 Hous. L. Rev. 281, 329 (2003) [8.08].

Berger, *Patient Confidentiality in a High Tech World*, 5 J. Pharmacy & L., 139, 141 (1996) [5.05].

Berger & Rosner, *Ethical Challenges Posed by Dementia and Driving*, 11 J. Clinical Ethics 304, 307, 308 (2000) [2.24].

Berger & Rosner, *The Ethics of Practice Guidelines*, 156 Arch. Intern. Med. 2051, 2053, 2056 (1996) [8.13].

Bernat, *Quality of Neurological Care: Balancing Cost Control and Ethics*, 54 Arch. Neurol. 1341, 1343, 1345 (1997) [8.032, 8.13].

Bernstein, *Out of the Frying Pan and Into the Fire: The Expert Witness Problem in Toxic Tort Litigation*, 10 Rev. Litigation 117, 143 (1990) [9.07].

Berrol, *Considerations for Management of the Persistent Vegetative State*, 67 Arch. Phys. Med. Rehabil. 283 (1986) [2.20].

Blair, *Lifting the Genealogical Veil: The Blueprint for Legislative Reform of the Disclosure of Health-Related Information in Adoption*, 70 No. Carolina L. Rev. 681, 692 (1992) [IV].

Bobinski, *Autonomy and Privacy: Protecting Patients from Their Physicians*, 55 U. Pitt. L. Rev. 291, 302, 313 (1994) [8.03, 8.15, 9.13].

Bobinski, *Patients and Providers in the Courts: Fractures in the Americans with Disabilities Act*, 61 Alb. L. Rev. 785, 790, 806 (1998) [9.131].

Bobinski & Epps, *Women, Poverty, Access to Health Care, and the Perils of Symbolic Reform*, 5 J. Gender, Race & Just. 233, 238 (2002) [9.122].

Bodenheimer & Grumbach, *Capitation or Decapitation: Keeping Your Head in Changing Times*, 276 JAMA 1025, 1031 (1996) [8.13].

Bond, *Diverse and Perverse Incentives In Managed Care: Where Will the Pendulum Stop?*, 1 Widener L. Symp. J. 141, 151, 154 (1996) [8.13].

Booker, *Physicians, Malpractice, and State Lines: A Guide to Personal Jurisdiction in Medical Malpractice Lawsuits*, 20 J. Legal Med. 385, 394 (1999) [5.02].

Boozang, *Death Wish: Resuscitating Self-Determination for the Critically Ill*, 35 Ariz. L. Rev. 23, 24, 28, 52 (1993) [2.22, 8.08].

Boozang, *Is the Alternative Medicine? Managed Care Apparently Thinks So*, 32 Conn. L. Rev. 567, 606 (2000) [II].

Bopp & Coleson, *The Constitutional Case Against Permitting Physician-Assisted Suicide for Competent Adults With Terminal Conditions*, 11 Issues in Law & Med. 239, 250 (1995) [2.211].

Botkin, *Prenatal Diagnosis and the Selection of Children*, 30 Fla. St. U. L. Rev. 265, 289 (2003) [2.12].

Bowser, *Eliminating Racial and Ethnic Disparities in Medical Care*, 30 Brief 24, 25 (Summer 2001) [9.121].

Bowser, *Racial Profiling in Health Care: An Institutional Analysis of Medical Treatment Disparities*, 7 Mich. J. Race & L. 79, 119 (2001) [9.121].

Boyle, *Managed Care in Mental Health: A Cure, or a Cure Worse Than the Disease?*, 40 St. Louis U. L. J. 437, 448 (1996) [8.13].

Brann, *Utah's Medical Malpractice Prelitigation Panel: Exploring State Constitutional Arguments Against a Nonbinding Inadmissible Procedure*, 2000 Utah L. Rev. 359, 399-400 (2000) [9.122].

Brennan, *Ensuring Adequate Health Care for the Sick: The Challenge of the Acquired Immunodeficiency Syndrome as an Occupational Disease*, 1988 Duke L. J. 29 (1988) [VI].

Brennan, *Transmission of the Human Immunodeficiency Virus in the Health Care Setting—Time for Action*, 324 New Eng. J. Med. 1504, 1505, 1506 (1991) [9.131].

Brock, *Voluntary Active Euthanasia*, 22 Hastings Center Rep. 10 (March/April 1992) [2.20, 2.21].

Brody, *Ethical Questions Raised by the Persistent Vegetative Patient*, 18 Hastings Center Rep. 33 (Feb./March 1988) [2.20].

Brody, *New Perspectives on Emergency Room Research*, 27 Hastings Center Rep. 7, 9 (Jan./Feb. 1997) [2.07].

Brody, *Special Ethical Issues in the Management of PVS Patients*, 20 Law, Med. & Health Care 104, 109 (1992) [2.20, 2.22].

Brody, *The Physician as Professional and the Physician as Honest Businessman*, 119 Arch. Otolaryngol. Head Neck Surg. 495, 496 (1993) [6.11].

Brooks, Smith, & Anderson, *Medical Apartheid: An American Perspective*, 266 JAMA 2746, 2748 (1991) [9.121].

Brown-Cranstoun, *Kringen v. Boslough and Saint Vincent Hospital: A New Trend for Healthcare Professionals Who Treat Victims of Domestic Violence?* 33 J. Health L. 629, 649, 650 (2000) [2.02].

Brownrigg, *Mother Still Knows Best: Cancer-Related Gene Mutations, Familial Privacy, and a Physician's Duty to Warn*, 26 Fordham Urb. L. J. 247 (1999) [IV].

Bruening, Andrew, & Smith, *Concurrent Care: An Ethical Issue for Family Physicians*, 36 J. Fam. Practice 606, 607 (1993) [Preamble].

Brunetti, Weiss, Studenski, & Clipp, *Cardiopulmonary Resuscitation Policies and Practices: A Statewide Nursing Home Study*, 150 Arch. Intern. Med. 121, 122 (1990) [2.20, 2.22].

Bruns & Wolman, *Morality of the Privacy of Genetic Information: Possible Improvements of Procedures*, 19 Med. Law 127, 129 (2000) [2.132].

Buchanan, *Medical Ethics at the Millennium: A Brief Retrospective*, 26 Colo. Law. 141, 142, 143, 144, 145 (1997) [5.05, 5.057, 7.01, 8.115, 8.12, 8.13, 9.12, 9.131, 10.01].

Buckles, *Electronic Formulary Management and Medicaid: Maximizing Economic Efficiency and Quality of Care in the Age of Electronic Prescribing*, 11 U. Fla. J. L. & Pub. Pol'y 179, 182-83 (2000) [8.135].

Bulleit & Krause, *Kickbacks, Courtesies, or Cost-Effectiveness?: Application of the Medicare Antikickback Law to the Marketing and Promotional Practices of Drug and Medical Device Manufacturers*, 54 Food & Drug L. J. 279, 296 (1999) [8.061].

Burman, *Lawyers and Domestic Violence: Raising the Standard of Practice*, 9 Mich. J. Gender & L. 207, 254 (2003) [5.05].

Burris, *Dental Discrimination Against the HIV-Infected: Empirical Data, Law and Public Policy*, 13 Yale J. On Reg. 1, 41 (1996) [9.131].

Canning, *Privileged Communications in Ohio and What's New on the Horizon: Ohio House Bill 52 Accountant-Client Privilege*, 31 Akron L. Rev. 505, 550 (1998) [IV].

Cantor, *Discarding Substituted Judgment and Best Interests: Toward a Constructive Preference Standard for Dying, Previously Competent Patients Without Advance Instructions*, 48 Rutgers L. Rev. 1193, 1234, 1247 (1996) [2.17].

Cantor, *My Annotated Living Will*, 18 Law, Med. & Health Care 114 (1990) [2.20].

Cantor, *The Permanently Unconscious Patient, Non-Feeding and Euthanasia*, XV Am. J. Law & Med. 381 (1989) [2.20].

Cantor & Thomas, *The Legal Bounds of Physician Conduct Hastening Death*, 48 Buff. L. Rev. 83, 110, 131, 158 (2000) [2.21, 2.211, 2.18, 2.20].

Caplan, Cooper, Garcia-Prats, & Brody, *Diffusion of Innovative Approaches to Managing Hypoplastic Left Heart Syndrome*, 150 Arch. Pediatr. Adolesc. Med. 487, 490 (1996) [2.162].

Capron, *Ethics: Public and Private*, 24 Hastings Center Rep. 26, 27 (Nov./Dec. 1994) [2.162].

Carter, *Health Information Privacy: Can Congress Protect Confidential Medical Information in the "Information Age"?*, 25 Wm. Mitchell L. Rev. 223, 236, 273 (1999) [5.05, 7.02, 7.05].

Casagrande, *Children Not Meant to Be: Protecting the Interests of the Child When Abortion Results in Live Birth*, 6 Quinnipiac Health L.J. 19, 44, 45, 47-48 (2002) [Preamble; I, III; 2.035, 2.20, 2.215].

Casarez, *Public Forums, Selective Subsidies, and Shifting Standards of Viewpoint Discrimination*, 64 Alb. L. Rev. 501, 558 (2000) [8.08].

Casell, *Lengthening the Stem: Allowing Federally Funded Researchers to Derive Human Pluripotent Stem Cells From Embryos*, 34 U. Mich. J. L. Ref. 547, 563 (2001) [2.141].

Caveney, *Going, Going, Gone … The Opportunities and Legal Pitfalls of Online Surgical Auctions*, 103 W. Va. L. Rev. 591, 607 (2001) [9.12].

Cerminara, *Protecting Participants in and Beneficiaries of ERISA-Governed Managed Health Care Plans*, 29 U. Mem. L. Rev. 317, 324 (1999). [2.20, 2.225].

Cerminara, *The Class Action Suit As a Method of Patient Empowerment in the Managed Care Setting*, 24 Am. J. Law & Med. 7, 16, 17, 23 (1998) [8.13, 8.132].

Chen, *Organ Allocation and the States: Can the States Restrict Broader Organ Sharing?*, 49 Duke L. J. 261, 273 (1999) [2.16].

Chen, Mueller, Prasad, Greinwald, Manaligod, Muilenburg, Verhoeven, Van Camp, & Smith, *Presymptomatic Diagnosis of Nonsyndromic Hearing Loss by Genotyping*, 124 Arch. Otolaryngol. Head Neck Surg. 20, 23 (1998) [2.12].

Cherry, *Polymorphic Medical Ontologies: Fashioning Concepts of Disease*, 25 J. Med. & Phil. 519, 532 (2000) [2.03].

Childress, *Ethics, Public Policy, and Human Fetal Tissue Transplantation Research*, 1 Kennedy Inst. Ethics J. 93, 116 (June 1991) [2.10].

Childress, *The Failure to Give: Reducing Barriers to Organ Donation*, 11 Kennedy Inst. Ethics J. 1, 13, 14 (2001) [2.155].

Chopko, *Responsible Public Policy at the End of Life*, 75 U. Det. Mercy L. Rev. 557, 573 (1998) [2.211].

Chouhan & Draper, *Modified Mandated Choice for Organ Procurement*, 29 J. Med. Ethics 157, 162 (2003) [2.155].

Christensen & Orlowski, *Iatrogenic Cardiopulmonary Arrests in DNR Patients*, 11 J. Clinical Ethics 14, 15, 20 (2000) [2.22].

Clark, *Autonomy and Death*, 71 Tul. L. Rev. 45, 89 (1996) [2.21, 2.211].

Clark, *Confidential Communications in a Professional Context: Attorney, Physician, and Social Worker*, 24 J. Legal Prof. 79, 92 (2000) [5.05].

Closen, *HIV-AIDS, Infected Surgeons and Dentists, and the Medical Profession's Betrayal of Its Responsibility to Patients*, 41 N.Y.L. Sch. L. Rev. 57, 65, 71-72, 129 (1996) [9.131].

Cohen, *Holistic Health Care: Including Alternative and Complementary Medicine in Insurance and Regulatory Schemes*, 38 Ariz. L. Rev. 83, 92 (1996) [3.01].

Cohen, *The Open Door: Will the Right to Die Survive Washington v. Glucksberg and Vacco v. Quill?*, 16 In Pub. Interest 79, 94 (1998) [2.20, 2.211].

Cohen, *Toward a Bioethics of Compassion*, 28 Ind. L. Rev. 667, 673, 681-82, 683 (1995) [2.01, 2.211, 8.18].

Cohen-Almagor, *A Critique of Callahan's Utilitarian Approach to Resource Allocation in Health Care*, 17 Issues L. & Med. 247, 261 (2002) [2.037].

Cohen & Cohen, *Required Reconsideration of "Do-Not-Resuscitate" Orders in the Operating Room and Certain Other Treatment Settings*, 20 Law, Med. & Health Care 354, 356 (1992) [2.22].

Cohn, Berger, Holzman, Lockhart, Reuben, Robertson, & Selbst, *Guidelines for Expert Witness Testimony in Medical Liability Cases*, 94 Pediatrics 755, 756 (1994) [9.07].

Coker, Smith, Bethea, King, & McKeown, *Physical Health Consequences of Physical and Psychological Intimate Partner Violence*, 9 Arch. Fam. Med. 451, 456, 457 (2000) [2.02].

Cole, *Beyond Unconstitutional Conditions: Charting Spheres of Neutrality in Government-Funded Speech*, 67 N.Y.U. L. Rev. 675, 744 (1992) [8.08].

Coleman, *Brother, Can You Spare a Liver? Five Ways to Increase Organ Donation*, 31 Val. U.L. Rev. 1, 30, 31 (1996) [2.06].

Coleson, *The Glucksberg & Quill Amicus Curiae Briefs: Verbatim Arguments Opposing Assisted Suicide*, 13 Issues in Law & Med. 3, 67 (1997) [2.211].

Collett, *Protecting Our Daughters: The Need for the Vermont Parental Notification Law*, 26 Vt. L. Rev. 101, 106-07 (2001) [2.015].

Colletti, Mulholland, & Sonnad, *Perceived Obstacles to Career Success for Women in Academic Surgery*, 135 Arch. Surg. 972, 976 (2000) [9.035].

Comment, *A Right to Die: Can a Massachusetts Physician Withdraw Artificial Nutrition and Hydration From a Persistently Vegetative Patient Following Cruzan v. Director, Missouri Department of Health?*, 26 New Eng. L. Rev. 199, 216, 220 (1991) [2.20].

Comment, *AIDSphobia: Forcing Courts to Face New Areas of Compensation for Fear of a Deadly Disease*, 39 Vill. L. Rev. 241, 277 (1994) [9.13, 9.131].

Comment, *Alliances for the Future: Cultivating a Cooperative Environment for Biotech Success*, 11 Berkeley Tech. L. J. 311, 344 (1996) [8.031].

Comment, *An Illinois Physician-Assisted Suicide Act: A Merciful End to a Terminally Ill Criminal Tradition*, 28 Loy. U. Chi. L. J. 763, 775 (1997) [2.20].

Comment, *Artificial Nutrition and the Terminally Ill: How Should Washington Decide?*, 61 Wash. L. Rev. 419 (1986) [2.20].

Comment, *Beyond Autonomy: Judicial Restraint and the Legal Limits Necessary to Uphold the Hippocratic Tradition and Preserve the Ethical Integrity of the Medical Profession*, 9 J. Contemp. Health L. & Pol'y 451, 467, 468 (1993) [2.20, 10.01].

Comment, *Curing the Health Care Industry: Government Response to Medicare Fraud and Abuse*, 5 J. Contemp. Health L. & Pol'y 175 (1989) [8.03].

Comment, *Dangerous Relations: Doctors and Extracorporeal Embryos, The Need For New Limits To Medical Inquiry*, 7 J. Contemp. Health L. & Pol'y 307, 309 (1991) [2.10, 2.14].

Comment, *Ethical Considerations in Resuscitation*, 268 JAMA 2282, 2283, 2287 (1992) [2.20, 2.22].

Comment, *From the Land of Lincoln a Healing Rule: Proposed Texas Rule of Civil Procedure Prohibiting Ex Parte Contact Between Defense Counsel and a Plaintiff's Treating Physician*, 25 Tex. Tech L. Rev. 1081, 1081, 1082 (1994) [II, IV; 5.05].

Comment, *Hold On Courts: May a Comatose Patient Be Denied Food and Water*, 31 St. Louis Univ. L. J. 749 (1987) [2.20].

Comment, *Medical Use of Marijuana: Legal and Ethical Conflicts in the Patient-Physician Relationship*, 30 U. Rich. L. Rev. 249, 268-69 (1996) [2.17].

Comment, *Noncompetition Clauses in Physician Employment Contracts in Oregon*, 76 Or. L. Rev. 195, 204-06 (1997) [Preamble; 6.11, 9.02, 9.06].

Comment, *Nonconsensual HIV Testing in the Health Care Setting: The Case for Extending the Occupational Protections of California Proposition 96 to Health Care Workers*, 26 Loy. L.A. L. Rev. 1251, 1269 (1993) [VI; 9.131].

Comment, *One Step Forward, Two Steps Back: A Constitutional and Critical Look at Ohio's New Living Will Statute*, 54 Ohio St. L. J. 445, 447, 460, 470 (1993) [2.20].

Comment, *Physician Assisted Suicide and the Right to Die With Assistance*, 105 Harvard L. Rev. 2021, 2027, 2035 (1992) [2.20].

Comment, *Physician-Assisted Suicide: Should Texas Be Different?*, 33 Hous. L. Rev. 1475, 1480, 1488 (1997) [2.21, 2.211].

Comment, *Physician Gag Clauses—The Hypocrisy of the Hippocratic Oath*, 21 So. Ill. U. L. J. 313, 318, 320 (1997) [8.13].

Comment, *Physician Retaliation: Can the Physician-Patient Relationship Be Protected?*, 94 Dickinson L. Rev. 965, 986 (1990) [9.131].

Comment, *Protecting Children Exposed to Domestic Violence in Contested Custody and Visitation Litigation*, 6 B.U. Pub. Int. L. J. 501, 502, 505 (1997) [2.02].

Comment, *Regulating Physician Investment and Referral Behavior in the Competitive Health Care Marketplace of the '90s—An Argument for Decentralization*, 65 Wash. L. Rev. 657, 658 (1990) [8.03].

Comment, *Right to Die: Oklahoma's Position on Nutrition and Hydration: Confusing or Unconstitutional?*, 43 Okla. L. Rev. 143, 151 (1990) [2.20].

Comment, *Shielding the Plaintiff and Physician: The Prohibition of Ex Parte Contacts With a Plaintiff's Treating Physician*, 13 Campbell L. Rev. 233, 243, 248 (1991) [IV; 5.06].

Comment, *Statutory Immunity for Volunteer Physicians: A Vehicle for Reaffirmation of the Doctor's Beneficent Duties—Absent the Rights Talk*, 1 Widener L. Symp. J. 425, 448, 449 (1996) [9.065, 10.01].

Comment, *Surrogate Health Care Decision Making: The Pennsylvania Supreme Court Recognizes the Right of an Individual in a Permanent Vegetative State to Refuse Life-Sustaining Measures through a Surrogate Decision Maker*, 35 Duq. L. Rev. 849, 859-60 (1997) [2.20].

Comment, *Taking Tarasoff Where No One Has Gone Before: Looking at Duty to Warn Under the AIDS Crisis*, 15 St. Louis U. Pub. L. Rev. 471, 499 (1996) [2.23, 5.057].

Comment, *The Hospice Movement: A Renewed View of the Death Process*, 4 J. Contemp. Health L. & Pol'y 295 (1988) [2.20].

Comment, *The Living Will: Preservation of the Right-To-Die Demands Clarity and Consistency*, 95 Dickinson L. Rev. 209, 217 (1990) [2.20].

Comment, *The Right to Refuse Life Sustaining Medical Treatment and the Nonterminally Ill Patient: An Analysis of Abridgment and Anarchy*, 17 Pepperdine L. Rev. 461, 462 (1990) [2.20].

Comment, *The Role of the Family in Medical Decision making for Incompetent Adult Patients: A Historical Perspective and Case Analysis*, 48 Univ. Pittsburgh L. Rev. 539 (1987) [2.20].

Comment, *Tort Reform to Ensure the Inclusion of Fertile Women in Early Phases of Commercial Drug Research*, 3 U. Chi. L. Sch. Roundtable 355, 359 (1996) [9.035].

Comment, *Who's in Charge: The Doctor or the Dollar?, Assessing the Relative Liability of Third Party Payors and Doctors After Wickline and Wilson*, 18 J. Contemp. L. 285, 301, 302 (1992) [2.03].

Comment, *Withholding Lifesaving Treatment From Defective Newborns: An Equal Protection Analysis*, 29 St. Louis Univ. L. J. 853 (1985) [2.17].

Cooper, *Restrictive Covenants*, 248 JAMA 3091 (1982) [9.02].

Crabtree, Pelletier, Gleason, Pruett, & Sawyer, *Gender-Dependent Differences in Outcome after the Treatment of Infection in Hospitalized Patients*, 282 JAMA 2143, 2148 (1999) [9.122].

Cramton & Knowles, *Professional Secrecy and its Exceptions: Spaulding v. Zimmerman Revisited*, 83 Minn. L. Rev. 63, 98 (1998) [5.09].

Crane, *The Problem of Physician Self-Referral Under the Medicare and Medicaid Antikickback Statute: The Hanlester Network Case and the Safe Harbor Regulation*, 268 JAMA 85, 89, 90 (1992) [8.032].

Cranford, *Neurologic Syndromes and Prolonged Survival: When Can Artificial Nutrition and Hydration Be Foregone?*, 19 Law, Med. & Health Care 13, 14, 16, 17 (1991) [2.20].

Crespi, *Overcoming the Legal Obstacles to the Creation of a Futures Market in Bodily Organs*, 55 Ohio St. L. J. 1, 74 (1994) [2.15].

Crossley, *Infants with Anencephaly, the ADA, and the Child Abuse Amendments*, 11 Issues in Law & Med. 379, 385, 409 (1996) [2.162, 2.17].

Crossley, *Infected Judgment: Legal Responses to Physician Bias*, 48 Vill. L. Rev. 195, 239, 297 (2003) [9.121, 9.122].

Crossley, *Of Diagnoses and Discrimination: Discriminatory Nontreatment of Infants With HIV Infection*, 93 Columbia L. Rev. 1581, 1620, 1621 (1993) [2.09, 2.17, 2.20, 2.22, 4.04, 8.03].

Cultice, *Medical Futility: When Is Enough, Enough?*, 27 J. Health & Hosp. Law 225, 230, 256 (1994) [2.03, 2.035, 2.095, 2.17, 2.19, 2.20, 2.22].

Cuzmanes & Orlando, *Automation of Medical Records: The Electronic Superhighway and Its Ramifications for Health Care Providers*, 6 J. Pharmacy & L. 19, 27 (1997) [IV].

Daar, *A Clash at the Bedside: Patient Autonomy v. a Physician's Professional Conscience*, 44 Hastings L. J. 1241, 1257, 1268, 1286 (1993) [2.20, 2.22].

Daar, *Medical Futility and Implications for Physician Autonomy*, XXI Am. J. Law & Med. 221, 234 (1995) [2.035].

Dahm, *Using DNA Profile as the Unique Patient Identifier in the Community Health Information Network: Legal Implications*, 15 J. Marshall J. Computer & Info. L. 227, 266, 275 (1997) [5.05].

Dalton, *Domestic Violence, Domestic Torts and Divorce: Constraints and Possibilities*, 31 New. Eng. L. Rev. 319, 354 (1997) [2.02].

Daniels, *Duty to Treat or Right to Refuse?*, 21 Hastings Center Rep. 36, 37, 42 (March/April 1991) [VI; 9.131].

Daugherty, *"Synthetic Sanity": The Ethics and Legality of Using Psychotropic Medications to Render Death Row Inmates Competent for Execution*, 17 J. Contemp. H. L. & Pol'y 715, 730 (2001) [2.06].

Davis & Grimaldi, *Sexual Confusion: Attorney-Client Sex and the Need for a Clear Ethical Rule*, 7 Notre Dame J. Law, Ethics, & Pub. Pol. 57, 61 (1993) [8.14].

Deady, *Cyberadvice: The Ethical Implications of Giving Professional Advice over the Internet*, 14 Geo. J. Legal Ethics 891, 905 (2001) [10.01].

Deftos, *Genomic Torts: The Law of the Future— The Duty of Physicians to Disclose the Presence of a Genetic Disease to the Relatives of Their Patients with the Disease*, 32 USF. L. Rev. 105, 130 (1997) [10.01].

Dehlendorf & Wolfe, *Physicians Disciplined for Sex-Related Offenses*, 279 JAMA 1883 (1998) [8.14].

DeLair, *Ethical, Moral, Economic and Legal Barriers to Assisted Reproductive Technologies Employed by Gay Men and Lesbian Women*, 4 DePaul J. Health Care L. 147, 150 (2000) [VI].

Dellinger & Vickery, *When Staff Object to Participating In Care*, 28 J. Health & Hospital Law 269, 272, 276 (1995) [I, VI; 1.02, 2.035, 9.055].

Delmonico, Arnold, Scheper-Hughes, Siminoff, Kahn & Youngner, *Ethical Incentives—Not Payment—for Organ Donation*, 346 New Eng. J. Med. 2002, 2005 (2002) [2.155].

DeMuro, *A Review of Key Legal Requirements Affecting Ambulatory Surgical Centers*, 11 Health Law. 1, 7 (1999) [8.032].

DeNatale & Parrish, *Health Care Workers' Ability to Recover in Tort for Transmission or Fear of Transmission of HIV from a Patient*, 36 Santa Clara L. Rev. 751, 782-83, 787 (1996) [IV; 9.131].

Dennis, *Promotion of Devices: An Extension of FDA Drug Regulation or a New Frontier?*, 48 Food & Drug L. J. 87 (1993) [8.061].

Denno, *Getting to Death: Are Executions Constitutional?*, 82 Iowa L. Rev. 319, 385-86 (1997) [2.06].

Denno, *When Legislatures Delegate Death: The Troubling Paradox Behind State Uses of Electrocution and Lethal Injection and What it Says About Us*, 63 Ohio St. L.J. 63, 112-13 (2002) [2.06].

Devettere, *The Imprecise Language of Euthanasia and Causing Death*, 1 J. Clinical Ethics 268, 268 (1990) [2.20].

DeVita, *Honestly, Do We Need a Policy on Truth?* 11 Kennedy Inst. Ethics J. 157, 158 (2001) [II; 8.12, 10.01].

Dickey, *Euthanasia: A Concept Whose Time Has Come?*, 8 Issues in Law & Med. 521, 523, 524 (1993) [2.17, 2.20].

Dillon, *Contingent Fees and Medical-Legal Consulting Services: Economical or Unethical?*, 11 J. Legal Med. 93, 101, 111 (1990) [6.01, 6.05, 9.07].

Dixon, *Conant v. McCaffrey: Physicians, Marijuana, and the First Amendment*, 70 U. Colo. L. Rev. 975, 977 (1999) [2.17].

Dowell, *The Corporate Practice of Medicine Prohibition: A Dinosaur Awaiting Extinction*, 27 J. Health & Hospital Law 369, 370 (1994) [VI].

Doyal, *Human Need and the Right of Patients to Privacy*, 14 J. Contemp. Health L. & Pol'y 1, 3 (1997) [IV].

Draper, *Preventive Law by Corporate Professional Team Players: Liability and Responsibility in the Work of Company Doctors*, 15 J. Contemp. Health L. & Pol'y. 525, 564 (1999) [2.132].

Dresser, *Relitigating Life and Death*, 51 Ohio St. L. J. 425, 436 (1990) [2.20].

Dresser, *Wanted: Single, White Male for Medical Research*, 22 Hastings Center Rep. 24, 28 (Jan./Feb. 1992) [9.122].

DuBois, *Non-Heart-Beating Organ Donation: A Defense of the Required Determination of Death*, 27 J. Law, Med. & Ethics 126, 128 (1999) [2.06, 2.162].

Duncan & Lubin, *The Use and Abuse of History in Compassion in Dying*, 20 Harv. J.L. & Pub. Pol'y 175, 183 (1996) [2.211].

Durst, *Cutting Through Pennsylvania's Medical Informed Consent Statute: A Reasonable Interpretation Abolishing the Surgical Requirement*, 104 Dick. L. Rev. 197, 225 (1999) [8.08].

Ehrlich, *Grounded in the Reality of Their Lives: Listening to Teens Who Make the Abortion Decision without Involving Their Parents*, 18 Berkeley Women's L. J. 61, 72, 84-85, 175-76 (2003) [2.015].

Ehrlich, *Journey Through the Courts: Minors, Abortion and the Quest for Reproductive Fairness*, 10 Yale J. L. & Feminism 1, 19 (1998) [2.015].

Ehrlich, *Minors as Medical Decision Makers: The Pretextual Reasoning of the Court in the Abortion Cases*, 7 Mich. J. Gender & L. 65, 91 (2000) [2.015].

Ehrlich, *Shifting Boundaries: Abortion, Criminal Culpability and the Indeterminate Legal Status of Adolescents*, 18 Wis. Women's L.J. 77, 105 (2003) [2.015].

Eisenstat, *An Analysis of the Rationality of Mandatory Testing for the HIV Antibody: Balancing the Governmental Public Health Interests With the Individual's Privacy Interest*, 52 Univ. Pittsburgh L. Rev. 327, 347 (1991) [9.131].

Eitel, Hegeman, & Evans, *Medicine on Trial: Physicians' Attitudes about Expert Medical Witnesses*, 18 J. Legal Med. 345, 355, 358 (1997) [II, VI; 9.07].

Elsas, *A Clinical Approach to Legal and Ethical Problems in Human Genetics*, 39 Emory L. J. 811, 816, 820 (1990) [5.05].

Emanuel, *Do Physicians Have an Obligation to Treat Patients With AIDS?*, 318 New Eng. J. Med. 1686 (1988) [9.12].

Emanuel, *Justice and Managed Care: Four Principles for the Just Allocation of Health Care Resources*, 30 Hastings Center Rep. 8, 16 (May/June 2000) [8.032].

Emanuel & Goldman, *Protecting Patient Welfare in Managed Care: Six Safeguards*, 23 J. Health Pol. Pol'y & L. 635, 641 (1998) [8.061].

Emanuel, Barry, Stoeckle, Ettelson, & Emanuel, *Advance Directives for Medical Care—A Case for Greater Use*, 324 New Eng. J. Med. 889 (1991) [2.20].

Emanuel, Emanuel, Stoeckle, Hummel, & Barry, *Advance Directives: Stability of Patients' Treatment Choices*, 154 Arch. Intern. Med. 209, 217 (1994) [2.20].

Emanuel, von Gunten, & Ferris, *Advance Care Planning*, 9 Arch. Fam. Med. 1181, 1181 (2000) [2.225].

Etzioni, *Organ Donation: A Communitarian Approach*, 13 Kennedy Inst. Ethics J. 1, 3, 4, 16 (March 2003) [2.15, 2.155].

Falk & Cary, *Death-Defying Feats: State Constitutional Challenges to New York's Death Penalty*, 4 J. L. & Pol'y 161, 233, 234 (1995) [2.06].

Fallek, *The Pain Relief Promotion Act: Will It Spell Death to "Death With Dignity" or Is It Unconstitutional?* 27 Fordham Urb. L. J. 1739, 1755 (2000) [2.20].

Farber, Davis, Weiner, Jordan, Boyer, & Ubel, *Physicians' Attitudes About Involvement in Lethal Injection for Capital Punishment*, 160 Arch. Intern. Med. 2912, 2912 (2000) [2.06].

Farber, Novack, & O'Brien, *Love, Boundaries, and the Physician-Patient Relationship*, 157 Arch. Intern. Med. 2291, 2292, 2293, 2294 (1997) [8.14].

Farley, *The Medicare Antifraud Statute and Safe Harbor Regulations: Suggestions for Change*, 81 Georgetown L. J. 167, 184 (1992) [8.032].

Fedder, *To Know or Not to Know: Legal Perspectives on Genetic Privacy and Disclosure of an Individual's Genetic Profile*, 21 J. Legal Med. 557, 563 (2000) [2.139].

Ferguson, *Ethical Postures of Futility and California's Uniform Health Care Decisions Act*, 75 S. Cal. L. Rev. 1217, 1252-53 (2002) [2.037].

Fernandez, *Is AIDS Different?*, 61 Alb. L. Rev. 1053 (1998) [2.23].

Field, *New Ethical Relationships Under Health Care's New Structure: The Need for a New Paradigm*, 43 Vill. L. Rev. 467, 468 (1998) [I].

Field, *Overview: Computerized Medical Records Create New Legal and Business Confidentiality Problems*, 11 HealthSpan 3, 4 (1994) [5.05].

Field, *Testing for AIDS: Uses and Abuses*, XVI Am. J. Law & Med. 34, 50 (1990) [9.131].

Fiestal, *A Solomonic Decision: What Will be the Fate of Frozen Preembryos?* 6 Cardozo Women's L. J. 103, 110 (1999) [2.141].

Fine, *Exploitation of the Elite: A Case for Physician Unionization*, 45 St. Louis L. J. 207, 207 (2001) [I].

Finks, *Lethal Injection: An Uneasy Alliance of Law and Medicine*, 4 J. Legal Med. 383 (1983) [2.06].

Fischer, Alpert, Stoeckle, & Emanuel, *Can Goals of Care Be Used to Predict Intervention Preferences in an Advance Directive?*, 157 Arch. Intern. Med. 801, 807 (1997) [2.20, 2.21].

FitzGibbon, *The Failure of the Freedom-Based and Utilitarian Arguments for Assisted Suicide*, 42 Am. J. Juris. 211, 252 (1997) [2.211].

FitzGibbon & Lai, *The Model Physician-Assisted Suicide Act and the Jurisprudence of Death*, 13 Issues in Law & Med. 173, 203-04 (1997) [2.211].

Flick, *The Due Process of Dying*, 79 Cal. L. Rev. 1121, 1152 (1991) [2.22].

Forrester, *AIDS: The Responsibility to Care*, 34 Vill. L. Rev. 799, 811 (1989) [VI; 9.131].

Forster, *The Legal and Ethical Debate Surrounding the Storage and Destruction of Frozen Human Embryos: A Reaction to the Mass Disposal in Britain and the Lack of Law in the United States*, 76 Wash. U. L.Q. 759, 766-67, 770 (1998) [2.141].

Freedman, *Health Professions, Codes, and the Right to Refuse to Treat HIV-Infectious Patients*, 18 Hastings Center Rep. 20 (Supp.) (April/May 1988) [VI; 8.11, 9.12].

Freedman & Halpern, *The Erosion of Ethics and Morality in Medicine: Physician Participation in Legal Executions in the United States*, 41 N.Y.L. Sch. L. Rev. 169, 174 (1996) [2.06].

Freeman, *Dealing with Doctors*, 13 S. C. Law 11, 11 (July/Aug. 2001) [5.05].

Freiman, *The Abandonment of the Antiquated Corporate Practice of Medicine Doctrine: Injecting a Dose of Efficiency into the Modern Health Care Environment*, 47 Emory L. J. 697, 712 (1998) [VI].

Friedland, *HIV Confidentiality and the Right to Warn— The Health Care Provider's Dilemma*, 80 Mass. L. Rev. 3, 4 (March 1995) [IV; 5.05, 10.01].

Friedland, *Managed Care and the Expanding Scope of Primary Care Physicians' Duties: A Proposal to Redefine Explicitly the Standard of Care*, 26 J. Law, Med. & Ethics 100, 104 (1998) [I].

Friedland, *Physician-Patient Confidentiality: Time to Re-Examine a Venerable Concept in Light of Contemporary Society and Advances in Medicine*, 15 J. Legal Med. 249, 257, 264, 276 (1994) [I, IV; 5.05].

Frye, *The International Bill of Gender Rights vs. the Cider House Rules: Transgenders Struggle with the Courts Over What Clothing They Are Allowed to Wear on the Job, Which Restroom They are Allowed to Use on the Job, Their Right to Marry, and the Very Definition of Their Sex*, 7 Wm. & Mary J. Women & L. 133, 149 (2000) [2.132, 2.135, 2.137, 5.08, 5.09].

Frye & Meiselman, *Same-Sex Marriages Have Existed Legally in the United States for a Long Time Now*, 64 Alb. L. Rev. 1031, 1053 (2001) [2.132, 2.135, 2.137, 5.08, 5.09].

Furman, *Genetic Test Results and the Duty to Disclose: Can Medical Researchers Control Liability?* 23 Seattle Univ. L. R. 391, 408-09 (1999) [2.07].

Furrow, *Doctor's Dirty Little Secrets: The Dark Side of Medical Privacy*, 37 Washburn L. Rev. 283, 290 (1998) [9.131].

Furrow, *Incentivizing Medical Practice: What (If Anything) Happens to Professionalism?*, 1 Widener L. Symp. J. 1, 9 (1996) [2.03].

Garris, *The Case for Patenting Medical Procedures*, XXII Am. J. Law & Med. 85, 93, 94-95 (1996) [9.08, 9.09, 9.095].

Gatter, *Protecting Patient-Doctor Discourse: Informed Consent and Deliberative Autonomy*, 78 Or. L. Rev. 941, 956 (1999) [Preamble; 8.03].

Gauthier, *Active Voluntary Euthanasia, Terminal Sedation, and Assisted Suicide*, 12 J. Clinical Ethics 43, 43-44, 49 (2001) [2.20, 2.21].

Gelein, *Are Online Consultations a Prescription for Trouble? The Uncharted Waters of Cybermedicine*, 66 Brook. L. Rev. 209, 239 (2000) [10.01].

Gellman, *Prescribing Privacy: The Uncertain Role of the Physician in the Protection of Patient Privacy*, 62 No. Carolina L. Rev. 255 (1984) [5.03, 5.04, 5.06, 5.07, 5.08, 5.09].

Gerbert, Bleecker, Miyasaki, & Maguire, *Possible Health Care Professional-to-Patient HIV Transmission: Dentists' Reactions to a Centers for Disease Control Report*, 265 JAMA 1845, 1846, 1847 (1991) [9.131].

Gerbert, Maguire, Bleecker, Coates, & McPhee, *Primary Care Physicians and AIDS: Attitudinal and Structural Barriers to Care*, 266 JAMA 2837, 2838 (1991) [9.131].

Gilmore, *Employment Protection for Lesbians and Gay Men*, 6 L. & Sex. 83, 95 (1996) [9.03].

Gimbel & Zaremski, *Medical Restrictive Covenants in Illinois: At the Crossroads of Carter-Shields and Prairie Eye Center*, 12 Annals Health L. 1, 12 (2003) [9.02].

Gittler & Rennart, *HIV Infection Among Women and Children and Antidiscrimination Laws: An Overview*, 77 Iowa L. Rev. 1313, 1363 (1992) [VII; 9.131].

Glynn, *Multidisciplinary Representation of Children: Conflicts Over Disclosures of Client Communications*, 27 J. Marshall L. Rev. 617, 625, 626, 630-32, 637, 639, 643 (1994) [III, IV; 1.02, 2.02, 5.05, 10.01].

Glynn, *Turning to State Legislatures to Legalize Physician-Assisted Suicide for Seriously Ill, Non-Terminal Patients After Vacco v. Quill and Washington v. Glucksberg*, 6 J. L. & Pol'y. 329, 345 (1997) [2.211].

Godoy, *Where is Biotechnology Taking the Law? An Overview of Assisted Reproductive Technology, Research on Frozen Embryos and Human Cloning*, 19 J. Juv. L. 357, 363 (1998) [2.141].

Goldberg, *Sex and the Attorney-Client Relationship: An Argument for a Prophylactic Rule*, 26 Akron L. Rev. 45 (1992) [8.14].

Goldman, *Revising Iowa's Life-Sustaining Procedures Act: Creating a Practical Guide to Living Wills in Iowa*, 76 Iowa L. Rev. 1137, 1149 (1992) [2.20].

Gorsuch, *The Right to Assisted Suicide and Euthanasia*, 23 Harv. J. L. & Pub. Pol'y 599, 653, 707 (2000) [2.20, 2.21, 2.211].

Gostin, *Deciding Life and Death in the Courtroom: From Quinlan to Cruzan, Glucksberg, and Vacco—A Brief History and Analysis of Constitutional Protection of the Right to Die,'* 278 JAMA 1523, 1525, 1528 (1997) [2.211].

Gostin, *Drawing a Line Between Killing and Letting Die: The Law, and Law Reform, on Medically Assisted Dying*, 21 J. Law, Med. & Ethics 94, 98 (1993) [2.20].

Grabois, *The Liability of Psychotherapists for Breach of Confidentiality*, 12 J. Law & Health 39, 53-54 (1998) [5.05, 5.06, 5.07, 5.08, 5.09].

Gray, *Trust and Trustworthy Care in the Managed Care Era*, 16 Health Affairs 34, 38, 47-48 (1997) [8.03].

Graybill, *Assisting Minors Seeking Abortions in Judicial Bypass Proceedings: A Guardian ad Litem is No Substitute for an Attorney*, 55 Vand. L. Rev. 581, 583 (2002) [2.015].

Greely, *Direct Financial Incentives in Managed Care: Unanswered Questions*, 6 Health Matrix 53, 81 (1996) [8.13].

Green, *NHGRI's Intramural Ethics Experiment*, 7 Kennedy Inst. of Ethics J. 181, 185, 188 (1997) [2.138].

Green & Thomas, *DNA: Five Distinguishing Features for Policy Analysis*, 11 Harv. J. L. & Tech. 571, 582-83 (1998) [2.138].

Green, Haggerty, & Hale, *Community-Based Plan for Treating Human Immunodeficiency Virus-Infected Individuals Sponsored by Local Medical Societies and an Acquired Immunodeficiency Syndrome Service Organization*, 151 Arch. Intern. Med. 2061, 2064 (1991) [9.131].

Gross, *Wagging the Watchdog: Law and the Emergence of Bioethical Norms*, 21 Med. & L. 687, 702 (2002) [2.20].

Guise, *Expansion of the Scope of Disclosure Required Under the Informed Consent Doctrine: Moore v. The Regents of the University of California*, 28 San Diego L. Rev. 455, 462 (1991) [Preamble].

Gutheil, Jorgenson, & Sutherland, *Prohibiting Lawyer-Client Sex*, 20 Bull. Am. Acad. Psychiatry Law 365 (1992) [8.14].

Hackler & Hiller, *Family Consent to Orders Not To Resuscitate: Reconsidering Hospital Policy*, 264 JAMA 1281, 1282 (1990) [2.17].

Haddon, *Baby Doe Cases: Compromise and Moral Dilemma*, 34 Emory L. J. 545 (1985) [2.20].

Hafemeister, *End-of-Life Decision Making, Therapeutic Jurisprudence, and Preventive Law: Hierarchical v. Consensus-Based Decision-Making Model*, 41 Ariz. L. Rev. 329 (1999) [2.20].

Halberstam, *Commercial Speech, Professional Speech, and the Constitutional Status of Social Institutions*, 147 U. Pa. L. Rev. 771, 857 (1999) [III].

Halevy & Brody, *Acquired Immunodeficiency Syndrome and the Americans with Disabilities Act: A Legal Duty to Treat*, 96 Am. J. Med. 282, 283, 284 (1994) [VI; 9.12, 9.131].

Halevy, *AIDS, Surgery, and the Americans with Disabilities Act*, 135 Arch. Surg. 51, 52, 53 (2000) [9.13, 9.131].

Hall, *A Theory of Economic Informed Consent*, 31 Ga. L. Rev. 511, 521, 524-25 (1997) [8.13].

Hall, *Bargaining with Hippocrates: Managed Care and the Doctor-Patient Relationship*, 54 S.C. L. Rev. 689, 696, 735 (2003) [VII; 8.03].

Hall, *Confidentiality as an Organizational Ethics Issue*, 10 J. Clinical Ethics 230, 232 (1999) [5.05].

Hall, *Law, Medicine, and Trust*, 55 Stan. L. Rev. 463, 471 (2002) [II; 8.12].

Hall, *Rationing Health Care at the Bedside*, 69 N.Y.U. L. Rev. 693, 704 (1994) [2.03].

Hall, *Third-Party Payor Conflicts of Interest in Managed Care: A Proposal for Regulation Based on the Model Rules of Professional Conduct*, 29 Seton Hall L. Rev. 95, 96, 107, 108, 109, 110, 111, 112, 134, 135, 136 (1998) [Preamble; 2.07, 2.08, 2.132, 4.04, 5.01, 8.03, 8.13, 9.06, 10.01].

Halpern, Ubel, & Caplan, *Solid-Organ Transplantation in HIV-Infected Patients*, 347 New Eng. J. Med. 284, 287 (2002) [2.16, 9.131].

Hamilton, Edwards, Boehnlein, & Hamilton, *The Doctor-Patient Relationship and Assisted Suicide: A Contribution from Dynamic Psychiatry*, 19 Am. J. Forensic Psychiatry 59, 60 (1998) [2.211].

Hammes & Webster, *Professional Ethics and Managed Care in Dermatology*, 132 Arch. Dermatol. 1070, 1072, 1073 (1996) [8.13].

Hanlon, Weiss, & Rees, *British Community Pharmacists' Views of Physician-Assisted Suicide (PAS)*, 26 J. Med. Ethics 363, 367, 369 (2000) [2.211].

Hanson, *Informed Consent and the Scope of a Physician's Duty of Disclosure*, 77 N.D. L. Rev. 71, 89, 91 (2001) [8.13].

Hardaway, Peterson, & Mann, *The Right to Die and the Ninth Amendment: Compassion and Dying after Glucksberg and Vacco*, 7 Geo. Mason L. Rev. 313, 342 (1999) [2.211].

Haroun & Morris, *Weaving a Tangled Web: The Deceptions of Psychiatrists*, 10 J. Contemp. Leg. Issues 227, 235 (1999) [II, III].

Harris, *The Regulation of Managed Care: Conquering Individualism and Cynicism in America*, 6 Va. J. Soc. Pol'y. & L. 315, 329 (1999) [2.16].

Harris & Foran, *The Ethics of Middle-Class Access to Legal Services and What We Can Learn from the Medical Profession's Shift to a Corporate Paradigm*, 70 Fordham L. Rev. 775, 817, 821, 822, 823, 824 (2001) [VI; 2.03, 2.09, 8.02, 8.021, 8.03, 8.05, 8.051, 8.054, 8.13, 8.132].

Hartog, *The Psychological Impact of AIDS on Real Property and a Real Estate Broker's Duty to Disclose*, 36 Ariz. L. Rev. 757, 772 (1994) [9.13, 9.131].

Harvey, *Confidentiality: A Measured Response to the Failure of Privacy*, 140 Univ. Pa. L. Rev. 2385, 2454 (1992) [8.08].

Hashimoto, *The Future Role of Managed Care and Capitation in Workers' Compensation*, XXII Am. J. Law & Med. 233, 258, 259 (1996) [8.13].

Hasko, *Persuasion in the Court: Nonlegal Materials in US Supreme Court Opinions*, 94 Law Libr. J. 427, 444, 453 (2002) [2.20, 2.211].

Haut, *Divorce and the Disposition of Frozen Embryos*, 28 Hofstra L. Rev. 493, 519 (1999) [2.141].

Healey & Dowling, *Controlling Conflicts of Interest in the Doctor-Patient Relationship: Lessons From Moore v. Regents of the University of California*, 42 Mercer L. Rev. 989, 997, 998 (1991) [2.19, 8.032, 8.06].

Hecht, *Legal and Ethical Aspects of Sports-Related Concussions: The Merril Hoge Story*, 12 Seton Hall J. Sport L. 17, 42-43 (2002) [10.015].

Helft, Siegler, & Lantos, *The Rise and Fall of the Futility Movement*, 343 New Eng. J. Med. 293, 294 (2000) [2.037].

Hermer, *Paradigms Revised: Intersex Children, Bioethics & the Law*, 11 Annals Health L. 195, 221 (2002) [10.01].

Hillerich, Ellerin, & Frieder, *Selecting and Presenting a Failure to Diagnose Breast Cancer Case*, 20 Am. J. Trial Advoc. 253, 271 (1996-97) [5.05, 5.06].

Hirshfeld, *Defining Full and Fair Disclosure in Managed Care Contracts*, 60 The Citation 67 (1990) [8.03, 8.032, 8.132].

Hirshfeld, *Economic Considerations in Treatment Decisions and the Standard of Care in Medical Malpractice Litigation*, 264 JAMA 2004, 2007 (1990) [2.03, 2.09].

Hirshfeld, *Should Ethical and Legal Standards for Physicians Be Changed to Accommodate New Models for Rationing Health Care?*, 140 Univ. Pa. L. Rev. 1809, 1816 (1992) [2.03, 2.09, 4.04].

Hirshfeld, *Should Third Party Payors of Health Care Services Disclose Cost Control Mechanisms to Potential Beneficiaries?*, 14 Seton Hall Legis. J. 115 (1990) [2.03, 2.09, 2.19, 4.04, 4.06, 8.03, 8.032].

Hirshfeld & Thomason, *Medical Necessity Determinations: The Need for a New Legal Structure*, 6 Health Matrix 3, 8-9 (1996) [I, II, III, IV, V, VI, VII; 2.03].

Ho, *Patents, Patients, and Public Policy: An Incomplete Intersection at 35 U.S.C. § 287(c)*, 33 U.C. Davis L. Rev. 601, 603, 623, 624, 625, 631 (2000) [V; 8.03, 9.08, 9.09, 10.01].

Hodges, Tolle, Stocking, & Cassel, *Tube Feeding: Internists' Attitudes Regarding Ethical Obligations*, 154 Arch. Intern. Med. 1013, 1020 (1994) [2.20].

Hoffman, *Preplacement Examinations and Job-Relatedness: How to Enhance Privacy and Diminish Discrimination in the Workplace*, 49 U. Kan. L. Rev. 517, 534, 535, 556, 565 (2001) [2.132, 2.139].

Hoffman, *The Use of Placebos in Clinical Trials: Responsible Research or Unethical Practice?* 33 Conn. L. Rev. 449, 454-55, 496 (2001) [2.075].

Hoge, *APA Resource Document: I. The Professional Responsibilities of Psychiatrists in Evolving Health Care Systems*, 24 Bull. Am. Acad. Psychiatry Law 393, 405 (1996) [2.095, 8.13, 8.132].

Hoge, *APA Resource Document: II. Regulatory Guidelines for Protecting the Interests of Psychiatric Patients in Emerging Health Care Systems*, 24 Bull. Am. Acad. Psychiatry Law 407, 412, 418 (1996) [8.13].

Hoge, *Proposed Federal Legislation Jeopardizes Patient Privacy*, 23 Bull. Am. Acad. Psychiatry Law 495, 498, 500 (1995) [IV; 5.07].

Holland, *Should Parents Be Permitted to Authorize Genetic Testing for Their Children?*, 31 Fam. L. Q. 321, 346-47 (1997) [2.132].

Holliday, *Traditional Medicines in Modern Societies: An Exploration of Integrationist Options through East Asian Experience*, 28 J. Med. & Phil. 373, 387 (2003) [Preamble; V].

Horan & Grant, *The Legal Aspects of Withdrawing Nourishment*, 5 J. Legal Med. 595 (1984) [2.20].

Horstman, *Commuting Death Sentences of the Insane: A Solution for a Better, More Compassionate Society*, 36 USF.L. Rev. 823, 848 (2002) [2.06].

Hughes, *The Uniform Mediation Act: To the Spoiled Go the Privileges*, 85 Marq. L. Rev. 9, 26 (2001) [5.05].

Hyams, *Expert Psychiatric Evidence in Sexual Misconduct Cases Before State Medical Boards*, XVIII Am. J. Law & Med. 171, 173, 174 (1992) [8.14].

Hyams, Shapiro, & Brennan, *Medical Practice Guidelines in Malpractice Litigation: An Early Retrospective*, 21 J. Health Pol. Pol'y & L. 289, 298 (1996) [8.16].

Hyman & Silver, *Just What the Patient Ordered: The Case for Result-Based Compensation Arrangements*, 29 J. L. Med. & Ethics 170, 170 (2001) [6.01].

Hyman & Silver, *You Get What You Pay For: Result Based Compensation for Health Care*, 58 Wash. & Lee L. Rev. 1427, 1459, 1460, 1461, 1481-82 (2001) [6.01, 9.121, 9.122].

Iheukwumere, *Doctor, are You Experienced? The Relevance of Disclosure of Physician Experience to a Valid Informed Consent*, 18 J. Contemp. Health L. & Pol'y 373, 376-77 (2002) [II; 8.12].

Iheukwumere, *HIV-Positive Medical Practitioners: Legal and Ethical Obligations to Disclose*, 71 St. John's L. Rev. 715, 732-34 (1997) [9.13, 9.131].

Ikemoto, *The Fuzzy Logic of Race and Gender in the Mismeasure of Asian American Women's Health Needs*, 65 U. Cin. L. Rev. 799, 800, 804, 810 (1997) [9.121, 9.122].

Ile, *Should Physicians Treat Patients Who Seek Second Opinions?*, 266 JAMA 273, 274 (1991) [6.11, 9.02, 9.06, 9.12].

Isaacman & Miller, *Neonatal HIV Seroprevalence Studies*, 14 J. Legal Med. 413, 428 (1993) [2.07].

Jacobi, *Patients at a Loss: Protecting Health Care Consumers through Data Driven Quality Assurance*, 45 U. Kan. L. Rev. 705, 720, 721, 759 (1997) [2.03, 2.09, 8.13].

Jacobs & Goodman, *Splitting Fees or Splitting Hairs? Fee Splitting and Health Care—The Florida Experience*, 8 Annals Health L. 239, 244 (1999) [6.02].

Jecker, *Genetic Testing and the Social Responsibility of Private Health Insurance Companies*, 21 J. Law, Med. & Ethics 109, 112 (1993) [2.132].

Jecker, *Privacy Beliefs and the Violent Family: Extending the Ethical Argument for Physician Intervention*, 269 JAMA 776, 778, 779 (1993) [IV; 5.05, 8.14, 9.131].

Jecker & Schneiderman, *An Ethical Analysis of the Use of "Futility" in the 1992 American Heart Association Guidelines for Cardiopulmonary Resuscitation and Emergency Cardiac Care*, 153 Arch. Intern. Med. 2195, 2197 (1993) [2.22].

Jensen, *Organ Procurement: Various Legal Systems and Their Effectiveness*, 22 Hous. J. Int'l L. 555, 578 (2000) [2.15].

Jerdee, *Breaking Through the Silence: Minnesota's Pregnancy Presumption and the Right to Refuse Medical Treatment*, 84 Minn. L. Rev. 971, 980 (2000) [2.20].

Johnson, *ERISA Doctor in the House? The Duty to Disclose Physician Incentives to Limit Health Care*, 82 Minn. L. Rev. 1631, 1639, 1649, 1655 (1998) [8.13, 8.132].

Johnson, *Harm to the "Fabric of Society" as a Basis for Regulating Otherwise Harmless Conduct: Notes on a Theme from Ravin v. State*, 27 Seattle U. L. Rev. 41, 55 (2003) [2.211].

Johnson, *HIV Testing of Health Care Workers: Conflict Between the Common Law and the Centers for Disease Control*, 42 Am. Univ. L. Rev. 479, 518 (1993) [9.131].

Johnson, *Judicial Review of Disciplinary Action for Sexual Misconduct in the Practice of Medicine*, 270 JAMA 1596 (1993) [8.14].

Johnson, *Minnesota's "Crack Baby" Law: Weapon of War or Link in a Chain?*, 8 Law & Ineq. 485, 494, 495, 496 (1990) [8.08].

Johnson, *The Death-Prolonging Procedures Act and Refusal of Treatment in Missouri*, 30 St. Louis Univ. L. J. 805 (1986) [2.19].

Johnson, Gibbons, Goldner, Wiener, & Eton, *Legal and Institutional Policy Responses to Medical Futility*, 30 J. Health & Hosp. L. 21, 26, 31, 35, 36 (1997) [2.035, 2.22].

Jones, *Battered Spouses' Damage Actions Against Non-Reporting Physicians*, 45 DePaul L. Rev. 191 (1996) [2.02].

Jones, *Kentucky Tort Liability for Failure to Report Family Violence*, 26 N. Ky. L. Rev. 43, 58 (1999) [2.02].

Jones, *Primum Non Nocere: The Expanding "Honest Services" Mail Fraud Statute and the Physician-Patient Fiduciary Relationship*, 51 Vand. L. Rev. 139, 161, 164 (1998) [2.03, 8.03, 8.06].

Joralemon, *Shifting Ethics: Debating the Incentive Question in Organ Transplantation*, 27 J. Med. Ethics 30, 31, 34 (2001) [2.15].

Jordan, *Financial Conflicts of Interest in Human Subjects Research: Proposals for a More Effective Regulatory Scheme*, 60 Wash. & Lee L. Rev. 15, 23 (2003) [9.095].

Jost & Davies, *The Empire Strikes Back: A Critique of the Backlash Against Fraud and Abuse Enforcement*, 51 Ala. L. Rev. 239, 240 (1999) [II].

Joynt, *Neurology*, 263 JAMA 2660 (1990) [2.161].

Jozefowicz, *The Case Against Having Professional Privilege in the Physician-Patient Relationship*, 16 Med. & L. 385, 386-87, 391 (1997) [Preamble; IV; 5.05].

Judge, *Issues Surrounding the Patenting of Medical Procedures*, 13 Santa Clara Computer & High Tech. L. J. 181, 202-03 (1997) [9.08, 9.095].

Jurevic, *Disparate Impact Under Title VI: Discrimination, By Any Other Name, Will Still Have the Same Impact*, 15 St. Louis U. Pub. L. Rev. 237, 253 (1996) [2.03].

Jurevic, *When Technology and Health Care Collide: Issues with Electronic Medical Records and Electronic Mail*, 66 UMKC L. Rev. 809, 819-20 (1998) [5.05, 5.07].

Kalt, *Death, Ethics, and the State*, 23 Harv. J. L. & Pub. Pol'y 487, 537, 539 (2000) [2.211].

Kamisar, *On the Meaning and Impact of the Physician-Assisted Suicide Cases*, 82 Minn. L. Rev. 895, 909, 918 (1998) [2.211].

Kamisar, *When is There A Constitutional "Right to Die"? When is There No Constitutional "Right to Live"?*, 25 Georgia L. Rev. 1203, 1207, 1208, 1222 (1991) [2.20].

Kane, *Driving into the Sunset: A Proposal for Mandatory Reporting to the DMV by Physicians Treating Unsafe Elderly Drivers*, 25 U. Haw. L. Rev. 59, 59, 61, 62, 67, 69, 82, 83 (2002) [1.02, 2.24, 5.05, 10.01].

Kane, *Information is the Key to Patient Empowerment*, 11 Annals Health L. 25, 29-30, 44 (2002) [V; 10.01, 10.02].

Kao & Linden, *Direct-to-Consumer Advertising and the Internet: Informational Privacy, Product Liability and Organizational Responsibility*, 46 St. Louis U. L.J. 157, 170 (2002) [5.015].

Kapp, *Legal Standards for the Medical Diagnosis and Treatment of Dementia*, 23 J. Legal Med. 359, 382 (2002) [2.24].

Kapp, *Physicians' Legal Duties Regarding the Use of Genetic Tests to Predict and Diagnose Alzheimer Disease*, 21 J. Legal Med. 445, 456-57, 465-66 (2000) [2.132, 2.139, 8.032].

Kapp, *Placebo Therapy and the Law: Prescribe With Care*, 8 Am. J. Law & Med. 371 (1983) [8.08, 8.12].

Kass & Lund, *Physician-Assisted Suicide, Medical Ethics and the Future of the Medical Profession*, 35 Duq. L. Rev. 395, 404 (1996) [2.211].

Kassel, *Counterpoint . . . Defense Counsel's Ex Parte Communication with Plaintiff's Doctors: A Bad One-Sided Deal*, 9 S.C. Law. 42, 43 (Sept./Oct. 1997) [IV; 5.05].

Kassirer, *Managing Care' Should We Adopt a New Ethic?*, 339 New Eng. J. Med. 397 (1998) [8.13].

Katner, *The Ethical Dilemma Awaiting Counsel Who Represent Adolescents with HIV/AIDS: Criminal Law and Tort Suits Pressure Counsel to Breach the Confidentiality of the Clients' Medical Status*, 70 Tul. L. Rev. 2311, 2341 (1996) [5.05].

Katz, *Informed Consent—Must It Remain a Fairy Tale?*, 10 J. Contemp. Health L. & Pol'y 69, 80 (1994) [8.08].

Katz, *The Pregnant Child's Right to Self-Determination*, 62 Alb. L. Rev. 1119, 1142 (1999) [2.015].

Keim, *Physicians for Professional Sports Teams: Health Care Under the Pressure of Economic and Commercial Interests*, 9 Seton Hall. J. Sport L. 196, 218-19 (1999) [3.06].

Kelley, *The Meanings of Professional Life: Teaching Across the Health Professions*, 27 J. Med. & Phil. 475, 485, 490, 491 (2002) [2.161, 8.13].

Kelly, *The "Right to Die" in America: The Ninth Circuit's Decision in Compassion in Dying v. The State of Washington*, 29 J. Health & Hosp. L. 246, 255 (1996) [2.211].

Kenworthy, *The Austrian Psychotherapy Act: No Legal Duty to Warn*, 11 Ind. Int'l & Comp. L. Rev. 469, 480-81, 485, 490, 496 (2001) [2.23, 5.05, 5.06].

Kerr, Hays, Mittman, Siu, Leake, & Brook, *Primary Care Physicians' Satisfaction with Quality of Care in California Capitated Medical Groups*, 278 JAMA 308, 312 (1997) [8.13].

Keyes, *The Choice of Participation by Physicians in Capital Punishment*, 22 Whittier L. Rev. 809, 810-11, 838 (2001) [2.06].

Khanna, Silverman, & Schwartz, *Disclosure of Operating Practices by Managed-Care Organizations to Consumers of Healthcare: Obligations of Informed Consent*, 9 J. Clinical Ethics 291, 293, 296 (1998) [8.13].

Kibler, *Administrative Law*, 38 U. Rich. L. Rev. 39, 47 (2003) [8.181].

Kinney, *Procedural Protections for Patients in Capitated Health Plans*, XXII Am. J. Law & Med. 301, 319-20 (1996) [8.13].

Kinney, *Tapping and Resolving Consumer Concerns About Health Care*, 26 Am. J. Law & Med. 335, 337, 375 (2000) [VI; 8.13, 9.065].

Kinney & Selby, *History and Jurisprudence of the Physician-Patient Relationship in Indiana*, 30 Ind. L. Rev. 263, 269, 272, 276 (1997) [2.20, 8.08, 9.06, 9.12].

Kirschenbaum & Kuhlik, *Federal and State Laws Affecting Discounts, Rebates, and Other Marketing Practices for Drugs and Devices*, 47 Food & Drug L. J. 533, 560 (1992) [8.06, 8.061].

Kleinman, *Health Care in Crisis: A Proposed Role for the Individual Physician as Advocate*, 265 JAMA 1991 (1991) [9.121].

Koniak, *The Law Between the Bar and the State*, 70 No. Carolina L. Rev. 1389, 1396 (1992) [1.02].

Kramer, Gruenberg, & Fidler, *Psychiatrists' Attitudes toward Physician-Assisted Suicide: A Survey*, 19 Am. J. Forensic Psychiatry 81, 87, 90 (1998) [2.06, 2.20].

Krause, *"Promises to Keep": Health Care Providers and the Civil False Claims Act*, 23 Cardozo L. Rev. 1363, 1365 (2002) [I, II, IV].

Krause, *The Brief Life of the Gag Clause: Why Antigag Clause Legislation Isn't Enough*, 67 Tenn. L. Rev. 1, 4, 43 (1999) [8.13].

Krishnan, Diette, Skinner, Clark, Steinwachs, & Wu, *Race and Sex Differences in Consistency of Care With National Asthma Guidelines in Managed Care Organizations*, 161 Arch. Intern. Med. 1660, 1660 (2001) [9.122].

Krumm, *Genetic Discrimination: Why Congress Must Ban Genetic Testing in the Workplace*, 23 J. Legal Med. 491, 506 (2002) [2.20].

Kruse, *A Call for New Perspectives for Living Wills (You Might Like It Here)*, 37 Real Prop., Prob. & Tr. J. 545, 550 (2002) [2.035].

Kumar & Kinney, *Indiana Lawmakers Face National Health Policy Issues*, 25 Indiana L. Rev. 1271, 1275, 1276 (1992) [2.20].

Kurfirst, *The Duty to Disclose HMO Physician Incentives*, 13 (3) Health Law. 18, 18, 22 (2001) [8.132].

Kurtz, *The Law of Informed Consent: From "Doctor is Right" to "Patient has Rights,"* 50 Syracuse L. Rev. 1243, 1245 (2000) [8.08].

Kutzko, Boyer, Thoman, & Scott, *HIPAA in Real Time: Practical Implications of the Federal Privacy Rule*, 51 Drake L. Rev. 403, 408 (2003) [5.05, 5.055, 5.057, 5.06, 5.07, 5.075, 5.08, 5.09].

Labowitz, *Beyond Tarasoff: AIDS and the Obligation to Breach Confidentiality*, 9 St. Louis Univ. Pub. L. Rev. 495, 514 (1990) [2.23].

Lafferty, *Statutory and Ethical Barriers in the Patenting of Medical and Surgical Procedures*, 29 J. Marshall L. Rev. 891, 912 (1996) [9.08].

Langwell & Moser, *Strategies for Medicare Health Plans Serving Racial and Ethnic Minorities*, 23 Health Care Financing Rev. 131, 134, 146 (2002) [9.121].

Larson, *Prescription for Death: A Second Opinion*, 44 DePaul L. Rev. 461, 472 (1995) [2.21, 2.211]. Larson, *Tales of Death: Storytelling in the Physician-Assisted Suicide Litigation*, 39 Washburn L. J. 159, 177 (2000) [2.211].

Laurie, *Challenging Medical-Legal Norms: The Role of Autonomy, Confidentiality, and Privacy in Protecting Individual and Familial Group Rights in Genetic Information*, 22 J. Legal Med. 1, 24 (2001) [IV; 10.01].

Law, *Silent No More: Physicians' Legal and Ethical Obligations to Patients Seeking Abortions*, 21 N.Y.U. Rev. L. & Soc. Change 279, 289, 290, 300 (1994) [3.04, 8.04].

Lazzarini, *An Analysis of Ethical Issues in Prescribing and Dispensing Syringes to Injection Drug Users*, 11 Health Matrix 85, 107, 119 (2001) [III; 1.02, 5.05].

LeBlang, *Obligations of HIV-Infected Health Professionals to Inform Patients of Their Serological Status: Evolving Theories of Liability*, 27 J. Marshall L. Rev. 317, 318 (1994) [9.131].

LeDoux, *Interspousal Liability and the Wrongful Transmission of HIV-AIDS: An Argument for Broadening Legal Avenues for the Injured Spouse and Further Expanding Children's Rights to Sue Their Parents*, 34 New Eng. L. Rev. 392, 411 (2000) [9.131].

Lee, *35 U.S.C. §287(C)— The Physician Immunity Statute*, 79 J. Pat. & Trademark Off. Soc'y 701, 702-04 (1997) [9.095].

Leflar, *Advance Health Care Directives Under Arkansas Law*, 1994 Ark. L. Notes 37, 42. [2.20].

LeGros & Pinkall, *The New JCAHO Patient Safety Standards and the Disclosure of Unanticipated Outcomes*, 35 J. Health L. 189, 203 (2002) [8.12].

Levine, *Medicalization of Psychoactive Substance Use and the Doctor-Patient Relationship*, 69 Milbank Quarterly 623, 624 (1991) [III].

Levitt & Ryan, *Not Competent to Be Executed: Dilemmas Faced By Psychiatrists and Attorneys*, 23 Am. J. Forensic Psych. 39, 47 (July 2002) [2.06].

Levy, *Because Judges Went to Law School, Not Medical School: Restrictive Covenants in the Practices of Law and Medicine*, 30 J. Health & Hosp. L. 89, 92, 101 (1997) [9.02].

Levy, *Collective Bargaining in the Elite Professions– Doctors' Application of the Labor Law Model to Negotiations with Health Plan Providers*, 13 U. Fla. J.L. & Pub. Pol'y 269, 277 (2002) [II].

Lieberman & Derse, *HIV-Positive Health Care Workers and the Obligation to Disclose: Do Patients Have a Right to Know?*, 13 J. Legal Med. 333, 353, 354, (1992) [8.03, 8.032, 9.131].

Liner, *Physician Deselection: The Dynamics of a New Threat to the Physician-Patient Relationship*, 23 Am. J. Law & Med. 511, 513, 527 (1997). [I, III; 8.05, 8.13]

Lipschitz, *Psychiatry and Consent for Physician-Assisted Suicide*, 19 Am. J. Forensic Psychiatry 91, 103, 104 (1998) [2.06, 2.211].

Livingston, *When Libido Subverts Credo: Regulation of Attorney-Client Sexual Relations*, 62 Fordham L. Rev. 5, 55 (1993) [8.14].

Lockhart, *The Safest Care is to Deny Care: Implications of Corporate Health Insurance, Inc. v. Texas Department of Insurance on HMO Liability in Texas*, 41 S. Tex. L. Rev. 621, 628, 634 (2000) [8.13].

Loeser, *The Legal, Ethical, and Practical Implications of Noncompetition Clauses: What Physicians Should Know Before They Sign*, 31 J.L. Med. & Ethics 283, 286, 287, 290 (2003) [9.02, 9.06, 10.01, 10.015].

Loftus, Paddock, & Guernsey, *Patient-Psychotherapist Privilege: Access to Clinical Records in the Tangled Web of Repressed Memory Litigation*, 30 U. Rich L. Rev. 109, 127 (1996) [IV; 5.05].

Lonchyna, *To Resuscitate or Not . . . In the Operating Room: The Need for Hospital Policies for Surgeons Regarding DNR Orders*, 6 Annals Health L. 209, 215, 217 (1997) [2.22, 8.08].

Loue, *Access to Health Care and the Undocumented Alien*, 13 J. Legal Med. 271, 291 (1992) [VI, VII].

Loue, *Intimate Partner Violence: Bridging the Gap Between Law and Science*, 21 J. Legal Med. 1, 18 (2000) [2.02].

Lubet, *Expert Witnesses: Ethics and Professionalism*, 12 Geo. J. Legal Ethics 465, 466 (1999) [IV].

Luna, *Sovereignty and Suspicion*, 48 Duke L. J. 787, 884 (1999) [2.132].

Lund, *The President as Client and the Ethics of the President's Lawyers*, 61 L. & Contemp. Probs. 65, 68 (1998) [IV].

Lundmark, *Surgery by an Unauthorized Surgeon as a Battery*, 10 J. L. & Health 287, 293 (1996) [8.16].

MacDonald, *Organ Donation: The Time Has Come to Refocus the Ethical Spotlight*, 8 Stan. L. & Pol'y Rev. 177, 179, 185 (1997) [2.155].

Madow, *Forbidden Spectacle: Executions, the Public and the Press in Nineteenth Century New York*, 43 Buff. L. Rev. 461, 475 (1995) [2.06].

Mahoney, *The Market for Human Tissue*, 86 Va. L. Rev. 163, 179 (2000) [2.15].

Mahowald, *Aren't We All Eugenicists? Commentary on Paul Lombardo's "Taking Eugenics Seriously"* 30 Fla. St. U. L. Rev. 219, 234 (2003) [2.12].

Makar, *Domestic Violence: Why the Florida Legislature Must Do More to Protect the "Silent" Victims*, 72 Fla. Bar J. 10, 16 (Nov. 1998) [2.02].

Malinowski, *Capitation, Advances in Medical Technology, and the Advent of a New Era in Medical Ethics*, XXII Am. J. Law & Med. 331, 337 (1996) [2.09].

Malinowski, *Conflicts of Interest in Clinical Research: Legal and Ethical Issues: Institutional Conflicts and Responsibilities in an Age of Academic-Industry Alliances*, 8 Wid. L. Symp. J. 47, 70 (2001) [8.031].

Malinowski, *Law, Policy, and Market Implications of Genetic Profiling in Drug Development*, 2 Hous. J. Health L. & Pol'y 31, 51 (2002) [8.031].

Malone, *Medical Authority and Infanticide*, 1 J. Law & Health 77 (1985-86) [2.17].

Mancino, *New GCM Suggests Rules for Ventures Between Nonprofit Hospitals and Doctors*, 76 J. Taxation 164, 167 (1992) [8.032].

Mars, *The Corporate Practice of Medicine: A Call for Action*, 7 Heath Matrix 241, 267 (1997) [VI].

Marsh, *Sacrificing Patients for Profits: Physician Incentives to Limit Care and ERISA Fiduciary Duty*, 77 Wash. U. L. Q. 1323, 1332 (1999) [8.03].

Marshall, O'Keefe, Fisher, Caruso, & Surdukowski, *Patients' Fear of Contracting the Acquired Immune Deficiency Syndrome From Physicians*, 150 Arch. Intern. Med. 1501, 1505 (1990) [9.131].

Martens, *Necessity of Adapting Psychiatric Treatment to Relevant Ethical Guidelines*, 20 Med. Law 393, 394 (2001) [VII].

Martin, *Legal Malpractice: Negligent Referral as a Cause of Action*, 29 Cumb. L. Rev. 679, 686 (1999) [8.132].

Martin, *Patentability of Methods of Medical Treatment: A Comparative Study*, 82 J. Pat. & Trademark Off. Soc'y 381, 383-84, 388, 423 (2000) [9.08, 9.09, 9.095].

Martin, *Tessie Hutchinson and the American System of Capital Punishment*, 59 Md. L. Rev. 553, 565 (2000) [2.06].

Martin & Bjerknes, *The Legal and Ethical Implications of Gag Clauses in Physician Contracts*, XXII Am. J. Law & Med. 433, 465-66 (1996) [Preamble; II, V, VI, 10.01].

Martin & Lagod, *The Human Preembryo, the Progenitors, and the State: Toward a Dynamic Theory of Status, Rights, and Research Policy*, 5 High Tech. L. J. 257, 304 (1990) [2.141].

Marzen, *Out, Out Brief Candle: Constitutionally Prescribed Suicide for the Terminally Ill*, 21 Hastings Const. L.Q. 799, 821 (1994) [2.06, 2.211].

Mayer, *Bergman v. Chin: Why an Elder Abuse Case is a Stride in the Direction of Civil Culpability for Physicians Who Undertreat Patients Suffering from Terminal Pain*, 37 New Eng. L. Rev. 313, 340 (2003) [2.20].

Mayo, *Sex, Marriage, Medicine, and Law: "What Hope of Harmony?"* 42 Washburn L.J. 269, 271 (2003) [2.162].

McAbee, *Improper Expert Medical Testimony: Existing and Proposed Mechanisms of Oversight*, 19 J. Legal Med. 257, 265 (1998) [6.01, 8.04, 9.07].

McConnell, *Confidentiality and the Law*, 20 J. Med. Ethics 47, 47 (1994) [IV; 10.01].

McConnell, *The Right to Die and the Jurisprudence of Tradition*, 1997 Utah L. Rev. 665, 703-04 (1997) [2.211].

McCormick, *Pharmaceutical Manufacturer's Duty to Warn of Adverse Drug Interactions*, 66 Def. Couns. J. 59, 61 (1999) [9.032].

McCullough, *A Basic Concept in the Clinical Ethics of Managed Care: Physicians and Institutions as Economically Disciplined Moral Co-Fiduciaries of Populations of Patients*, 24 J. Med. Phil. 77, 82-83, 87, 89, 91, 96 (1999) [8.13].

McFarlane, *Mandatory Reporting of Domestic Violence: An Inappropriate Response for New York Health Care Professionals*, 17 Buff. Pub. Int. L. J. 1, 29 (1998) [2.02].

McGonnigal, *This is Who Will Die When Doctors Are Allowed To Kill Their Patients*, 31 J. Marshall L. Rev. 95, 103 (1997) [2.211].

McGrath, *Raising the "Civilized Minimum" of Pain Amelioration for Prisoners to Avoid Cruel and Unusual Punishment*, 54 Rutgers L. Rev. 649, 657, 660 (2002) [V; 2.20].

McGuire, *AIDS and the Sexual Offender: The Epidemic Now Poses New Threats to the Victim and the Criminal Justice System*, 96 Dickinson L. Rev. 95, 109, 110 (1991) [5.05].

McIntyre, *Loosening Criteria for Withholding Prehospital Cardiopulmonary Resuscitation*, 153 Arch. Intern. Med. 2189, 2190 (1993) [2.22].

McKnight & Bollis, *Foregoing Life-Sustaining Treatment for Adult Developmentally Disabled, Public Wards: A Proposed Statute*, XVIII Am. J. Law & Med. 203, 206, 220, 227 (1992) [2.20].

McLean & Richards, *Managed Care Liability for Breach of Fiduciary Duty after Pegram v. Herdrich: The End of ERISA Preemption for State Law Liability for Medical Care Decision Making*, 53 Fla. L. Rev. 1, 38 (2001) [8.06].

McMullen, *Equitable Allocation of Human Organs: An Examination of the New Federal Regulations*, 20 J. Legal Med. 405, 412 (1999) [2.03].

McNaughton & McNaughton, *Divided Loyalty: The Dilemma of the Treating Physician Advocate*, 22 Okla. City U. L. Rev. 1051, 1052, 1054, 1056, 1058, 1059, 1062 (1997) [5.05, 5.07, 5.08, 7.02, 8.02, 8.03, 9.07].

McNoble, *The Cruzan Decision—A Surgeon's Perspective*, 20 Memphis State Univ. L. Rev. 569, 581, 600, 601 (1990) [2.20].

Mechanic, *The Functions and Limitations of Trust in the Provision of Medical Care*, 23 J. Health Pol. Pol'y & Law 661, 667 (1998) [6.02, 8.03].

Mehlman, *How Will We Regulate Genetic Enhancement?*, 34 Wake Forest L. Rev. 671, 693-94, 695 (1999) [2.11, 2.138, 9.065].

Mehlman, *Medical Advocates: A Call for a New Profession*, 1 Widener L. Symp. J. 299, 314 (1996) [2.03].

Mehlman, *Rationing Expensive Lifesaving Medical Treatments*, 1985 Wisconsin L. Rev. 239, 250, 260 (1985) [2.03].

Mehlman, *The Law of Above Averages: Leveling the New Genetic Enhancement Playing Field*, 85 Iowa L. Rev. 517, 527-28, 559 (2000) [2.11, 2.12].

Mehlman, *The Patient-Physician Relationship in an Era of Scarce Resources: Is There a Duty to Treat?*, 25 Conn. L. Rev. 349 (1993) [2.09].

Mehlman & Massey, *The Patient-Physician Relationship and the Allocation of Scarce Resources: A Law and Economics Approach*, 4 Kennedy Inst. Ethics J. 291, 292 (1994) [2.09, 2.095].

Meisel, *A Retrospective on Cruzan*, 20 Law, Med. & Health Care 340, 345 (1992) [2.20].

Meisel, *Barriers to Forgoing Nutrition and Hydration in Nursing Homes*, XXI Am. J. Law & Med. 335, 353-54 (1995) [2.20].

Meisel, *Legal Myths About Terminating Life Support*, 151 Arch. Intern. Med. 1497, 1499 (1991) [2.20].

Meisel, *Lessons from Cruzan*, 1 J. Clinical Ethics 245, 248 (1990) [2.20].

Meisel, *The Legal Consensus About Forgoing Life-Sustaining Treatment: Its Status and Its Prospects*, 2 Kennedy Inst. Ethics J. 309, 325 (1992) [2.20].

Menikoff, *Organ Swapping*, 29 Hastings Center Rep. 28, 32 (Nov./Dec. 1999) [2.15].

Merkatz, *Women in Clinical Trials: An Introduction*, 48 Food & Drug L. J. 161, 163 (1993) [9.122].

Merz, *Psychosocial Risks of Storing and Using Human Tissues in Research*, 8 Risk: Health Safety & Env't 235, 236 (1997) [2.132].

Merz, Sankar, & Yoo, *Hospital Consent for Disclosure of Medical Records*, 26 J. Law, Med. & Ethics 241, 248 (1998) [IV; 5.05].

Michalos, *Medical Ethics and the Executing Process in the United States of America*, 16 Med. & Law 125, 131, 133 (1997) [2.06].

Michels & Rothman, *Update on Unethical Use of Placebos in Randomised Trials*, 17 Bioethics 188, 200 (2003) [2.075].

Milani, *Better Off Dead Than Disabled?: Should Courts Recognize a Wrongful Living Cause of Action When Doctors Fail to Honor Patients' Advance Directives?*, 54 Wash. & Lee L. Rev. 149, 151-52 (1997) [2.22].

Miles, *Medical Futility*, 20 Law, Med. & Health Care 310, 311, 313 (1992) [2.20, 2.21, 2.22].

Miles, *On a New Charter to Defend Medical Professionalism: Whose Profession is it Anyway?* 32 Hastings Center Rep. 46, 47 (May/June 2002) [2.06].

Miles, *What Are We Teaching about Indigent Patients?*, 268 JAMA 2561, 2562 (1992) [9.131].

Miller, *Managed Care Regulation: In the Laboratory of the States*, 278 JAMA 1102, 1104, 1108-09 (1997) [8.13].

Miller, *Trusting Doctors: Tricky Business When It Comes to Clinical Research*, 81 B.U.L. Rev. 423, 427-28 (2001) [IV; 8.032].

Miller & Sage, *Disclosing Physician Financial Incentives*, 281 JAMA 1424, 1425 (1999). [8.032, 8.13, 8.132]

Miller-Rice, *The "Insane" Contradiction of Singleton v. Norris: Forced Medication in a Death Row Inmate's Medical Interest Which Happens to Facilitate His Execution*, 22 U. Ark. Little Rock L. Rev. 659, 673 (2001) [2.06].

Minor, *Identity Cards and Databases in Health Care: The Need for Federal Privacy Protections*, 28 Colum. J.L. & Soc. Probs. 253, 279 (1995) [5.05].

Mishu, Schaffner, Horan, Wood, Hutcheson, & McNabb, *A Surgeon With AIDS: Lack of Evidence of Transmission to Patients*, 264 JAMA 467 (1990) [9.131].

Misocky, *The Patients' Bill of Rights: Managed Care Under Siege*, 15 J. Contemp. Health L. & Pol'y 57, 73 (1998) [8.13].

Mitchell, *Physician-Assisted Suicide: A Survey of the Issues Surrounding Legalization*, 74 N.D. L. Rev. 341, 349 (1998) [2.20, 2.211, 8.08].

Mitchell & Scott, *Evidence on Complex Structures of Physician Joint Ventures*, 9 Yale J. Regulation 489, 503 (1992) [8.032].

Mitchell & Scott, *New Evidence of the Prevalence and Scope of Physician Joint Ventures*, 268 JAMA 80, 84 (1992) [8.032].

Mitchell & Scott, *Physician Ownership of Physical Therapy Services: Effects on Charges, Utilization, Profits, and Service Characteristics*, 268 JAMA 2055, 2058 (1992) [8.032].

Mitchell & Sunshine, *Consequences of Physicians' Ownership of Health Care Facilities—Joint Ventures in Radiation Therapy*, 327 New Eng. J. Med. 1497, 1500 (1992) [8.032].

Mitten, *Team Physicians and Competitive Athletes: Allocating Legal Responsibility for Athletic Injuries*, 55 U. Pitt. L. Rev. 129, 140 (1993) [3.06].

Modlin, *Forensic Psychiatry and Malpractice*, 18 Bull. Am. Acad. Psychiatry Law 153, 161 (1990) [II, IV].

Moore, *Physician-Assisted Suicide: Does "The End" Justify the Means?*, 40 Ariz. L. Rev. 1471, 1472, 1481-82, 1491 (1998) [2.20, 2.211].

Moore, *What Doctors Can Learn from Lawyers about Conflicts of Interest*, 81 B.U.L. Rev. 445, 447, 449-50 (2001) [Preamble; IV; 2.07, 8.03, 8.031, 10.01].

Morgan & Sutherland, *Last Rights? Confronting Physician-Assisted Suicide in Law and Society: Legal Liturgies on Physician-Assisted Suicide*, 26 Stetson L. Rev. 481, 484 (1996) [2.20, 2.21, 2.211].

Morgan, Marks, & Harty-Golder, *The Issue of Personal Choice: The Competent Incurable Patient and the Right to Commit Suicide?*, 57 Mo. L. Rev. 1, 44, 45 (1992) [2.21, 2.211].

Morley, *Increasing the Supply of Organs for Transplantation Through Paired Organ Exchanges*, 21 Yale L. & Pol'y Rev. 221, 255 (2003) [2.15].

Morreim, *Am I My Brother's Warden? Responding to the Unethical or Incompetent Colleague*, 23 Hastings Center Rep. 19, 23 (May/June 1993) [II; 8.14, 9.031].

Morreim, *Blessed Be the Tie That Binds? Antitrust Perils of Physician Investment and Self-Referral*, 14 J. Legal Med. 359, 367, 374, 377, 394, 409 (1993) [8.032].

Morreim, *Diverse and Perverse Incentives of Managed Care: Bringing Patients into Alignment*, 1 Widener L. Symp. J. 89, 129 (1996) [8.13].

Morreim, *Economic Disclosure and Economic Advocacy: New Duties in the Medical Standard of Care*, 12 J. Legal Med. 275, 306 (1991) [8.08, 8.12].

Morreim, *Patient-Funded Research: Paying the Piper or Protecting the Patient?*, 13 IRB 1, 2 (May/June 1991) [8.031].

Morreim, *Physician Investment and Self-Referral: Philosophical Analysis of a Contentious Debate*, 15 J. Med. & Phil. 425, 428, 429, 430, 431 (1990) [8.032].

Morreim, *Redefining Quality by Reassigning Responsibility*, 20 Am. J. Law & Med. 79, 103 (1994) [10.02].

Morris, *Dissing Disclosure: Just What the Doctor Ordered*, 44 Ariz. L. Rev. 313, 344, 349, 362, 363, 366 (2002) [VII; 8.03, 8.053, 8.054, 8.08].

Moskowitz, *Saving Granny from the Wolf: Elder Abuse and Neglect—The Legal Framework*, 31 Conn. L. Rev. 77, 116, 120, 121, 122 (1998) [2.02, 5.05].

Mossinghoff, *Remedies Under Patents on Medical and Surgical Procedures*, 78 J. Pat. & Trademark Off. Soc'y 789, 790 (1996) [9.095].

Mowery, *A Patient's Right of Privacy in Computerized Pharmacy Records*, 66 U. Cin. L. Rev. 697, 717 (1998) [5.05].

Mullins, *The Need for Guidance in Decision making for Terminally Ill Incompetents: Is the Ohio Legislature in a "Persistent Vegetative State?,"* 17 Ohio No. Univ. L. Rev. 827, 844 (1991) [2.20].

Munoz, Nichols, Okata, Pitt, & Seager, *The Two Faces of Gag Provisions: Patients and Physicians in a Bind*, 17 Yale L. & Pol'y Rev. 249, 258 (1998) [II].

Murphy, *Expert Witnesses at Trial: Where are the Ethics?* 14 Geo. J. Legal Ethics 217, 231-32 (2000) [I, II, III, V; 1.02, 6.01, 9.07].

Myers, Sonenshein, & Hofstein, *To Regulate or Not To Regulate Attorney-Client Sex? The Ethical Question in Pennsylvania*, 69 Temp. L. Rev. 741, 780 (1996) [II].

Naccasha, *The Permissibility of Routine AIDS Testing in the Health Care Context*, 5 Notre Dame J.L. Ethics & Pub. Pol'y, 223, 241 (1990) [VI; 9.131].

Nandi, *Ethical Aspects of Clinical Practice*, 135 Arch. Surg. 22, 23 (2000) [Preamble].

Napoli, *The Doctrine of Informed Consent and Women: The Achievement of Equal Value and Equal Exercise of Autonomy*, 4 J. Gender & L. 335, 336 (1996) [9.122].

National Council on Disability, *Assisted Suicide: A Disability Perspective*, 14 Issues L. & Med. 273, 292 (1998) [2.20].

Needell, *Legal Ethics in Medicine: Are Medical Ethics Different from Legal Ethics?* 14 St. Thomas L. Rev. 31, 35, 50 (2001) [II; 5.02].

Nelson & Cranford, *Legal Advice, Moral Paralysis and the Death of Samuel Linares*, 17 Law, Med. & Health Care 316 (1989) [2.20].

Newdick, *Public Health Ethics and Clinical Freedom*, 14 J. Contemp. Health L. & Pol'y 335, 336, 339, 356, 359, 361 (1998) [8.13].

Newman, *Baby Doe, Congress and the States: Challenging the Federal Treatment Standard for Impaired Infants*, XV Am. J. Law and Med. 1 (1989) [2.17].

Nidich, *Zinermon v. Burch and Voluntary Admissions to Public Hospitals: A Common Sense Proposal for Compromise*, 25 N. Ky. L. Rev. 699, 710 (1998) [I, III].

Noah, *Adverse Drug Reactions: Harnessing Experimental Data to Promote Patient Welfare*, 49 Cath. U. L. Rev. 449, 477, 497-98 (2000) [V; 5.05, 9.032].

Noah, *Death of a Salesman: To What Extent Can the FDA Regulate the Promotional Statements of Pharmaceutical Sales Representatives?*, 47 Food & Drug L. J. 309, 316 (1992) [8.061].

Noah, *Informed Consent and the Elusive Dichotomy Between Standard and Experimental Therapy*, 28 Am. J.L. & Med. 361, 394, 395 (2002) [2.07, 9.032].

Noah, *Medicine's Epistemology: Mapping the Haphazard Diffusion of Knowledge in the Biomedical Community*, 44 Ariz. L. Rev. 373, 404, 447, 448 (2002) [V; 9.08, 9.095].

Noah, *Pigeonholing Illness: Medical Diagnosis as a Legal Construct*, 50 Hastings L. J. 241, 301, 302 (1999) [II; 9.07].

Noah, *Triage in the Nation's Medicine Cabinet: The Puzzling Scarcity of Vaccines and Other Drugs*, 54 S.C. L. Rev. 741, 755 (2003) [2.16].

Noah & Brushwood, *Adverse Drug Reactions in Elderly Patients: Alternative Approaches to Postmarket Surveillance*, 33 J. Health L. 383, 400, 445 (2000) [V; 9.032].

Nodzenski, *HIV-Infected Health Care Professionals and Informed Consent*, 2 S. Cal. Interdisciplinary L. J. 299, 327 (1993) [9.13].

Noonan, *Patenting Medical Technology*, 11 J. Legal Med. 263, 268 (1990) [9.09].

Northern, *Procreative Torts: Enhancing the Common-Law Protection for Reproductive Autonomy*, 1998 U. Ill. L. Rev. 489, 525 (1998) [8.08].

Note, A Case Study of New Textualism in State Courts: Doe v. Marselle and the Confidentiality of HIV-Related Information, 30 Conn. L. Rev. 295, 297 (1997) [5.05].

Note, Administrative Agencies Get Their Way Over Constitutional Rights in Rust v. Sullivan, 28 Willamette L. Rev. 173, 193 (1991) [8.08].

Note, Aid-in-Dying: Should We Decriminalize Physician-Assisted Suicide and Physician-Committed Euthanasia?, XVIII Am. J. Law & Med. 369, 370 (1992) [2.211].

Note, AIDS: Establishing a Physician's Duty to Warn, 21 Rutgers L. J. 645, 652 (1990) [5.05].

Note, Constitutional Aspects of Physician-Assisted Suicide After Lee v. Oregon, XXIII Am. J. Law & Med. 69 (1997) [2.211].

Note, Constitutional Law—Judicial Deference— Supreme Court Will Defer to "Reasonable" Abortion Restrictions, 14 Univ. Ark. Little Rock 557, 573 (1992) [8.08].

Note, Contingent Expert Witness Fees: Access and Legitimacy, 64 So. Cal. L. Rev. 1363, 1374, 1382 (1991) [8.04].

Note, Covenants Not to Compete and Liquidated Damages Clauses: Diagnosis and Treatment for Physicians, 46 S.C. L. Rev. 505, 514 (1995) [9.02, 9.06].

Note, Cruzan v. Director, Missouri Department of Health: To Die or Not to Die: That is the Question— But Who Decides?, 51 Louisiana L. Rev. 1307, 1327, 1333 (1991) [2.20].

Note, Denial of Coverage for "Experimental" Medical Procedures: The Problem of De Novo Review Under ERISA, 79 Kentucky L. J. 801, 824 (1990-91) [? 03, 2.09].

Note, Ethics and AIDS: A Summary of the Law and a Critical Analysis of the Individual Physician's Ethical Duty to Treat, XVI Am. J. Law & Med. 249, 262 (1990) [VI].

Note, Exercising the Right to Die: North Carolina's Amended Natural Death Act and the 1991 Health Care Power of Attorney Act, 70 No. Carolina L. Rev. 2108, 2116 (1992) [2.20].

Note, Healer-Patient Privilege: Extending the Physician-Patient Privilege to Alternative Health Practitioners in California, 48 Hastings L. J. 633, 657 (1997) [5.05].

Note, Health Care Proxies: New York's Attempt to Resolve the Right to Die Dilemma, 57 Brooklyn L. Rev. 145, 168 (1991) [2.20].

Note, HIV and Dentistry, 29 Val. U.L. Rev. 297, 317 (1994) [9.131].

Note, HMO Exclusion of Chiropractors, 66 So. Cal. L. Rev. 807, 823 (1993) [3.04].

Note, I Have a Conscience, Too: The Plight of Medical Personnel Confronting the Right to Die, 65 Notre Dame L. Rev. 699, 706 (1990) [2.20].

Note, Informed Choice: Physicians' Duty to Disclose Nonreadily Available Alternatives, 43 Case W. Res. L. Rev. 491, 491, 498-99, 508, 509 (1993) [I, II, III, IV, V; 8.08].

Note, Patenting Medical Procedures: A Search for a Compromise Between Ethics and Economics, 18 Cardozo L. Rev. 1527, 1544, 1547, 1554 (1997) [9.08, 9.09, 9.095].

Note, Perry v. Louisiana: Medical Ethics on Death Row—Is Judicial Intervention Warranted?, 4 Georgetown J. Legal Ethics 707, 714 (1991) [2.06].

Note, Physician-Patient Sexual Contact: The Battle Between the State and the Medical Profession, 50 Wash. & Lee L. Rev. 1725, 1725-26, 1734, 1752 (1993) [8.14].

Note, Physicians, Bound and Gagged: Federal Attempts to Combat Managed Care's Use of Gag Clauses, 21 Seton Hall Legis. J. 567, 601-02 (1997) [II, V; 8.13, 10.01].

Note, Preventing Patient Dumping: Sharpening the COBRA's Fangs, 61 N. Y. U. L. Rev. 1186 (1986) [VI; 8.11].

Note, Professional Ethics Codes in Court: Redefining the Social Contract Between the Public and the Professions, 25 Georgia L. Rev. 1327, 1335, 1351 (1991) [II; 2.19].

Note, Redefining the Right to Die in Illinois, 15 So. Ill. Univ. L. J. 1261, 1273 (1991) [2.20].

Note, Restricting Ex Parte Interviews With Nonparty Treating Physicians: Crist v. Moffatt, 69 No. Carolina L. Rev. 1381, 1391, 1392 (1991) [5.50].

Note, Rust on the Constitution: Politics and Gag Rules, 37 How. L. J. 83, 96 (1993) [8.08].

Note, Sexual Conduct Within the Physician-Patient Relationship: A Statutory Framework for Disciplining this Breach of Fiduciary Duty, 1 Widener L. Symp. J. 501, 507 (1996) [II; 8.14].

Note, Something Worth Writing Home About: Clear and Convincing Evidence, Living Wills, and Cruzan v. Director, Missouri Department of Health, 22 Univ. Toledo L. Rev. 871, 879 (1991) [2.20].

Note, *State Natural Death Acts: Illusory Protection of Individuals' Life-Sustaining Treatment Decisions*, 29 Harvard J. Legis. 175, 186, 194, 195, 201 (1992) [2.20, 2.22].

Note, *Stop Gagging Physicians!*, 7 Health Matrix 187, 193, 200, 208-09 (1997) [8.13].

Note, *The Americans With Disabilities Act: Magic Bullet or Band-Aid for Patients and Health Care Workers Infected With the Human Immunodeficiency Virus?*, 57 Brooklyn L. Rev. 1277, 1279, 1305 (1992) [9.131].

Note, *The Economic Wisdom of Regulating Pharmaceutical "Freebies,"* 1991 Duke L. J. 206, 216, 233, 234 (1991) [8.061, 8.08].

Note, *The Informed-Consent Policy of the International Conference on Harmonization of Technical Requirements for Registrations of Pharmaceuticals for Human Use: Knowledge is the Best Medicine*, 30 Cornell Int'l L. J. 203, 209 (1997) [2.07].

Note, *The New Patent Infringement Liability Exception for Medical Procedures*, 23 J. Legis. 265, 268 (1997) [9.095].

Note, *The Ohio Physician-Patient Privilege: Modified, Revised, and Defined*, 49 Ohio St. L. J. 1147 (1989) [II, IV; 5.05].

Note, *The Policy Against Federal Funding for Abortions Extends Into the Realm of Free Speech After Rust v. Sullivan*, 19 Pepperdine L. Rev. 637, 681 (1992) [8.08].

Note, *Torts: Defining the Duty Imposed on Physicians by the Doctrine of Informed Consent*, 22 Wm. Mitchell L. Rev. 149, 160 (1996) [9.13].

Note, *Toward a More Perfect Union: A Federal Cause of Action for Physician Aid-In-Dying*, 27 U. Mich. J.L. Ref. 521, 538 (1994) [I, III; 2.06].

Note, *Who Decides if There is Triumph in the Ultimate Agony? Constitutional Theory and the Emerging Right to Die With Dignity*, 37 Wm. & Mary L. Rev. 827, 829 (1996) [2.20, 2.211].

Noyes, *Higher Penalties for Failing to Pay Child Support: A Look at Medical License Revocation*, 19 J. Legal Med. 127, 138 (1998) [5.05, 9.02, 9.06].

Obade, *Whisper Down the Lane: AIDS, Privacy, and the Hospital Grapevine*, 2 J. Clinical Ethics 133, 133 (1991) [5.05].

Oberman, *Mothers and Doctors' Orders: Unmasking the Doctor's Fiduciary Role in Maternal-Fetal Conflicts*, 94 Nw. U. L. Rev. 451, 456, 462, 493 (2000) [8.08, 8.13, 10.01].

Oddi, *Reverse Informed Consent: The Unreasonably Dangerous Patient*, 46 Vand. L. Rev. 1417, 1449, 1463, 1465, 1479 (1993) [IV, VI; 8.11, 9.131].

Ogbogu, Fleischer, Brodell, Bhalla, Draelos, & Feldman, *Physicians' and Patients' Perspectives on Office-Based Dispensing: The Central Role of the Physician-Patient Relationship*, 137 Arch. Dermatol. 151, 151 (2001) [8.06].

Oken, *Curing Healthcare Providers' Failure to Administer Opioids in the Treatment of Severe Pain*, 23 Cardozo L. Rev. 1917, 1925-26, 1952, 1954 (2002) [2.20, 2.21, 2.211].

Olson, *Physician Specialty Advertising: The Tendency to Deceive?*, 11 J. Legal Med. 351, 354 (1990) [5.02].

O'Neill, *Surrogate Health Care Decisions for Adults in Illinois—Answers to the Legal Questions That Health Care Providers Face on a Daily Basis*, 29 Loy. Univ. Chi. L. J. 411, 445, 448 (1998) [2.035, 2.22, 8.11].

Oppenheim, *Physicians as Experts Against Their Own Patients? What Happened to the Privilege?*, 63 Def. Couns. J. 254, 257, 261 (1996) [IV; 5.05].

Orenstein, *Apology Excepted: Incorporating a Feminist Analysis into Evidence Policy Where You Would Least Expect It*, 28 S.W. U. L. Rev. 221, 264 (1999) [I, II].

Orentlicher, *Advance Medical Directives*, 263 JAMA 2365 (1990) [2.20].

Orentlicher, *Cloning and the Preservation of Family Integrity*, 59 La. L. Rev. 1019, 1022 (1999) [2.147].

Orentlicher, *Denying Treatment to the Noncompliant Patient*, 265 JAMA 1579, 1581 (1991) [VI; 9.12].

Orentlicher, *Health Care Reform and the Patient-Physician Relationship*, 5 Health Matrix 141, 143, 148 (1995) [5.05, 10.01].

Orentlicher, *HIV-Infected Surgeons: Behringer v. Medical Center*, 266 JAMA 1134, 1136 (1991) [8.032, 9.131].

Orentlicher, *Paying Physicians More to Do Less: Financial Incentives to Limit Care*, 30 U. Rich. L. Rev. 155, 167 (1996) [8.13].

Orentlicher, *The Illusion of Patient Choice in End-of-Life Decisions*, 267 JAMA 2101, 2102 (1992) [2.20, 2.22, 9.121].

Orentlicher, *The Influence of a Professional Organization on Physician Behavior*, 57 Alb. L. Rev. 583, 592, 593, 594, 595, 596 (1994) [1.01, 1.02, 8.061, 9.04, 9.131].

Orentlicher, *The Legalization of Physician Assisted Suicide: A Very Modest Revolution*, 38 B.C.L. Rev. 443, 459-60 (1997) [2.211].

Ornish, Mills, & Ornish, *Prearraignment Forensic Evaluations: Toward a New Policy*, 24 Bull. Am. Acad. Psychiatry Law 453, 454, 469 (1996) [Preamble; IV; 5.05].

Orr & Bishop, *Why Psychiatrists Should Not Participate in Euthanasia and Physician-Assisted Suicide*, 19 Am. J. Forensic Psychiatry 35, 36 (1998) [2.211].

Orr & Hook, *Stem Cell Research: Magical Promise v Moral Peril*, 2 Yale J. Health Pol'y, Law & Ethics 189, 197 (2001) [2.30].

Orr, Johnston, Ashwal, & Bailey, *Should Children with Severe Cognitive Impairment Receive Solid Organ Transplants?* 11 J. Clinical Ethics 219, 222-23, 228 (2000) [2.16].

O'Shaughnessy, *The Worst of Both Worlds?: Parental Involvement Requirements and the Privacy Rights of Mature Minors*, 57 Ohio St. L. J. 1731, 1764-65 (1996) [2.015].

O'Sullivan & Borcherding, *Informed Consent for Medication in Persons with Mental Retardation and Mental Illness*, 12 Health Matrix 63, 75, 86, 87, 88 (2002) [Preamble; I, III, IV, VIII, IX; 8.08].

O'Toole, *HIV-Specific Crime Legislation: Targeting an Epidemic for Criminal Prosecution*, 10 J.L. & Health 183, 195, 199 (1995) [2.23].

Packer, *Ethics and Medical Patents*, 117 Arch. Ophthalmol. 824, 825 (1999) [9.08].

Paltrow, *The War on Drugs and the War on Abortion: Some Initial Thoughts on the Connections, Intersections and the Effects*, 28 S.U. L. Rev. 201, 219 (2001) [10.01].

Park, *Physician-Assisted Suicide: State Legislation Teetering at the Pinnacle of a Slippery Slope*, 7 Wm. & Mary Bill Rts. J. 277, 292, 293 (1998) [2.211].

Parker, *Corporate Practice of Medicine: Last Stand or Final Downfall?*, 29 J. Health & Hosp. L. 160, 167, 173 (1996) [VI].

Parmet, *The Supreme Court Confronts HIV: Reflections on Bragdon v. Abbott*, 26 J. Law, Med. & Ethics 225 (1998) [9.131].

Partlett, *Misuse of Genetic Information: The Common Law and Professionals' Liability*, 42 Washburn L.J. 489, 503 (2003) [2.132].

Patterson, *Conflicts of Interest in Scientific Expert Testimony*, 40 Wm. & Mary L. Rev. 1313, 1330, 1332, 1335, 1371 (1999) [8.061, 9.07].

Patterson, *Planning for Health Care Using Living Wills and Durable Powers of Attorney: A Guide for the South Carolina Attorney*, 42 So. Carolina L. Rev. 525, 535, 541, 547, 548 (1991) [2.20].

Patton, *A Call for Common Sense: Organ Donation and the Executed Prisoner*, 3 Va. J. Soc. Pol'y & L. 387, 404, 405, 407-10 (1996) [VII; 2.06, 2.162].

Pearlman, Cain, Patrick, Appelbaum-Maizel, Starks, Jecker, & Uhlmann, *Insights Pertaining to Patient Assessments of States Worse than Death*, 4 J. Clinical Ethics 33, 40 (1993) [2.20, 2.21].

Pearson, Kahn, Harrison, Rubenstein, Rogers, Brook, & Keeler, *Differences in Quality of Care for Hospitalized Elderly Men and Women*, 268 JAMA 1883 (1992) [9.122].

Peccarelli, *A Moral Dilemma: The Role of Judicial Intervention in Withholding or Withdrawing Nutrition and Hydration*, 23 John Marshall L. Rev. 537, 539, 540, 541 (1990) [Preamble; I, II, III, IV, V, VI, VII; 2.20].

Perales, *Rethinking the Prohibition of Death Row Prisoners as Organ Donors: A Possible Lifeline to Those on Organ Donor Waiting Lists*, 34 St. Mary's L. J. 687, 721, 725 (2003) [VII; 2.06].

Perdue & Binion, *A License to Kill: The Unintended (?) Consequence of Milo on Kramer*, 41 S. Tex. L. Rev. 293, 309 (2000) [8.12].

Pereira & Pearson, *Patient Attitudes toward Physician Financial Incentives*, 161 Arch. Intern. Med. 1313, 1316, 1317 (2001) [8.132].

Pergament, *Internet Psychotherapy: Current Status and Future Regulation*, 8 Health Matrix 233, 253 (1998) [9.12].

Perkin & Resnik, *The Agony of Agonal Respiration: Is the Last Gasp Necessary?* 28 J. Med. Ethics 164, 169 (2002) [2.211].

Persels, *Forcing the Issue of Physician-Assisted Suicide: Impact of the Kevorkian Case on the Euthanasia Debate*, 14 J. Legal Med. 93, 115 (1993) [2.06, 2.20].

Petrila, *Ethics, Money, and the Problem of Coercion in Managed Behavioral Health Care*, 40 St. Louis U. L. J. 359, 377 (1996) [2.03, 4.04].

Phan, *Physician Unionization: The Impact on the Medical Profession*, 20 J. Legal Med. 115, 136, 137 (1999) [9.025].

Pierucci, Kirby, & Leuthner, *End-of-Life Care for Neonates and Infants: The Experience and Effects of a Palliative Care Consultation Service*, 108 Pediatrics 653, 659 (2001) [2.215].

Pittman, *Any Willing Provider Laws and ERISA's Saving Clause: A New Solution for an Old Problem*, 64 Tenn. L. Rev. 409, 416 (1997) [8.13].

Pittman, *Physician-Assisted Suicide in the Dark Ward: The Intersection of the Thirteenth Amendment and Health Care Treatments Having Disproportionate Impacts on Disfavored Groups*, 28 Seton Hall L. Rev. 774, 784 (1998) [2.211].

Plambeck, *Divided Loyalties: Legal and Bioethical Considerations of Physician-Pregnant Patient Confidentiality and Prenatal Drug Abuse*, 23 J. Legal Med. 1, 8, 25 (2002) [IV; 10.01].

Polsky, *Winning Medicine: Professional Sports Team Doctors' Conflicts of Interest*, 14 J. Contemp. Health L. & Pol'y 503, 505 (1998) [VI].

Pope, *The Maladaptation of Miranda to Advance Directives: A Critique of the Implementation of the Patient Self-Determination Act*, 9 Health Matrix 139, 178 (1999) [2.20].

Porter, *Physician Advertising—What is Legal? What is Ethical? What is Acceptable?*, 80 Ohio State Med. J. 437 (1984) [5.02].

Post, *Subsidized Speech*, 106 Yale L. J. 151, 173 (1996) [8.08].

Post, Blustein, Gordon, & Dubler, *Pain: Ethics, Culture, and Informed Consent to Relief*, 24 J. Law, Med. & Ethics 348, 349, 356 (1996) [2.20].

Potter, *Failure to Disclose HMO Incentives and the Breach of Fiduciary Duty: Is a New Cause of Action Against Physicians the Best Solution?*, 34 USF. L. Rev. 733, 753 (2000) [8.132].

Povenmire, *Do Parents Have the Legal Authority to Consent to the Surgical Amputation of Normal, Healthy Tissue from their Infant Children?: The Practice of Circumcision in the United States*, 7 Am. U. J. Gender Soc. Pol. & L. 87, 96 (1999) [IV].

Pratt, *Too Many Physicians: Physician-Assisted Suicide After Glucksberg/Quill*, 9 Alb. L. J. Sci. & Tech. 161, 208 (1999) [2.20, 2.21, 2.211].

Prentice, *Clinical Trial Results, Physicians, and Insider Trading*, 20 J. Legal Med. 195, 221 (1999) [8.032].

Preston, *Baby Spice: Lost Between Feminine and Feminist*, 9 Am. U. J. Gender Soc. Pol'y & L. 541, 590 (2001) [9.122].

Price, *Between Scylla and Charybdis: Charting a Course to Reconcile the Duty of Confidentiality and the Duty to Warn in the AIDS Context*, 94 Dickinson L. Rev. 435, 477 (1990) [2.23].

Pritts, *Altered States: State Health Privacy Laws and the Impact of the Federal Health Privacy Rules*, 2 Yale J. Health Pol'y, L. & Ethics 327, 351 (2002) [10.02].

Pronovost & Williams, *Telemedicine and End-of-Life Care: What's Wrong with This Picture?* 12 J. Clinical Ethics 64, 68 (2001) [2.20].

Puglise, *"Calling Dr. Love": The Physician-Patient Sexual Relationship as Grounds for Medical Malpractice B Society Pays While the Doctor and Patient Play*, 14 J. L. & Health 321, 324-25, 349 (2000) [8.14].

Pugno, *Hospital Privileges for Family Physicians: Rights, Rationale, and Resources*, 17 J. Fam. Practice 77 (1983) [9.05].

Quill & Cassel, *Nonabandonment: A Central Obligation for Physicians*, 10 Trends in Health Care, Law & Ethics 25, 27 (Winter/Spring 1995) [8.11].

Quill, Cassel, & Meier, *Care of the Hopelessly Ill: Proposed Clinical Criteria for Physician-Assisted Suicide*, 327 New Eng. J. Med. 1380, 1381 (1992) [2.20].

Quinn, *The Best Interests of Incompetent Patients: The Capacity for Interpersonal Relationships as a Standard for Decisionmaking*, 76 Cal. L. Rev. 897 (1988) [2.20].

Rabeneck, McCullough, & Wray, *Ethically Justified, Clinically Comprehensive Guidelines for Percutaneous Endoscopic Gastrostomy Tube Placement*, 349 Lancet 496, 497, 498 (1997) [2.17].

Radelet, *Capital Punishment in Colorado: 1859-1972*, 74 U. Colo. L. Rev. 885, 940 (2003) [2.06].

Rai, Siegler, & Lantos, *The Physician as a Health Care Proxy*, 29 Hastings Center Rep. 14, 19 (Sep./Oct. 1999) [2.03].

Reardon, *American Medical Association Perspective on Physician Assisted Suicide*, 75 U. Det. Mercy L. Rev. 515 (1998) [2.211].

Rediger, *Living in a World with HIV: Balancing Privacy, Privilege and the Right to Know Between Patients and Health Care Professionals*, 21 Hamline J. Pub. L. & Pol'y 443, 456-57, 461, 472 (2000) [2.23, 9.13, 9.131].

Regan, *Regulating the Business of Medicine: Models for Integrating Ethics and Managed Care*, 30 Colum. J.L. & Soc. Probs. 635, 651, 656, 657 (1997) [Preamble; I, II, III, IV, V; 8.13].

Reisman, *Physicians and Surgeons as Inventors: Reconciling Medical Process Patents and Medical Ethics*, 10 High Tech. L. J. 355, 356, 368-70, 385 (1995) [VII; 9.08, 9.09, 9.095].

Reiss, *Commentary on Payment and Reimbursement Issues Affecting the Marketing of Drugs, Medical Devices, and Biologics, with Emphasis on the Anti-Kickback Statute and Stark II*, 52 Food & Drug L. J. 99, 107 (1997) [8.061].

Relman, *"Self-Referral"—What's at Stake?*, 327 New Eng. J. Med. 1522, 1524 (1992) [8.032].

Resnik, *DNA Patents and Human Dignity*, 29 J. L. Med. & Ethics 152, 158, 159 (2001) [2.105].

Reuland, *Health Maintenance Organizations and Physician Financial Incentive Plans: Should Physician Disclosure be Mandatory?* 27 Iowa J. Corp. L. 293, 312 (2002) [8.13].

Reutenauer, *Medical Malpractice Liability in the Era of Genetic Susceptibility Testing*, 19 QLR 539, 571 (2000) [10.01].

Reza, *Religion and the Public Defender*, 26 Fordham Urb. L. J. 1051, 1062, 1063 (1999) [VI; 8.11, 9.06, 9.12].

Rheinstein, *MedWatch: The FDA Medical Products Reporting Program*, 48 Am. Fam. Physician 636, 636 (1993) [9.032].

Rice, *The Superior Orders Defense in Legal Ethics: Sending the Wrong Message to Young Lawyers*, 32 Wake Forest L. Rev. 887, 908-09 (1997) [9.055].

Rich, *A Prescription for the Pain: The Emerging Standard of Care for Pain Management*, 26 Wm. Mitchell L. Rev. 1, 35-36, 85 (2000) [V; 2.20, 9.011].

Rich, *Advance Directives: The Next Generation*, 19 J. Legal Med. 63, 79 (1998) [2.20].

Rich, *Prognostication in Clinical Medicine: Prophecy or Professional Responsibility?* 23 J. Legal Med. 297, 299, 318, 327 (2002) [IV; 8.12, 10.01].

Rich, *The Assault on Privacy on Healthcare Decision making*, 68 Denver L. Rev. 1, 10 (1991) [2.20].

Richards & Wolf, *Medical Confidentiality and Disclosure of Paternity*, 48 S.D. L. Rev. 409, 411, 412, 413 (2003) [I, II, IV, V; 1.02, 5.05, 5.055, 10.01].

Rie, *The Limits of a Wish*, 21 Hastings Center Rep. 24 (July/August 1991) [2.20].

Risley, *Ethical and Legal Issues in the Individual's Right to Die*, 20 Ohio N.U.L. Rev. 597, 605 (1993) [2.20].

Rivo & Satcher, *Improving Access to Health Care Through Physician Workforce Reform*, 270 JAMA 1074, 1075 (1993) [9.121].

Roach, *Paradox and Pandora's Box: The Tragedy of Current Right-to-Die Jurisprudence*, 25 Univ. Mich. J. Law Reform 133, 137, 158 (1991) [2.20].

Roberts, *Rust v. Sullivan and the Control of Knowledge*, 61 Geo. Wash. L. Rev. 587, 641 (1993) [8.08].

Roberts, Roberts, Warner, Solomon, Hardee, & McCarty, *Internal Medicine, Psychiatry, and Emergency Medicine Residents' Views of Assisted Death Practices*, 157 Arch. Intern. Med. 1603, 1609 (1997) [2.211].

Robertson, *Dilemma in Danville*, 11 Hastings Center Rep. 5 (Oct. 1981) [2.17].

Robertson, *Prior Agreements for Disposition of Frozen Embryos*, 51 Ohio St. L. J. 407, 419 (1990) [2.141]. Robertson, *The Dead Donor Rule*, 29 Hastings Center Rep. 6, 13 (Nov./Dec. 1999) [2.162].

Rodes, *On Law and Chastity*, 76 Notre Dame L. Rev. 643, 675 (2001) [8.14].

Rodriguez, *Suing Health Care Providers for Saving Lives: Liability for Providing Unwanted Life-Sustaining Treatment*, 20 J. Legal Med. 1, 62 (1999) [2.20].

Rodwin, *Strains in the Fiduciary Metaphor: Divided Physician Loyalties and Obligations in a Changing Health Care System*, XXI Am. J. Law & Med. 241, 246, 250 (1995) [Preamble; 8.032].

Rodwin & Okamoto, *Physicians' Conflicts of Interest in Japan and the United States: Lessons for the United States*, 25 J. Health Pol. Pol'y & L. 343, 355, 358 (2000) [8.032, 8.061].

Rosato, *The Ultimate Test of Autonomy: Should Minors Have a Right to Make Decisions Regarding Life-Sustaining Treatment?*, 49 Rutgers L. Rev. 1, 80-81, 82 (1996) [2.20].

Rosato, *Using Bioethics Discourse to Determine When Parents Should Make Health Care Decisions for their Children: Is Deference Justified?* 73 Temp. L. Rev. 1, 40, 44 (2000) [2.20].

Rose, *Financial Conflicts of Interest: How Are We Managing?* 8 Wid. L. Symp. J. 1, 24 (2001) [8.03, 8.031].

Rosenfeld, *Assisted Suicide, Depression, and the Right to Die,* 6 Psychol. Pub. Pol'y & L. 467, 469 (2000) [2.21, 2.211].

Rosner, Cassell, Friedland, Landolt, Loeb, Numann, Ora, Risemberg, & Sordillo, *Ethical Considerations of Reproductive Technologies,* 87 N.Y. State J. Med. 398 (1987) [2.04, 2.05, 2.14, 2.18].

Rosoff, *Breach of Fiduciary Duty Lawsuits Against MCOs,* 22 J. Legal Med. 55, 65 (2001) [8.0132].

Rosoff, *The Changing Face of Pharmacy Benefits Management: Information Technology Pursues a Grand Mission,* 42 St. Louis U. L. J. 1, 25-26 (1998) [5.05].

Roth & Levin, *Dilemma of Tarasoff: Must Physicians Protect the Public or Their Patients?,* 11 Law, Med. & Health Care 104 (1983) [IV].

Rothenberg, *Gestational Surrogacy and the Health Care Provider: Put Part of the IVF Genie Back Into the Bottle,* 18 Law, Med. & Health Care 345, 346 (1990) [2.18].

Rothenberg, *Who Cares? The Evolution of the Legal Duty to Provide Emergency Care,* 26 Houston L. Rev. 21 (1989) [VI].

Rothstein, *The Role of IRBs in Research Involving Commercial Biobanks,* 30 J. Law, Med. & Ethics 105, 106, 108 (2002) [8.031].

Rothstein & Hoffman, *Genetic Testing, Genetic Medicine, and Managed Care,* 34 Wake Forest L. Rev. 849, 883 (1999) [2.23].

Rothstein, Gelb, & Craig, *Protecting Genetic Privacy by Permitting Employer Access Only to Job-Related Employee Medical Information: Analysis of a Unique Minnesota Law,* 24 Am. J. Law & Med. 399, 400 (1998) [2.132].

Rugg, *An Old Solution to a New Problem: Physician Unions Take the Edge Off Managed Care,* 34 Colum. J. L. & Soc. Probs. 1, 41 (2000) [VI, VII; 10.01].

Sabo, *Limiting a Surrogate's Authority to Terminate Life-Support for an Incompetent Adult,* 79 N.C.L. Rev. 1815, 1815 (2001) [2.20].

Sadoff, *Ethical Obligations for the Psychiatrist: Confidentiality, Privilege, and Privacy in Psychiatric Treatment,* 29 Loy. L.A. L. Rev. 1709, 1710, 1711 (1996) [IV; 5.05].

Safriet, *Closing the Gap Between Can and May in Health-Care Providers' Scopes of Practice: A Primer for Policymakers,* 19 Yale J. on Reg. 301, 311 (2002) [I, II].

Sage, *Physicians as Advocates,* 35 Hous. L. Rev. 1529, 1537, 1541, 1542, 1552-53, 1554, 1556, 1557, 1559, 1561-62, 1564, 1571, 1574, 1576, 1580 (1999) [IV, VI; Elements (2), (4), (6); 2.03, 2.07, 2.09, 2.16, 2.19, 3.06, 4.01, 4.04, 6.01, 7.02, 8.02, 8.03, 8.13, 8.132, 9.06, 9.07, 9.131, 10.01, 10.02].

Sage, *Regulating Through Information: Disclosure Laws and American Health Care,* 99 Colum. L. Rev. 1701, 1753, 1758, 1760 (1999) [8.032, 8.051, 8.13].

Sanematsu, *Taking a Broader View of Treatment Disputes Beyond Managed Care: Are Recent Legislative Efforts the Cure?* 48 UCLA L. Rev. 1245, 1258, 1284 (2001) [2.035, 2.037, 2.17, 2.22].

Sangree, *Control of Childbearing by HIV-Positive Women: Some Responses to Emerging Legal Policies,* 41 Buff. L. Rev. 309, 362 (1993) [8.08].

Santayana, *The Michigan Legislature Persists in Prohibiting Assisted Suicide,* 77 U. Det. Mercy L. Rev. 875, 886 (2000) [2.211].

Sargent, *Treating the Condemned to Death,* 16 Hastings Center Rep. 5 (Dec. 1986) [I; 2.06].

Schawbel, *Are You Taking Any Prescription Medication?: A Case Comment on Weld v. CVS Pharmacy, Inc.,* 35 New Eng. L. Rev. 909, 957 (2001) [5.05].

Schiff, *The Lawyer's Role in Restoring Adolescents' Abortion Rights,* 44 Fed. Law. 60, 62 (May 1997) [2.015].

Schlesinger, Gray, & Perreira, *Medical Professionalism under Managed Care: The Pros and Cons of Utilization Review,* 16 Health Affairs 106, 119, 120, 124 (1997) [8.13, 9.031].

Schmid, *Protecting the Physician in HIV Misdiagnosis Cases,* 46 Duke L. J. 431, 458 (1996) [IV].

Schmidt, *Professional Courtesy Discounts Under Siege—Part II,* 29 Colo. Law. 59, 62 (Jan. 2000) [6.12, 6.13].

Schneider, *Adverse Impact of Predisposition Testing on Major Life Activities: Lessons from BRCA1/2 Testing,* 3 J. Health Care L. & Pol'y 365, 380 (2000) [2.132].

Schneiderman, Teetzel, & Kalmanson, *Who Decides Who Decides? When Disagreement Occurs Between the Physician and the Patient's Appointed Proxy About the Patient's Decision-Making Capacity*, 155 Arch. Intern. Med. 793, 796 (1995) [2.20].

Schnibbe, *Recent Legislative Developments in Utah Law: Family Law*, 1996 Utah L. Rev. 1335, 1394 (1996) [8.08].

Schoenholtz, Freedman, & Halpern, *The Legal Abuse of Physicians in Deaths in the United States: The Erosion of Ethics and Morality in Medicine*, 42 Wayne L. Rev. 1505, 1542 (1996) [2.06].

Schwartz, *Privacy and the Economics of Personal Health Care Information*, 76 Tex. L. Rev. 1, 59 (1997) [5.07].

Schwartz & Gibson, *Defining the Role of the Physician: Medical Education, Tradition, and the Legal Process*, 18 Houston L. Rev. 779 (1981) [IV].

Sciarrino, *Ferguson v. City of Charleston: "The Doctor Will See You Now, Be Sure to Bring Your Privacy Rights in With You!"* 12 Temp. Pol. & Civ. Rts. L. Rev. 197, 213, 215, 220, 221, 222 (2002) [Preamble; VIII, IX; 2.136, 5.05, 10.01].

Scott, *Cybermedicine and Virtual Pharmacies*, 103 W. Va. L. Rev. 407, 441, 451 (2001) [5.05, 6.02, 6.03].

Scott, *Is Too Much Privacy Bad for Your Health? An Introduction to the Law, Ethics, and HIPAA Rule on Medical Privacy*, 17 Ga. St. U. L. Rev. 481, 494 (2000) [10.01].

Severyn, *Jacobson v. Massachusetts: Impact on Informed Consent and Vaccine Policy*, 5 J. Pharmacy & L. 249, 253, 274 (1996) [8.08, 10.01].

Shapiro, *On the Possibility of "Progress" in Managing Biomedical Technologies: Markets, Lotteries, and Rational Moral Standards in Organ Transplantation*, 31 Cap. U. L. Rev. 13, 29 (2003) [2.16].

Shepherd, *HIV, the ADA, and the Duty to Treat*, 37 Hous. L. Rev. 1055, 1061, 1083-84 (2000) [Preamble; VI; 9.131].

Shepherd, *Sophie's Choices: Medical and Legal Responses to Suffering*, 72 Notre Dame L. Rev. 103, 106, 133 (1996) [VI; 2.162].

Shewmon, *Active Voluntary Euthanasia: A Needless Pandora's Box*, 3 Issues in Law and Med. 219 (1987) [2.06, 8.11, 9.06].

Shimm & Spece, *Conflict of Interest and Informed Consent in Industry-Sponsored Clinical Trials*, 12 J. Legal Med. 477, 481, 507, 510 (1991) [8.031].

Shin, *Redressing Wounds: Finding a Legal Framework to Remedy Racial Disparities in Medical Care*, 90 Cal. L. Rev. 2047, 2056, 2057, 2100 (2002) [9.121].

Shiner, *Medical Futility: A Futile Concept?*, 53 Wash. & Lee L. Rev. 803, 834 (1996) [10.01].

Shorr, *AIDS, Judaism, and the Limits of the Secular Society*, 20 Second Opinion 23, 24, 27 (1995) [5.05, 9.131].

Shultz, *From Informed Consent to Patient Choice: A New Protected Interest*, 95 Yale L. J. 219 (1985) [II, IV; 6.02, 8.03, 8.032].

Sigman, Kraut, & La Puma, *Disclosure of a Diagnosis to Children and Adolescents When Parents Object*, 147 Am. J. Diseases Children 764, 766 (1993) [II].

Silver, *From Baby Doe to Grandpa Doe: The Impact of the Federal Age Discrimination Act on the Hidden Rationing of Medical Care*, 37 Catholic Univ. L. Rev. 993 (1988) [2.03].

Silver, *Love, Hate, and Other Emotional Interference in the Lawyer/Client Relationship*, 6 Clinical L. Rev. 259, 266 (1999) [8.14].

Silverstein & Speitel, *"Honey, I Have No Idea": Court Readiness to Handle Petitions to Waive Parental Consent for Abortion*, 88 Iowa L. Rev. 75, 116, 117 (2002) [2.015].

Simon, *Treatment Boundary Violations: Clinical, Ethical, and Legal Considerations*, 20 Bull. Am. Acad. Psychiatry Law 269, 282 (1992) [6.07].

Singleton, *Privacy Versus the First Amendment: A Skeptical Approach*, 11 Fordham Intell. Prop. Media & Ent. L. J. 97, 122 (2000) [5.05].

Sirmon & Kreisberg, *The Invisible Patient*, 334 New Eng. J. Med. 908, 910, 911 (1996) [8.12].

Skiver & Hickey, *AIDS: Legal Issues 1992*, 19 Ohio No. Univ. L. Rev. 839, 860 (1993) [5.05].

Sklansky, *Neonatal Euthanasia: Moral Considerations and Criminal Liability*, 27 J. Med. Ethics 5, 8, 9 (2001) [2.215].

Skobeloff, Spivey, St. Clair, & Schoffstall, *The Influence of Age and Sex on Asthma Admissions*, 268 JAMA 3437, 3439, 3440 (1992) [9.122].

Smith, *Euphemistic Codes and Tell-Tale Hearts: Humane Assistance in End-of-Life Cases*, 10 Health Matrix 175, 177 (2000) [2.22].

Smith, *Ignorance Is not Bliss: Why a Ban on Human Cloning is Unacceptable*, 9 Health Matrix 311, 330, 331 (1999) [2.162].

Smith, *Legal Recognition of Neocortical Death*, 71 Cornell L. Rev. 850 (1986) [2.20].

Smith, *Murder, She Wrote or Was It Merely Selective Nontreatment?*, 8 J. Contemp. Health L. & Pol'y 49, 53 (1992) [2.17, 2.20].

Smith, *Our Hearts Were Once Young and Gay: Health Care Rationing and the Elderly*, 8 U. Fla. J.L. & Pub. Pol'y 1, 21 (1996) [2.09].

Sneed, May, & Stencel, *Physicians' Reliance on Specialists, Therapists, and Vendors When Prescribing Therapies and Durable Medical Equipment for Children with Special Health Care Needs*, 107 Pediatrics 1283, 1287, 1288, 1289 (2001) [8.06, 9.132].

Snyder, *Artificial Feeding and the Right to Die: The Legal Issues*, 9 J. Legal Med. 349 (1988) [2.20].

Solomon & Asaro, *Community-Based Health Care: A Legal and Policy Analysis*, 24 Fordham Urb. L. J. 235, 276-77 (1997) [9.065, 10.01].

Solove, *Digital Dossiers and the Dissipation of Fourth Amendment Privacy*, 75 S. Cal. L. Rev. 1083, 1155 (2002) [5.05].

Sontag, *Are Clinical Ethics Consultants in Danger? An Analysis of the Potential Legal Liability of Individual Clinical Ethicists*, 151 U. Pa. L. Rev. 667, 679 (2002) [9.11].

Spector, *Managed Healthcare Liability Issues*, 32 Cumb. L. Rev. 311, 335-36 (2002) [8.132].

Spielberg, *On Call and Online: Sociohistorical, Legal, and Ethical Implications of E-mail for the Patient-Physician Relationship*, 280 JAMA 1353, 1356 (1998) [5.04, 5.05, 5.057, 5.07, 5.075, 5.08].

Spielberg, *Online Without a Net: Physician-Patient Communication by Electronic Mail*, 25 Am. J. Law & Med. 267, 284-85 (1999) [5.04, 5.05, 5.06, 5.07].

Spielman, *After the Gag Episode: Physician Communication in Managed Care Organizations*, 22 Seton Hall Legis. J. 437, 453, 461, 463 (1998) [8.13].

Spielman, *Managed Care Regulation and the Physician-Advocate*, 47 Drake L. Rev. 713, 717, 719 (1999) [8.13].

Spielman, *Professionalism in Forensic Bioethics*, 30 J.L. Med. & Ethics 420, 425, 427, 436 (2002) [9.07].

Sprung, *Changing Attitudes and Practices in Forgoing Life-Sustaining Treatments*, 263 JAMA 2211, 2213 (1990) [2.20].

Staihar, *The State's Unqualified Interest in Preserving Life: A Critique of the Formulations of Life's Sanctity in Washington v. Glucksberg*, 34 Idaho L. Rev. 401, 415 (1998) [2.211].

Stark, *Bio-Ethics and Physician Liability: The Liability Effects of Developing Pain Management Standards*, 14 St. Thomas L. Rev. 601, 631 (2002) [2.21, 2.211].

Steinbrook & Lo, *Artificial Feeding—Solid Ground, Not a Slippery Slope*, 318 New Eng. J. Med. 286 (1988) [2.20].

Stone & Winslade, *Physician-Assisted Suicide and Euthanasia in the United States: Legal and Ethical Observations*, 16 J. Legal Med. 481, 483, 490, 497, 498, 499 (1995) [III, IV, VI; 2.20, 2.21, 8.11, 9.12].

Stonefield, *Lawyer Discrimination Against Clients: Outright Rejection—No; Limitations on Issues and Arguments—Yes*, 20 W. New Eng. L. Rev. 103, 112 (1998) [9.12].

Storey, *Does Ethics Make Good Law? A Case Study*, 19 Cardozo Arts & Ent. L.J. 467, 470 (2001) [1.02].

Strasser, *The Futility of Futility?: On Life, Death, and Reasoned Public Policy*, 57 Md. L. Rev. 505, 523, 552, 553 (1998) [2.22].

Strong, *Consent to Sperm Retrieval and Insemination After Death or Persistent Vegetative State*, 14 J.L. & Health 243, 248 (2000) [2.22].

Sugarman & Yarashus, *Admissibility of Managed Care Financial Incentives in Medical Malpractice Cases*, 34 Tort & Ins. L. J. 735, 743, 746, 759 (1999) [8.13, 8.132].

Sullivan & Reynolds, *Where Law and Bioethics Meet . . . and Where They Don't*, 75 U. Det. Mercy L. Rev. 607, 612 (1998) [8.08, 8.115].

Sulmasy, Geller, Faden, & Levine, *The Quality of Mercy: Caring for Patients With "Do Not Resuscitate" Orders*, 267 JAMA 682 (1992) [2.22].

Sulmasy & Pellegrino, *The Rule of Double Effect: Clearing Up the Double Talk* 159 Arch. Intern. Med. 545, 550 (1999) [2.20].

Sundram, *In Harm's Way: Research Subjects Who are Decisionally Impaired*, 1 J. Health Care L. & Pol'y 36, 43-44 (1998) [2.07].

Svoboda, Van Howe, & Dwyer, *Informed Consent for Neonatal Circumcision: An Ethical and Legal Conundrum*, 17 J. Contemp. Health L. & Pol'y 61, 67, 73, 82 (2000) [8.03, 8.03, 9.011].

Swedlow, Johnson, Smithline, & Milstein, *Increased Costs and Rates of Use in the California Workers' Compensation System as a Result of Self-Referral By Physicians*, 327 New Eng. J. Med. 1502 (1992) [8.032].

Szczygiel, *Beyond Informed Consent*, 21 Ohio N.U.L. Rev. 171, 217, 218, 220, 225, 226, 256 (1994) [Preamble; I, II, III, IV, V, VI; 1.01, 1.02, 8.08, 10.01].

Tabor, *The Battle for Hospital Privileges*, 251 JAMA 1602 (1984) [9.05].

Tadd & Bayer, *Commentary: Medical Decision Making Based on Chronological Age–Cause for Concern*, 11 J. Clinical Ethics 328, 330 (2000) [2.035].

Talesh, *Breaking the Learned Helplessness of Patients: Why MCOs Should be Required to Disclose Financial Incentives*, 26 Law & Psychol. Rev. 49, 60-61, 63 (2002) [2.03, 8.13].

Tarantino, *Withdrawal of Life Support: Conflict Among Patient Wishes, Family, Physicians, Courts and Statutes, and the Law*, 42 Buff. L. Rev. 623, 638, 639, 646 (1994) [2.20].

Taslitz, *A Feminist Fourth Amendment?: Consent, Care, Privacy, and Social Meaning in Ferguson v. City of Charleston*, 9 Duke J. Gender L. & Pol'y 1, 18, 19 (2002) [II, IV; 10.01].

Taub, *Withholding Treatment From Defective Newborns*, 10 Law, Med. & Health Care 4 (Feb. 1982) [2.17].

Tenery, *Interactions Between Physicians and the Health Care Technology Industry*, 283 JAMA 391, 393 (2000) [8.061, 9.011].

Terry, *An eHealth Diptych: The Impact of Privacy Regulation on Medical Error and Malpractice Litigation*, 27 Am. J.L. & Med. 361, 402 (2001) [IV].

Terzian, *Direct-to-Consumer Prescription Drug Advertising*, 25 Am. J. Law & Med. 149, 165 (1999) [II, III].

Testa, *Sentenced to Life? An Analysis of the United States Supreme Court's Decision in Washington v. Glucksberg*, 22 Nova L. Rev. 821, 839 (1998) [2.211].

Thomasma, *When Physicians Choose to Participate in the Death of Their Patients: Ethics and Physician-Assisted Suicide*, 24 J. Law, Med. & Ethics 183, 184, 195 (1996) [2.211].

Thompson, *Understanding Financial Conflicts of Interest*, 329 New Eng. J. Med. 573 (1993) [8.032].

Toll, *For My Doctor's Eyes Only: Ferguson v. City of Charleston*, 33 Loy. U. Chi. L.J. 267, 305 (2001) [5.05].

Trew, *Regulating Life and Death: The Modification and Commodification of Nature*, 29 U. Tol. L. Rev. 271, 292 (1998) [2.162].

Trunkey, Cahn, Lenfesty, & Mullins, *Management of the Geriatric Trauma Patient at Risk of Death: Therapy Withdrawal Decision Making*, 135 Arch. Surg. 34, 35 (2000) [2.037].

Truog, *Futility in Pediatrics: From Case to Policy*, 11 J. Clinical Ethics 136, 139, 141 (2000) [2.037].

Truog & Brennan, *Participation of Physicians in Capital Punishment*, 329 New Eng. J. Med. 1346 (1993) [2.06].

Tsai, *Cheaper and Better: The Congressional Administrative Simplification Mandate Facilitates the Transition to Electronic Medical Records*, 19 J. Legal Med. 549, 570, 581 (1998) [IV; 5.07, 5.075, 8.061].

Turkington, *Medical Record Confidentiality Law, Scientific Research, and Data Collection in the Information Age*, 25 J. Law, Med. & Ethics 113, 126 (1997) [IV].

Underwood & Cadle, *Genetics, Genetic Testing, and the Specter of Discrimination: A Discussion Using Hypothetical Cases*, 85 Ky. L. J. 665, 684 (1996-97) [2.12].

Urofsky, *Justifying Assisted Suicide: Comments on the Ongoing Debate*, 14 Notre Dame J. L. Ethics & Pub. Pol'y 893, 918, 923 (2000) [2.06, 2.211].

Urofsky, *Leaving the Door Ajar: The Supreme Court and Assisted Suicide*, 32 U. Rich. L. Rev. 313, 336 (1998) [2.211].

Van Der Goes, *Opportunity Lost: Why and How to Improve the HHS-Proposed Legislation Governing Law Enforcement Access to Medical Records*, 147 U. Pa. L. Rev. 1009, 1063 (1999) [IV].

Veatch, *Abandoning Informed Consent*, 25 Hastings Center Rep. 5, 6 (March/April 1995) [8.08].

Veatch, *Doctor Does Not Know Best: Why in the New Century Physicians Must Stop Trying to Benefit Patients*, 25 J. Med. & Phil. 701, 710, 711 (2000) [II; 8.08].

Veatch, *Why Liberals Should Accept Financial Incentives for Organ Procurement*, 13 Kennedy Inst. Ethics J. 19, 34 (March 2003) [2.15].

Virmani, Schneiderman, & Kaplan, *Relationship of Advance Directives to Physician-Patient Communication*, 154 Arch. Intern. Med. 909, 913 (1994) [2.20].

Vital, *Mandatory Reporting Statutes and the Violence Against Women Act: An Analytical Comparison*, 10 Geo. Mason U. Civ. Rts. L. J. 171, 189 (2000) [2.02].

Volkert, *Telemedicine: RX for the Future of Health Care*, 6 Mich. Telecomm. & Tech. L. Rev. 147, 214, 225 (2000) [5.05, 5.07].

Wallace, *Incompetency for Execution: The Supreme Court Challenges the Ethical Standards of the Mental Health Professions*, 8 J. Legal Med. 265 (1987) [2.06].

Waller & Fulton, *The Electronic Chart: Keeping it Confidential and Secure*, 26 J. Health & Hosp. L. 104, 105 (April 1993) [IV; 5.07].

Walters, *Life-Sustaining Medical Decisions Involving Children: Father Knows Best*, 15 T. M. Cooley L. Rev. 115, 128, 138, 151 (1998) [2.20].

Walters & Ashwal, *Organ Prolongation in Anencephalic Infants: Ethical and Medical Issues*, 18 Hastings Center Rep. 19 (Oct./Nov. 1988) [2.20].

Walzer, *Impaired Physicians: An Overview and Update of the Legal Issues*, 11 J. Legal Med. 131, 174, 192 (1990) [IV; 4.07].

Wanzer, Federman, Adelstein, Cassel, Cassem, Cranford, Hook, Lo, Moertel, Safar, Stone, & Van Eys, *The Physician's Responsibility Toward Hopelessly Ill Patients: A Second Look*, 320 New Eng. J. Med. 844 (1989) [2.20].

Warren, *Pennsylvania Medical Informed Consent Law: A Call to Protect Patient Autonomy Rights By Abandoning the Battery Approach*, 38 Duq. L. Rev. 917, 925 (2000) [IV; 8.08, 10.01].

Watson, *Medicaid Physician Participation: Patients, Poverty, and Physician Self-Interest*, XXI Am. J. Law & Med. 191, 218 (1995) [VI].

Watson, *Race, Ethnicity and Quality of Care: Inequalities and Incentives*, 27 Am. J. L. & Med. 203, 206 (2001) [9.121].

Wazana, *Physicians and the Pharmaceutical Industry: Is a Gift Ever Just a Gift?* 283 JAMA 373, 380 (2000) [8.061].

Wear, Coles, Szczygiel, McEvoy, & Pegels, *Patenting Medical and Surgical Techniques: An Ethical-Legal Analysis*, 23 J. Med. Phil. 75, 76, 87 (1998) [9.08, 9.095].

Weiner & Wettstein, *Confidentiality of Patient-Related Information*, 112 Arch. Ophthalmology 1032, 1033 (1994) [IV; 10.01].

Weinstock, Leong, & Silva, *Opinions by AAPL Forensic Psychiatrists on Controversial Ethical Guidelines: A Survey*, 19 Bull. Am. Acad. Psychiatry Law 237, 238 (1991) [1.02, 5.09].

Weir & Gostin, *Decisions to Abate Life-Sustaining Treatment for Nonautonomous Patients: Ethical Standards and Legal Liability for Physicians After Cruzan*, 264 JAMA 1846, 1849, 1850 (1990) [2.20].

Wentz, Osteen, & Gannon, *Continuing Medical Education: Unabated Debate*, 268 JAMA 1118 (1992) [8.061, 9.011].

Wentz, Osteen, & Gannon, *Refocusing Support and Direction*, 266 JAMA 953 (1991) [8.061, 9.011].

Wertheimer, *Ockham's Scalpel: A Return to a Reasonableness Standard*, 43 Vill. L. Rev. 321, 327 (1998) [8.13].

Westfall, McCabe, & Nicholas, *Personal Use of Drug Samples by Physicians and Office Staff*, 278 JAMA 141, 142 (1997) [8.061].

White, *Health Care Professionals and Treatment of HIV-Positive Patients*, 20 J. Legal Med. 67, 86 (1999) [VI; 2.23, 9.131].

White & Zimbelman, *Abandoning Informed Consent: An Idea Whose Time Has Not Yet Come*, 23 J. Med. Phil. 477, 496 (1998) [Preamble].

Widmer, *South Dakota Should Follow Public Policy and Switch to the Preponderance Standard for Medical License Revocation After In Re the Medical License of Dr. Reuben Setliff, M.D.*, 48 S.D. L. Rev. 388, 396-97, 402 (2003) [II, III, IV; 1.02, 9.07].

Wilcox, *Enforcing Lawyer Non-Competition Agreements While Maintaining the Profession: The Role of Conflict of Interest Principles*, 84 Minn. L. Rev. 915, 966 (2000) [9.02].

Wilde, *Air Force Women's Access to Abortion Services and the Erosion of 10 U.S.C. § 1093*, 9 Wm. & Mary J. Women & L. 351, 371 (2003) [8.08, 10.01].

Williams & Rucker, *Understanding and Addressing Racial Disparities in Health Care*, 21 Health Care Fin. Rev. 75, 88 (2000) [9.122].

Windsor, *Disposition of Cryopreserved Preembryos After Divorce*, 88 Iowa L. Rev. 1001, 1026 (2003) [2.141].

Winn, *Confidentiality in Cyberspace: The HIPAA Privacy Rules and the Common Law*, 33 Rutgers L.J. 617, 622 (2002) [5.05].

Wolf, *Health Care Reform and the Future of Physician Ethics*, 24 Hastings Center Rep. 28, 32, 40 (March/April 1994) [2.03, 2.09, 4.04, 5.01, 8.03, 9.121, 9.122].

Wolf, *Toward a Systemic Theory of Informed Consent in Managed Care*, 35 Hous. L. Rev. 1631, 1641, 1658, 1661, 1662, 1679 (1999) [2.03, 8.03, 8.032, 8.051, 8.13, 8.132].

Wolfson, *A Quality of Mercy: The Struggle of the AIDS-Afflicted to Use Marijuana as Medicine*, 22 T. Jefferson L. Rev. 1, 24 (1999) [2.17].

Woodward, *Medical Record Confidentiality and Data Collection: Current Dilemmas*, 25 J. Law, Med. & Ethics 88, 90, 95 (1997) [5.07].

Wusthoff, *Medical Mistakes and Disclosure: The Role of the Medical Student*, 286 JAMA 1080, 1080 (2001) [8.12].

Yang & Gorman, *What's Yours is Mine: Protection and Security in a Digital World*, 36 Md. B.J. 24, 28-29 (Nov./Dec. 2003) [5.05].

Young, *Telemedicine: Patient Privacy Rights of Electronic Medical Records*, 66 UMKC L. Rev. 921, 926 (1998) [IV; 5.05].

Zer-Gutman, *Revising the Ethical Rules of Attorney-Client Confidentiality: Towards a New Discretionary Rule*, 15 Loy. L. Rev. 669, 683-84, 699, 709, 718 (1999) [IV; 5.05, 5.07].

Ziegler, Mosier, Buenaver, & Okuyemi, *How Much Information About Adverse Effects of Medication Do Patients Want From Physicians?*, 161 Arch. Intern. Med. 706, 710 (2001) [10.01].

Zwirn, *Professionalism, Mental Disability, and the Death Penalty*, 41 N.Y.L Sch. L. Rev. 163, 165 (1996) [2.06].